CSI-NIC

Manual of Interventional Cardiology

CSI-NIC
Manual of Interventional Cardiology

Editor

Prathap Kumar
MD DM FIC
Chief Interventional Cardiologist
Department of Cardiology
Meditrina Hospital
Kollam, Kerala, India

Co-Editors

Manu Rajendran
MD DM
Senior Interventional Cardiologist
Department of Cardiology
Meditrina Hospital
Kollam, Kerala, India

Blessvin Jino
MD DM FNB
Consultant Interventional Cardiologist
Department of Cardiology
Meditrina Hospital
Kollam, Kerala, India

Forewords

Gerald S Werner
Imad Sheiban
Ramesh Daggubati

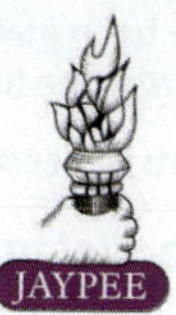

JAYPEE BROTHERS MEDICAL PUBLISHERS
The Health Sciences Publisher
New Delhi | London

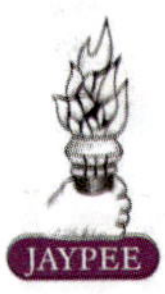

Jaypee Brothers Medical Publishers (P) Ltd

Headquarters
EMCA House, 23/23-B
Ansari Road, Daryaganj
New Delhi 110 002, India
Landline: +91-11-23272143, +91-11-23272703
+91-11-23282021, +91-11-23245672
e-mail: jaypee@jaypeebrothers.com

Corporate Office
4838/24, Ansari Road, Daryaganj
New Delhi 110 002, India
Phone: +91-11-43574357
Fax: +91-11-43574314
e-mail: jaypee@jaypeebrothers.com

Overseas Office
JP Medical Ltd.
83, Victoria Street, London
SW1H 0HW (UK)
Phone: +44-20 3170 8910
e-mail: info@jpmedpub.com

EU GPSR Authorised Representative
Logos Europe, 9 rue Nicolas Poussin
17000, La Rochelle, France
Phone: +33 (0) 6 67 93 73 78
e-mail: contact@logoseurope.eu

Website: www.jaypeebrothers.com
Website: www.jaypeedigital.com

Inquiries for bulk sales may be solicited at: jaypee@jaypeebrothers.com

CSI-NIC Manual of Interventional Cardiology

First Edition: **2025**

ISBN: 978-93-5696-733-5

Printed at Officenow India

Contributors

A Sreenivas Kumar MD DM FACC
Senior Consultant Cardiologist and Director
Department of Cardiology and Clinical Research
Apollo Hospitals
Hyderabad, Telangana, India

Abhishek Rathore MD DM PDF
Consultant Cardiologist and Electrophysiologist
Department of Cardiology
Apollo Hospitals
Indore, Madhya Pradesh, India

Achukatla Kumar Pharm D
Senior Research Consultant
Department of Cardiology
Apollo Hospitals
Indore, Madhya Pradesh, India

Aditya Kapoor MD DM
Professor and Head
Department of Cardiology
Sanjay Gandhi Postgraduate Institute of Medical Sciences
Lucknow, Uttar Pradesh, India

Ajay J Swamy MD DM FACC FACAI
Senior Consultant Interventional Cardiologist
Department of Cardiology
KIMS Hospitals
Secunderabad, Telangana, India

Ajith R Bhagawat
MD DM FACC FSCAI FESC FISE FCSI
DIPLOMATE, American Board of Cardiology
Director
Cath Lab and Interventional Cardiology
Department of Cardiology
Kamalnayan Bajaj Hospital and Marathwada Medical and Research Institute (MMRI)
Aurangabad, Maharashtra, India

(Col) Anil Dhall
Sena Medal MD (Medicine) DM (Cardiology) FACC FESC FAHA FRCP (Edinburgh) FSCAI FHRS FCSI
Professor and Head
Department of Cardiology
Janakpuri Super Speciality Hospital
New Delhi, India

Arun Gopi MD DM DNB
Senior Interventional Cardiologist and Electrophysiologist
Department of Cardiology
Metromed International Cardiac Centre
Kozhikode, Kerala, India

Arun Mohanty MD DM FESC FACC
Professor
Department of Cardiology
Sir Ganga Ram Hospital
New Delhi, India

Ashish Kumar Mandalay MD DM
Senior Interventional Cardiologist
Department of Cardiology
Myhart, Starcare Hospital
Kozhikode, Kerala, India

Ashraf SM MD DM FACC
Professor and Head
Department of Cardiology
Government Medical College
Kannur, Kerala, India

Atul Mathur
MD (Medicine) DM (Cardiology)
Chairman and Head
Department of Cardiology
Fortis Escorts Heart Institute
New Delhi, India

AV Ganesh Kumar
MD DNB DM (Cardiology)
Head
Department of Cardiology
Dr LH Hiranandani Hospital
Mumbai, Maharashtra, India

Ayush Malhotra
MD (Medicine) DrNB (Cardiology)
Consultant Cardiologist
Department of Cardiology
Janakpuri Super Speciality Hospital
New Delhi, India

Bagirath Raghuraman
MBBS MD DNB (General Medicine) DM (Cardiology) FESC FSCAI FHFA
Senior Consultant Cardiologist and Director Heart Transplant
Department of Cardiology
Narayana Institute of Cardiac Sciences, Narayana Health City
Bengaluru, Karnataka, India

Blessvin Jino
MD DM FNB
Consultant Interventional Cardiologist
Department of Cardiology
Meditrina Hospital
Kollam, Kerala, India

Byju Cheriya Kacheri
MD DM (Cardiology)
Director
Department of Cardiology
HMS Hospital
Palathara, Kerala, India

C Raghu
MD DM FACC FESC FSCAI
Cath Lab Director
Department of Cardiology
Yashoda Hospitals
Hyderabad, Telangana, India

Debabrata Roy
MD DM (Cardiology) FACC FESC FSCAI FAHA
Senior Consultant
Interventional Cardiologist and Academic Co-ordinator
NH-Rabindranath Tagore International Institute of Cardiac Sciences
Kolkata, West Bengal, India

Deepak Davidson
DM (Cardiology) MD (General Medicine) DNB (General Medicine)
Senior Interventional Cardiologist
Department of Cardiology
Caritas Heart Institute
Kottayam, Kerala, India

Dibya Kumar Baruah
MD DM FACC FSCAI FAPSC FCSI
Senior Consultant and Director
Catheterization Laboratory
Apollo Hospitals, Health City
Visakhapatnam, Andhra Pradesh, India

Dilip Kumar
MD DM FACC FRCP (Glasgow) FSCAI FESC FICC FHRS FHFA CCDS
Director—Cardiac Cath Lab Services
Senior Consultant, Interventional Cardiologist and Electrophysiologist
Chief Academic, Co-ordinator
Medica Institute of Cardiac Science
Kolkata, West Bengal, India

Haresh Mehta
MD (Medicine) DNB (Cardiology) FACC FESC FSCAI
Director—Interventional and Structural Cardiology
SL Raheja—Fortis Hospital
Mumbai, Maharashtra, India

Harikrishnan S DM FACC FRCP FAMS
Professor and Head
Department of Cardiology
Sree Chitra Tirunal Institute for Medical Sciences and Technology
Thiruvananthapuram, Kerala, India

J Ezhilan
MD DM (Cardio) DNB (Cardio) MNAMS FSCAI FNB (Int. Cardio)
Director—Endo and Peripheral Vascular
Department of Cardiology
Madras Medical Mission Hospital
Chennai, Tamil Nadu, India

K Sivaprasad MD DM DNB FESC FSCAI
Professor and Head
Department of Cardiology
Government Medical College
Thiruvananthapuram, Kerala, India

Keshava Ramaiah
MD DM DNB (Cardiology)
Director
Department of Cardiology
Fortis Hospital
Bengaluru, Karnataka, India

Kritika Arora MSc
Research Scholar
Asia Pacific Vascular Society
Indraprastha Apollo Hospital
New Delhi, India

Lais Muhammed
MBBS MD (Internal Medicine) DM (Cardiology)
Assistant Professor
Department of Cardiology
Government Medical College
Thiruvananthapuram, Kerala, India

Madhu Sreedharan
MD DM MRCP (UK) FRCP FACC FESC
Director
Department of Cardiology
NIMS Heart Foundation
Thiruvananthapuram, Kerala, India

Mahesh Nalin Kumar
MD DrNB FACC FESC
Head and Senior Consultant Cardiology
St Gregorios Medical Mission Hospital
Parumala, Kerala, India

Manoj Sivaraman
MBBS MD (General Medicine) DNB (General Medicine) DM (Cardiology) DNB (Cardiology)
MNAMS FACC FSCAI
Senior Consultant and Interventional Cardiologist
Department of Cardiology
Kauvery Hospital
Chennai, Tamil Nadu, India

Manu Rajendran MD DM
Senior Interventional Cardiologist
Department of Cardiology
Meditrina Hospital
Kollam, Kerala, India

Mathew Iype
MBBS MD and DNB (Internal Medicine) DM and DNB (Cardiology)
Professor
Department of Cardiology
Government Medical College
Thiruvananthapuram, Kerala, India

Mrinal Kanti Das
MD DM FICP FICC FCSI FACC FESC
Consultant Cardiologist
CK Birla Hospitals (BMB/CMRI)
Kolkata, West Bengal, India

NN Khanna
MD DM FRCP (London Glasgow, Edinburgh)
FACC FSCAI FESC FAPSIC FCCP FEISI FICC FCSI
Senior Consultant Cardiologist
Indraprastha Apollo Hospital
New Delhi, India

Pankaj Manoria
MD DM FESC FACC FSCAI FAPSIC
Chief Interventional Cardiologist and Director
Department of Cardiology
Manoria Heart Hospital
Bhopal, Madhya Pradesh, India

PK Asokan
MD DM FRCP FCSI FICC FSCAI FESC FACC
Chief Consultant Cardiologist
Fathima Hospital
Kozhikode, Kerala, India

Placid Sebastian MD DM FACC FSCAI
Senior Consultant Interventional Cardiologist
Department of Cardiology
Aster MIMS
Kannur, Kerala, India

Prasant Kr Sahoo
MD DM FRCP (Lond. & Glasg) FACC FSCAI FESC FAPSIC FCSI FICC
Director, Interventional Cardiology
Department of Cardiology
Apollo Hospitals
Bhubaneswar, Odisha, India

Prathap Kumar MD DM FIC
Chief Interventional Cardiologist
Department of Cardiology
Meditrina Hospital
Kollam, Kerala, India

Praveen Chandra
MD DM FACC FESC FSCAI FAPSIC
Chairman
Division of Interventional Cardiology
Medanta—The Medicity
Gurugram, Haryana, India

Praveen Velappan
MBBS MD (Internal Medicine) DM (Cardiology)
Associate Professor
Department of Cardiology
Government Medical College
Thiruvananthapuram, Kerala, India

Radhapriya Yalamanchi
MBBS DNB (Gen Med) DrNB (Cardio)
Consultant
Department of Cardiology
Apollo Main Hospital
Chennai, Tamil Nadu, India

Rajesh Vijayvergiya
MD DM FSCAI FACC FESC FISES
Professor
Department of Cardiology
Postgraduate Institute of Medical Education and Research
Chandigarh, India

Ramesh Natarajan
MD DM DNB FESC MNAMS
Senior Consultant Cardiologist
Department of Cardiology
KIMS Health
Thiruvananthapuram, Kerala, India

Ravinder Singh Rao MD DM FACC
Chairman, RHL Heart Center
Rajasthan Hospital
Jaipur, Rajasthan, India

Refai Showkathali
MBBS MRCP (UK) FRCP (Lon) FESC FACC
Senior Consultant
Department of Cardiology
Apollo Main Hospital
Chennai, Tamil Nadu, India

Rishi Sethi
MD DM FACC FESC FRCP (Edinburgh, London) FSCAI FAPSIC FAMS FCSI FISC
Professor
Department of Cardiology
King George's Medical University
Lucknow, Uttar Pradesh, India

Roopali Khanna
MD DM FACC FSCAI FCSI
Professor
Department of Cardiology
Sanjay Gandhi Postgraduate Institute of Medical Sciences
Lucknow, Uttar Pradesh, India

Roshan Rao
MD DM FACC FESC FSCAI
Senior Interventional Cardiologist and Head
Department of Cardiology
Apollo Hospitals
Indore, Madhya Pradesh, India

S Selvamani
DNB (Cardiology)
Senior Consultant and Interventional Cardiologist
Meenakshi Mission Hospital and Research Centre
Madurai, Tamil Nadu, India

Sabarish Sankaran
MBBS MD DM FNB (Interventional Cardiology)
Fellow in Interventional Cardiology
Department of Cardiology
Narayana Institute of Cardiac Sciences
Bengaluru, Karnataka, India

Sajan Narayanan
MD (Internal Medicine) DM (Cardiology) FESC
Senior Consultant and Interventional Cardiologist
Little Flower Hospital and Research Institute
Kochi, Kerala, India

Sanjay Kumar Chugh
MBBS MD (General Medicine) MRCPI D, Cardiology DM (Cardiology, AIIMS, New Delhi) FACC FSCAI
Head, Cardiology and Chief Interventional Cardiologist
Department of Cardiology
Meditrina Heart Center, Civil Hospital
Gurugram, Haryana, India

Sarita Rao MD DM FACC FSCAI
Senior Interventional Cardiologist and Director, Cath Lab
Department of Cardiology
Apollo Hospitals
Indore, Madhya Pradesh, India

Saurabh Bhardwaj MD DNB
Junior Consultant
Cardiology
Indraprastha Apollo Hospital
New Delhi, India

Sharath Reddy Annam
MD DM FSCAI FACC FAHA
Director—Cath Lab
Department of Cardiology
Medicover Hospitals
Hyderabad, Telangana, India

Siva Kumar DrNB (Cardio)
Senior Interventional Cardiologist
Department of Cardiology
Meenakshi Mission Hospital and Research Centre
Madurai, Tamil Nadu, India

Sridhar Kasturi
MBBS MD DM
Head and Senior Interventional Cardiologist
Department of Cardiology and Cardiothoracic Surgery
KIMS Sunshine Heart Institute
Hyderabad, Telangana, India

Stalin Roy J
MBBS MD DM
Senior Consultant Cardiologist
Department of Cardiology
Kauvery Hospital
Chennai, Tamil Nadu, India

Sunita Chugh
MBBS MASE
Principal MO
Department of Cardiology
Fortis Memorial Research Institute
Gurugram, Haryana, India

Surya Prakash
MD DM FACC FESC FSCAI
Senior Interventional Cardiologist and Head
Department of Cardiology
Care Hospitals
Hyderabad, Telangana, India

Yashasvi Chugh MD
Cardiologist
Department of Interventional and Structural Cardiology
Baylor, Scott and White Heart Center
Texas, USA

Foreword

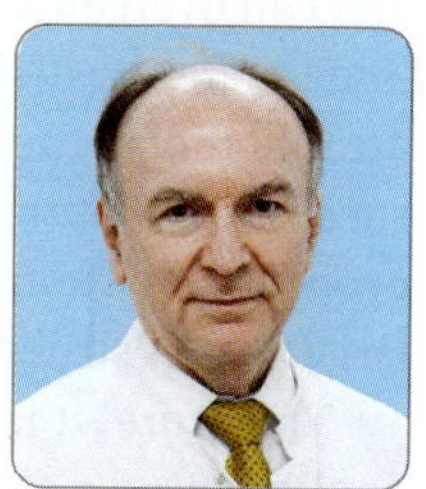

Interventional therapy of coronary artery disease has developed rapidly over the past decades, with improved outcomes in even more complex situations. When Grüntzig conceived the percutaneous approach for treatment of coronary artery disease, he right away identified the problems the pioneers faced such as total closures of arteries and calcifications. On the other side of treating coronary artery disease bypass surgery had already established itself as superior to medical treatment with proven long-term survival benefits. Grüntzig early on understood that percutaneous coronary intervention is at a disadvantage compared to surgery as it must resolve the coronary obstructions in their anatomic setting while the bypass quality depends only on the quality of the peripheral vessel and circumvents the obstructions.

The Achilles' heel of coronary intervention is the passing of complex lesions, especially total long-standing obstructions, but above all to keep these lesions open with a long-term patency comparable to surgery. Even though 20 years ago, coronary intervention already had solved some problems with the advent of drug-eluting stents, but in the first and unfortunately until today last direct comparison of surgery and intervention, in the SYNTAX study surgery was superior in most endpoints especially out to ten years follow-up. However, today we know that coronary intervention was not yet perfectly represented in this study as interventional therapy presents itself today.

One of the major setbacks in that study was the low success of opening total chronic coronary occlusions, and the lack of understanding how essential intravascular imaging is to achieve an optimal outcome, and intracoronary physiology to avoid treating irrelevant lesions and not overlook clinically relevant lesions. In addition, the main "enemy" of the interventionist, "calcium", was only treatable by rotational atherectomy, while in the last decade many more options were added like orbital atherectomy and lithoplasty to prepare lesions for a perfect stent result.

And the journey is not at its end, despite some setbacks on the way like the promising but finally disappointing first appearance of bioresorbable scaffolds. The underlying concept of the scaffold would be leaving behind a restored anatomy including biological viability of the vessel function. While such a concept would not be applicable to severely calcified lesions, for many patients this would allow the restoration of vessel function. This concept receives new appeal from the growing experience with drug-eluting balloons outside the setting of stent restenosis treatment, and we can look ahead to interesting results from these new developments.

It appears today, that we have conquered most of the problems of coronary artery disease with multiple tools available for all these problems and can overcome even the most difficult situations, but this requires a deep understanding of the "toolbox" and knowledge of pitfalls and dangers which are inherent in the ever-increasing complexity of these devices. Following the success in treating of coronary artery disease, cardiac intervention naturally evolved into the treatment of other fields of cardiac disease, specifically the large area of structural disorders.

Therefore, it is a commendable effort undertaken by the Cardiological Society of India to create this Manual for aspiring interventionists and it will be of value even for those with a long career in intervention who can relate to this manual as a valuable reference outside their own expertise. The wide scope of the topics represents all of today's interventional therapy of heart disease beyond coronary artery disease alone.

Over many years of interacting with the leading interventional cardiologist in India I know that the expertise in all fields represented in this manual is abundantly present in this nation, at institutes that can compete with any around the World. In addition, Indian companies have entered the field with great international success.

I am sure that this manual written by Indian experts for Indian experts and fellows will be a great success and addition to our resources of improved training in ever complex interventions.

Gerald S Werner
MD PhD FESC FSCAI FACC
Klinikum Darmstadt
Darmstadt, Germany

Foreword

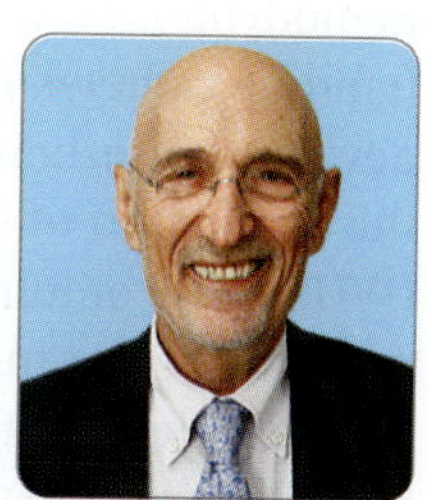

Since its introduction into daily clinical practice, percutaneous coronary interventions (PCI) have continued to grow exponentially due to the continuous technological refinement and development and introduction of new adjunctive devices that improve the efficacy and safety of the procedure. Particular impact was provided by intravascular imaging as well as devices for the debulking of calcified lesions (rotational atherectomy, cutting balloons, laser, high pressure balloons, IVL), which allow interventional cardiologists to further improve their experience and technical optimization of the procedure with a significant positive impact on clinical outcome.

Nevertheless, with the advent of drug-coated stents (DES) and consequently the dramatic reduction of restenosis and the need for new revascularization procedures supported by a huge number of well-conducted randomized studies led to an expansion of clinical indications to more and more complex cases and scenarios, pushing interventional cardiology further, thus becoming globally the first approach in managing coronary artery disease.

Moreover, in the last two decades interventional cardiology has also expanded its boundaries beyond the coronary arteries to include structural interventions (ASD/VSD/PFO closure, valvular interventions: TAVI, TMVI, TTVI) making possible today to treat the greatest number of cardiac diseases percutaneously without resorting to conventional cardiac surgery.

This book has been compiled by bringing together a group of renowned and experienced interventional cardiologists led by Dr Prathap Kumar to provide an update in this ever-developing and growing field of interventional cardiology and to provide tips and tricks from these expert operators learned from their own experience to deal with the technical difficulties encountered in daily practice and can be of great help for young interventional cardiologists at their early clinical activity and career.

I know Dr Prathap Kumar well from about 20 years, since he had his fellowship in Interventional Cardiology at my Cath Lab at the University of Turin, and he stayed with us for 18 months, so we had the opportunity to work and discuss together different strategies and complex approaches, and I followed his exponential growth upon his return to India, becoming at the present time, one of the most experienced operators not only at a national level but also internationally. His dedication and passion for interventional cardiology as well as his constant commitment guarantee the high quality of this book dedicated to all cardiologists who wish to deepen and grow in interventional cardiology starting from the basic elements such as clinical indication and continuing with other important topics such as vascular access, hemodynamics, coronary angiography, basic materials for PCI procedures (guiding catheter, guides, balloons, stents, drug-coated balloons, additional devices, i.e., atherectomy, cutting balloon, intravascular lithotripsy...) for the evaluation of coronary lesions to be treated by intravascular imaging (IVUS-OCT) or functional evaluation (FFR, iFR, CFR), the drugs used during procedures and in emergency situations. Lesion-specific approaches using different debulking devices, bifurcation lesion techniques and strategies, ostial lesions, and total occlusion antegrade and retrograde interventions are described and discussed in detail.

More importantly, complications in Cath Lab during PCI and how to address them and their management are emphasized and described in detail, both to do the best for patient safety but also to do everything possible to prevent complications.

Structural interventional procedures are also described step-by-step with possible complications and how to address them, as well as peripheral interventional procedures.

It is a comprehensive manual covering all fields of percutaneous interventions written by experienced and renowned operators. A practical and applicable manual to a variety of procedures in interventional cardiology, keeping up to date with the advancements in percutaneous coronary, structural, and peripheral interventions. The authors have done their best to identify areas that have significantly developed and offer step-by-step user guides for the latest cardiac intervention techniques for the treatment of various conditions and the use of devices. An ideal manual for use by practicing and trainee cardiologists seeking an easily accessible reference to apply in their everyday clinical practice. Undoubtedly, this book will be a reference resource for all those working in this field, and I am sure that it will be an important support for further growth of Interventional Cardiology.

I have had a unique opportunity to follow the development of interventional cardiology in India over the last 15 years. Giant strides and an amazing job have been taken in these years by Indian Cardiologists and their scientific societies, and I'm proud to have given my modest personal contribution together with them.

Imad Sheiban
MD FSCAI
Associate Professor of Cardiology
Pederzoli Hospital, Italy

Foreword

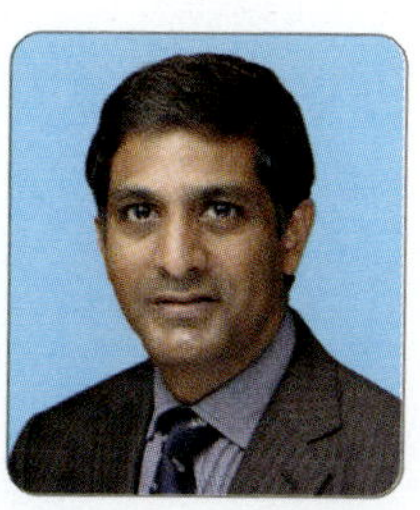

Interventional cardiology stands at the forefront of modern cardiovascular medicine, representing a dynamic and rapidly evolving field that has revolutionized the diagnosis, treatment, and management of a wide range of cardiovascular diseases. From the development of coronary angioplasty to the more recent innovations in structural heart interventions, interventional cardiology has continually reshaped the landscape of patient care.

This manual by Dr Prathap Kumar serves as a comprehensive and indispensable guide for both seasoned practitioners and those beginning their journey in this specialized domain. It provides not only the technical knowledge necessary for performing complex procedures but also offers insights into the clinical decision-making, patient selection, and post-procedural care that are critical for achieving optimal outcomes.

This manual addresses the full spectrum of interventional cardiology—from diagnostic coronary angiography to advanced interventions like transcatheter aortic valve replacement (TAVR) and left atrial appendage closure—focusing on both the procedural steps and the underlying principles that guide them.

Written by experts in the field, this work integrates the latest advancements in technology, procedural techniques, and evidence-based practices, ensuring that readers are equipped with the most up-to-date knowledge. Beyond the techniques themselves, the manual emphasizes the importance of a multidisciplinary approach, the collaboration between cardiologists, surgeons, radiologists, and other healthcare professionals, and the vital role of patient-centered care in achieving the best outcomes.

I am confident that this manual will serve as an invaluable reference for interventional cardiologists at all stages of their careers, offering both practical guidance and clinical wisdom. May it inspire continued excellence in the practice of interventional cardiology and contribute to the ongoing advancement of cardiovascular care worldwide.

Ramesh Daggubati
MD FACC FSCAI
Vice Chair of Cardiology
Chief of Interventional Cardiology
West Virginia University

Preface

The field of interventional cardiology has changed colossally ever since the first coronary angioplasty performed by Gruentzig in 1977. The coronary angioplasty was once considered a major procedure with high failure rates. However, with the availability of dual lumen microcatheters, dedicated CTO wires, atherectomy devices, coronary lithotripsy, excimer laser, and intracoronary imaging like IVUS and OCT, the procedural success has increased even in complex coronary lesions. In the last three decades, coronary angioplasty has evolved significantly to the extent that modern cardiologists attempt to open even the most complex tortuous calcified long segment chronic total occlusions. Similarly, percutaneous mechanical circulatory support devices help to attempt complex PCI in high-risk populations. According to the CSI NIC 2023 data, more than 10 lakhs PCI were performed in India during 2023. Along with PCI, the number of structural heart interventions has also increased. Newer technologies in transcatheter heart valves keep expanding the indications of transcatheter heart valve implantations and reducing the complication rates. Similar to transcatheter heart valve implantations, mitral and tricuspid valve edge-to-edge repairs have reduced mortality and morbidity significantly in high-risk patients. Newer advances in the field of interventional cardiology have given better longevity and quality of life to high-risk patients.

In this manual of interventional cardiology, we have carefully selected topics to give practical tips for interventional cardiologists who are in their early stages of the career. All the authors have attempted to provide the most updated knowledge in their respective topics. We have included topics on coronary, structural heart, and peripheral arterial interventions that are done in our routine clinical practice. I believe that this manual will serve as good reference material for fellows and young cardiologists.

Prathap Kumar
Chairman and Managing Director
Meditrina Group of Hospitals, India

Acknowledgments

I am indebted to all the authors who have helped me to prepare this manual. This manual would not have been possible without their sincere efforts. I thank Dr Manu Rajendran and Dr Blessvin Jino for helping me to edit this book. I also thank M/s Jaypee Brothers Medical Publishers (P) Ltd, New Delhi, India, especially Himani Pandey, Pragati Singh and Chetna Malhotra, for developing, proofreading and delivering the book in a better manner.

I am thankful for my teachers and mentors who have inspired me throughout my career in interventional cardiology. I also thank my colleagues and patients for supporting me to improve my interventional skills. Finally, I would like to thank my wife Manju Prathap and my children, Arya and Aditya, for their constant support and sacrifices, which boosted me to achieve more in my profession.

Contents

CHAPTER 1

Catheter Selection and Angiographic Views for Anomalous Coronary Arteries: A Practical Guide

Aditya Kapoor

INTRODUCTION

The exponential surge in the coronary interventions has resulted in an increased number of anomalous coronary encounters. This leads to an excessive radiation exposure to the operator and a large amount of contrast usage to the patient. Anomalous coronary arteries (ACAs) have been variously classified and described by their site of origin and course. The more common ones are those involving the abnormal aortic origin of coronaries and clinically relevant ones are anomalous coronaries arising from opposite sinus (ACAOS). Their significance lies in the fact that often they are difficult to engage with the diagnostic catheters and sometimes present a technical challenge for even the most experienced operators.[1,2]

There is a set of principles to be followed while cannulating a coronary:

- Anticipated site of coronary origin
- Appropriate angiographic projections
- Catheter selection

ANTICIPATED SITE OF CORONARY ORIGIN

Distribution of epicardial coronary arteries forms a water-tight system such that if the left circumflex (LCX) artery is narrow caliber vessel, supplying a small myocardial area, then right coronary artery (RCA) has to have appropriately large myocardial area supply. Similarly, if posterior descending artery (PDA) is arising from LCX, then RCA has to be more or less nondominant. *An important corollary is that "while hooking left main coronary artery (LMCA), if there is a very long left main stem and LCX is not visualized and RCA is also not superdominant then it is likely that we are missing out on separately originating anomalous LCX"* and what appears as long left main stem is actually left anterior descending (LAD) artery originating separately from aortic root. Therefore, a conscious thought of what we see on angiogram, merely a close observation may help suspect coronary anomaly.[3]

Practical Tip

No area of cardiac myocardium on fluoroscopy can be without an arterial supply. If there is, then we must search for the artery supplying its territory.

APPROPRIATE ANGIOGRAPHIC PROJECTIONS

Though cannulation of LMCA is often done in anterior–posterior (AP) view, the left anterior oblique (LAO) projection carries certain merits compared to cannulation in the AP view. LAO view separates the left coronary sinus and right coronary sinus position, simplifying the visualization of two, with left sinus seen on patient left side and right one on patient's right. So, whenever, we have a difficult LMCA hooking, it is wise to switch to LAO view. Additionally, by nonselective contrast puffs or nonselective root aortogram, it is possible to identify right and left cusps and respective coronaries origin.

The anomalous right coronary originating from left sinus (R-ACAOS) which is more common than left ACAOS (L-ACAOS) is often delineated in LAO when there is failure to cannulate RCA from right sinus and contrast opacification of right sinus does not opacify RCA.

Practical Tip

When RCA cannot be cannulated using work-house catheter in LAO, and LCX is nondominant, we should consider taking a nonselective root aortogram to look for dominant RCA arising from anomalous site.

Similarly left ACAOS can be appropriately anticipated if in LAO projection, operator finds no coronary arising from left coronary cusp with contrast puff or on root aortogram. For identifying the course of a L-ACAOS, Ishikawa has described *"using two orthogonal angiographic views"*. LAO view provides information about cranial or caudally originating stem, while right anterior oblique (RAO) gives idea about anteriorly or posteriorly situated stem.[4] This generates four permutations for L-ACAOS course as shown in **Table 1**. These are retroaortic, interarterial, septal, or free wall courses. Among these, the interarterial course often carries high-risk features like ostial stenosis and intramural course and hence considered malignant.

CATHETER SELECTION

In the beginnings, coronary catheters were hand crafted for different shapes of aorta. In the current era, different preshaped industry-manufactured

TABLE 1: Permutations for the L-ACAOS course.

Course of loop in LAO	*Course of loop in RAO*	*Name of course*
Cranial	Anterior	Free wall course
Cranial	Posterior	Interarterial course
Caudal	Anterior	Septal course
Caudal	Posterior	Retroaortic (most common)

(L-ACAOS: left coronary originating from left sinus; LAO: left anterior oblique; RAO: right anterior oblique)

catheters are readily available for both right and left coronary artery cannulation. Moreover, nowadays, when transradial coronary interventions are preferred over femoral interventions due to lower hospital stay and complications, single diagnostic catheter concept has emerged, obviating the need for exchange. The TIG catheter (manufactured by Terumo) is one such catheter, which is more or less a passive universal diagnostic catheter, used for cannulating both left and the right coronary arteries. After entering via retroaortic route and reaching distalmost part of aortic root [which is usually right coronary cusp (RCC)], its brought from this distal position in RCC to a more proximal one in LCC by pulling back (considered as first jump) and further pull back hooks the LMCA (considered as second jump) **(Fig. 1)**. Only sometimes slight rotation or torque in clockwise manner is required to get its distal tip closer to the LMCA origin (for shorter ascending aorta). For the RCA cannulation, TIG catheter is dehooked from LMCA by push or pull and pushed distally to reach RCC and then rotated in a clockwise manner with slight pull to cannulate the RCA.

These maneuvers work well, when the coronary arteries are normal in origin.

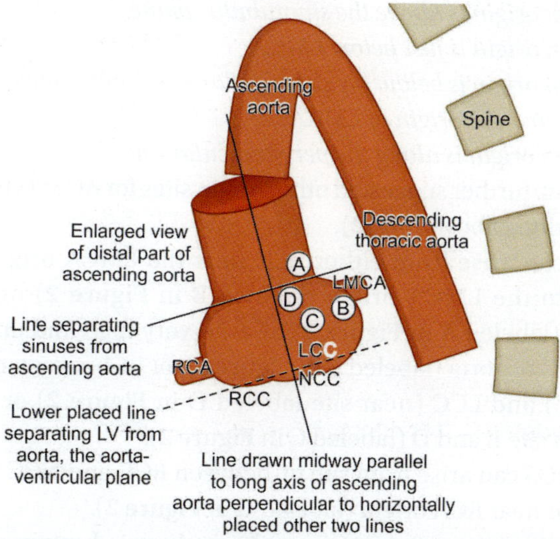

Fig. 1: A pictorial illustration showing enlarged view of ascending aorta in LAO projection showing left coronary cusp (LCC) on patient's left and right coronary cusp (RCC) on patient's right along with origins of left main coronary artery (LMCA) and right coronary artery (RCA). There are two horizontal lines, the superiorly placed horizontal line (solid) separates sinuses from ascending aorta and inferiorly placed line (dotted) represents aortoventricular plane. The third line is placed midway along the long axis of ascending aorta intersecting the other two horizontal lines perpendicularly. Together these landmarks can be used to describe origin sites of anomalous coronaries. These sites are labeled here as A, B, C, and D. (LAO: left anterior oblique; LV: left ventricle; NCC: noncoronary cusp)

If an experienced operator is unable to cannulate LMCA or RCA using these routine manners, suspicion for anomalous origin of coronaries should immediately arise. One important thing to realize is that TIG catheter can be easily employed for cannulating ACAOS also. Sometimes, however, to have a better aortic root support, Amplatzer left (AL), which is an active catheter, may be required.[5]

In order to develop a better understanding of catheter selection for various origin sites of ACAOS, we can systematically categorize the sites of anomalous coronary origin using the concept of sinus aortic and aortoventricular planes as suggested by work of Sarkar et al. They proposed that if we assume left ventricular outflow and aorta as cylindrical object with bulge in lower middle representing aortic sinuses, and divide the aortic sinuses from aorta with an imaginary horizontal line and further divide the aortic cusps from the ventricular outflow tract with another lower placed horizontal line (shown as dotted line in **Figure 1**) and finally draw a line parallel to long axis of ascending aorta intersecting the sinoaortic plane (solid horizontal line in **Figure 1**) and aortoventricular planes (dotted horizontal line in **Figure 1**) perpendicularly, the various origin sites of ACAOS can be objectively defined in relation to these planes (*see* **Fig. 1**).[6]

- *Site A: When origin is above the sinotubular plane.*
- *Site B: When origin is just below LMCA.*
- *Site C: When origin is below the sinotubular plane but somewhere between the midline and the origin of LMCA.*
- *Site D: When origin is along the perpendicular line.*

Ben Dor et al. further suggested other origin sites for ACAOS besides these four sites described above **(Fig. 2)**.

- *R-ACAOS* can arise from either LCC near the LMCA origin, or a little inferiorly to the LMCA origin (labeled B in **Figure 2**) or sometimes superiorly (labeled A in **Figure 2**) or even very high and anterior along the long axis of aorta (labeled E in **Figure 2**), or in-between noncoronary cusp (NCC) and LCC (near site labeled D in **Figure 2**) or somewhere in-between site B and D (labeled C in **Figure 2**).[7]
- The *L-ACAOS* can arise from site in-between RCC and NCC (labeled F in **Figure 2**) or near RCA origin (labeled G in **Figure 2**).[7]

The fact that origin of R-ACAOS can be such varied, supports reasoning that we should be using different catheters for differently originating R-ACAOS. If so, then, we should also consider adding 2–3 more catheters for L-ACAOS. In fact, there are numerous catheters available in market that are shaped for various anomalous positions but the concept is simple.[7]

The more leftward the origin of anomalous vessel, more is the curve length (i.e., distance between primary and secondary curve of the catheter) required with the catheter selected and if this curve length is shorter than required then we need to manipulate or give more torque, clockwise

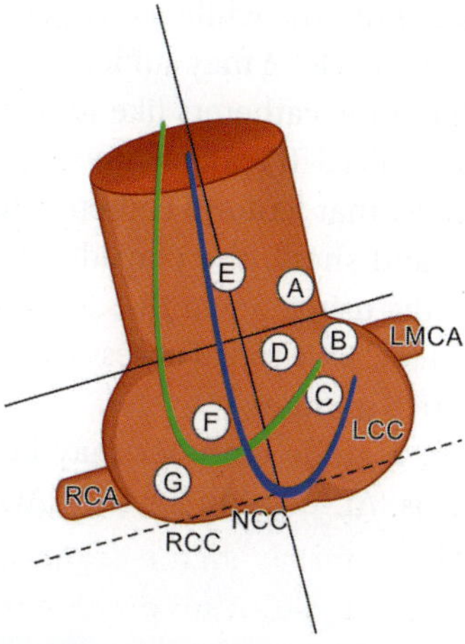

Fig. 2: An illustration showing relative position of coronary cusps and landmark planes represented by two horizontal lines (solid one represents sinoaortic plane and dotted one represents aortoventricular plane) and one vertical line (along long axis of aorta), to precisely localize various sites of origin of anomalous coronaries. R-ACAOS can origin from sites A, B, C, D, and E while L-ACAOS can take origin from site F and G. There two curved color lines representing coronary catheters course via retroaortic route and exemplifying the fact that the catheter with more curve length engages a superiorly originating vessel (represented by green-colored thick line) one having shorter curve engages an inferiorly originating coronary (blue-colored thick line). (R-ACAOS: right anomalous coronaries arising from opposite sinus; LCC: left coronary cusp; LMCA: left main coronary artery; NCC: noncoronary cusp; RCC: right coronary cusp)

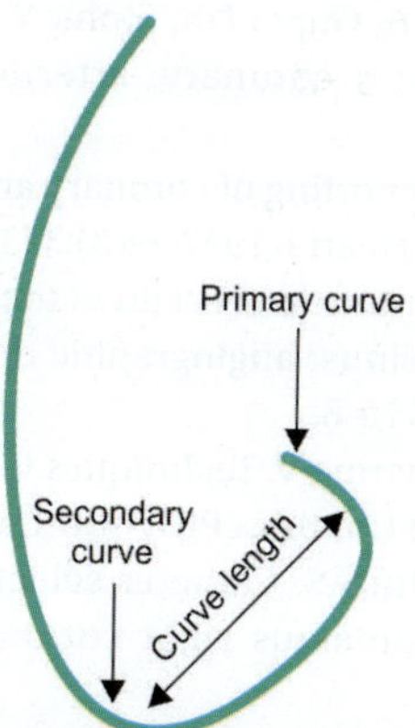

Fig. 3: Concept of "curve length" in a Judkins right catheter.

for leftward or forward movement and counter-clockwise for backward movement of the catheter tip **(Figs. 2 and 3)**.

Practical Tip

Thus, for R-ACAOS, with origin around LCC, Amplatzer left (AL)-2 or TIG-4.5 (instead of regular TIG-4) or Judkins left (JL)-5 is preferred, which has more curve for superiorly placed origins while as we move on toward inferiorly placed origins, AL-1 or regular TIG-4 may suffice.

For L-ACAOS, smaller curve catheters like Judkins right (JR)-3.5 or ECR catheters or smaller TIG-3.5 (TIG-II) can be utilized.

It is worthwhile to know that femoral catheters like JL and JR work well even from radial access and should be considered wherever required. In fact, in a prospective study, using single JR-3.5 catheter, it was possible to cannulate both RCA and LMCA via radial access itself in 94% cases and mean procedural time was about 6 minutes.[8]

Sometimes, however, a guide catheter may be required for hooking ACAOS. In such scenarios, AL-2 guide for R-ACAOS and JR-3.5 guide for L-ACAOS will do the trick.

CONCLUSION

Suspicion of anomalous coronaries arises whenever there is nonvisualization of supply to a part of myocardium or when routine maneuvers of coronary cannulation fail. A nonselective aortic root angiogram may often reveal the site of anomalous coronary origin. Selecting appropriate view and catheter helps with the successful cannulation.

REFERENCES

1. Gentile F, Castiglione V, De Caterina R. Coronary Artery Anomalies. Circulation. 2021;144(12):983-96.
2. Garg N, Tewari S, Kapoor A, Gupta DK, Sinha N. Primary congenital anomalies of the coronary arteries: a coronary: arteriographic study. Int J Cardiol. 2000;74(1):39-46.
3. Goel PK. A relook at the reporting of coronary angiograms in the interventional era: a perspective. Indian Heart J. 1997;49(3):323-6.
4. Ishikawa T, Brandt PW. Anomalous origin of the left main coronary artery from the right anterior aortic sinus: angiographic definition of anomalous course. Am J Cardiol. 1985;55(6):770-6.
5. Chawla R, Ahamad W, Sharma V. Techniques to Overcome Difficulty in Device Deliverability to Lesion in Complex PCI. Curr Cardiol Rev. 2020;16(2):117-24.
6. Sarkar K, Sharma SK, Kini AS. Catheter selection for coronary angiography and intervention in anomalous right coronary arteries. J Interv Cardiol. 2009;22(3):234-9.
7. Ben-Dor I, Weissman G, Rogers T, Slack M, Pichard A, Ben-Dor N, et al. Catheter Selection and Angiographic Views for Anomalous Coronary Arteries: A Practical Guide. JACC Cardiovasc Interv. 2021;14(9):995-1008.
8. Rondán J, Lozano I, Morís C, Martín M, Avanzas P, Suárez E. Cateterismo cardíaco por vía radial derecha con catéter Judkins izquierdo. Estudio prospectivo [Cardiac catheterization via the right radial artery with a Judkins left catheter. A prospective study]. Rev Esp Cardiol. 2005;58(7):868-71.

CHAPTER 2

Femoral Artery Approach: Access Techniques, Challenges, and Complications

Debabrata Roy

INTRODUCTION

The femoral artery access approach, initially described by Ivar Seldinger, has historically been the primary method of vascular access for coronary catheterization procedures. While several randomized trials have demonstrated the superiority of radial access over femoral access in terms of bleeding and vascular complications,[1-6] transradial access has now become the predominant route for coronary angiography and percutaneous coronary interventions. However, transfemoral access remains essential for selected complex percutaneous coronary interventions, mechanical circulatory support, and structural heart procedures requiring large bore access. The integration of adjunctive technology and techniques such as ultrasound guidance and micropuncture combined with fluoroscopy and palpation can improve outcomes associated with femoral vascular access.

INDICATIONS

- Access site for coronary angiography and intervention, particularly for procedures requiring larger sheath sizes
- Access site for percutaneous structural heart procedures (e.g., balloon valvuloplasty, percutaneous valves)
- Access site for peripheral vascular angiography
- Access for intra-aortic balloon pump/TandemHeart/extracorporeal membrane oxygenation (ECMO)/Impella device placement for hemodynamic support.
- Port for arterial access for invasive hemodynamic monitoring (radial access preferred)
- Patients with prior difficult radial access.

PRECAUTIONS AND PROPER PATIENT SELECTION

Vascular access site complications are common during coronary angiography and intervention and can be prevented by adhering to good access techniques, starting with appropriate patient selection based on a thorough history and physical examination.

- *Thorough history:* Assessing factors such as peripheral artery disease (PAD), prior interventions for PAD, recent femoral access, presence of active groin infection, prior groin surgeries or radiation therapy, iliac or aortoiliac aneurysms, difficulties during prior femoral access, and risk factors for complications.
- *Physical examination:* Inspecting the groin for signs of infection or swelling, palpating for femoral and distal arterial pulses, and auscultating for bruits.
- *Basic laboratory values:* Including hemoglobin, platelet count, coagulation panel, electrolyte panel, and creatinine.

TECHNIQUES

The most secure location for puncturing is the common femoral artery (CFA) due to its substantial size and the ability to compress it over the femoral head. Originating from the external iliac artery, the CFA traverses beneath the inguinal ligament and divides distally into the superficial (SFA) and profunda (PFA) femoral arteries (*see* **Fig. 1**).[7] The optimal puncture site lies in the segment of the CFA situated above the bifurcation of the SFA and PFA and below the inferior epigastric branch, ensuring compressibility against the femoral head.

- *Access using anatomical landmarks* **(Table 1)**
- *Fluoroscopic guided access* **(Table 2)**
- *Ultrasound-guided approach* **(Table 3)**
- *Utilizing a micropuncture needle* **(Table 4)**
    - In fully anticoagulated patients, obtaining femoral access with a smaller gauge needle (micropuncture needle—21-gauge) is preferable to minimize access site complications.

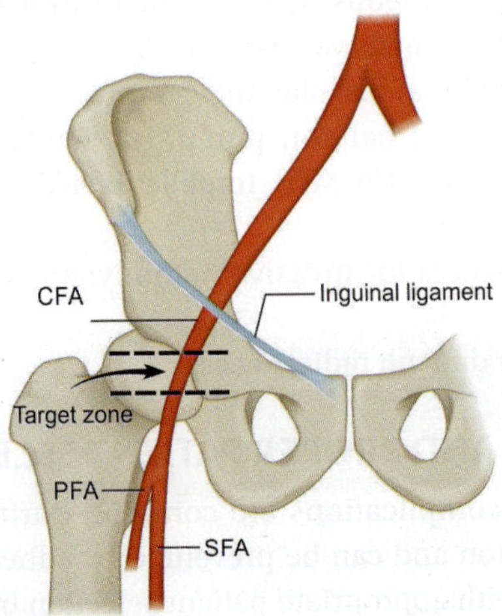

Fig. 1: Anatomical landmarks for femoral access.[8] (CFA: common femoral artery; PFA: profunda femoral artery; SFA: superficial femoral artery)

TABLE 1: Access using anatomical landmarks.

Steps	*Advantages*	*Disadvantages*
• Identify the anterior superior iliac spine laterally and the symphysis pubis as a landmark for the inguinal ligament • Obtain access 2–3 centimeters below the midpoint between these landmarks • Needle to be aimed toward the area of strongest pulse. Angle of needle with skin should be 30–45°	Based on traditional teaching and most familiar method	• Inguinal crease is an unreliable marker for location of inguinal ligament • Difficult to appreciate the location of the inguinal ligament with palpation, especially in obese patients • Anatomical variations—high bifurcation, calcification, and plaque and obesity diminish the accuracy of this technique[9] • Low access increases the risk for bleeding and hematoma due to lack of a compressible site, and pseudoaneurysm[10,11] • High access (above the inguinal ligament) increases the risk of a retroperitoneal bleed and adverse outcomes[12]

TABLE 2: Fluoroscopic guided access.

Steps	*Advantages*	*Disadvantages*
Tip of the hemostat to be placed at the inferior border of the femoral head under fluoroscopic guidance: • Enter the skin with a needle at this site **(Figs. 2A and B)** • The CFA overlying the middle third of the femoral head should be aimed for puncture	Rapid access especially in cases with weak pulse • The presence and extent of vessel calcification can be noted	• Mismatch between skin entry site and location of inferior border of femoral head may occur after infiltration of skin with local anesthetic • Cannot account for a high CFA bifurcation (superior to the inferior border of the femoral head but inferior to the midpoint of the femoral head) or a very high bifurcation (superior to the midpoint of the femoral head)[13]

(CFA: common femoral artery)

- The micropuncture kit typically comprises a 21-gauge stainless steel needle, a 0.018-inch guidewire with a soft flexible tapered tip, and a 4 Fr × 10 cm micropuncture sheath with a dilator.

TABLE 3: Ultrasound-guided approach.

Steps	*Advantages*	*Disadvantages*
• Position the vascular ultrasound (US) probe (5–10 Hz) above the palpated pulsation in the groin • Ensure the US probe is perpendicular to the course of the femoral artery, observing a clear and complete circle on the screen • Scan the artery by moving the US probe caudally along the skin to follow the course of the femoral artery and identify the bifurcation of the common femoral artery • Note that the vein is compressible, while the artery is typically pulsatile and not collapsible • Identify an anterior wall segment of the artery that is free of atherosclerotic disease or calcification • Locate the marker on the probe that corresponds to the marker on the ultrasound machine screen	• Enables the operator to identify and avoid plaque, calcification, and a pulsatile femoral vein • Prevents back-wall and side-wall punctures	• Operator training and experience are necessary • There is a risk of high puncture if the US probe slides cranially or if the needle trajectory is shallow and close to the US probe • There may be underestimation of the needle tip depth • Bony landmarks are challenging to visualize in ultrasound
• Align both as this is used to direct the needle as it traverses the skin and subcutaneous tissue. The common femoral vein is medial to the artery • Adjust the needle skin puncture site according to the depth of the femoral artery by puncturing away from the probe at a distance similar to the artery's depth • Continuously visualize the needle tip as it traverses the subcutaneous tissue. Ensure the ultrasound probe and beam remain stable while adjusting the needle direction in the subcutaneous tissue. Aim to puncture the anterior arterial wall of the segment and monitor the tip entering the artery • Exercise extreme caution to avoid moving the probe or left hand • Once access is achieved, maintain the probe in place until a wire is introduced through the needle and into the vessel		

TABLE 4: Utilizing a micropuncture needle.

Steps	*Advantages*	*Disadvantages*
• Advance the micropuncture needle in a manner similar to that of a standard gauge needle • Once the artery is cannulated, ensure adequate blood flow. Insert and advance the 0.018-inch guidewire, preferably under fluoroscopic guidance • Remove the micropuncture needle over the guidewire and exchange it for the 4-Fr micropuncture sheath and dilator • Note brisk pulsatile arterial flow at this stage • Utilize a 0.035-inch J-tip guidewire through the micropuncture sheath and exchange the sheath for a regular 5–8-Fr femoral artery sheath	• Facilitates femoral angiography before inserting a larger caliber catheter, confirming the safety of the puncture site • Abandoning puncture sites with micropuncture access enables easier hemostasis afterward due to the smaller puncture size	• The guidewire's highly flexible tip reduces the tactile feedback during advancement compared to traditional spring-tip guidewires • Smaller caliber guidewires may inadvertently enter small branches, coupled with reduced tactile feedback, potentially leading to aggressive advancement into a small branch, causing perforation, a large hematoma, and other access site complications. This risk can be mitigated by closely monitoring the micropuncture guidewire advancement under fluoroscopy

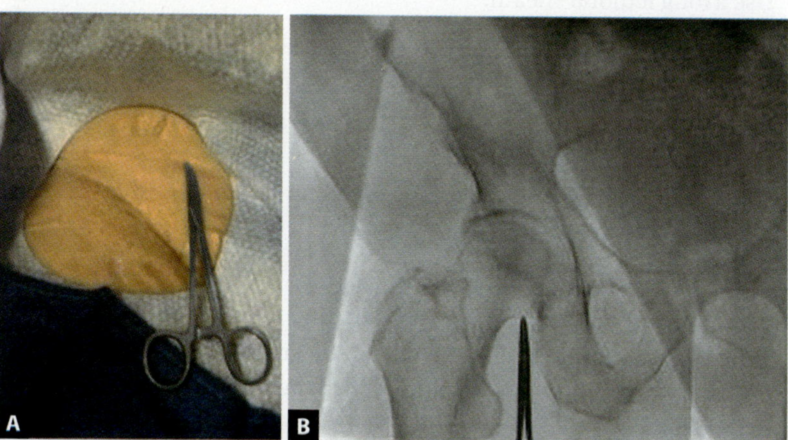

Figs. 2A and B: Correct location of skin entry based on the location of the inferior border of the femoral head.[13]

CHALLENGES

Navigating tortuous and diseased iliac arteries:

- Common in the elderly

- After gaining access, it is crucial to assess the extent of the access wire within the femoral/iliac vessel.
- If the J-wire encounters resistance due to tortuosity or stenotic disease in the iliac arteries, consider placing a micropuncture sheath and then exchanging the J-wire for a soft angled glidewire. Avoid inserting the glidewire directly through the introducer needle to prevent stripping off its hydrophilic coat into the vessel.
- Once the wire reaches the aorta, switch to a long (25–45 cm) femoral sheath inserted over the wire under fluoroscopic visualization to bypass possible resistance points hindering catheter manipulation.
- If encountering resistance, reassess for the possibility of being subintimal or in a dissection plane, particularly in the presence of significant plaque. In cases of a tortuous aorta, a 45–90-cm sheath may be necessary, preferably placed over a stiff 0.035″ guidewire.

Access through femoral graft:

- Utilize ultrasound guidance to identify the anastomosis site and the optimal puncture site.
- Employ a micropuncture needle.
- Exercise caution when directing the wire into the graft and aorta (fluoroscopy guidance aids).
- Minimize manipulation within the graft.
- Serial dilation may be required.
- Use a long femoral sheath.

Patient on oral anticoagulants (OAC):

- Patients on OAC and fully anticoagulated [international normalized ratio (INR) >1.6] have similar 30-day major adverse event rates compared to those not anticoagulated.[14]
- To mitigate complications, employ micropuncture.
- Avoid heparin use if INR >2.5.
- Prefer radial access.

Anomalous femoral artery:

- Typically, the groin vein lies medial to the artery. However, in rare cases, the artery can be superficial to the vein at the base of the femoral triangle in the groin.[15]
- In such situations, prefer an ultrasound-guided approach to prevent AV fistula or retroperitoneal hematoma.

COMPLICATIONS[7,16-19]

Table 5 describes the complications and their management of a femoral arterial puncture.

TABLE 5: Complications of a femoral arterial puncture and their management.

Complication	*Incidence*	*Risk factors*	*Management*
Hematoma	<3%	Low femoral puncture, multiple punctures, puncturing through an overlying vein, large sheath size, ineffective manual compression, female gender, anticoagulant and antifibrinolytic therapy and hypertension	• Small hematoma—manual compression • Large hematoma—rapid internal balloon tamponade, covered stent, or surgical correction
Pseudoaneurysm	1–3%	Low puncture	• <2 cm—no intervention • >2 cm and narrow neck—USG-guided compression or thrombin injection • >2 cm and wide neck—surgical closure
Dissection	1%	Occurs during withdrawal of shaped catheters, or large devices	• Retrograde dissection—conservative • Antegrade dissection—if flow limiting—femoral artery stenting
Arteriovenous (AV) fistula	<1%	Same as hematoma	Prolonged bandage, coil embolization, surgery
Retroperitoneal hemorrhage	<3%	High puncture, use of glycoprotein IIb–IIIa inhibitors, posterior wall puncture	• Intravenous fluid/blood transfusion • Reversal of anticoagulation • Angiography with selective embolization of active bleeding • Covered stent placement • Open surgical repair
Acute limb ischemia	<1%	Inadequate anticoagulation, delayed sheath removal	• Rutherford class I and IIa—endovascular techniques (percutaneous catheter-directed thrombolysis, thromboaspiration with or without thrombolytic therapy, mechanical thrombectomy) • Rutherford class IIb—open revascularization

CONCLUSION

A combined strategy of fluoroscopic assessment of bony landmarks and ultrasound-guided arterial puncture in a segment without significant atherosclerotic burden can help target the ideal common femoral puncture site while ensuring safe transfemoral access. Micropuncture access followed by femoral angiography by hand injection enhances spatial orientation of the access site, contributing to improved outcomes.

REFERENCES

1. Bernat I, Horak D, Stasek J, Mates M, Pesek J, Ostadal P, et al. ST-segment elevation myocardial infarction treated by radial or femoral approach in a multicenter randomized clinical trial: the STEMI-RADIAL trial. J Am Coll Cardiol. 2014;63:964-72.
2. Chiarito M, Cao D, Nicolas J, Roumeliotis A, Power D, Chandiramani R, et al. Radial versus femoral access for coronary interventions: An updated systematic review and meta-analysis of randomized trials. Catheter Cardiovasc Interv. 2021;97:1387-96.
3. Jhand A, Atti V, Gwon Y, Dhawan R, Turagam MK, Mamas MA, et al. Meta-Analysis of Transradial vs Transfemoral Access for Percutaneous Coronary Intervention in Patients with ST Elevation Myocardial Infarction. Am J Cardiol. 2021;141:23-30.
4. Jolly SS, Yusuf S, Cairns J, Niemelä K, Xavier D, Widimsky P, et al. Radial versus femoral access for coronary angiography and intervention in patients with acute coronary syndromes (RIVAL): a randomised, parallel group, multicentre trial. Lancet. 2011;377:1409-20.
5. Mehta SR, Jolly SS, Cairns J, Niemela K, Rao SV, Cheema AN, et al. Effects of Radial Versus Femoral Artery Access in Patients with Acute Coronary Syndromes with or without ST-Segment Elevation. J Am Coll Cardiol. 2012;60:2490-9.
6. Romagnoli E, Biondi-Zoccai G, Sciahbasi A, Politi L, Rigattieri S, Pendenza G, et al. Radial versus femoral randomized investigation in ST-segment elevation acute coronary syndrome: the RIFLE-STEACS (Radial Versus Femoral Randomized Investigation in ST-Elevation Acute Coronary Syndrome) study. J Am Coll Cardiol. 2012;60:2481-9.
7. Bangalore S, Bhatt DL. Femoral Arterial Access and Closure. Circulation. 2011;124:e147-56.
8. Bhatty S, Cooke R, Shetty R, Jovin IS. Femoral vascular access-site complications in the cardiac catheterization laboratory: Diagnosis and management. Interv Cardiol. 2011;3(4):503-14.
9. Garrett PD, Eckart RE, Bauch TD, Thompson CM, Stajduhar KC. Fluoroscopic localization of the femoral head as a landmark for common femoral artery cannulation. Catheter Cardiovasc Interv. 2005;65:205-7.
10. Altin R, Flicker S, Naidech H. Pseudoaneurysm and arteriovenous fistula after femoral artery catheterization: Association with low femoral punctures. Am J Roentgenol. 1989;152:629-31.
11. Rapoport S, Sniderman KW, Morse SS, Proto MH, Ross GR. Pseudoaneurysm: A complication of faulty technique in femoral arterial puncture. Radiology. 1985;154:529-30.

12. Kwok CS, Kontopantelis E, Kinnaird T, Potts J, Rashid M, Shoaib A, et al. Retroperitoneal Hemorrhage after Percutaneous Coronary Intervention: Incidence, Determinants, and Outcomes as Recorded by the British Cardiovascular Intervention Society. Circ Cardiovasc Interv. 2018;11:e005866.
13. Pitta S, Bagai J, Swaminathan RV, Latif F. (2020). Safe femoral access: Using all the tools in the toolbox. [online] Available from https://scai.org/safe-femoral-access-using-all-tools-toolbox. [Last accessed August, 2024].
14. Shammas NW, Shammas GA, Jones-Miller S, Gumpert MR, Gumpert MJ, Harb C, et al. Predictors of common femoral artery access site complications in patients on oral anticoagulants and undergoing a coronary procedure. Ther Clin Risk Manag. 2017;13:401-6.
15. Sahin B, Uzun A, Emirzeoglu M, Kosif R, Bilgic S. A deep femoral artery passing in front of the femoral vein. Folia Morphol (Warsz). 2003;62:143-6.
16. Işık M, Tanyeli Ö, Dereli Y, Taban VB, Altınbaş Ö, Görmüş N. Gradual treatment of arteriovenous fistula in femoral vessels as a complication of coronary angiography. Rev Bras Cir Cardiovasc. 2018;33(6):631.
17. Martin K, Ma AD, Key NS. Molecular basis of hemostatic and thrombotic diseases. In: Molecular Pathology. Amsterdam: Elsevier; 2018. pp. 277-97.
18. Olinic DM, Stanek A, Tătaru DA, Homorodean C, Olinic M. Acute limb ischemia: An update on diagnosis and management. J Clin Med. 2019;8(8):1215.
19. Stinis CT. Avoiding and managing femoral access site complications. Promedicacme.com. Available from https://promedicacme.com/wp-content/uploads/2017/11/Stinis-Curtiss-Femoral-Access-Complications.pdf. [Last accessed August, 2024].

CHAPTER

3

Radial Access, Challenges, and Complications

Yashasvi Chugh, Sunita Chugh, Sanjay Kumar Chugh

INTRODUCTION

Radial access is now recommended for all percutaneous coronary interventions (PCIs), as per the recent European and American guidelines,[1,2] because of less bleeding and vascular complications, especially in the acute and sicker patients in whom transradial access has proven survival benefit over transfemoral access. In addition, it is patient friendly as the patient can mobilize early, sit up and eat immediately after procedure, and can be discharged home 4–6 hours after an angiogram and usually the day after an uncomplicated angioplasty, if the patient is stable.

PREPARATION FOR RADIAL CASE

The following must be available:

- Noninvasive blood pressure monitoring cuff and venous access, with fluid running according to patient's left ventricular function, on patient's contralateral arm.
- Fentanyl and anesthetist should be available for intravenous administration of fentanyl and/or midazolam, if patient begins to get spasm of radial artery or feels pain.
- Injection diltiazem or verapamil prepared as 1 mg per mL, injection nitroglycerin prepared as 100 µg/mL, injection Nikoran prepared as 1 mg per mL should be available for intra-arterial administration into radial artery by the operator.
- Injection Heparin 5,000 IU should be ready for intra-arterial administration. Which is the usual recommended dose for an average 70 kg person, the per kg bodyweight dose being 70–100 IU per kg for angiography and angioplasty.

RADIAL ACCESS: PUNCTURE

The puncture is done at the wrist, 2 cm proximal to styloid process mostly using a double puncture technique with a Terumo sheathed needle and radial kit. The sheathed needle is used to puncture the radial artery at 45° angle. After the needle punctures the radial artery, a drop of blood is visible in the hub, at which time, the needle is advanced to puncture and go beyond the posterior wall. Then the metallic needle is removed and the sheath of the needle is withdrawn slowly till it is intraluminal with the radial artery, when flow is noted through the sheath of the needle. At this point, a 0.018″ Teflon coated sheath glidewire is introduced into the needle sheath and the needle sheath is removed. Following this, a sheath with dilator is introduced into the artery over the wire, dilator is removed and sheath is flushed, and spasmolytics are administered intra-arterially into radial artery, as per the choice of the operator.

Alternatively, a metallic needle may be utilized to introduce a sheath using the Seldinger technique, as with femoral artery access. The Cook radial kit has a micropuncture needle and 0.018″ wire, while the cordis radial kit has a small metallic needle and a noncoated 0.021″ wire. A similar radial kit by Arrow is also available.

CHALLENGES

The challenges may arise from tortuosities along the course from radial to subclavian to reach the ascending aorta. Such tortuosities can be crossed using a Terumo glidewire; failing which a 0.014″ angioplasty wire can enable crossing. One has to be careful to reduce or modify the bevel or gap between the guide catheter (GC) and wire using a balloon or a 1F smaller multipurpose (MPA) or pigtail catheter introduced inside the guide catheter (e.g., a 5F pigtail or MPA catheter inside a 6F guide catheter).

In addition, a big breath always helps to negotiate subclavian tortuosity. Cubital loops can be negotiated by using 4F catheter and 0.014″ angioplasty wire. But because of risk of extravasation, European guidelines recommend using alternative access rather than risk complication of extravasation due to vessel injury.[3]

In patients with hypertension, severe aortic regurgitation and in the elderly, the anatomy of ascending aorta may get modified, with unfolding of aorta, rotation of sinuses and dilatation of ascending aorta which can make hooking of coronary arteries challenging.

In a retroesophageal right subclavian artery (RORSA) **(Fig. 1)**, the hooking of coronaries becomes difficult. The trick is to deflect a wire off the aortic knuckle into ascending aorta, then track a catheter over it to hook the coronaries. A JL 3 or XB 3 is best to hook left coronary artery (LCA) in RORSA; while for right coronary artery (RCA), a JR is adequate.

When the aorta is horizontal, the left coronary arises at 12 o'clock position and the right coronary arises from a 7 o'clock position.[4] While LCA can be hooked as usual, hooking of the RCA may be challenging and may require either the JR to be counter-clockwise rotated and pushed to engage the RCA or alternatively, an Amplatz catheter may be able to hook the RCA and give support for angioplasty. This is also true when better guide support is required for PCI in chronic total occlusion (CTO) or tortuosity of RCA. Incidentally, left radial provides better support for complex PCI of RCA.

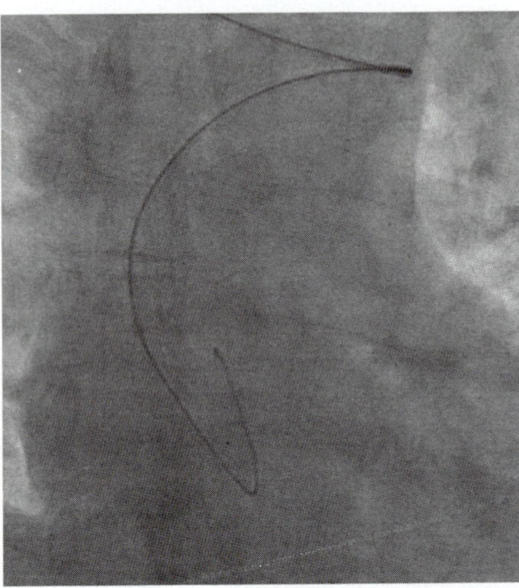

Fig. 1: Typical shape of angiographic guidewire and catheter in a patient with a retro-esophaeal right subclavian artery, the subclavian artery on the right side originates distally from the arch of aorta or rarely from the descending thoracic aorta and courses behind the esophagus.

For bypass graft angiography or angioplasty, left radial access is preferred. A TIG (Terumo) catheter can hook all grafts; internal mammary artery (IMA) catheter is better used for hooking left IMA graft.

Most angioplasty can be done using 6F GC, including kissing balloon, spider filter, 1.5-mm rotablation burr, guideliner, and intravascular ultrasound (IVUS).

A 7F GC is required for performing simultaneous kissing stent procedure, rotablation using 1.75 mm burr and also for many cases of CTO, especially where the retrograde approach is used.

For more details, including information on distal radial access, please refer to the Handbook of Transradial Interventions, published by Oxford University Press, edited by Dr. Sanjay Kumar Chugh.

COMPLICATIONS

The complications are listed below and described in detail in our award-winning paper in Indian Heart Journal:[5]

- Radial artery spasm (RAS)
- Radial artery occlusion (RAO)
- Bleeding, localized and remote (including radial artery perforation)
- Hematoma and compartment syndrome
- Rarer complications include radial pseudoaneurysm and arteriovenous fistula.
- *Radial artery spasm:* Radial artery is prone to spasm and spasm begets spasm; hence, it is important to prevent rather than treat RAS. Using a

sheath or catheter of a diameter greater than the diameter of the access radial artery can lead to stretch and initiation of RAS. Hence, it is important to size the sheath according to radial artery. Our sheath sizing protocol is useful for the purpose and was shown in the PRIMAFACIE TRI study to reduce spasm, procedure failure, and RAO.[6]

- *Radial artery occlusion:* Radial artery occlusion has been reported from 0.46[6] to 10% and the incidence depends on use of best practices[7] which include the following:
    - Preprocedure measurement of RA size and following sheath sizing protocol to minimize RA stretch by maintaining the ratio of sheath/ catheter size (mm) to radial artery size (mm) as close to 1:1 as possible
    - Adequate anticoagulation of 100 U/kg; and a minimum of 5,000 units for coronary angiography
    - Practice of patent hemostasis. In this, the hemostatic compression device is loosened just enough to stop it from bleeding but at the same time to allow antegrade flow through the radial artery, which is detected as a waveform on plethysmograph despite compression of ulnar.
    - Minimizing compression pressure to minimum required (feasible with TR band) and limiting compression time to under 2 hours for PCI while monitoring for hematoma. For angiograms, much shorter compression times (30–60 minutes) are often adequate.
    - Administration of additional intravenous heparin or use of compression of ulnar artery for situations where the pulse is lost early postprocedure.
    - Avoidance of balloon or catheter-assisted tracking.
- *Bleeding: localized and remote:* Access site bleed can lead to a hematoma in forearm if compression is not adequate. It is important to maintain compression for hemostasis both proximal and distal to puncture to prevent bleeding from collateral flow distal to puncture. Sometimes inadequate compression can lead to bleeding from posterior wall puncture of radial artery.

  Remote bleeding can occur from perforation of a branch by a coated glidewire.
- Radial artery perforation can occur from the edge of a guide catheter. Reduce this injury, which can occur especially when negotiating tortuosities and loops, a balloon-assisted tracking of a 1F smaller diagnostic catheter inside a GC may be useful in preventing the injury.

  If, however, a perforation is noted, the operator should continue working and the perforation seals off by the time the angioplasty is completed.
- *Hematoma and compartment syndrome:* Bleeding, if undetected, can lead to hematoma of forearm which could lead to the dreaded compartment

syndrome that can lead to hand ischemia, gangrene, and even death. This is best prevented by palpating the forearm to feel for collection, rather than just inspecting it. In case hematoma is developing, compression is applied by gauze balls placed along the length of the radial artery. In addition, a sphygmomanometer cuff is inflated to above systolic for 3 minutes, and deflated for 30 seconds to allow the hand to perfuse and presence of a good waveform on a plethysmograph connected to the index finger or thumb of the affected hand reflects adequate hand perfusion. The cuff is inflated again, thereafter. This process is continued usually for 2 hours, by which time the active bleed stops.

- *Rarer complications include radial pseudoaneurysm and arteriovenous fistula:* In the author's series, we reported[5] 1:14,330 incidence of radial pseudoaneurysm and the authors have seen only 1 radial arteriovenous fistula in 14,330 cases. While the latter requires surgery by a vascular surgeon, the former can be treated by manual compression and only rarely is surgery required to repair the vessel. This can be performed easily as a day care procedure under local anesthesia by a vascular surgeon.

CONCLUSION

In conclusion, transradial access is the recommended route for all diagnostic and interventional procedures, based on the evidence of lower risk of bleeding as well as of survival benefit; especially in the acute and sicker patients.

The only limitation for use of radial access, other than lack of experience and skill, is the use of wide bore access; since it is usually difficult to use greater than 7F sheaths or catheters via the radial artery, because of its smaller diameter.

Complications of radial access are rare and are easily preventable.

REFERENCES

1. Neumann FJ, Sousa-Uva M, Ahlsson A, Alfonso F, Banning AP, Benedetto U, et al. 2018 ESC/EACTS Guidelines on myocardial revascularization. Eur Heart J. 2019;40(2):87-165.
2. Lawton JS, Tamis-Holland JE, Bangalore S, Bates ER, Beckie TM, Bischoff JM, et al. 2021 ACC/AHA/SCAI Guideline for Coronary Artery Revascularization: Executive Summary: A Report of the American College of Cardiology/American Heart Association Joint Committee on Clinical Practice Guidelines. Circulation. 2022;145(3):e4-e17.
3. Hamon M, Pristipino C, Di Mario C, Nolan J, Ludwig J, Tubaro M, et al. Consensus document on the radial approach in percutaneous cardiovascular interventions: position paper by the European Association of Percutaneous Cardiovascular Interventions and Working Groups on Acute Cardiac Care and Thrombosis of the European Society of Cardiology. EuroIntervention. 2013;8:1242-51.

4. Chugh Y, Chugh S, Chugh SK. Tips and tricks for transradial interventions, Chapter 10. In: Chugh SK (Ed). Handbook of Transradial Interventions. Noida, UP: Oxford University Press; 2024. p. 213.
5. Chugh SK, Chugh Y, Chugh S. How to tackle complications in radial procedures: Tip and tricks. Indian Heart J. 2015;67(3):275-81.
6. Chugh SK, Chugh S, Chugh Y, Rao SV. Feasibility and utility of pre-procedure ultrasound imaging of the arm to facilitate transradial coronary diagnostic and interventional procedures (PRIMAFACIE-TRI). Catheter Cardiovasc Interv. 2013;82(1):64-73.
7. Chugh Y, Chugh S, Chugh SK. Distal radial artery access (DRA) vs. Transradial access (TRA): Current evidence. Int J Med Res Rev. 2022;10(5):147-53.

CHAPTER 4

Techniques to Enhance the Guide Catheter Support During Coronary Interventions

Mrinal Kanti Das

INTRODUCTION

The last three decades have the golden era for effective, evidence-based management of coronary artery disease which is increasing year by year. Percutaneous coronary interventions (PCIs) have been such a modality which has changed the natural history of the disease significantly. With the increase in number of PCI, there has been more and more challenging cases being taken up. These cases though during the case presentation scenario appear to be simple and easy, but lot of preprocedure strategies are needed to execute the whole procedure. Out of these strategies, guidewire selection and appropriate guide catheter for support are the most important ones. With the advancement of the time, the technological development of guidewires in terms of flexibility, torque control, trackability, torque control, steerability, pushability, radio-opacity, hydrophilic or hydrophobic quality, crossability, tactile feeling ability, etc. has remarkably increased support on their own. The next step is of course the guide catheter selection. There are conditions like anomalous origin and course of the coronary arteries, chronic total occlusion (CTO), long tortuous arteries, complex bifurcation lesions, tight calcified arteries, etc., which require extraordinary guide catheter support. The following article aims to galvanize the conceptual basis of the supporting systems with no further details on guidewires.[1]

GUIDE CATHETER[1]

A guide catheter has a stiffer shaft and larger internal diameter as compared to the diagnostic catheter. The three layers reinforcing the catheter are: (1) Outer layer with polyurethane or polyethylene to increase the radial strength, (2) middle layer with matrix for easy torque, and (3) the inner layer with Teflon coating for uninterrupted gliding of the various hardware. It has also nontapered shorter tip and more open primary curve.

This is basically a conduit for delivery of the various hardware for PCI apart from injecting the contrast. The hardware could be a balloon, a stent, microcatheter, hemodynamic monitoring device for fractional flow reserve (FFR), imaging devices like intravascular ultrasound (IVUS) or optical coherence tomography (OCT), rotablation bar, and shockwave balloon or devices delivering LASER.

For getting proper support, the selection of the proper type of guidewire is the first step followed by selection of the guide catheter (guide). Usually 5F or 6F guides are enough to perform most of the PCI procedures through radial or femoral routes. Only occasionally 7F or 8F guides may be required during double kissing technique or PCI on left main coronary artery. Guide catheters with side holes are much more useful in the ostioproximal lesions of the right coronary artery (RCA), where the chances of contrast induced dissection are higher due to noncoaxial guide catheter engagement.[2]

To have the support during delivery of different hardware, shaft of the guide catheters is anchored in the aorta and the tip is negotiated to the coronary ostium. The support is ensured with either different shapes of the guidewire or softly negotiating the tip of the catheter deep inside the artery, also called deep seating or throttling.

TYPES OF THE SUPPORT

- *Active support:* This uses the aortic root to ensure the desired shape which may be accomplished by performer's active manipulation to have the coaxial position. The examples of catheters for this type of use are Mach 1, Sherpa, Zuma 2, Wise guide, etc.
- *Passive support:* This is almost automatic and without any active manipulation. This is achieved by selecting appropriate size and shape of the guide conforming with the anatomy, size of the aorta, and the tip is engaged to the ostium. The examples of catheters for this type of use are Zuma, etc.
- *Balanced support:* This will be achieved by depending on properties of the shaft and tip. The flexible distal segment may be manipulated for extra backup. The examples of catheters for this type of use are Vistabrite, Launcher, etc.

CHOOSING GUIDE CATHETERS[1]

They are mostly Judkins (JL for left and JR for right), extra back up (EBU), and Amplatz (AL for left and AR for right).

- For left anterior descending (LAD) → one can use JL 3.5 or 4; EBU; Voda left; XB-LAD
- For right coronary artery (RCA) → JR3.5 or 4; Voda right; Hockey stick; AL2. For anomalous RCA either high, posterior or left sinus origin or Shepherd-crook RCA with initial upward direction, short-tip with side hole Amplatz guide is a good choice. The latter is also useful for RCA CTO.[2] However, JL guide with secondary curve one size larger than that is used for LMCA and an EBU guide with preshaped configuration can also be used.
- For left circumflex (LCX) → JL4, EBU; Voda left or AL2

- For left main coronary artery (LMCA) → JL guide is the default catheter. In most of the cases, JL4, JL3, or 3.5 for small aorta or anteriorly placed LAD; JL5 for dilated aorta may suffice. EBU can be used with long LMCA as the longer tip of the catheter reduces a long LMCA to a short LMCA. For ostial LMCA PCI → here the guide should not seat exactly in the LMCA, but should be loosely engaged.
- For saphenous venous graft (SVG) PCI → JR3.5 or JR4; AL or multipurpose for left coronary bypass. For SVG to RCA, JR or MP with deep throats may serve the purpose.
- For left internal mammary artery (LIMA) → JR is the initial choice. Minimum manipulation and coaxial position of the tip are asked for to prevent concertina effect and trauma.

SPECIAL GUIDE CATHETERS FOR TRANSRADIAL PERCUTANEOUS CORONARY INTERVENTION

With more and more radial interventions being taken up, there has been quantum jump in the development of the transradial intervention hardware. The same guide catheters used for transfemoral approach can be used satisfactorily. Guide catheters like Fajadet, Ikari, Kimmy or Barbeau, etc. could not withstand the test of time. One of the most commonly encountered problems faced during transradial PCI is the unfolded aorta causing the brachiocephalic artery to move toward the left of the spine causing difficulty to engage the left coronary artery (LCA). The trick could be to make a loop on the right aortic wall with the hard end of 0.035 inch guidewire and then to manipulate unlooping of the total system and thus engaging the LMCA.

SPECIAL MEASURES FOR GUIDE SUPPORT

- *Balloon:* A small diameter balloon over a guidewire is inflated proximal to the tip and kept there, thereby getting good support during CTO-PCI or where not a strong support is achieved during stent delivery.
- *Mother and child technique or five-in-six guide technique:*[3,4] Many a time, a lesion cannot be crossed by a balloon or a stent in the usual 6F guide, this technique is attempted. First the balloon or stent is taken away and a 5F guide is introduced inside the 6F guide keeping the tip of 5F guide away from that of the 6F guide and then the 5F guide is connected to the Y-connector and procedure is restarted. Then the balloon catheter is advanced into the target lesion before the 5F guide is advanced in the target artery and keeping the tension on the balloon catheter, the 5F guide is pushed out slowly. This reduces the chance of injury to the vessel by the tip of the 5F guide.
- *Microcatheter:* A microcatheter put inside the guide catheter has given extraordinary support in many situations, exactly in the same fashion like the above technique when the Guideliner is not available on the table.

- *Guideliner or Guidezilla:*[5] Guide extensions like Guideliner or Guidezilla are innovative devices to improve upon the mother and child technique. Guideliner is a flexible monorail with length of 20 cm and 135 cm working length, straight and soft tipped silicon-coated tube, and it is 1F size smaller than the guide. It has a rapid-exchange design and is advanced over the guidewire. This needs to be negotiated through the Y-connector and passed on the wire as a rapid exchange balloon deep inside the coronary artery beyond the guide. It allows coaxial alignment and offers extra support in coronaries with difficult anatomy or coronary with unusual take-off. Deep vessel engagement can be enhanced by putting a balloon catheter over the primary wire into the distal vessel. Then low-pressure balloon inflation is carried out. This works like an anchor and support advancement of the Guideliner gently. A Guideliner can be of also of other different sizes like 6F, 7F, and 8F. Usually 5F works for most of the cases. Guideliner is contraindicated in arteries with size less than 2.5 mm diameter. **Figures 1A to C** depict graphical representation of the use of Guidezilla and a case of anomalous origin of the RCA from left coronary cusp with significant mid-segment lesion. The successful deployment of the stent was achieved using guide support with EBU followed by introducing Guidezilla. This case was presented in the CSI-NIC conference.

Indications for the use of Guideliner are:[6,7]

- Chronic total occlusion
- Long tortuous arteries
- Severely calcified arteries
- Anomalous origin of the RCA
- *Long sheath:*[4] Many a time, good support cannot be achieved during transfemoral PCI because of the tortuous iliac arteries. In this situation, 40 or 60 cm long arterial sheath may offer the desired support. Apart from the iliac artery, even for complex coronary interventions, a long sheath may offer stiffness and support to the guide depending on the closeness of the tip of the guide. The increased closeness offers more support. The sheath size will be guided by the height of the patient and the requirement of more support. The greater the size, greater is the support. The sheath is advanced high up in the ascending aorta. Then as per the requirement, it may be further advanced. It thereby straightens the secondary and tertiary curves of the guide facilitating the tip of the guide to go forward easily. Guides with simple curves like Amplatz, EBU, or multipurpose are more suited for the purpose. In all the steps of advancement of the sheath and the guide, continuous monitoring of the tip with the fluoroscopy is warranted to avoid unnecessary injury to the vessel. After the PCI is complete, one great tip is that the long sheath should be removed

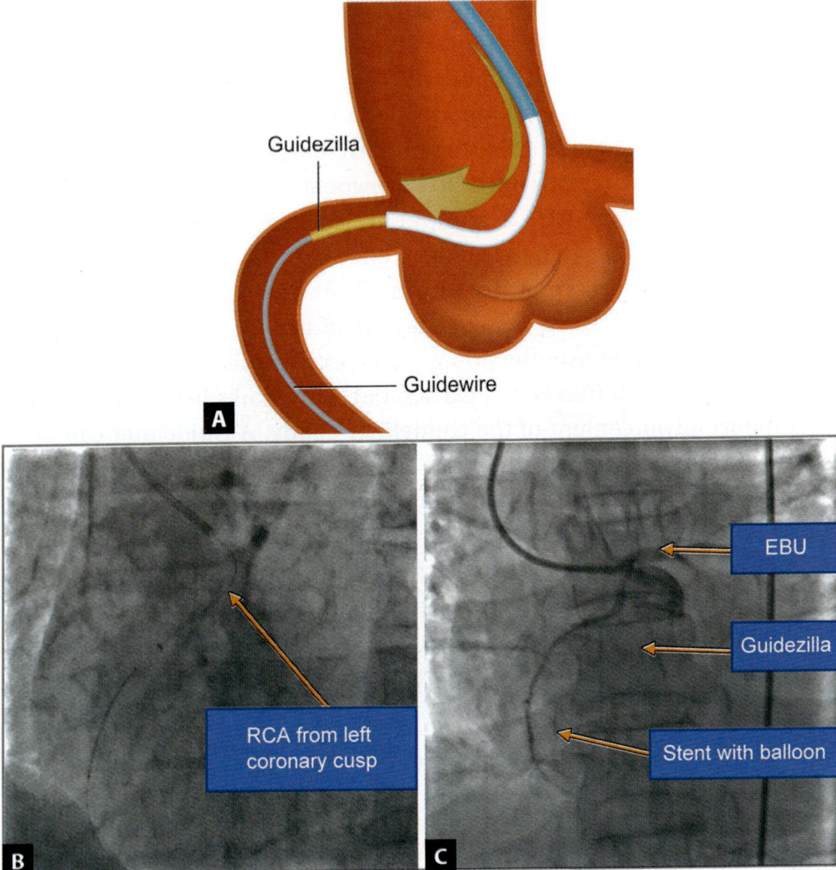

Figs. 1A to C: (A) Mother-in-child technique as graphical representation. Guidezilla introduced inside guide catheter over the same guidewire; (B) Anomalous origin of the RCA from left coronary cusp with long segment lesion at mid-RCA; (C) PCI done with EBU and Guidezilla and stent in balloon was deployed in the mid-RCA lesion successfully. (EBU: extra back up; PCI: percutaneous coronary intervention; RCA: right coronary artery)

first and brought near descending aorta keeping the guide fixed at the ostium under monitoring. After the sheath has been positioned there in descending aorta or lower down, the guide tip can be disengaged. The withdrawal of the sheath will then ease pulling out the guide.

- *Buddy wire technique:*[8] Buddy wire technique can also offer more support in case of unstable guide. A second angioplasty floppy wire is advanced parallel to the first wire **(Fig. 2)**. It provides better support and straightens the tortuous artery. It can be put in a side branch allowing better anchoring of the guide, preventing retraction. It also prevents the guide being "sucked in" beyond the left main after deploying the balloon and stents or after the poststent dilation. If a second wire does not work,

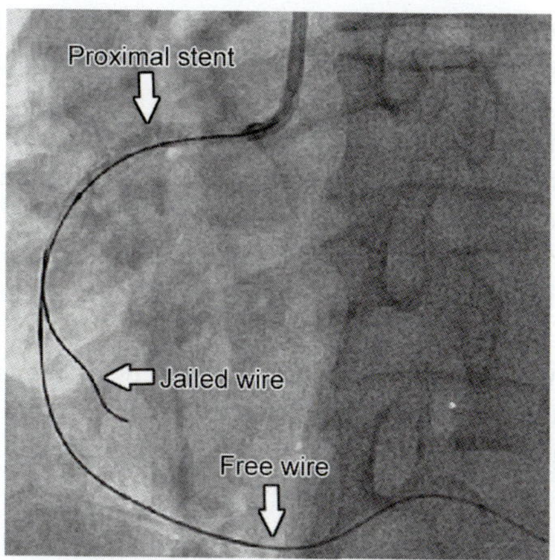

Fig. 2: Two parallel wires (Buddy wire technique) for stabilization and support during PCI. (PCI: percutaneous coronary intervention)

a third wire can be also used rarely for more stabilization, albeit with more risk of injury to the target or nondiseased artery.

CONCLUSION

Guide catheter support is of prime importance during all kinds of PCI especially in challenging cases like anomalous origin of coronary arteries, CTOs, severely calcified or tortuous arteries. The support is all the more required during additional procedures like imaging, hemodynamic study with FFR, rotablation, or orbital atherectomy. The bigger size intravascular balloon lithotripsy also warrants good support. An easy looking procedure during seminars may not be all that easy on the table and, therefore, all the hardware need to be present at the shelf and all kinds of standard preparations and precautions are highly recommended.

REFERENCES

1. Nguyen T, Hu D, Chen SL, Kim MH, Saito S, Grines CL, et al. Practical Handbook of Advanced Interventional Cardiology: Tips and Tricks, 4th edition. Hoboken: Wiley-Blackwell; 2012.
2. De Bruyne B, Stockbroeckx J, Demoor D, Heyndrickx GR, Kern MJ. Role of side holes in guide catheters: Observations on coronary pressure and flow. Catheter Cardiovasc Diag. 1994;33:145-52.
3. Takahasi S, Saito S, Tanaka S, Miyashita Y, Shiono T, Arai F, et al. New method to increase a backup support of a 6 French guiding coronary catheter. Catheter Cardiovasc Interv. 2004;63:452-6.
4. Hynes B, Dollard J, Murphy G, O'Sullivan J, Ruggiero N, Margey R, et al. Enhancing back-up support during difficult coronary stent delivery: single centre case series of experience with Hearrail II catheter. J Invasive Cardiol. 2011;23:E43-6.

5. Cola C, Miranda F, Vaqerizo B, Fantuzzi A, Bruguera J. The Guideliner™ catheter for stent delivery in difficult cases: Tips and tricks. J Interv Cardiol. 2011;24:450-61.
6. Topaz O, Disciascio G, Goudreau E, Cowley MJ, Nath A, Kohli RS, et al. Coronary angioplasty of anomalous coronary arteries: Notes on technical aspects. Catheter Cardiovasc Diag. 1990;21:106-11.
7. Sarkar K, Sharma SK, Kini AS. Catheter selection for coronary angiography and intervention in anomalous right coronary arteries. J Interv Cardiol. 2009;22:234-9.
8. Burzotta F, Trani C, Mazzari MA, Mongiardo R, Rebuzzi AG, Buffon A, et al. Use of a second buddy wire during percutaneous coronary interventions: a simple solution for some challenging situations. J Invasive Cardiol. 2005;17(3):171-4.

CHAPTER 5

Guide Catheter Extensions: Utility, Deployment Techniques, and Troubleshooting

Mathew Iype, Praveen Velappan, Lais Muhammed

INTRODUCTION

Complex angioplasties, especially done via the radial route, require good support. One option for increasing the guide support is the guide catheter extension. Guide catheter extension is used as an extension from the guiding catheter to deep intubate the coronary artery. This increases the guide catheter support. The whole system of the guide catheter along with guide catheter extension is referred to as "Mother and Child" technique. Guide catheter extensions are thus a valuable asset to improve the success of percutaneous coronary angioplasty.

BASIC ARCHITECTURE OF GUIDE CATHETERS EXTENSIONS

It is composed of a proximal portion, a mid-push shaft portion and a distal extension.[1] It is passed over the guidewire in a rapid exchange fashion. The guide extension portion is usually 25-cm long. The guide extension is 1F smaller than the guide catheter and is designed to minimize trauma to the coronary artery. The proximal end of the extension is attached to a thin stainless-steel pushrod, which is used to push and pull the system independent of the guide catheter. Guide extension catheters can be used in both femoral and radial approach. These can be inserted inside compatible guides over monorail support without the need to exchange the system. The commonly used guide extensions are shown in **Table 1**. The manufacturers are shown in **Table 2**.

TABLE 1: Commonly used guide extensions.

Guide extension	*Total length*	*Distal extension length*	*6F system—distal extension inner diameter*
Guideliner V3	150 cm	25 cm	0.057 inch
Guidezilla II	150 cm	25 cm	0.057 inch
Telescope	150 cm	25 cm	0.057 inch
TrapLiner	150 cm	13 cm	0.056 inch

TABLE 2: Commonly used guide catheter extensions and their manufacturers.

Guide extension	*Manufacturer*	*Year of FDA approval*
Guideliner V3	Vascular Solutions	2009
Guidezilla II	Boston Scientific	2013
Telescope	Medtronic	2019
TrapLiner	Vascular Solutions	2017

SOME SALIENT FEATURES OF THE COMMONLY USED GUIDE CATHETER EXTENSIONS

- *Guideliner V3:* The distal extension is 25 cm long and is silicon coated. The proximal end of the extension is attached to a thin pushrod. The pushrod is flat rectangular cross-section stainless steel.
- *Guidezilla II:* The distal extension is 25-cm long and has a 1 × 1 braid design to facilitate extra back-up support for complex or tortuous coronary anatomy without overstraightening the coronary arteries. The proximal end of the extension is attached to a thin pushrod. The pushrod is made of hollow, round cross-section stainless steel.
- *Telescope:* The distal extension is 25-cm long, wire reinforced to improve flexibility and deliverability and has a hydrophilic coating that improves deliverability. The distal extension is polytetrafluoroethylene (PTFE) lined so has low friction. The proximal end of the extension is attached to a pushrod that is solid and round made up of stainless-steel reinforced coil. The solid pushrod of telescope is in contrast to the rectangular pushrod of Guideliner V3 and the round and hollow pushrod of Guidezilla guide extension.
- *TrapLiner:* TrapLiner has the added feature of an integrated balloon for trapping a standard 0.014-inch guidewire within a guide catheter. There is no need of an additional trapping balloon. The trapping balloon is flowed by a 3-cm half pipe. The half pipe is followed by the 13-cm guide extension. The proximal part is the pushrod of 130 cm. The pushrod is made of rectangular cross-section stainless steel.

HOW TO DELIVER THE GUIDE CATHETER EXTENSION?

To deliver a guide catheter extension, the essential prerequisite is a guide catheter and a wire in the artery. The guide catheter extension monorail portion is passed over the wire and advanced into the hemostatic valve. The pushrod is used to pass the extension to the tip of the GC, avoiding crossing or twisting of the pushrod and the wire. It is always safe to advance the guide extension over a balloon catheter inside the coronary.

There are different techniques of advancing guide extension within the coronary artery:

- *Balloon-assisted tracking technique (BTT):* In BTT, a balloon is placed distally inside the coronary. The guide catheter extension is then advanced by pushing it forward while holding the inflated balloon in place. When it reaches the balloon edge, it is deflated and the catheter is advanced over it.
- *Balloon surfing technique (BST):* Small balloon is inflated at the end of the guide extension catheter, partially protruding into the artery to form a soft tip.
- *Inchworm technique:* If there is significant disease or a stenosis of the proximal vessel, inflate a balloon in this area, and then push the guide extension, while the balloon is being deflated. This is done sequentially in a stepwise fashion to gradually advance the extension bit by bit distally into the vessel. This maneuver is called inchworm technique.

UTILITY OF GUIDE CATHETER EXTENSION IN DIAGNOSTIC CORONARY ANGIOGRAPHY

Guide extensions can be used to cannulate aberrant origin coronaries and grafts when it cannot be engaged by a usual guide. Take a guide or diagnostic catheter close to the ostium and wire the coronary. If the wire is delivered through a diagnostic catheter, the wire should be a supportive 300-cm wire that is kept distal in the coronary and used to exchange for a guide placed in the aorta. A guide catheter extension is advanced to the tip of the guide. A balloon is passed into the artery and inflated and this balloon is used as an anchor to allow delivery of the guide extension into the target vessel, and the percutaneous coronary intervention (PCI) can then be completed.

UTILITY OF GUIDE CATHETER EXTENSION IN CONVENTIONAL CORONARY INTERVENTIONS

The main utility of a guide catheter extension is to increase backup force. We may have difficulty in advancing equipment and stents in the coronary artery in some cases. This is especially true when the guide support is poor. Guide catheter extension provides good backup force. Guide catheter extensions are also used to bypass segments with calcification and tortuosity. In many cases, it may not be possible to take stents to more distal sites in a coronary due to calcification and tortuosity of proximal segments. In that case, a guide extension can be taken across the zone of calcification and tortuosity and advanced to the stent landing zone (*see* **Fig. 1**). In patients with renal insufficiency and heart failure, placing a guide extension distally may reduce the need for larger volumes of contrast.

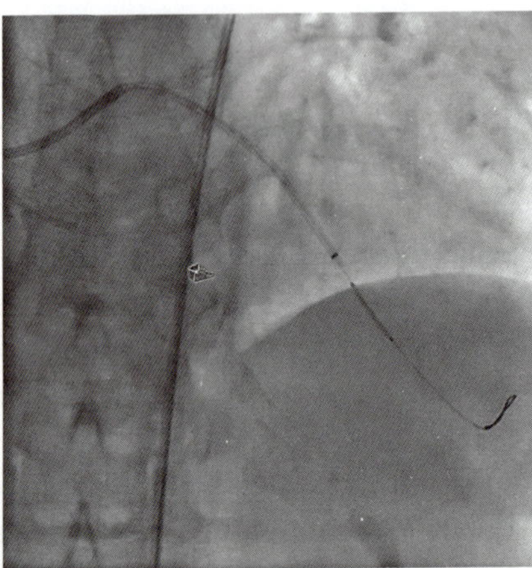

Fig. 1: Guide extension catheter deeply intubated into the left anterior descending coronary artery to advance a stent into the distal part of the artery.

UTILITY OF GUIDE CATHETER EXTENSION IN CHRONIC TOTAL OCCLUSION CORONARY INTERVENTIONS

In Reverse Controlled Antegrade and Retrograde Tracking (Reverse CART) chronic total occlusion (CTO) attempt, a guide catheter extension is useful. The extension is passed into the subintimal space in an antegrade fashion using the inchworm technique. The retrograde wire is then advanced into the extension, rather than requiring reentry into the guide catheter. This allows antegrade balloon inflation to be performed just ahead of the extension, thus minimizing the length of subintimal space to traverse with the retrograde wire.[2] Using a guide catheter extension during reverse CART also allows for a standard-length retrograde guide by shortening the total distance for the retrograde microcatheter. Use of the guide catheter extension during reverse CART also avoids the risk of extending the dissection into the aorta or dissecting past and occluding a major side branch.

UTILITY OF GUIDE CATHETER EXTENSION IN PRIMARY PERCUTANEOUS CORONARY INTERVENTIONS

In primary PCI on a heavily thrombus-laden coronary, when a thrombus aspiration catheter fails, a guide extension can be used to facilitate more effective aspiration.

UTILITY OF GUIDE CATHETER EXTENSION IN BIFURCATION PERCUTANEOUS CORONARY INTERVENTION

Another important use in rotablation cases is in bifurcation PCI where maintaining two wires at a time can be feasible with employment of guide extension.

UTILITY OF GUIDE CATHETER EXTENSION IN TRANSCATHETER AORTIC VALVE REPLACEMENT

Guide catheter extensions may be useful in accessing coronary arteries after transcatheter aortic valve replacement (TAVR) implant. The guide will not engage the coronary ostia. So wire the coronary through a standard guide and then take a guide extension. This may engage the coronary well.

PRECAUTIONS IN THE USE OF GUIDE CATHETER EXTENSIONS

Never advance a guide extension catheter without a balloon. Avoid injections through the guide extension catheter if possible. It can rarely cause spiral dissections. Remove the guide extension system as soon as the intended use is over. Always look out for complications.

DRAWBACKS OF GUIDE CATHETER EXTENSIONS

The main disadvantages are risk of dissecting the proximal coronary artery and ischemia, due to the extension within the coronary lumen.[3] Large stents of 4 mm may not pass through guide extensions. Sometimes, the pushrod and wire may intertwine and can result in inability to pass stents into the coronary artery. So, it is important to maintain separation of the guidewire and pushrod. Use of an additional wire is challenging. The second wire can pass outside the guide extension. So the second wire, if required, should be carefully introduced. Keep the collar, which has a marker, in view and manipulate the wire into the guide extension.

COMPLICATIONS

The most common complications due to use of guide catheter extensions are coronary artery ischemia, coronary dissection, and stent damage on advancement or withdrawal into the guide extension.

CONCLUSION

Guide catheter extensions form an essential component of the tool kit required to successfully execute a complex angioplasty. When used with caution, guide catheter extensions are relatively safe. They have widened the horizon of coronary anatomies amenable for angioplasty.

REFERENCES

1. Chandra S, Tiwari A, Choudhary G, Yadav R. A Guide catheter extension systems: Hype or a need? Indian Heart J. 2021;3(5):535-8.
2. Hellig F, van Wyk P, Moosa MZ. (2020). The Dos and Don'ts of Guide Catheter Extensions. [online] Available from https://assets.bmctoday.net/citoday/pdfs/cit0920_F5_Hellig.pdf. [Last accessed August, 2024].
3. Waggoner T, Desai H, Sanghvi K. A unique complication of the GuideZilla guide extension support catheter and the risk of stent stripping in interventional and endovascular interventions. Indian Heart J. 2015;67(4):381-4.

CHAPTER 6

Dual Lumen Microcatheters for Complex Percutaneous Coronary Intervention

PK Asokan

INTRODUCTION

Dual lumen microcatheters (DLMs) have a growing role and are expected to further expand as the complexity of percutaneous coronary intervention (PCI) increases. They are particularly beneficial in the treatment of bifurcation lesions, chronic total occlusions (CTOs), and a combination of both. Currently, there are various DLMs available, each with its own unique design characteristics. However, they all share a common feature of having two distinct lumens, which enables the accurate manipulation of two separate guidewires.[1]

DUAL LUMEN MICROCATHETERS

Most modern DLMs have two lumens: (1) A rapid exchange (RX) lumen with the distal port at the tip of the catheter and (2) an OTW lumen with the distal port located more proximally. The distance between the catheter tip (RX port) and OTW port varies depending on the specific catheter. To identify the exit ports of both lumens, two radiopaque markers are positioned. All current DLMs are compatible with 5F guiding catheters and feature a hydrophilic coating to enhance delivery.

Twin-Pass and Twin-Pass Torque (Teleflex), NHancer Rx (IMDS), Sasuke (Asahi Intecc USA, Inc.), ReCross (IMDS), FineDuo (Terumo Europe), and the Crusade (Kaneka) are some of the available DLMs **(Figs. 1A to F)**.

Table 1 provides an overview of the key features and distinctions among the various DLMs available. The Twin-Pass Torque microcatheter stands out with its stainless-steel braided shaft, which improves torque control and delivery. On the other hand, the NHancer Rx boasts a distal shaft design that offers the smallest dual lumen crossing profile (2.3F), enabling catheter trapping using a conventional balloon in a 6F guide. Lastly, the ReCross microcatheter is unique in that it has two OTW lumens, allowing for guidewire exchange.

There are two lumens, both of which have different features. One of the lumens has two exit ports that are positioned 180° apart. This specific characteristic enables the advancement of guidewires in various directions, which can be helpful in achieving true lumen reentry when crossing

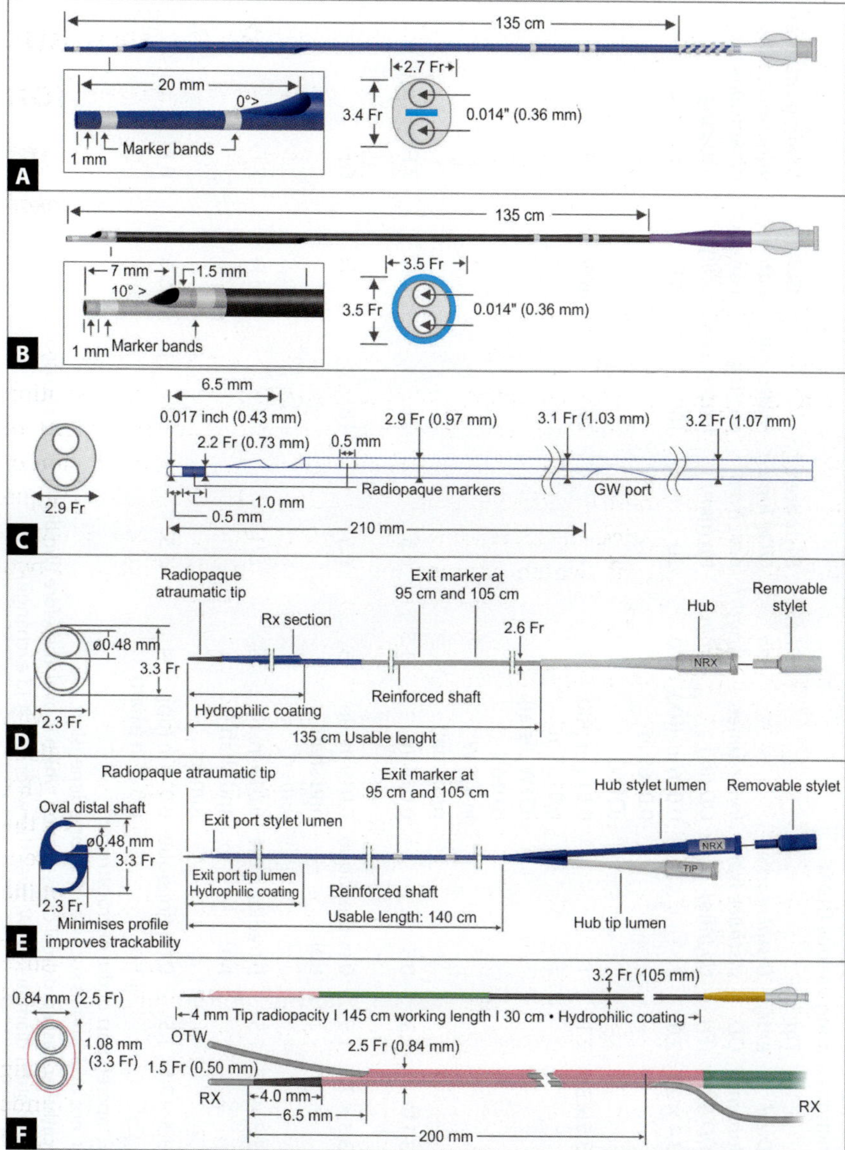

Figs. 1A to F: (A) Twin-Pass (Teleflex); (B) Twin-Pass Torque (Teleflex); (C) FineDuo (Terumo); (D) NHancer Rx (IMDS); (E) ReCross (IMDS); (F) Sasuke (Asahi Intecc). (GW: guidewire; OTW: over-the-wire; RX: rapid exchange)

subintimal guidewires. DLMs with a larger outer diameter have bigger crossing profiles, but they also provide improved back-up and stability.

All current DLMs are compatible with the standard 6F guiding catheters and can accommodate 0.014-inch guiding wires through both the RX and OTW ports. Larger-bore guiding catheters (≥7F) should be considered to provide additional support to allow larger device delivery.

TABLE 1: Key features and distinctions among various DLMs.

	Length (cm)	*Proximal OD (Fr)*	*Dual lumen OD (Fr)*	*Tip entry OD (Fr)*	*Distal marker distance from tip (mm)*	*Inner lumen OD (in.)*	*Distal tip length* (mm)*	*Distance of OTW lumen port from tip (mm)*	*Hydrophilic coating length (cm)*	*Guiding catheter compati-bility*	*Guiding catheter minimal luminal dimensions for trapping*
Twin-Pass	135	29	3.4 × 2.7	2.0	1	0.016 in. (RX) 0.0165 in (OTW)	20	20	18	6 Fr	7 Fr
Twin-Pass Torque	135	3.1	3.5 × 3.5	2.1	1	0.015 in (RX) 0.0155 in. (OTW distal) 0.0165 in (OTW proximal)	7	7	25	6 Fr	7 Fr
Fine duo/ crusade	140	3.2	3.1**	1.3	0.5	0.014 in.	1.5	6.5	21	6 Fr	7 Fr
NHancer Rx	135	2.6	3.3 × 2.3	1.5	0 (radiopaque tip)	0.019 in. tip and shaft lumen	5	6.5	18	6 Fr	6 Fr
ReCross	140	3.4 × 2.6***	3.3 × 2.3	1.5	0 (radiopaque tip)	0.019 in. tip and shaft lumen	5	8/12	25	6 Fr	7 Fr
SASUKE	145	3.2	3.3 × 2.5	1.5	0 (radiopaque tip)	0.016 in (tip) 0.017 in (shaft)	4	6.5	38	6 Fr	6 Fr

Note: *Defined as length the distal tapered part of the microcatheter.

** The FineDuo/Crusade is circular, not oval, and as such has only one dimension.

***The ReCross dual lumen microcatheter has a proximal cross-section which is oval, therefore two dimensions are used.

(DLM: dual lumen microcatheter; OD: outer diameter; OTW: over-the-wire; RX: rapid exchange)

PROCEDURE STEPS

- Prepare the lesion to aid in advancement, and DLMs are advanced over the 0.014-inch guidewire through the RX.
- Advance the DLM over the guidewire.
- Once the catheter is in place, it can then be positioned such that the radiopaque marker identifying the OTW exit port is situated at the site where precise wiring is needed.
- The currently available DLMs have varying distances between the OTW lumen distal port and the tip of the catheter (RX port).
- Remove the DLM. Once the guidewire in the OTW port has successfully been placed in the target vessel, the DLM should ideally be removed with a trapping balloon technique.
- Alternatively, the DLM can be removed via the hydraulic technique, using OTW or a wire extension for short wires.
- Once removed, the DLM can be replaced with a workhorse microcatheter as needed.

DIFFERENT USES OF DUAL LUMEN MICROCATHETERS

The role of DLMs is expanding and is expected to further increase as PCI becomes more complex. They are particularly beneficial in the treatment of bifurcation lesions, CTOs, and a combination of both **(Table 1)**. The applications of DLM are given in **Table 2**.

TABLE 2: Applications of dual lumen microcatheter.

Bifurcations	Highly angulated (angles ≥150°) side branches	Reverse wiring technique; side branches with unfavorable take-off	Rewiring difficult side branches through prior stent struts
CTO		• Antegrade wiring of CTO when there is a side branch adjacent to the proximal cap • Side branch anchor technique	Wiring of difficult-to-access collaterals for retrograde approach
Bifurcation CTO lesions	Wiring of the distal true lumen without losing access to a side branch near or past the distal cap	Antegrade wiring of the distal true lumen if the externalized retrograde guidewire crossed a collateral close to the distal cap	

(CTO: chronic total occlusion)

Bifurcations

Coronary bifurcation PCI represents around 20% of all PCI procedures and is linked to elevated procedural expenses, greater rates of complications, and poorer outcomes.[2]

This is especially true in cases involving bifurcations, where coronary bifurcation PCI procedures account for a significant portion of all PCI procedures. These procedures are known to have higher complication rates, worse outcomes, and increased procedural costs.[2] DLMs not only aid in navigating through prior stent struts but also provide additional support when rewiring difficult side branches. In this scenario, the subintimal wire acts as a guide and provides support to the second working wire, which can be manipulated to find the true lumen. DLMs can also be used to wire the distal true lumen without losing access to a distal side branch near the distal cap of a CTO.

To address the difficulties in wiring challenging side branches with highly angulated angles or unfavorable take-off angles, a microcatheter-assisted reverse wire (RW) technique can be utilized **(Fig. 2)**.[3]

This technique has been modified to incorporate DLMs to facilitate the wiring of narrow and angulated side branches.

Chronic Total Occlusion

In the case of CTOs, which remain one of the most challenging lesion subsets for percutaneous intervention, the inability to cross the CTO is often the primary cause of failure.[4] The complexity of these lesions is further increased when bifurcation lesions are present.[5] DLMs can be beneficial in antegrade CTO PCI procedures.

Parallel Wire Technique Dual Lumen Microcatheters

When initial wiring attempts are subintimal in CTO PCI, the parallel wire technique proves to be a useful technique for accessing the true lumen. The DLM is advanced over the subintimal wire via the RX lumen. The catheter is positioned proximal to where the first wire entered the subintimal space.

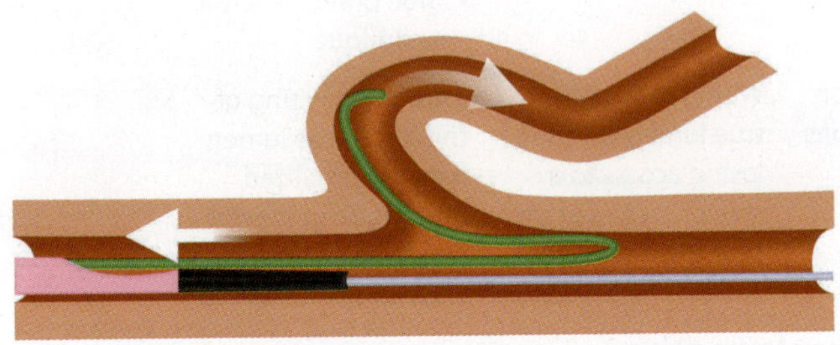

Fig. 2: Microcatheter-assisted reverse wire technique.

A second guidewire can then be advanced through the OTW lumen and the parallel wire technique employed.

For antegrade wiring of CTO with an adjacent side branch near the proximal CTO cap, a DLM is advanced in a side branch until the lateral port is at the level of the proximal cap. A CTO dedicated guidewire can then be advanced through the OTW lumen to engage the occlusion.

To access the side branch at the distal occlusion cap, the parallel wire technique is also used. The DLM is advanced through the collateral channel over a wire positioned in the side branch until the lateral port is at the level of the distal cap **(Fig. 3)**.

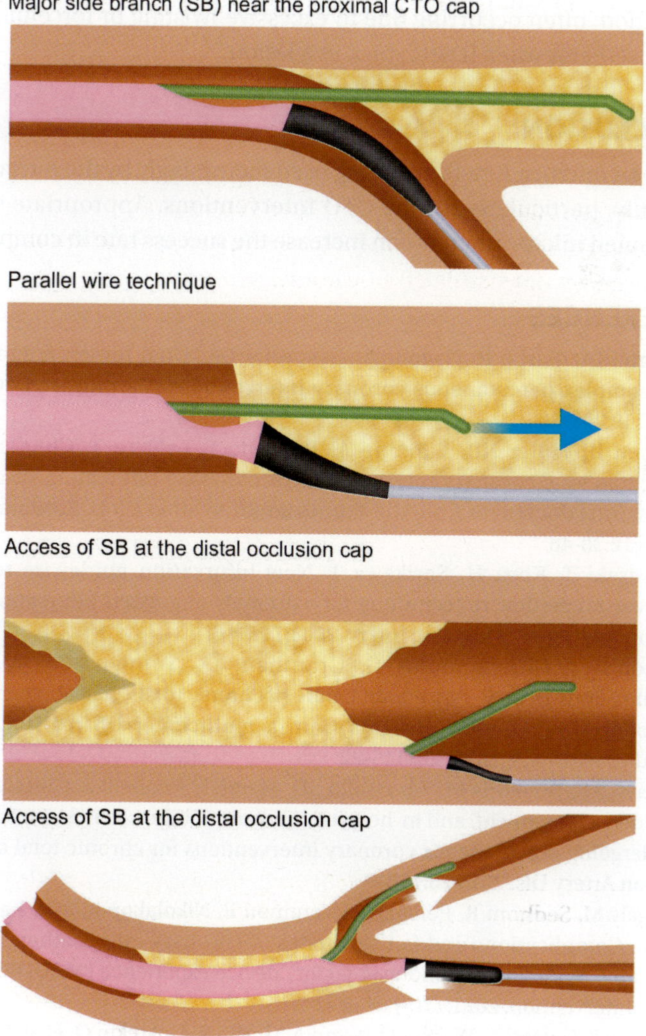

Fig. 3: Use of dual lumen microcatheters in CTO PCI. (CTO: chronic total occlusion; PCI: percutaneous coronary intervention)

Retrograde Chronic Total Occlusion

Difficult-to-access collaterals can pose a challenge when attempting a retrograde approach for wiring. In retrograde CTO PCI, once the CTO is traversed in a retrograde fashion and the guidewire is externalized, a DLM is then advanced antegrade on the externalized guidewire. A second "workhorse" guidewire is then advanced through the OTW lumen of the DLM to wire the true lumen of the vessel distally.

COMPLICATIONS

Tip fracture of the microcatheter is frequently reported as the main complication, often occurring due to excessive twisting or forcefully pulling the microcatheter when it gets stuck in a lesion.[6,7]

CONCLUSION

Dual lumen microcatheters are being used increasingly by the interventional community, particularly during CTO interventions. Appropriate selection of dual lumen microcatheters can increase the success rate in complex PCI.

REFERENCES

1. Oreglia JA, Garbo R, Gagnor A, Gasparini GL. Dual lumen microcatheters for complex percutaneous coronary interventions. Cardiovasc Revasc Med. 2018;19:298-305.
2. Lassen JF, Holm NR, Banning A, Burzotta F, Lefèvre T, Chieffo A, et al. Percutaneous coronary intervention for coronary bifurcation disease: 11th consensus document from the European Bifurcation Club. Eurointervention. 2016;12:38-46.
3. Kawasaki T, Koga H, Serikawa T. New bifurcation guidewire technique: a reversed guidewire technique for extremely angulated bifurcation—a case report. Catheter Cardiovasc Interv. 2008;71:73-6.
4. Sapontis J, Christopoulos G, Grantham JA, Wyman RM, Alaswad K, Karmpaliotis D, et al. Procedural failure of chronic total occlusion percutaneous coronary intervention: insights from a multicenter US registry. Catheter Cardiovasc Interv. 2015;85:1115-22.
5. Galassi AR, Boukhris M, Tomasello SD, Marzà F, Azzarelli S, Giubilato S, et al. Incidence, treatment, and in-hospital outcome of bifurcation lesions in patients undergoing percutaneous coronary interventions for chronic total occlusions. Coron Artery Dis. 2015;26:142-9.
6. Megaly M, Sedhom R, Pershad A, Vemmou E, Nikolakopoulos I, Karacsonyi J, et al. Complications and failure modes of coronary microcatheters: Insights from the manufacturer and user facility device experience (MAUDE) database. EuroIntervention. 2021;17(5):e436-8.
7. Pyxaras S, Galassi A, Werner G, Avran A, Garbo R, Goktekin O, et al. Dual lumen microcatheters for recanalisation of chronic total occlusions: a EuroCTO Club expert panel report: DLMC in CTO-PCI. EuroIntervention. 2021;17(12):e966-70.

CHAPTER

7

Intravascular Ultrasound in Interventional Practice

Sajan Narayanan

INTRODUCTION

- Coronary atherosclerosis is a diffuse process.
- During initial phases of atherosclerotic pathogenesis, vessel wall undergoes compensatory enlargement to accommodate plaque deposition preventing luminal compromise.
- Coronary angiogram (CAG) provides only a two-dimensional assessment of vessel lumen (essentially a luminogram) and does not reveal pathology in the vessel wall.
- Assessment of coronary stenosis on CAG is often based on assumption of adjacent "normal" segment, which may not be true due to diffuse nature of atherosclerotic process and has a high inter- and intraobserver variability.
- Intravascular ultrasound (IVUS) provides accurate assessment of vessel wall pathology and avoids ambiguity in analysis of vessel segments, especially at branch points, dilated segments, and tortuous calcified areas **(Fig. 1)**.
- Axial and longitudinal information of the vessel provided by IVUS helps in comprehensive analysis and treatment of lesions in the coronary arteries.

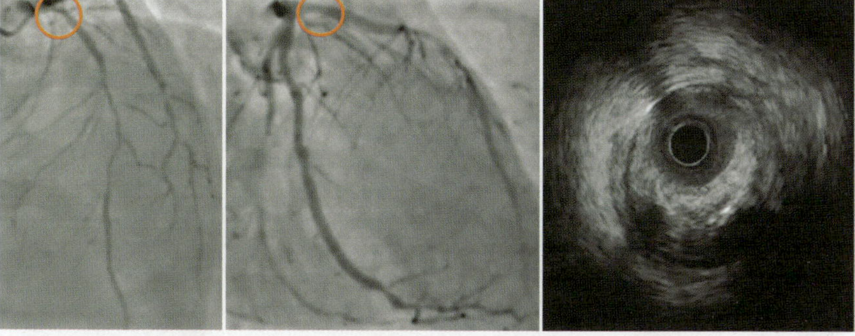

Fig. 1: *Importance of intravascular imaging*: A case with non-ST elevation ACS. Angiogram showed mid-LAD diffuse 90% lesion. IVUS assessment showed a lesion in proximal LAD (red circle) which had high-plaque burden and significant luminal narrowing which appeared insignificant on diagnostic angiogram. (ACS: acute coronary syndrome; IVUS: intravascular ultrasound; LAD: left anterior descending)

- Certain pathologies like spontaneous coronary dissection mimic acute coronary syndrome (ACS) and are difficult to distinguish on CAG. IVUS is very useful in identifying pathobiological mimics and helps in tailoring the treatment.

EVIDENCE FOR USE OF INTRAVASCULAR ULTRASOUND IN PERCUTANEOUS CORONARY INTERVENTION

- Multiple randomized controlled trials (RCTs) have confirmed the benefit of routine IVUS guidance during percutaneous coronary interventions (PCI) with regard to reduction in short- and long-term outcomes.
- The clinical benefit of IVUS guidance is seen not only in complex PCI subsets, but also in apparently noncomplex PCI subsets as well.
- Studies have shown that IVUS guidance during PCI reduces hard endpoints like cardiac death and incidence of myocardial infarction (MI) **(Tables 1 and 2)**.

BASIC PRINCIPLES OF INTRAVASCULAR ULTRASOUND EXAMINATION

- Intravascular ultrasound transducer is mounted at tip of a catheter where it emits and receives ultrasound signals.
- Transducers that emit ultrasound signals at frequencies of 20–60 MHz are available for commercial use.
- Ultrasound beams get partially reflected, refracted, and attenuated based on acoustic impedance properties of the tissues. Analysis of these acoustic characteristics helps to define normal and pathological structures in vivo.

TABLE 1: Risk ratio for cardiac death.

	Number of events/person years		
Study	***IVUS-guided arm***	***Angio-guided arm***	***Risk ratio***
AIR-CTO	3/230	5/230	0.6 (0.15–2.48)
AVIO	0/284	2/284	0.2 (0.01–4.15)
CTO-IVUS	0/201	2/201	0.2 (0.01–1.14)
IVUS-XPL	6/3,500	14/3,500	0.43 (0.16–1.11)
Liu et al.	3/167	10/169	0.3 (0.09–1.08)
RENOVATE	16/2,184	17/1,094	0.47 (0.24–0.93)
COMPLEX PCI	0/269	1/274	0.34 (0.01–8.3)
RESET	2/122	3/124	0.68 (0.12–3.98)
Tan et al.	15/2,142	19/2,127	0.78 (0.4–1.54)
ULTIMATE			

(CTO: chronic total occlusion; IVUS: intravascular ultrasound; PCI: percutaneous coronary intervention)

Source: Data obtained from randomized controlled trials comparing IVUS guided with angiography guided PCI.

TABLE 2: Risk ratio for myocardial infarction.

	Number of events/person years		
Study	*IVUS-guided arm*	*Angio-guided arm*	*Risk ratio*
AIR-CTO	20/230	15/230	1.33 (0.7–2.54)
AVIO	10/284	12/284	0.83 (0.37–1.9)
CTO-IVUS	0/201	2/201	0.2 (0.01–4.14)
HOME DES IVUS	1/157	4/157	0.25 (0.03–2.21)
IVUS-XPL	4/3,500	6/3,500	0.67 (0.19–2.36)
Liu et al.	19/167	23/169	0.84 (0.47–1.48)
MOZART	1/14	2/13	0.46 (0.05–4.53)
RENOVATE	43/2,184	32/1,094	0.67 (0.43–1.06)
COMPLEX PCI	0/269	2/274	0.2 (0.01–4.22)
RESET	1/122	2/124	0.51 (0.05–5.53)
Tan et al.	7/2,142	15/2,127	0.46 (0.129–1.13)
ULTIMATE	1/38	0/42	3.31 (0.14–78.84)
Wang et al.			

(CTO: chronic total occlusion; IVUS: intravascular ultrasound; PCI: percutaneous coronary intervention)

Source: Data obtained from randomized controlled trials comparing IVUS guided with angiography guided PCI.

INTRAVASCULAR ULTRASOUND EXAMINATION PROCEDURE

- Intravascular ultrasound catheters to be introduced only through a guide catheter.
- ACT to be maintained >250 s.
- Intracoronary vasodilators (e.g., nitroglycerin 100–200 μg) to be administered to avoid vasospasm while introducing catheter inside the coronaries.
- Mechanical system should be properly cleared off air bubbles inside sheath covering the transducer by flushing with heparinized saline.
- IVUS catheter to be introduced under fluoroscopic guidance. Examination may start from 5 to 10 mm distal to intended area of interest, where vessel appears normal (plaque burden <40% with no high-risk features) and end at least 5–10 mm proximal to the lesion (plaque burden <40% with no high-risk features).

ASSESSMENT OF VESSEL STRUCTURE AND PLAQUE MORPHOLOGY (FIG. 2)

The border between media and adventitia, i.e., external elastic lamina is the most well-defined landmark visualized on IVUS and is used as reference to determine vessel size and plaque area.

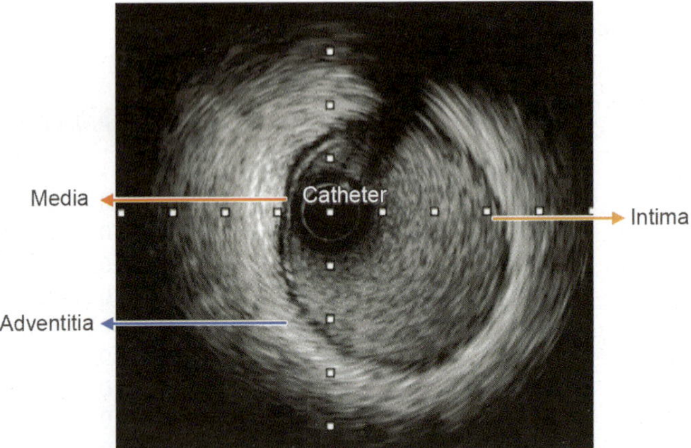

Fig. 2: Normal vessel wall on IVUS appears trilaminar in structure. Blood may be visualized as speckles. Intima is composed of single layer of endothelial cells and is in direct contact with blood in the lumen (orange arrow). Intima is separated from media by internal elastic lamina which is not visualized on IVUS. Media is composed of smooth muscle cells and is less echogenic than intima, but may appear thick due to signal attenuation and weak reflectivity of internal elastic lamina (red arrow). Adventitia is separated from media by external elastic membrane (EEM). Adventitia contain abundant collagen fibrils, fibroblasts, vasa vasorum, and nerve endings. Due to presence of collagen, they reflect ultrasound and appear bright (blue arrow).

Quantitative Assessment of Vessel Parameters

- Most well-demarcated boundary in the vessel wall of a normal arterial structure is between media and adventitia, which corresponds to position of external elastic membrane (EEM). When we draw a circle along this boundary, we get EEM-derived area, which corresponds to vessel area. Minimum and maximum diameters correspond to EEM-derived values which when averaged will provide mean vessel diameter at that site **(Fig. 3A)**.
- When we draw a circle along leading edge of the intima, we get luminal area (LA). Minimum and maximum diameters correspond to lumen-derived values which when averaged will provide the mean luminal diameter **(Fig. 3B)**.
- Atherosclerotic plaque accumulates in the subintimal space and hence plaque area cannot be assessed directly. So, we can subtract lumen area from vessel area which would provide plaque + media (P + M) area. Dividing P + M area with vessel area (EEM-derived area) and multiplying by 100 would provide plaque burden (PB) in percentage **(Fig. 3C)**.

Qualitative Assessment of Plaque Morphology

Assessment of plaque morphology on IVUS is important in planning plaque preparation. Some plaque types like calcified or fibrous lesions would need

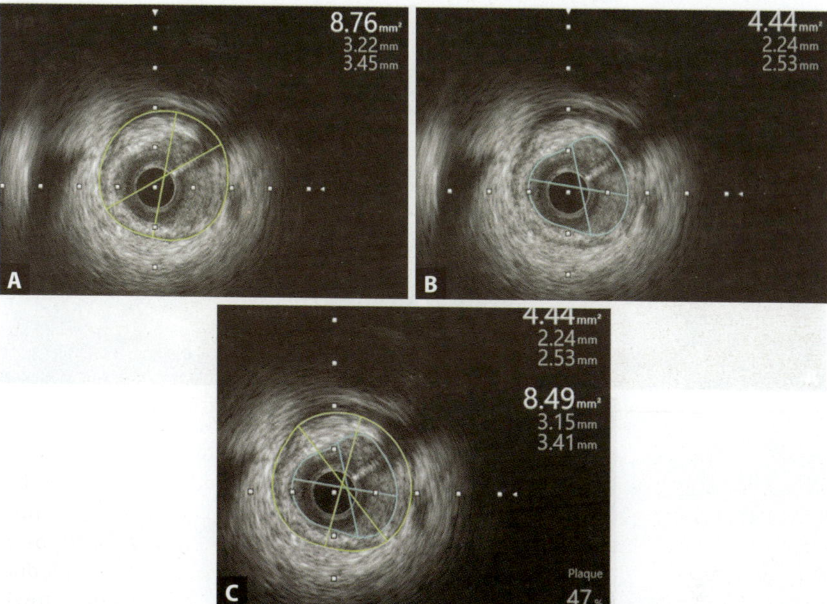

Figs. 3A to C: Pictures illustrating measurements of vessel area (A), lumen area (B), and plaque burden (C). Vessel area illustrated in picture C is 8.49 mm^2. Lumen area is 4.44 mm^2. Hence, plaque + media area (P + M) is 8.49 – 4.44 = 4.05 mm^2. PB is 4.05 mm^2/8.49 mm^2 × 100 = 47%. (PB: plaque burden)

aggressive plaque preparation prior to stent placement. Significant plaque attenuation and thrombus can create plaque embolism and be associated with slow flow after stent placement. Brightest structure in a normal IVUS is adventitia. Darkest structure is the media. All pathological plaque types are compared with these two structures in echogenicity to identify individual plaque types. Normally, ultrasound would travel beyond adventitia and can reveal structures outside vessel wall. Some plaque types will not allow ultrasound to penetrate and we may not be able to visualize structures beyond the plaque. So by noting the echogenicity and reflective/attenuation characteristics, we can identify different plaque types **(Figs. 4 to 7)**.

Pre-stent Assessment of the Vessel

- *Reference segment:* This is the area of vessel wall which appears normal or relatively normal. It encompasses the diseased segment which the operator plans to treat the vessel between these two points. A reference segment should have a plaque burden of <40% and should not have high-risk plaque characteristics like attenuation or calcium occupying more than two quadrants. Stent edges which show significant PB and high-risk features are associated with increased risk of recurrent stent failure. Distal reference segment should be a point at least 5 mm distal to intended distal

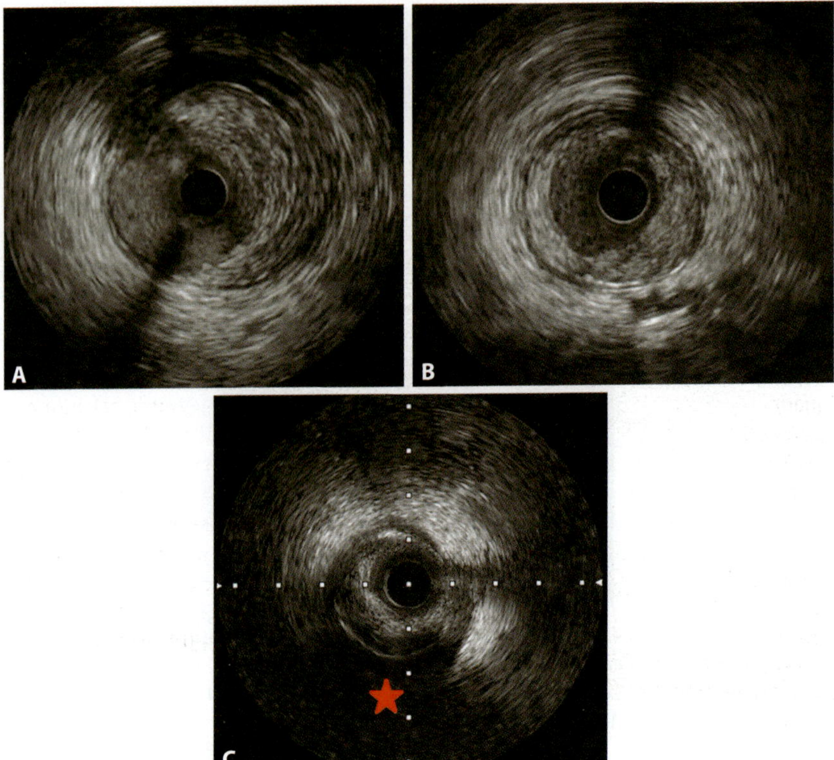

Figs. 4A to C: (A) Soft plaque; echogenicity is lower than that of adventitia. Soft plaques are lipid rich. *Importance:* We can attempt direct stenting and these plaque types may not need aggressive lesion preparation; (B) Fibrous plaques have intermediate echogenicity between soft echolucent plaque that of adventitia. *Importance:* We may need to prepare lesion especially at branch ostial points with modified balloons (e.g., scoring/cutting balloons); (C) Attenuated plaque visualized between 4 and 10 o'clock position (star). Defined as deep area of ultrasound attenuation with no overlying fibrous tissue/calcium. Attenuated plaque signifies lipid-rich plaque with confluent lipid pools. Lipid pools can attenuate ultrasound signals and we cannot see structures beyond the plaque. *Importance:* Can be associated with embolism and no reflow after stent placement.

stent edge, where there are no major side branches. Proximal reference segment is the point at least 5 mm proximal to intended proximal stent edge, where there are no major side branches.

- *Selection of stent size*: Stent diameter is selected according to *distal* reference segment diameter. We can select either according to EEM-based or lumen-based approach **(Figs. 8A to C)**.

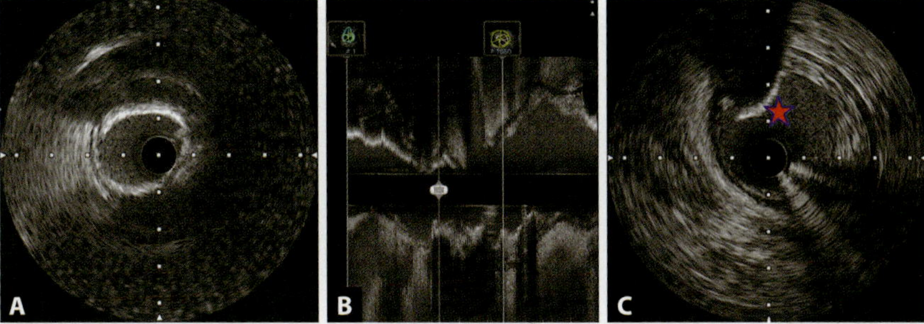

Figs. 5A to C: Calcified plaques appear highly echogenic (A). We cannot visualize structures behind the plaque since calcium reflects entire ultrasound beam and does not allow penetration. We can define degree of calcium by noting the number of quadrants occupied by the plaque (e.g., in Figure A, there is concentric calcium and hence 360°). In longitudinally reconstructed view (L-mode), we can estimate length of calcified plaque (B). Calcium reflects ultrasound and hence depth of calcification cannot be assessed on IVUS. Figure C illustrates calcified nodular protrusion (10–11 o'clock position). By noting these variables, we can construct well-described IVUS-derived calcium score—which has four variables: (1) Calcium arc >270° for every 5 mm—1 point, (2) 360° calcium—1 point, (3) presence of calcified nodule—1 point, (4) vessel diameter involved is <3.5 mm—1 point. A score of ≥2 predicts significant stent underexpansion without adequate plaque preparation. (IVUS: intravascular ultrasound)

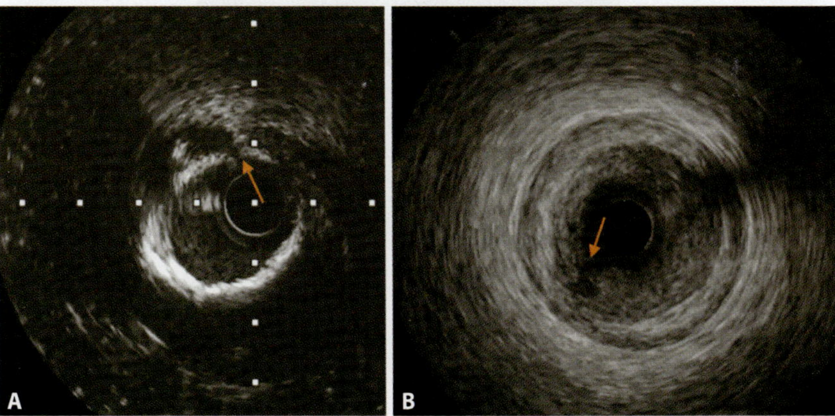

Figs. 6A and B: (A) *Ruptured plaque:* Note the breach in intima (arrow) with blood (black) inside the cavity extending to media; (B) *Plaque erosion*: Note the breach limited to intima (arrow) without extension into media. *Importance*: ACS with plaque erosion as etiology can be treated with DAPT and statins without need for stent placement. (ACS: acute coronary syndrome; DAPT: dual antiplatelet therapy)

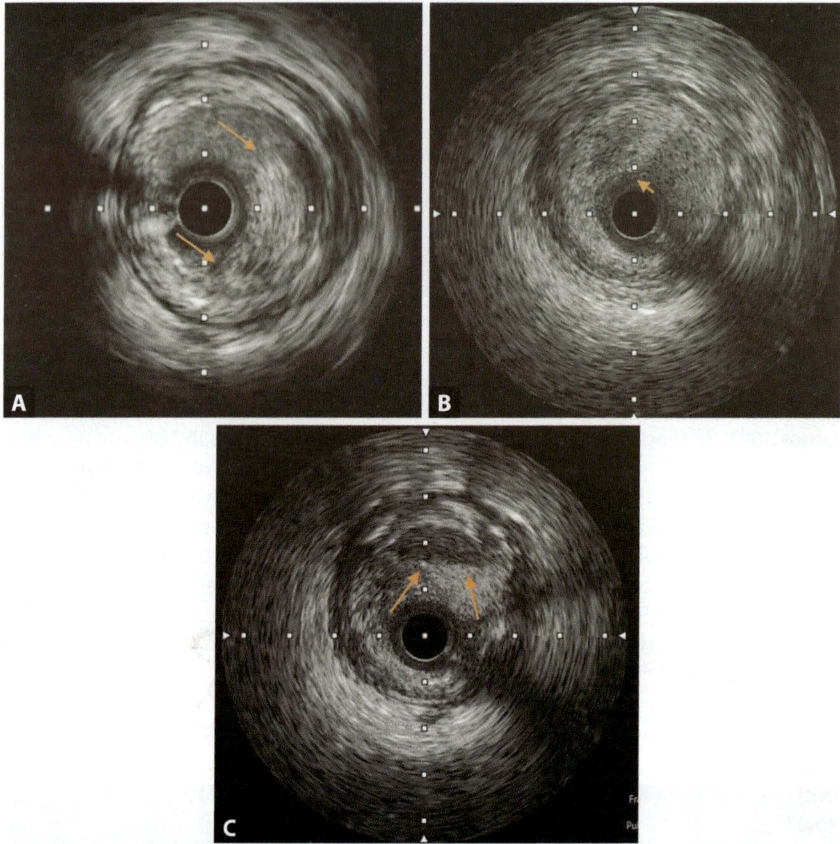

Figs. 7A to C: *Thrombus:* Thrombus appears as ill-defined variable echo densities within vessel lumen attached to intima. (A) Fresh thrombus is platelet rich and will reflect ultrasound—hence appears bright; (B) *Subacute thrombus*: As thrombus becomes older, proportion of RBCs in the clot increases and clot will appear heterogenous in echodensity with hyper- and hypoechoic areas within clot; (C) Organized clot—note the hypoechoic leading edge due to red clot.

Poststent Assessment

- Minimum stent area (MSA)—must be at least >5.5 mm^2 or >80% of average reference (proximal + distal/2) lumen area **(Table 3; Figs. 9A to C)**. MSA is single most important predictor of outcomes after PCI.
- Apposition—no significant gap (<400 μm) between stent strut and vessel wall **(Figs. 10A and B)**
- Edge complications **(Figs. 11 and 12)**
- Imaging checklist for patients undergoing IVUS-guided PCI is depicted in **Table 4**.

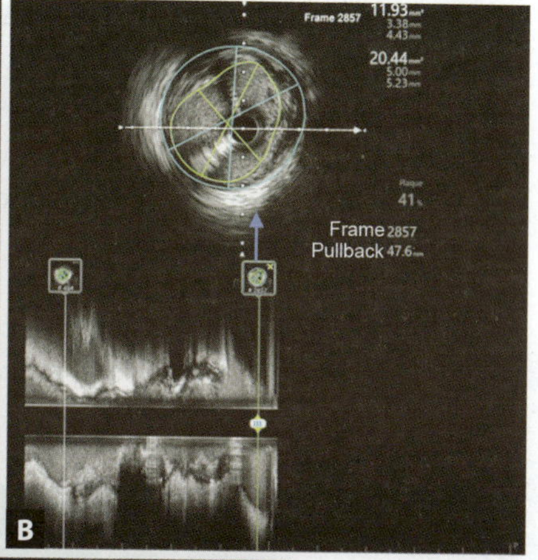

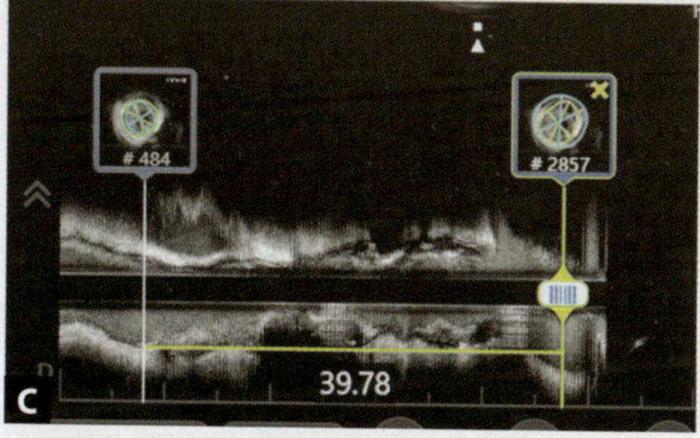

Figs. 8A to C: (A) Distal reference (orange arrow) segment. EEM-based average (green font) luminal diameter is 3.5 mm. Lumen-based average (blue font) diameter is 2.9 mm. Now if we go by EEM-based approach, stent size can be downsized by 0.25–0.5 mm from EEM-derived average diameter. So here stent diameter would be 3 mm. If we go by lumen-based approach, we can upsize average diameter by 0.25–0.5 mm to nearest available stent size. Here it would be 3 mm. Similarly, proximal stent diameter (B) to be approximated with POT balloon can be selected according to proximal reference diameter. Length of stent (between proximal and distal reference segments) can be estimated from L-mode (C). (EEM: external elastic membrane; POT: proximal optimization technique)

TABLE 3: Stent expansion criteria employed across different imaging studies.

Criteria	*Studies*	
MSA >distal RLA	• IVUS-XPL • CTO-IVUS	
MSA >80% average RLA	• RESIST • TULIP	• AIR-CTO • RENOVATE COMPLEX PCI
MSA >90% of average RLA	• SIPS • OPTICUS • AVID	• ILUMIEN III • ULTIMATE • ILUMIEN IV
Stent diameter >90% of RVD	• OCTOBER	

(MSA: minimum stent area; RLA: reference lumen area; RVD: reference vessel diameter)

Intravascular Ultrasound Assessment of Left Main Disease

- Intravascular ultrasound-guided PCI improves clinical outcomes in patients undergoing left main intervention.
- Intravascular ultrasound can be used in decision making, i.e., rule in and rule out left main lesions which appear ambiguous or of borderline significance on angiogram.
- Unlike in nonleft main segments, imaging criteria to rule in or rule out on IVUS in left main have robust correlation with fractional flow reserve (FFR) and carry prognostic significance.

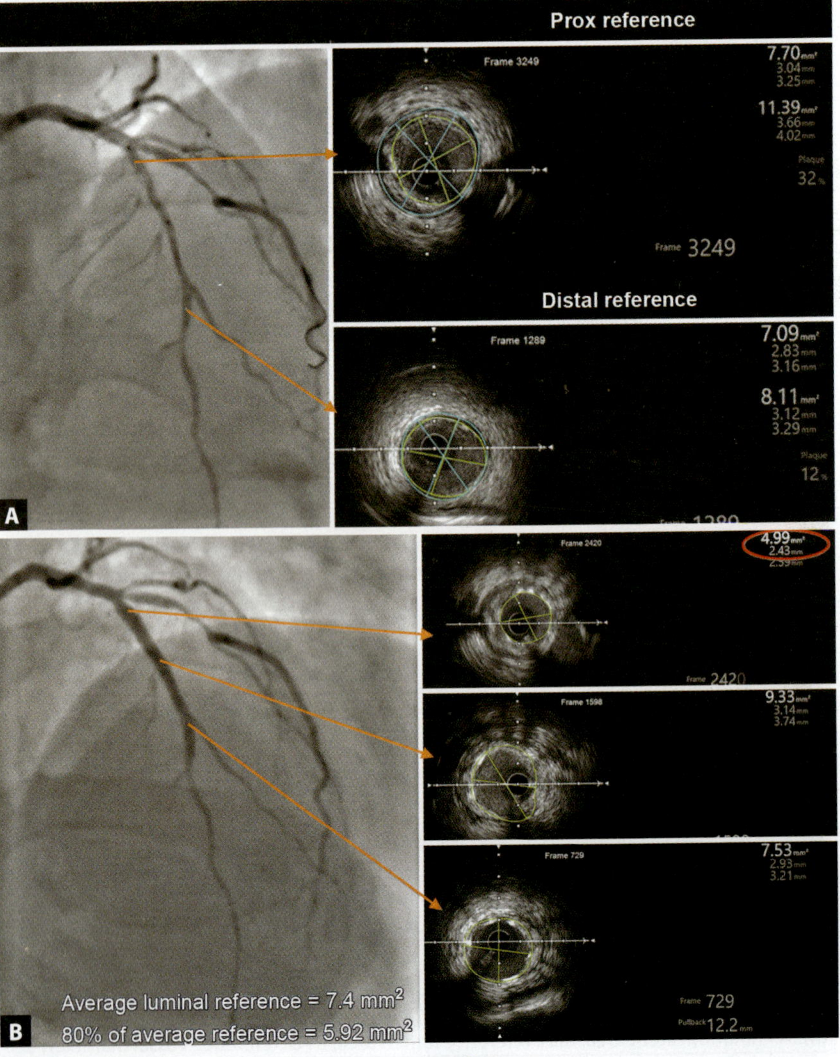

Figs. 9A and B

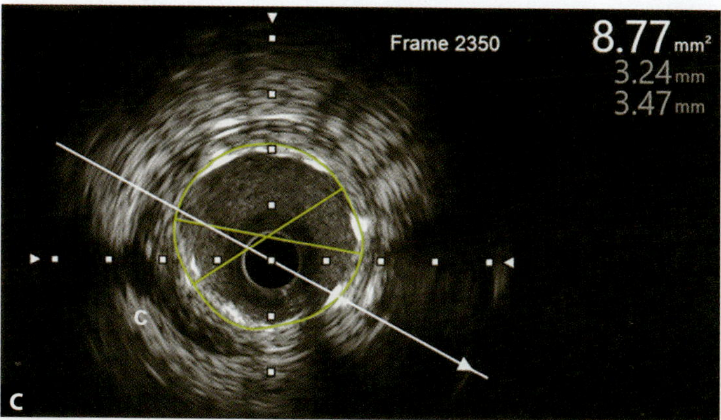

Fig. 9C

Figs. 9A to C: (A) Long segment lesion from first diagonal to distal LAD. Proximal reference lumen area = 7.7 mm^2. Distal reference lumen area at segment just beyond origin of second diagonal = 7.09 mm^2. Average reference lumen area = 7.7 + 7.09/2 = 7.4 mm^2. Hence, MSA should be at least >80% of 7.4 mm^2, i.e., 5.92 mm^2. Patient received 2.75 × 34 mm DES (B). POT was performed with 3.5-mm balloon. Proximal MSA = 4.99 mm^2 which is less than expected MSA—hence underexpanded. Figure C shows MSA after postdilatation with 3.5 mm NC balloon at 20 atm. Final MSA obtained was 8.77 mm^2 which is >80% of average reference vessel lumen area. (LAD: left anterior descending; MSA: minimum stent area)

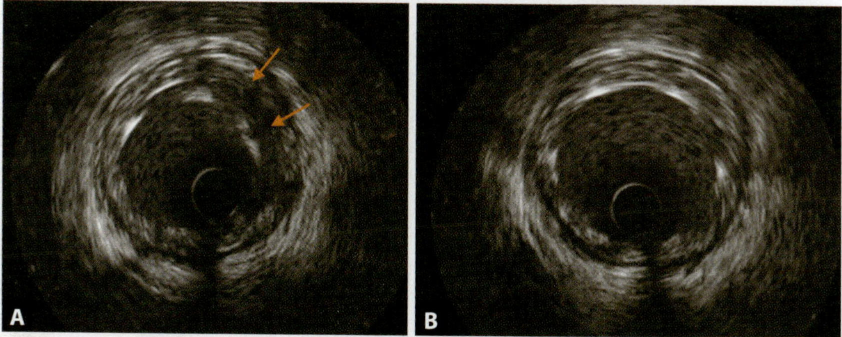

Figs. 10A and B: (A) Significant gap between stent struts and vessel wall between 12 and 3 o'clock position, signifying malapposition. A malapposition distance of >400 μm and extending along axial length of >1 mm must be corrected; (B) After postdilatation with a 4-mm semicompliant balloon.

Procedural Tips

- Always perform IVUS pullback from both left anterior descending (LAD) and left circumflex arteries (LCX).
- Disengage the guide catheter from left main (LM) ostium while interrogating ostioproximal segment **(Figs. 13A and B)**.

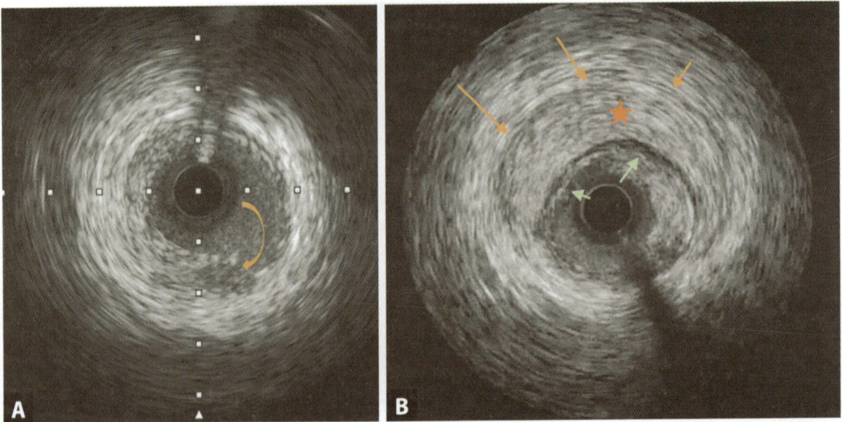

Figs. 11A and B: (A) Edge dissection at 5–6 o'clock position. A dissection flap occupying >60° and axial length of >2 mm should be treated with additional stent placement; (B) Stent edge intramural hematoma. Stagnant blood (star) seen separating media (green arrows) from adventitia (orange arrows).

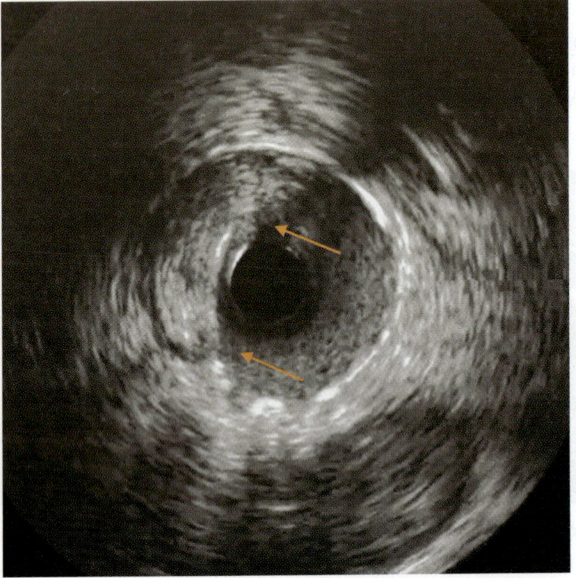

Fig. 12: Plaque prolapse. Note the protrusion of plaque material through stent struts between 7 and 12 o'clock position where stent struts just disappear. If final lumen area is <5.5 mm^2, plaque prolapse may be treated with semicompliant balloon dilatation sized to vessel diameter at site at nominal pressures.

- Left main size has to be assessed from the straighter branch. Pullback from angulated branch can overestimate LM size. When no straighter branch is available, always take smaller value of LM size (since we can only overestimate the LM size) **(Figs. 14A and B)**.

TABLE 4: Imaging checklist for patients undergoing PCI.

Pre-PCI	*Post-PCI*
Distal reference segment: • Average vessel diameter • Average lumen diameter • Lumen area • Plaque burden *Proximal reference segment:* • Average vessel diameter • Average lumen diameter • Lumen area • Plaque burden	*Minimum stent area:* • >5.5 mm^2 or • >80–90% of average RLA *Malapposition:* • <400 µm • Axial length <1 mm *Stent edge dissection:* • Not extending to media • <60° • Axial length <2 mm • No intramural hematoma • No significant plaque prolapse

(PCI: percutaneous coronary intervention; RLA: reference lumen area)

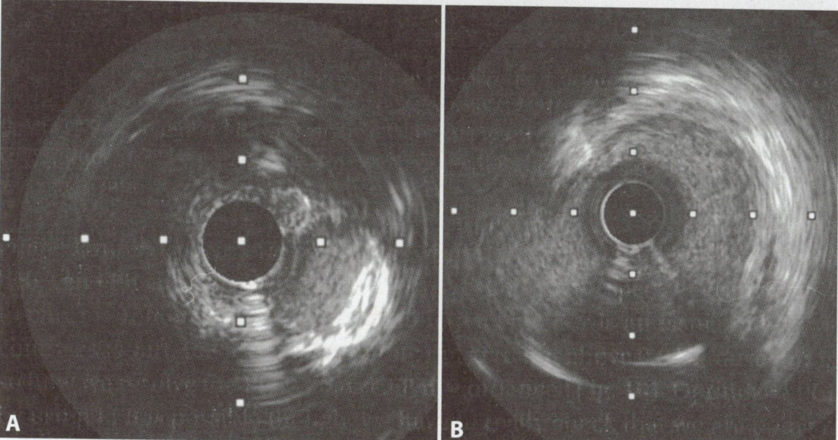

Figs. 13A and B: (A) Note artefactual appearance of critical lesion at left main ostium when guide catheter engages; (B) Ostium when IVUS run repeated after disengaging from ostium. (IVUS: intravascular ultrasound)

- Always assess side branch (SB) disease through a dedicated pullback from the branch concerned. SB disease assessment from main branch can be erroneous **(Figs. 15A and B)**.

Assessment of Severity of Left Main Disease

- Most important predictor of clinical outcomes in LM disease is the minimum lumen area (MLA). MLA correlates with FFR values. An MLA cutoff value of <4.5 mm^2 identifies patients who benefit from revascularization. A value of >6 mm^2 helps to defer revascularization in left main disease.

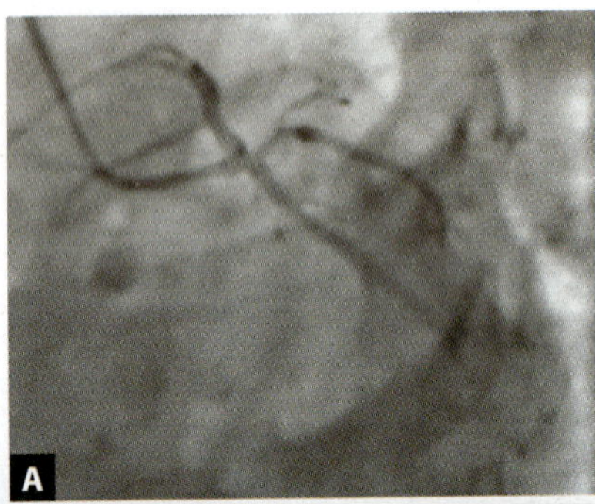

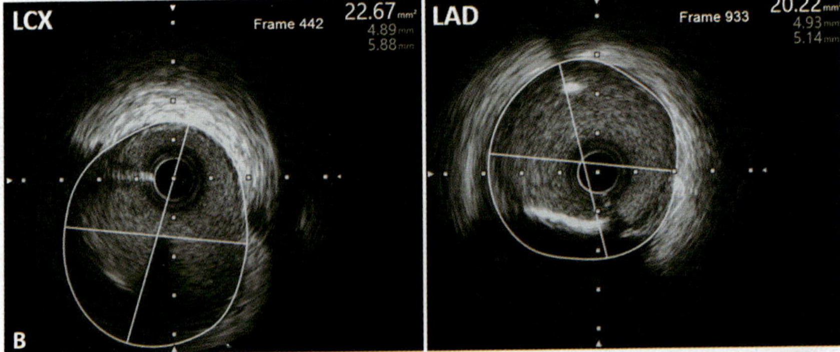

Figs. 14A and B: IVUS assessment from LCX (left) and LAD (right). Note overestimation of LM diameter from LCX pullback. (IVUS: intravascular ultrasound; LAD: left anterior descending; LCX: left circumflex artery)

- If LM MLA is between 4.5 and 6 mm^2, then we can decide on revascularization based on physiological significance and stenting strategy **(Figs. 16 and 17)**.

Poststent Assessment of Left Main

- Studies have shown that post-PCI MSA of at least >10 mm^2 at left main is associated with good short- and long-term outcomes **(Fig. 18)**.
- Stent should be well apposed with no edge dissection. In funnel-shaped LM (ostial LM having negative remodeling) and tapering LM (distal LM having negative remodeling), MSA must be at least 80% of the distal and proximal reference, respectively.

Intravascular Ultrasound Assessment in Stent Failure

- All cases of stent failure must be assessed with imaging to tailor the treatment **(Box 1)**.
- Assess three regions—proximal in-segment—i.e., proximal 5–10 mm of inflow region of stent implanted, in stent area and distal in-segment (5–10 mm distal to stent edge) portions.

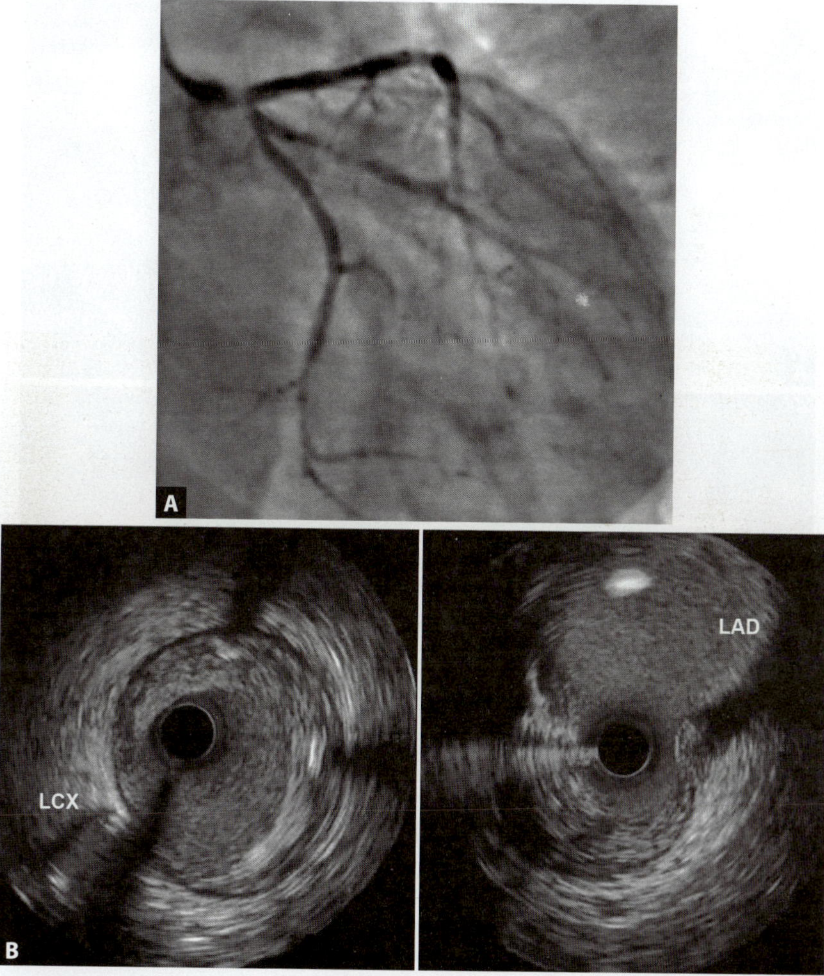

Figs. 15A and B: A 54-year-old gentleman presented with acute NSTEMI. Angiogram showed distal LM critical lesion. IVUS runs from LAD (left) and LCX (right) that are shown in lower panel. Run from LAD showed no significant plaque at LCX ostium (7 o'clock position), while run from LCX showed significant circumferential plaque with compromised ostial lumen of SB (right). (IVUS: intravascular ultrasound; LAD: left anterior descending; LCX: left circumflex artery; NSTEMI: non-ST-elevation myocardial infarction)

- At proximal and distal in-segment areas, look for progression of native disease, plaque type, and vessel sizes.
- In stent area, pattern of restenosis (neointimal hyperplasia vs. neoatherosclerosis), stent expansion and malapposition
- Case examples are illustrated in **Figures 19 and 20**.

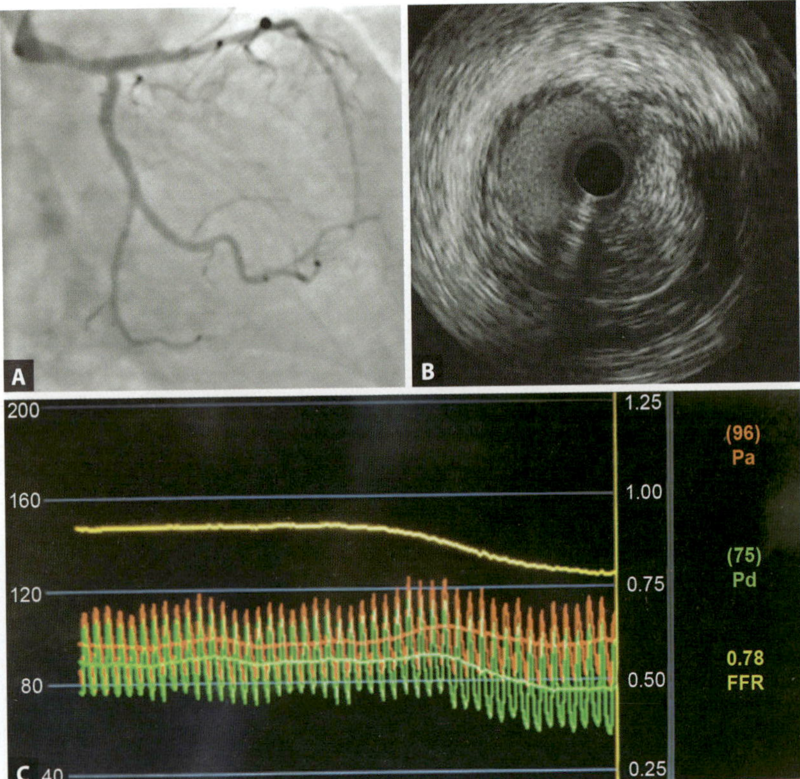

Figs. 16A to C: A 72-year-old lady who presented with acute inferior wall STEMI. Distal LCX was totally occluded. Underwent primary PCI to distal LCX. There was a mid-left main tubular 50–60% lesion on angiogram. IVUS assessment (right) showed MLA of 5.15 mm^2. Underwent FFR which was 0.78 confirming physiological significance of the lesion. (FFR: fractional flow reserve; IVUS: intravascular ultrasound; LCX: left circumflex artery; PCI: percutaneous coronary intervention; STEMI: ST-elevation myocardial infarction)

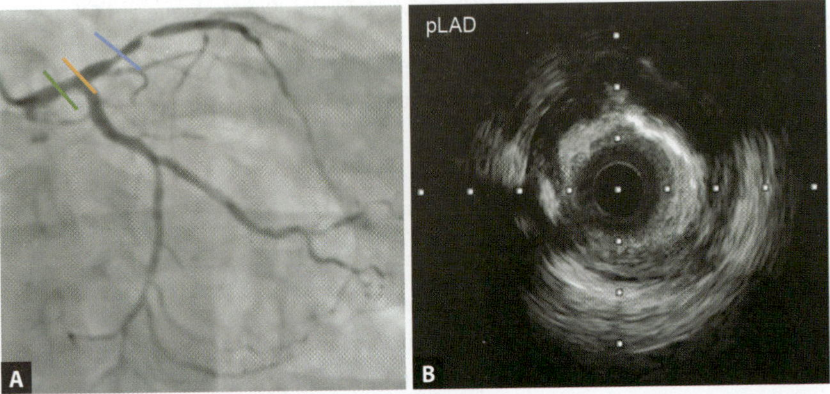

Figs. 17A and B

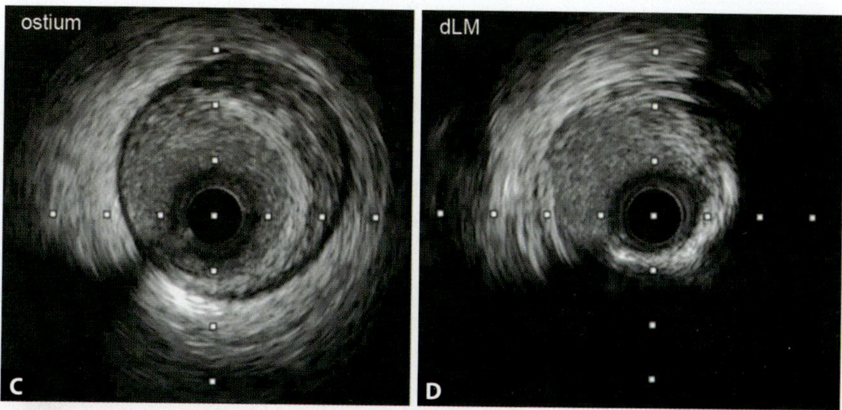

Figs. 17C and D

Figs. 17A to D: A 56-year-old gentleman, presented with acute NSTEMI. Angiogram showed two tandem lesions in proximal LAD. IVUS assessment shown in lower panel. LAD ostium had plaque burden of 60%. Distal left main showed significant plaque burden of 66% with MLA of 6.7 mm^2. Here, extending stent into proximal left main (i.e., crossover from LM into LAD vs. proximal LAD only) would be associated with good long-term outcomes rather than landing proximal stent edge at distal left main where there is significant PB. (IVUS: intravascular ultrasound; LAD: left anterior descending; MLA: minimum lumen area; NSTEMI: non-ST-elevation myocardial infarction; PB: plaque burden)

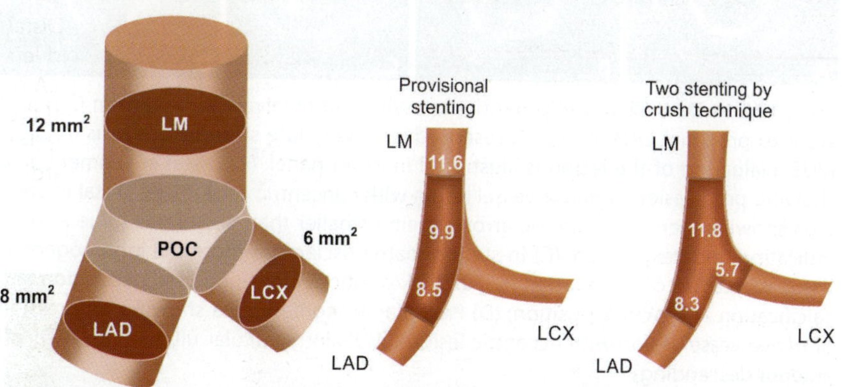

Fig. 18: 5-year MACE rates were lowest when MSA at LM was at least 12 mm^2, 8 mm^2 at proximal LAD, and 6 mm^2 at proximal LCX. MSA cutoffs which predicted outcomes in provisional and two-stent strategy are illustrated on right. (LAD: left anterior descending; LCX: left circumflex artery; MACE: major adverse cardiovascular event; MSA: minimum stent area)

BOX 1: Imaging checklist for stent failure.

- Distal RVD and RLA
- Distal in-segment lesion morphology
- *In-stent plaque morphology:*
  - Homogenous echo texture—neointimal hyperplasia
  - Heterogenous echo—neoatherosclerosis
- In-stent MLA
- Proximal in-segment plaque morphology
- Proximal RVD and MLA
- Length of the lesion

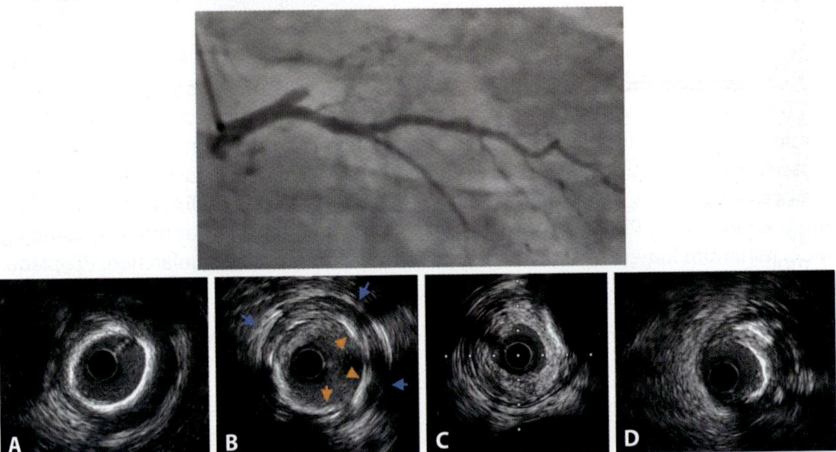

Figs. 19A to D: A 57-year-old gentleman who had received 3.5 × 18 mm Cypher™ stent to proximal LAD in 2006, presented with very late stent thrombosis in 2020. IVUS evaluation of the lesion is illustrated in lower panel. (A) Distal in-segment area showing progression of native vessel lesion with concentric calcium; (B) Distal in-stent area showing stent size (orange arrows) being smaller than vessel size (blue arrows) indicating underexpansion; (C) In-stent neoatherosclerosis—note the inhomogenous tissue with areas of attenuation (6–7 o'clock position) indicating lipid deposition and calcification at 2 o'clock position; (D) Proximal in-segment area showing progression of native vessel lesion with eccentric lesion. (IVUS: intravascular ultrasound; LAD: left anterior descending)

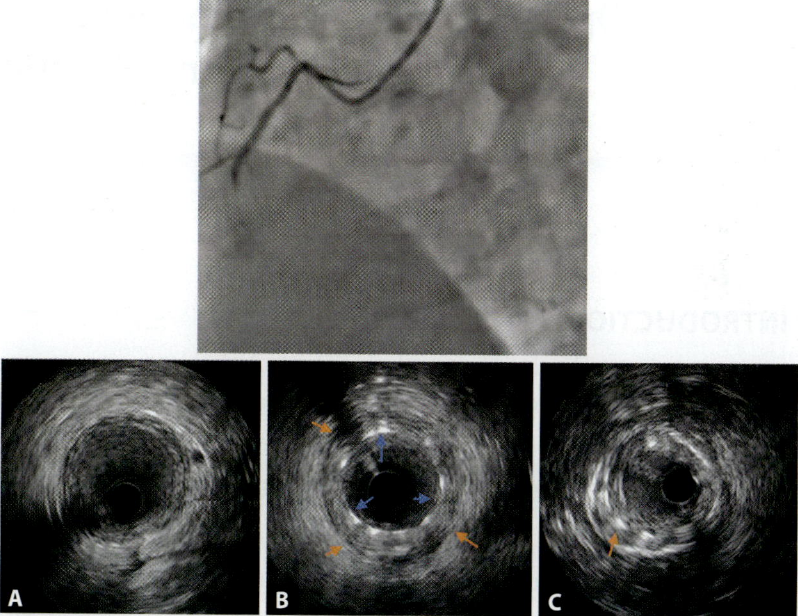

Figs. 20A to C: A 45-year-old lady underwent PCI to RCA with 2.75 × 34 mm DES, 3 months back. Now she presented with late-stent thrombosis. IVUS assessment illustrated in lower panel. (A) Distal reference segment showing EEM-derived vessel size being 3.75 mm, MLA was 10.08 mm^2; (B) Underexpanded stent (orange arrows indicate vessel size and blue arrows indicate stent outline). MSA was 5.05 mm^2; (C) Malposed stent struts between 6 and 9 o'clock position (orange arrows). (EEM: external elastic membrane; IVUS: intravascular ultrasound; MLA: minimum lumen area; MSA: minimum stent area; PCI: percutaneous coronary intervention; RCA: right coronary artery)

EUROPEAN SOCIETY OF CARDIOLOGY GUIDELINES ON USE OF INTRAVASCULAR ULTRASOUND (TABLE 5)

TABLE 5: European Society of Cardiology (ESC) guidelines on use of IVUS.

Indication	*Recommendation level*	*Level of evidence*
ACS* To guide PCI In ambiguous culprit lesions	 Class IIa Class IIb	
To optimize stent implantation#	Class IIa	B
To optimize treatment of unprotected LM lesions¶	Class IIa	B

(IVUS: intravascular ultrasound; PCI: percutaneous coronary intervention)
*2023 ESC guidelines for management of acute coronary syndromes
#,¶ 2018 ESC EACTS guidelines on myocardial revascularization

CONCLUSION

The benefit of IVUS as an adjunctive tool during complex PCI is supported by the results from multiple studies. Proper interpretation of the IVUS image helps in lesion preparation and stent optimization.

CHAPTER 8

Optical Coherence Tomography in Interventional Practice

S Selvamani

INTRODUCTION

Coronary angiography is commonly used to visually assess coronary anatomy and guide procedures like percutaneous coronary interventions (PCIs). However, its two-dimensional lumenogram does not show the vessel wall, hindering the evaluation of vessel size, plaque details, and direct assessment of stent implantation outcomes. Intracoronary imaging with intravascular ultrasound (IVUS) and optical coherence tomography (OCT) offers additional crucial information, helping optimize stent placement and reduce stent-related issues in clinical practice.[1,2]

METHODOLOGY

Pre-PCI OCT has a major role compared to post-PCI OCT. Pre-PCI OCT enables precise assessment of stenosis severity, extension, and plaque characteristics. It helps to identify suitable areas for stent placement, ensuring accurate selection of stent size and length. Additionally, it anticipates the need for postdilatation, specifying the type and size of the required balloon. Essentially, pre-PCI OCT imaging allows strategic planning for stent optimization. Following a successful angiographic outcome, post-PCI OCT verifies the results, determining if any additional adjustments are necessary.

Pre-Percutaneous Coronary Intervention OCT

To interpret OCT images accurately, it is crucial to understand how light interacts with vascular layers. When directed at tissue, some light passes through, while some is scattered or reflected. The brightness of tissue in OCT images depends on the amount of backscatter. Tissue attenuation, or the light absorbed during passage, determines OCT penetration depth. The intima and adventitia, rich in collagen and elastin, appear bright due to their backscattering properties. In contrast, the medial layer, with smooth muscle cells, appears dark. This "bright-dark-bright" pattern signifies a normal coronary artery, while atherosclerotic plaques disrupt this pattern[3] **(Figs. 1 and 2)**.

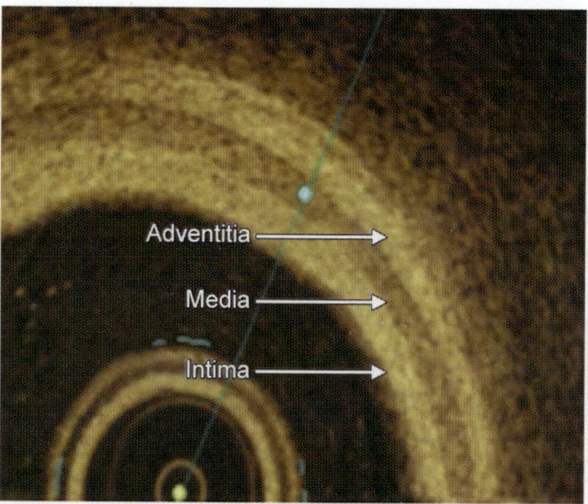

Fig. 1: Normal coronary artery.

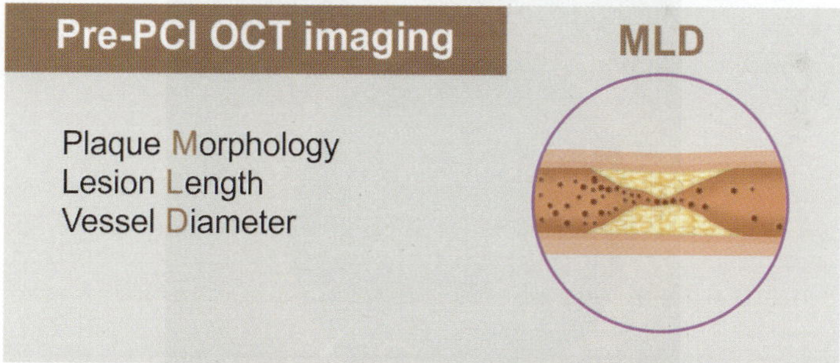

Fig. 2: Pre-PCI algorithm. (PCI: percutaneous coronary intervention; OCT: optical coherence tomography)

Plaque Morphology

Lipid-rich plaque (LRP): Plaques rich in lipids, known as lipid-rich plaques, are mainly composed of a necrotic lipid core covered by a fibrous cap, categorized as fibroatheromas. The risk of rupture is linked to the thickness of this cap, with those <65 μm (thin-cap fibroatheroma—TCFA) being especially prone to rupture. When dealing with significant blockages caused by mainly LRPs and TCFAs, direct stenting without predilatation can be an effective treatment approach **(Fig. 3)**.

Fibrotic plaque: Fibrotic plaques, abundant in collagen or smooth muscle cells, show a consistent and signal-rich backscatter on OCT. These are often considered stable plaques, and the risk of rupture relates to the extent of internal lipid deposition. When dealing with fibrotic lesions causing substantial blockages, cutting balloons or noncompliant balloons are used to prepare the vessel bed before stent deployment, ensuring optimal stent

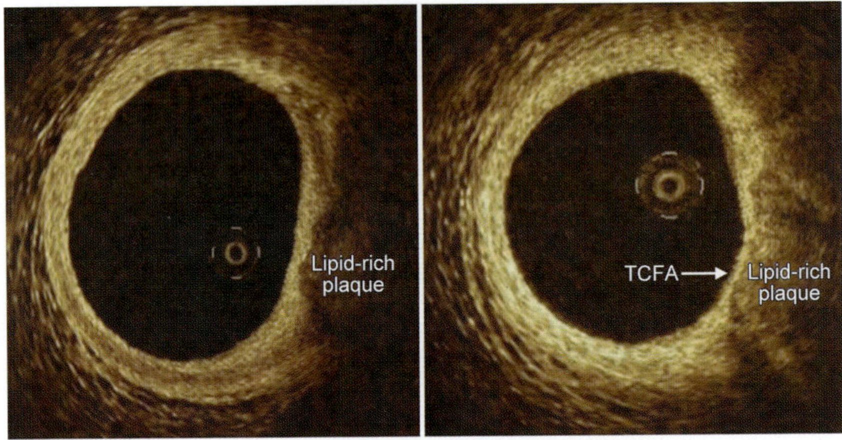

Fig. 3: Lipid-rich plaque and TCFA. (TCFA: thin-cap fibroatheroma)

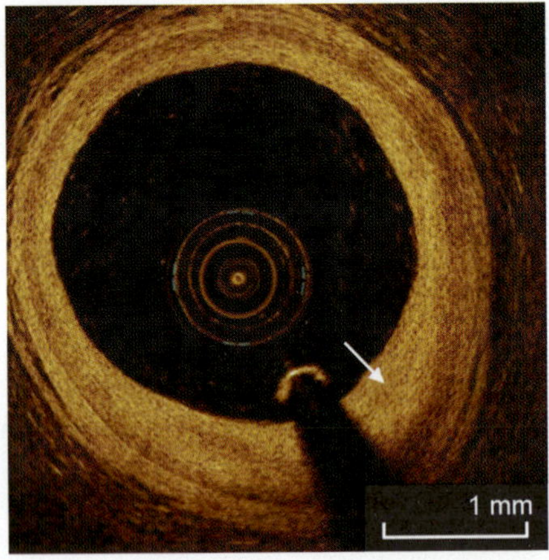

Fig. 4: Fibrous plaque.

expansion. For fibrofatty lesions with a predominant fatty composition, compliant balloons are preferred for bed preparation **(Fig. 4)**.

Calcific plaque: Calcific plaques are recognized by low attenuation, allowing light to penetrate deeply, revealing the underlying tissue. These plaques have distinct, well-defined edges, resembling islands or rocks. OCT categorizes calcium into three types—superficial, deep, and nodular—with each type having specific treatment implications[4] **(Figs. 5 to 8)**.

Vulnerable plaque: A vulnerable plaque is a lipid-rich one with a thin fibrous cap (thinnest part ≤65 μm), and the lipid part occupies at least two quadrants.[5] The risk of plaque rupture increases with the presence of cholesterol crystals, macrophages, and microchannels[6] **(Fig. 9 and Flowchart 1)**.

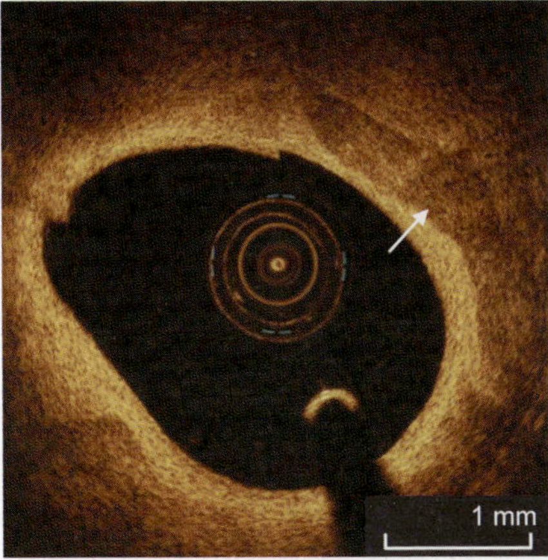

Fig. 5: Calcific plaque.

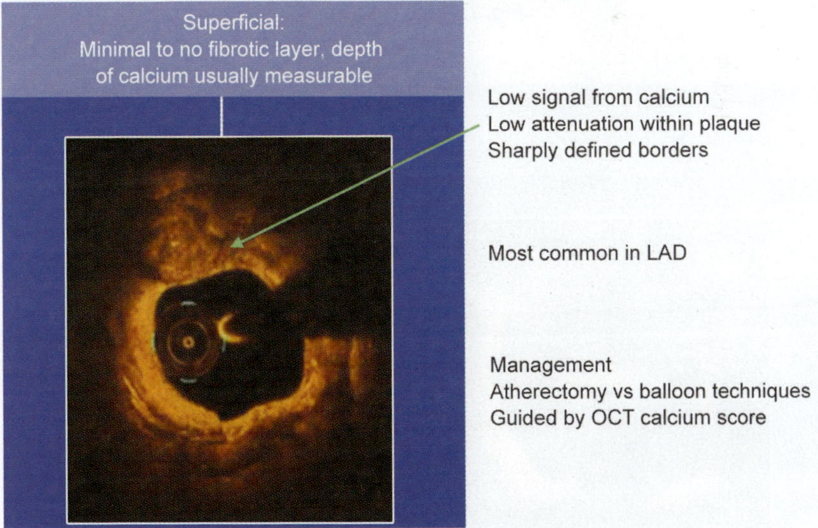

Fig. 6: Superficial calcium. (LAD: left anterior descending; OCT: optical coherence tomography)

Stent Length Estimation

To estimate length, the L-mode view of the OCT pullback uses pullback speed and frame rate calculations. Within 5 mm of the stenotic lesion, normal-appearing segments with preserved trilaminar morphology or minimal atherosclerotic distortion (<50% plaque burden) are chosen as proximal and distal stent landing zones. In diffusely diseased coronaries, landing zones are selected based on OCT markers indicating stable plaque, like thick fibrous cap atheroma, and calcified plaque.[7]

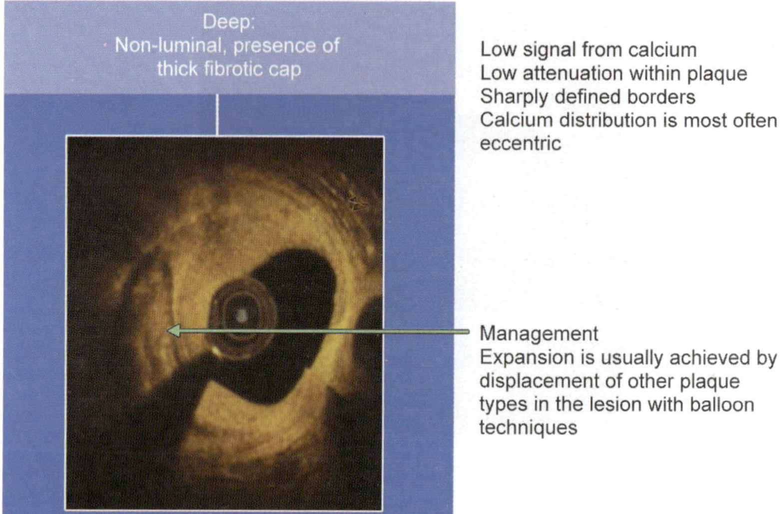

Fig. 7: Deep calcium.

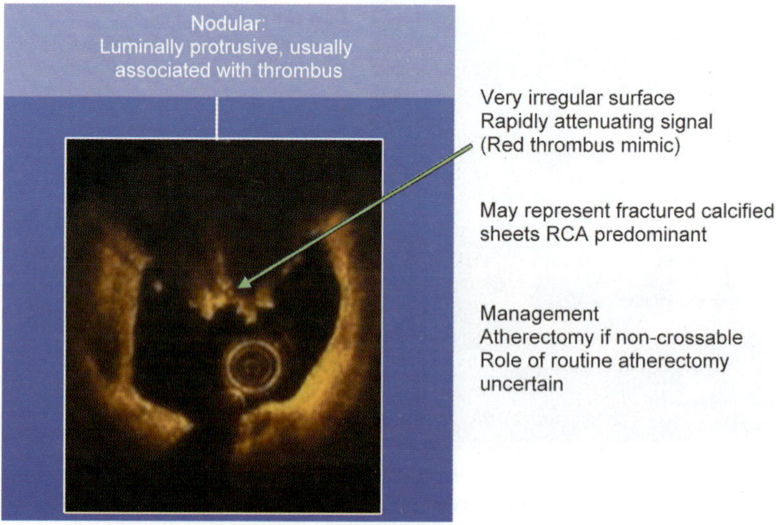

Fig. 8: Nodular calcium.

Stent Diameter Estimation

For sizing the stent at the distal landing zone, measurements based on the external elastic lamina (EEL) are recommended. Two separate diameter measurements, at least one quadrant apart, are taken, and their mean is rounded down by 0.25 mm to determine the appropriate stent size.[8] If the EEL is not clearly visible, the mean lumen diameter is used for sizing, and the stent size is rounded up between 0.25 and 0.5 mm[9] **(Fig. 10)**.

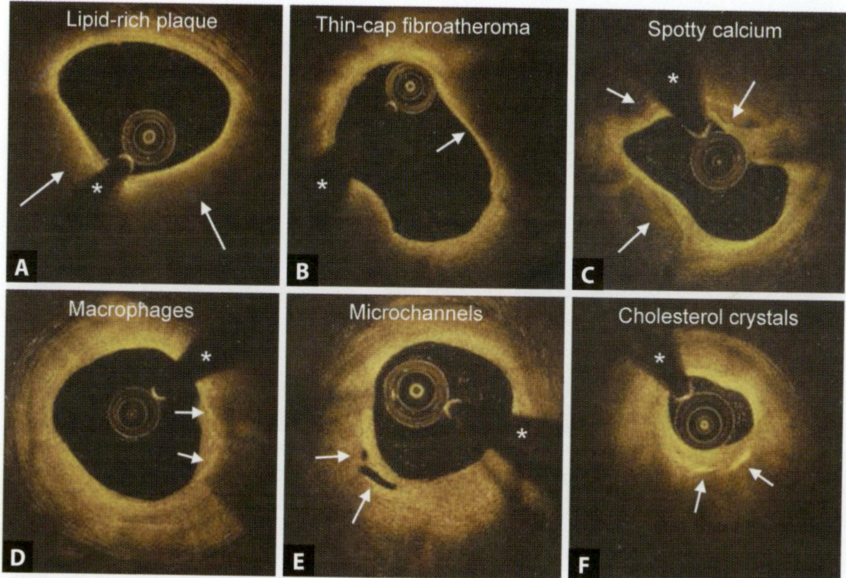

Figs. 9A to F: Vulnerable plaque.

Flowchart 1: Simplified algorithm for morphology assessment in OCT.

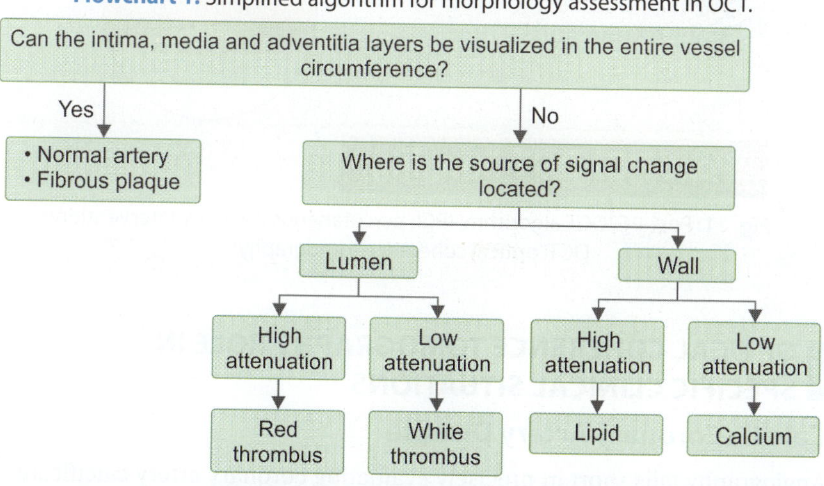

(OCT: optical coherence tomography)

Post-Percutaneous Coronary Intervention OCT

After stent placement, IVUS/OCT helps identify fixable issues concerning the stent and the vessel wall, including underexpansion, missed plaque areas, improper strut positioning, and dissection at the stent edges. These issues are linked to negative outcomes in PCI[1] **(Figs. 11 to 15)**.

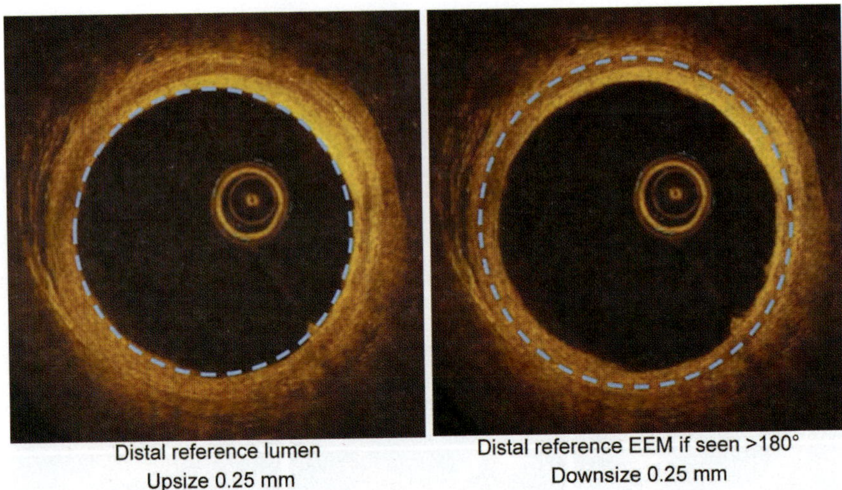

Fig. 10: Diameter estimation.

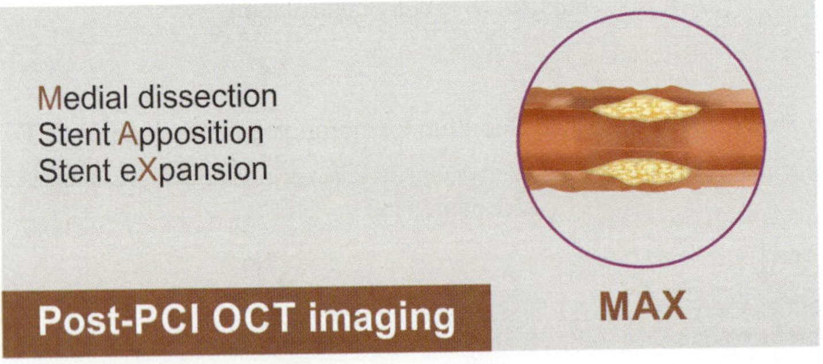

Fig. 11: Post-PCI OCT algorithm. (PCI: percutaneous coronary intervention; OCT: optical coherence tomography)

OPTICAL COHERENCE TOMOGRAPHY ROLE IN SPECIFIC CLINICAL SITUATIONS

Calcific Coronary Artery Disease

Angiography falls short in precisely evaluating coronary artery calcification, particularly when compared to OCT. OCT offers a detailed and accurate assessment of calcium burden, guiding effective prestent preparation based on morphology. An OCT-based calcium score has been developed and verified to predict the likelihood of stent underexpansion in calcified lesions[10] **(Fig. 16)**.

A score of 3 or lower ensures satisfactory stent expansion, while a score of 4 indicates lower expansion and suggests modifying calcium during lesion preparation. Focusing on calcium fractures, visible in OCT, improves stent

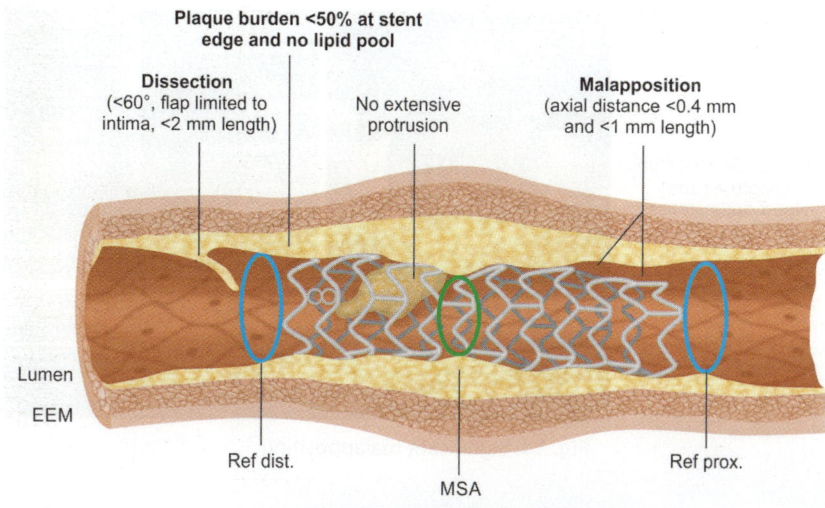

Fig. 12: Post-PCI optimization targets. (EEM: external elastic membrane; IVUS: intravascular ultrasound; MSA: minimum stent area; OCT: optical coherence tomography; PCI: percutaneous coronary intervention)

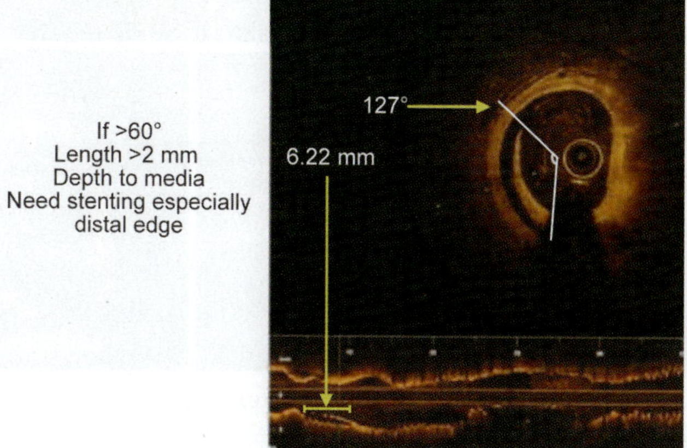

Fig. 13: Significant medial dissection.

expansion compared to dealing with calcified lesions without fractures[11] **(Flowchart 2)**.

Acute Coronary Syndrome

Approximately 4–10% of ST-elevation myocardial infarction (STEMI) patients and over 30% of non-ST-elevation myocardial infarction (NSTEMI) patients do not show a clear culprit lesion, and >10% may have multiple culprit

If distance >0.4 mm
Length >1 mm
Need optimization

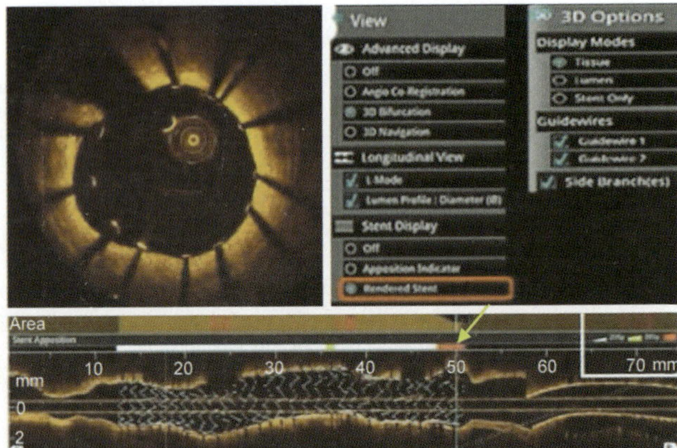

Fig. 14: Significant malapposition.

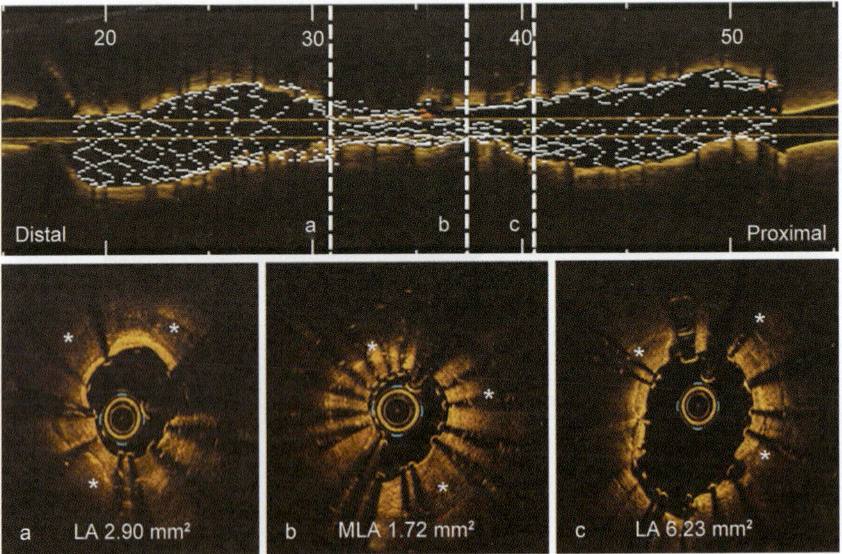

Fig. 15: Significant underexpansion.

lesions on angiography. OCT not only identifies these culprit lesions, especially when angiography results are unclear, but also sheds light on the underlying mechanisms in acute coronary syndrome (ACS). This information assists in making informed decisions about interventions[12] **(Flowchart 3).**

Plaque Rupture

The most frequent cause of ACS, accounting for 60–70% of cases, involves a rupture in the fibrous cap covering a lipid-rich core. When this rupture occurs, the contents of the core interact with the bloodstream, leading to

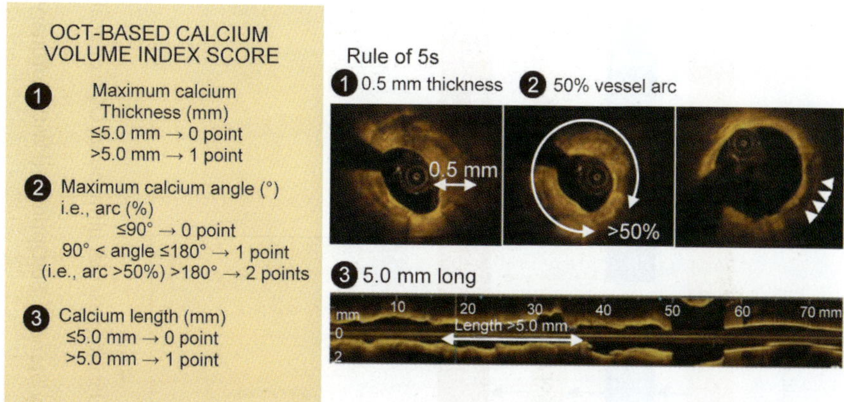

Fig. 16: Calcium score. (OCT: optical coherence tomography)

the formation of a fibrin-rich red thrombus, usually found near the ruptured plaque[13] **(Fig. 17)**.

Plaque Erosion

Plaque erosion contributes to about 20–30% of ACS cases, often affecting younger individuals, premenopausal women, current smokers, and those without traditional coronary risk factors. Typically, it involves a single-vessel disease with less severe lesions, larger vessel size, and lesions nearing bifurcations. Plaque erosion is identified by luminal surface irregularity without fibrous cap disruption. This type of ACS tends to have a lower white thrombus burden, maintains vascular structure, and results in a larger remaining lumen.[14] Treating plaque erosion with potent antithrombotic measures can eliminate the need for stent placement, preventing both immediate and delayed complications linked to stents[15] **(Fig. 18)**.

Calcified Lesions in ACS

In about 7–10% of ACS patients, calcified lesions with disrupted fibrous caps and no lipid core rupture are observed. Three types of culprit calcified plaques are identified in ACS patients: (1) Eruptive calcified nodules, involving small calcific nodules extruding into the lumen, (2) superficial calcific sheet, the most common type associated with poor baseline TIMI flow and reduced luminal diameter, and (3) calcified protrusion, characterized by a protruding calcific mass without eruptive nodules. All three calcific lesion types are easily identifiable with OCT and are linked to more complications during procedures and suboptimal PCI outcomes compared to noncalcified culprit plaques. Eruptive calcified nodules are often found in the mid-RCA, where cyclic heart movement may weaken calcified plaques, leading to fractures, while superficial calcific sheets are most frequently located in the left anterior descending artery[16] **(Fig. 19)**.

Flowchart 2: Algorithm in calcified coronary artery disease.

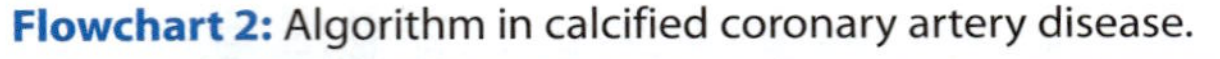

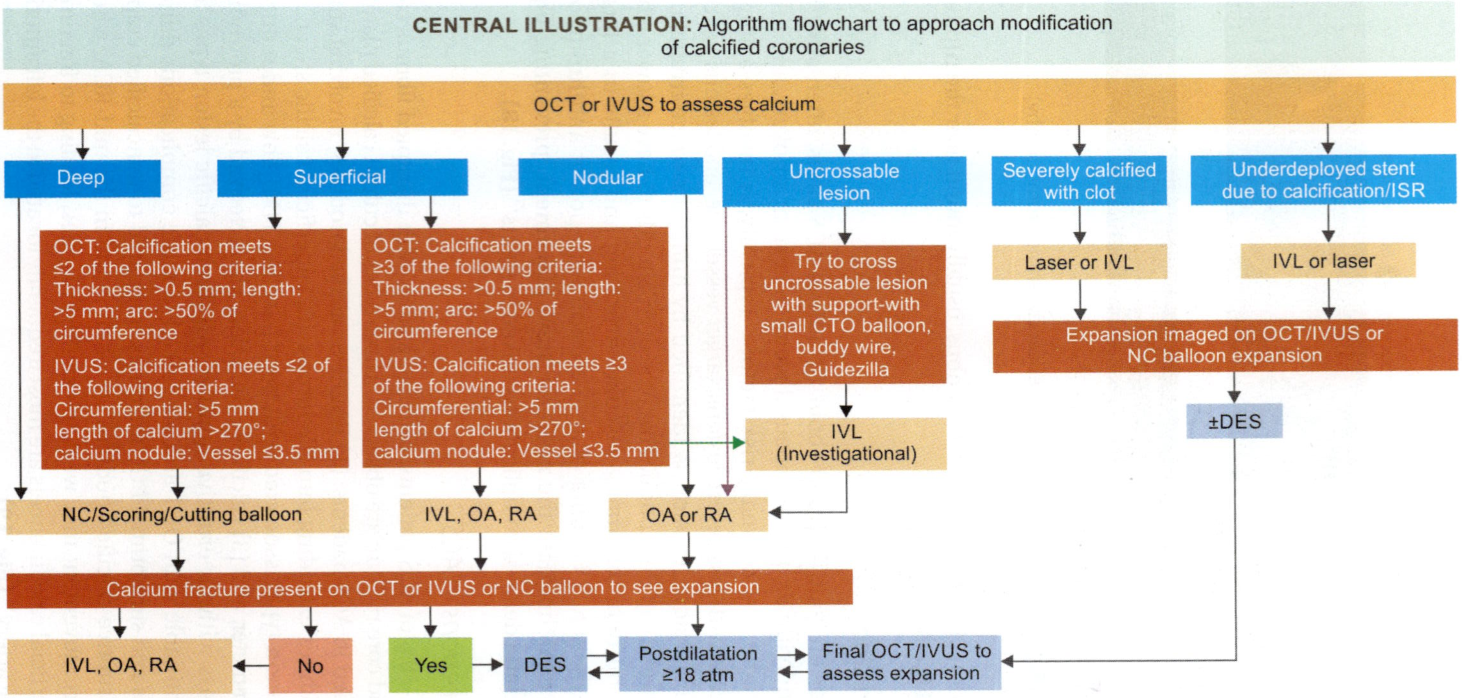

(CTO: chronic total occlusion; DES: drug-eluting stent; ISR: in-stent restenosis; IVL: intravascular lithotripsy; IVUS: intravascular ultrasound; OCT: optical coherence tomography; RA: rotational atherectomy)

Source: Mody R, Dash D, Mody B, Maligireddy AR, Agrawal A, Rastogi L, et al. Can Most Calcified Coronary Stenosis Be Optimized With Coronary Intravascular Lithotripsy? JACC Asia. 2023;3(2):185-97.

Flowchart 3: Algorithm in ACS.

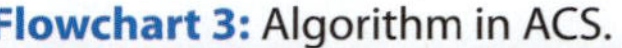

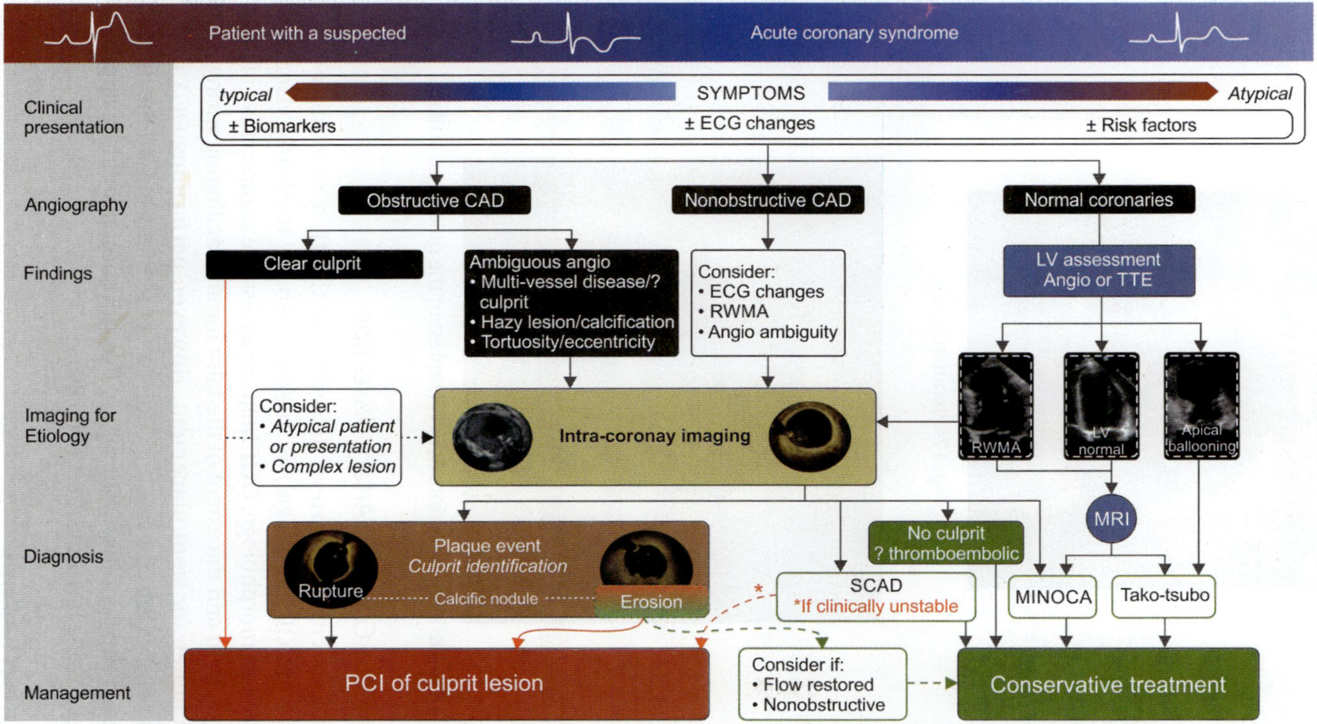

(ACS: acute coronary syndrome; CAD: coronary artery disease; ECG: electrocardiogram; LV: left ventricle; MINOCA: myocardial infarction with non-obstructive coronary arteries; MRI: magnetic resonance imaging; PCI: percutaneous coronary intervention; RWMA: regional wall motion abnormality; SCAD: spontaneous coronary artery dissection; TTE: transthoracic echocardiogram)

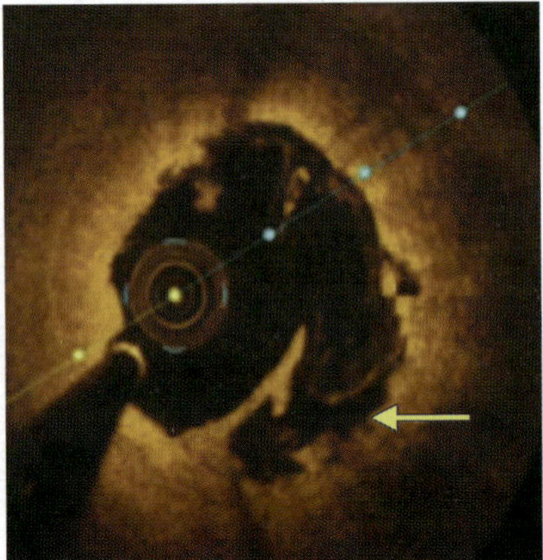

Fig. 17: Plaque rupture.

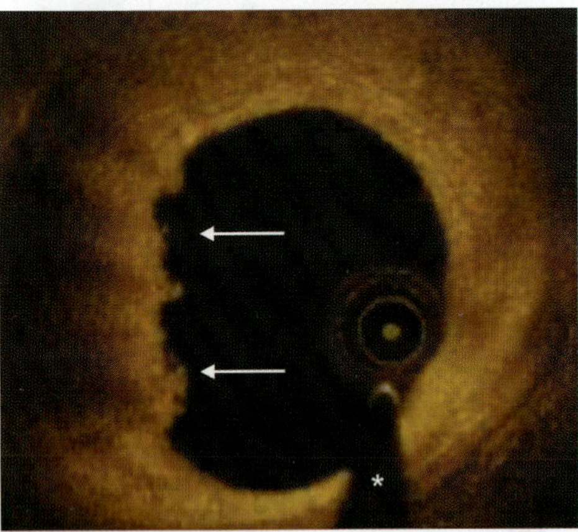

Fig. 18: Plaque erosion. Asterisk represent the guidewire artifact.

Spontaneous Coronary Artery Dissection

Spontaneous coronary artery dissection (SCAD), a rare cause of ACS, benefits from OCT in diagnosis due to its ability to clearly visualize the double lumen morphology. OCT helps to assess the compromise of the true coronary lumen and the extent of the false lumen, facilitating wiring through the true lumen for stent placement. However, performing OCT in SCAD involves risks, as the contrast injection can potentially extend the dissection and worsen the condition. Therefore, dye injection should be approached cautiously, using low-flow rates **(Fig. 20)**.

Bifurcation Lesions

Bifurcation lesions, making up 15–20% of PCI procedures, are typically complex and present distinct challenges in both the procedure itself and the

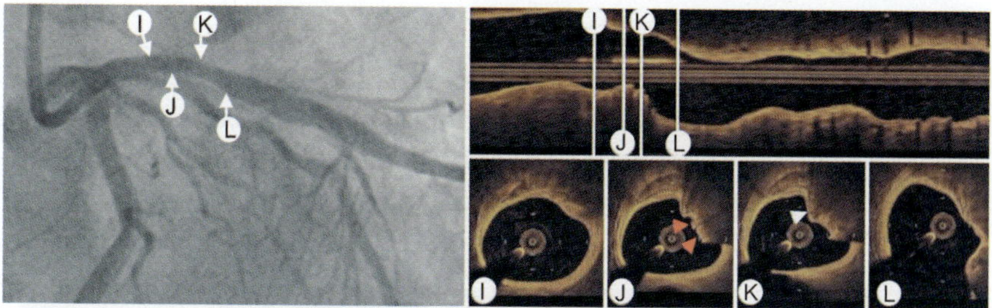

Fig. 19: Eruptive calcified nodule.

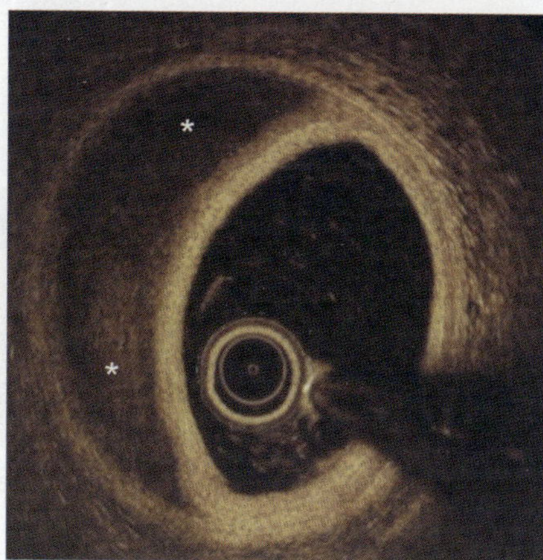

Fig. 20: Spontaneous coronary artery dissection (SCAD). Asterisks (*) represent the intramural hematoma.

expected outcomes.[17] In provisional bifurcation angioplasty, aside from the standard pre-PCI OCT evaluation, it is crucial to note three key parameters: the distribution of plaque concerning the side branch (SB) opening, the carina tip (CT) angle, and the length from CT to bifurcation point (BP). A CT angle <50° and a CT-BP length under 1.7 mm are identified as independent predictors of complications in the side branch during the provisional strategy.[18] A mostly calcified plaque opposite the SB opening predicts SB compromise after main branch (MB) stenting because of carinal shift. 3D reconstruction at the bifurcation precisely assesses stent struts around the SB opening, determines if the carina is link-free, and aids in distal guidewire recrossing. In cases where the carina is link-free, crossing the distal cell is linked to fully releasing the SB opening.[19] In a two-stent strategy, pre-PCI OCT examines both SB and main branch (MB). Post-final KBI, MB OCT pullback analyzes the SB opening. To prevent SB restenosis, check for hanging stent struts at the SB opening in 3D reconstruction, ensure minimal metallic carinal length in the L mode, and look for the dumbbell sign next to the native carina in cross-sectional view **(Figs. 21 to 23)**.

Stent Failure

Optical coherence tomography is the preferred method for evaluating stent failure, focusing on issues such as in-stent restenosis (ISR), stent thrombosis (ST), and scaffold thrombosis. By offering detailed insights into the failure mechanism, OCT aids in choosing the right management approach.

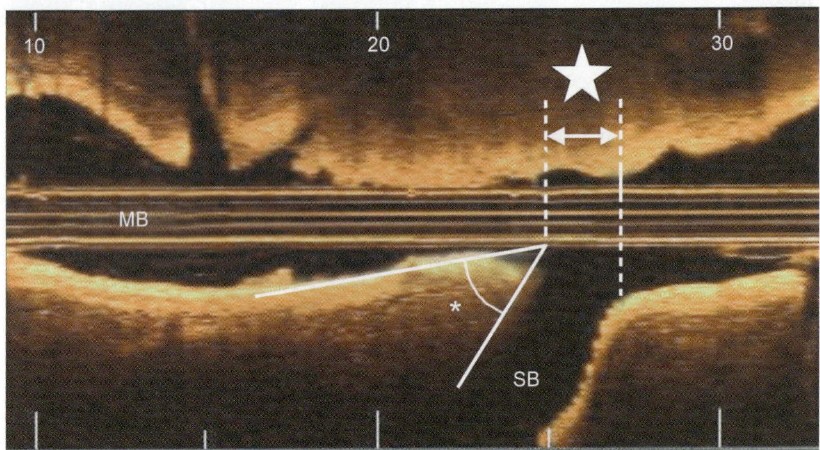

Fig. 21: Predictors of SB occlusion in provisional stenting. (MB: main branch; SB: side branch)

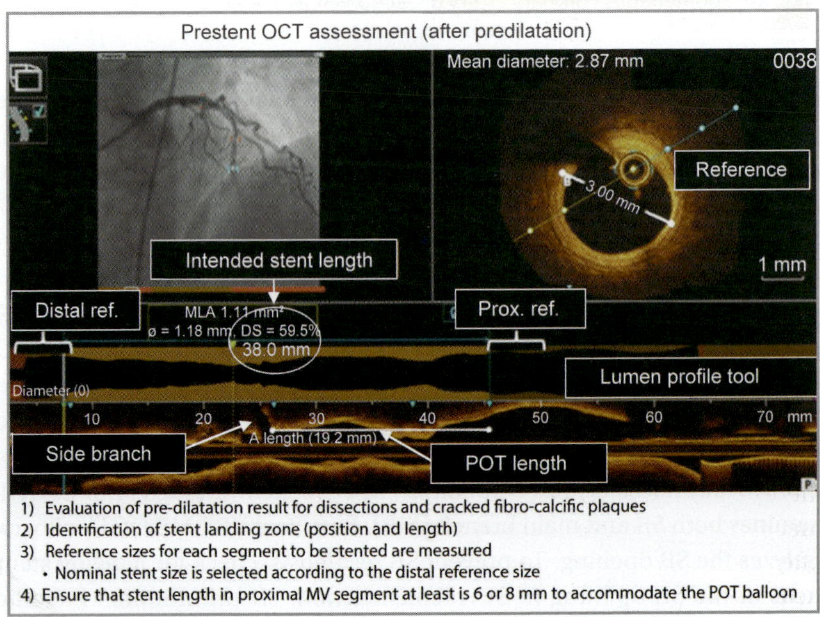

Fig. 22: Prestenting OCT algorithm in bifurcation stenting. (OCT: optical coherence tomography; POT: proximal optimization technique)

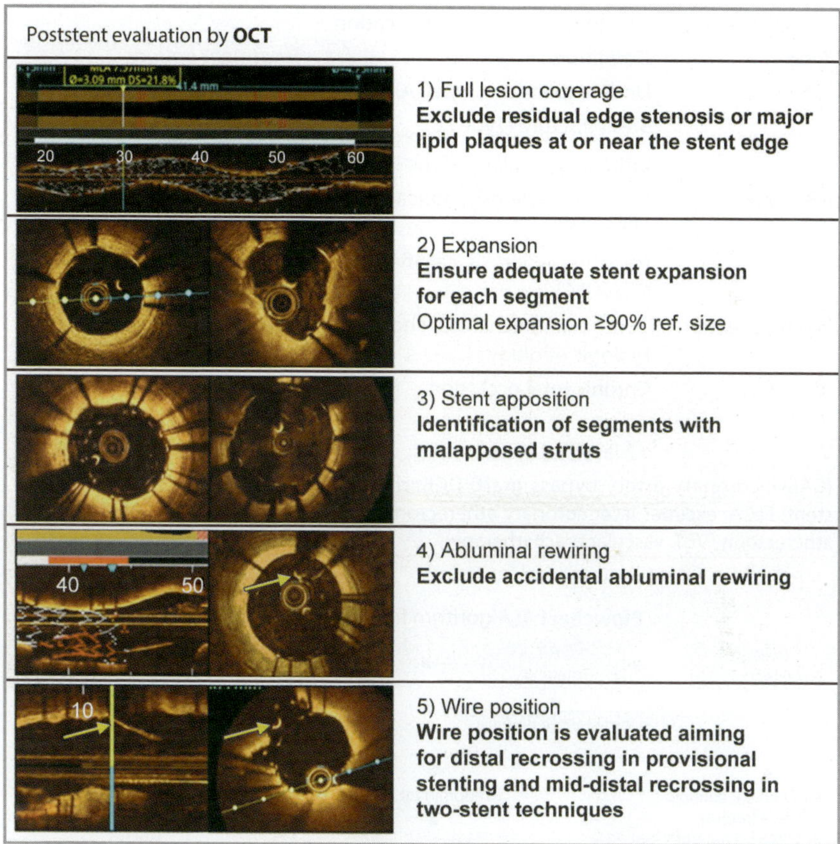

Fig. 23: Poststenting OCT algorithm in bifurcation stenting.
(OCT: optical coherence tomography)

In-stent Restenosis

Despite advancements in second-generation drug-eluting stent design and materials, ISR rates persist, posing a therapeutic challenge. OCT identifies ISR causes such as underexpansion, malapposition, or strut fracture, and characterizes ISR as either NIH or neoatherosclerosis[20] **(Table 1 and Flowchart 4)**.

Stent Thrombosis

Stent thrombosis is a serious complication of stent implantation, impacting life expectancy and causing heart attacks. OCT offers insights into the mechanistic processes behind ST. Uncovered and malapposed struts are often seen, and their prevalence decreases over time from the initial stenting. Acute/subacute ST is associated with uncovered struts and underexpansion, while late/very late ST is linked to uncovered struts and neoatherosclerosis[21] **(Flowchart 5)**.

TABLE 1: Waksman in-stent restenosis classification.

Type	*Definition*	*Treatment options*
I Mechanical	Underexpansion (Type I A)	High-pressure balloon
	Stent fracture (Type I B)	DES
II Biologic	Intimal hyperplasia (Type II A)	Balloon, DCB, DES, and VBT
	Neoatherosclerosis, noncalcified (Type II B)	DCB and DES
	Neoatherosclerosis, calcified (Type II C)	Scoring balloon, ELCA, and RA
III Mixed pattern	Combined mechanical and biologic etiology	High-pressure balloon with DCB, DES, or VBT
IV	Chronic total occlusion	DCB or DES, VBT for multiple layers, CABG as needed
V	>2 layers of stent	Balloon, DCB, VBT, and CABG

(CABG: coronary artery bypass graft; DCB: drug-coated balloon; DES: drug-eluting stent; ELCA: excimer laser coronary atherectomy; ISR: in-stent restenosis; RA: rotational atherectomy; VBT: vascular brachytherapy)

Flowchart 4: Algorithm for ISR management.

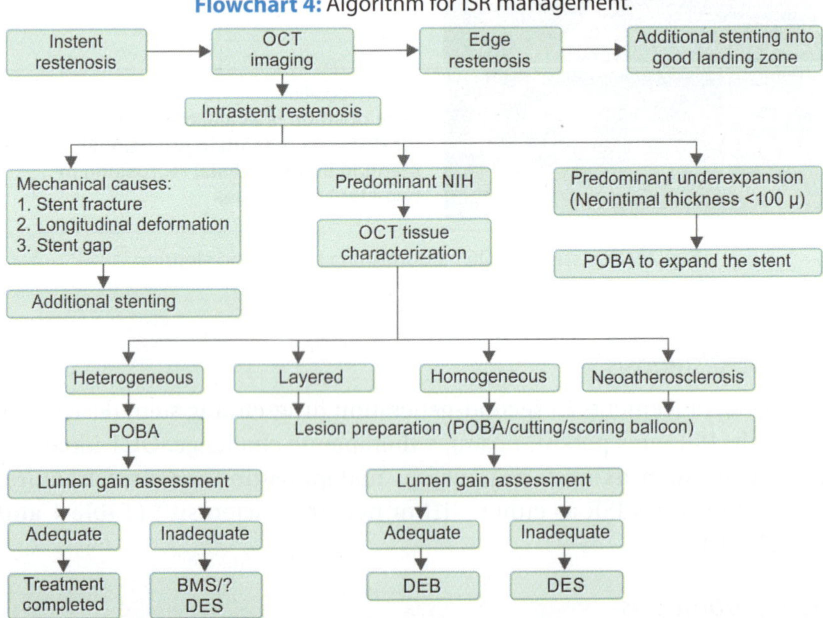

(BMS: bare metal stent; DEB: drug eluting balloon; DES: drug-eluting stent; ISR: in-stent restenosis; NIH: neo-intimal hyperplasia; OCT: optical coherence tomography; POBA: plain old balloon angioplasty)

Borderline Lesions

Cardiologists face a dilemma when deciding on PCI for intermediate lesions. The FORZA trial suggests considering PCI, if—(1) area stenosis (AS) is >75%,

Flowchart 5: Algorithm for stent thrombosis management.

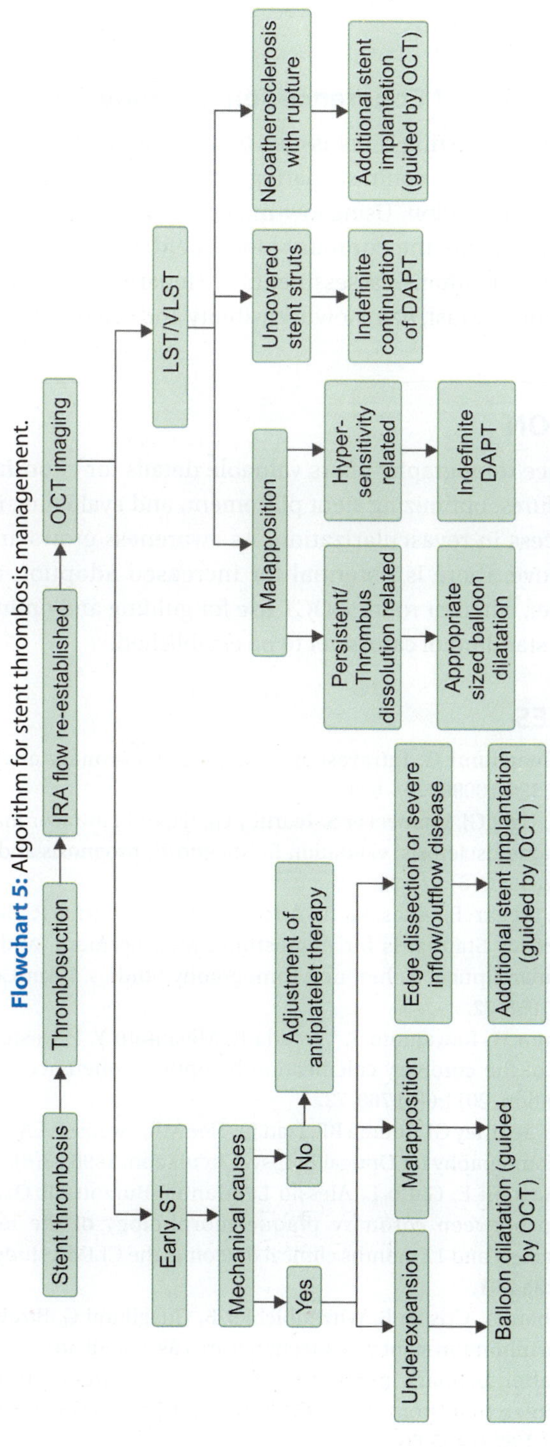

(DAPT: dual antiplatelet therapy; IRA: infarct related artery; LST: late stent thrombosis; OCT: optical coherence tomography; ST: stent thrombosis; VLST: very late stent thrombosis)

(2) AS is between 50 and 75% with MLA <2.5 mm^2, or (3) AS is between 50 and 75% with plaque rupture.[22]

Zero Contrast Optical Coherence Tomography

For patients with preexisting renal issues or a heightened risk of contrast-induced nephropathy, new contrast-sparing techniques allow the use of OCT in coronary revascularization. Using low-molecular-weight dextran (LMWD) instead of contrast clears the coronary blood field, achieving comparable image quality and quantitative assessment.[23,24] Heparinized saline, explored as an alternative to contrast, has shown feasibility and safety with satisfactory image quality.[25]

CONCLUSION

Optical coherence tomography offers valuable details for choosing lesions, planning procedures, optimizing stent placement, and evaluating immediate procedural success in revascularization. As awareness grows and clinical outcomes improve, there is potential for increased adoption of OCT in practice. However, whether routine OCT use for guiding and optimizing PCI will become the standard of care is yet to be established.

REFERENCES

1. Mintz GS, Guagliumi G. Intravascular imaging in coronary artery disease. Lancet. 2017;390(10096):793-809.
2. Koskinas KC, Ughi GJ, Windecker S, Tearney GJ, Räber L. Intracoronary imaging of coronary atherosclerosis: validation for diagnosis, prognosis and treatment. Eur Heart J. 2015;37(6):524-35.
3. Tearney GJ, Regar E, Akasaka T, Adriaenssens T, Barlis P, Bezerra HG, et al. Consensus Standards for Acquisition, Measurement, and Reporting of Intravascular Optical Coherence Tomography Studies. J Am Coll Cardiol. 2012;59(12):1058-72.
4. Kume T, Okura H, Kawamoto T, Yamada R, Miyamoto Y, Hayashida A, et al. Assessment of the coronary calcification by optical coherence tomography. EuroIntervention. 2011;6(6):768-72.
5. Brezinski ME, Tearney GJ, Bouma BE, Izatt JA, Hee MR, Swanson EA, et al. Optical Coherence Tomography for Optical Biopsy. Circulation. 1996;93(6):1206-13.
6. Prati F, Romagnoli E, Gatto L, Alessio La Manna, Burzotta F, Ozaki Y, et al. Relationship between coronary plaque morphology of the left anterior descending artery and 12 months clinical outcome: the CLIMA study. Eur Heart J. 2019;41(3):383-91.
7. Choi S, Maehara A, Cristea E, Witzenbichler B, Guagliumi G, Brodie BR, et al. Usefulness of minimum stent cross sectional area as a predictor of angiographic restenosis after primary percutaneous coronary intervention in acute myocardial infarction (from the HORIZONS-AMI Trial IVUS Substudy). Am J Cardiol. 2012;109(4):455-60.

8. Ali ZA, Maehara A, Généreux P, Shlofmitz RA, Fabbiocchi F, Nazif TM, et al. Optical coherence tomography compared with intravascular ultrasound and with angiography to guide coronary stent implantation (ILUMIEN III: OPTIMIZE PCI): a randomised controlled trial. Lancet. 2016;388(10060):2618-28.
9. Kubo T, Shinke T, Okamura T, Hibi K, Nakazawa G, Morino Y, et al. Optical frequency domain imaging vs. intravascular ultrasound in percutaneous coronary intervention (OPINION trial): one-year angiographic and clinical results. Eur Heart J. 2017;38(42):3139-47.
10. Fujino A, Mintz GS, Matsumura M, Lee T, Kim SY, Hoshino M, et al. A new optical coherence tomography-based calcium scoring system to predict stent underexpansion. EuroIntervention. 2018;13(18):2182-9.
11. Fujino A, Mintz GS, Lee T, Hoshino M, Usui E, Kanaji Y, et al. Predictors of Calcium Fracture Derived From Balloon Angioplasty and its Effect on Stent Expansion Assessed by Optical Coherence Tomography. JACC Cardiovasc Interv. 2018;11(10):1015-7.
12. Johnson TW, Räber L, Di Mario C, Bourantas CV, Jia H, Mattesini A, et al. Clinical use of intracoronary imaging. Part 2: acute coronary syndromes, ambiguous coronary angiography findings, and guiding interventional decision-making: an expert consensus document of the European Association of Percutaneous Cardiovascular Interventions. EuroIntervention. 2019;15(5):434-51.
13. Jia H, Abtahian F, Aguirre AD, Lee S, Chia S, Lowe H, et al. In vivo diagnosis of plaque erosion and calcified nodule in patients with acute coronary syndrome by intravascular optical coherence tomography. J Am Coll Cardiol. 2013;62(19):1748-58.
14. Kramer MCA, Rittersma SZH, de Winter RJ, Ladich ER, Fowler DR, Liang YH, et al. Relationship of thrombus healing to underlying plaque morphology in sudden coronary death. J Am Coll Cardiol. 2010;55(2):122-32.
15. Xing L, Yamamoto E, Sugiyama T, Jia H, Ma L, Hu S, et al. EROSION Study (Effective Anti-Thrombotic Therapy Without Stenting: Intravascular Optical Coherence Tomography-Based Management in Plaque Erosion). Circ Cardiovasc Interv. 2017;10(12):e005860.
16. Sugiyama T, Yamamoto E, Fracassi F, Lee H, Yonetsu T, Kakuta T, et al. Calcified plaques in patients with acute coronary syndromes. JACC Cardiovasc Interv. 2019;12(6):531-40.
17. Lassen JF, Holm NR, Stankovic G, Lefèvre T, Chieffo A, Hildick-Smith D, et al. Percutaneous coronary intervention for coronary bifurcation disease: Consensus from the first 10 years of the European Bifurcation Club meetings. EuroIntervention. 2014;10(5):545-60.
18. Watanabe M, Uemura S, Simon CH Yu, Ueda T, Soeda T, Takeda Y, et al. Side branch complication after a single-stent crossover technique. Coron Artery Dis. 2014;25(4):321-9.
19. Okamura T, Onuma Y, Yamada J, Iqbal J, Tateishi H, Nao T, et al. 3D optical coherence tomography: New insights into the process of optimal rewiring of side branches during bifurcational stenting. EuroIntervention. 2014;10(8):907-15.
20. Habara M, Terashima M, Nasu K, Kaneda H, Inoue K, Ito T, et al. Difference of tissue characteristics between early and very late restenosis lesions after bare-metal stent implantation. Circ Cardiovasc Interv. 2011;4(3):232-8.
21. Adriaenssens T, Joner M, Godschalk TC, Malik N, Alfonso F, Xhepa E, et al. Optical coherence tomography findings in patients with coronary stent thrombosis:

A Report of the PRESTIGE Consortium (Prevention of Late Stent Thrombosis by an Interdisciplinary Global European Effort). Circulation. 2017;136(11): 1007-21.

22. Burzotta F, Leone AM, Aurigemma C, Zambrano A, Zimbardo G, Arioti M, et al. Fractional flow reserve or optical coherence tomography to guide management of angiographically intermediate coronary stenosis. JACC Cardiovas Interv. 2020;13(1):49-58.
23. Ozaki Y, Kitabata H, Tsujioka H, Hosokawa S, Kashiwagi M, Ishibashi K, et al. Comparison of contrast media and low-molecular-weight dextran for frequency-domain optical coherence tomography. Circulation. 2012;76(4):922-7.
24. Vijayvergiya R, Ratheesh KJ, Gupta A. Low molecular weight Dextran: An alternative to radiographic contrast agent for Optical coherence tomography imaging. IHJ Cardiovasc Case Rep. 2017;1(1):10-1.
25. Mahesh NK, Gupta A, Barward P, Vijayvergiya R, Sharma P, Mahesh A. Study of saline optical coherence tomography-guided percutaneous coronary intervention (SOCT-PCI Study). Indian Heart J. 2020;72(4):239-43.

CHAPTER 9

Image-based Optimization of Stent Implantation

Rajesh Vijayvergiya

INTRODUCTION

Coronary angiography is primarily a luminogram and hence, has some inherent shortcomings. Tortuosity or overlapping of vessels may prevent an accurate assessment of lesion severity. Calcification of lesions may be underestimated by angiography alone. Intravascular imaging is more accurate in assessing lesion severity, plaque characteristics, and calcification quantification. These modalities help in planning coronary lesion management strategy and stent optimization. Various large, randomized control trials (RCTs) and meta-analyses have shown that the use of intravascular imaging to guide percutaneous coronary intervention (PCI) is associated with reduced major adverse cardiovascular events (MACE).

Several intravascular imaging modalities have been developed which include angioscopy, optical coherence tomography (OCT), intravascular ultrasound (IVUS), virtual histology IVUS, and near-infrared spectroscopy (NIR). IVUS and OCT are the most well-studied and frequently used imaging modalities in routine clinical practice. IVUS uses ultrasound waves with a frequency between 20 and 60 MHz. Cross-sectional images are generated from the reflected waves based on the differential acoustic impedance of various tissues. The axial resolution is 40–60 µm, and depth penetration is up to 10 mm. The intima and adventitia appear as echogenic layers while the media is echo lucent. OCT uses infrared electromagnetic rays for image acquisition. OCT has a higher resolution (axial 10–20 µm); however, in-depth penetration is less than IVUS. A flush medium is required for OCT. **Table 1** enumerates the fundamental differences between the two modalities. The structure of a normal vessel, as seen in IVUS and OCT, is shown in **Figures 1A to D**.

PREINTERVENTION EVALUATION

Lesion Assessment

Characterization of plaque morphology like fibrotic, lipid-rich or calcific plaque and quantification of calcium can be done with intravascular imaging. A good understanding of plaque morphology helps in appropriate plaque modification techniques and stent optimization. Lipid-rich and

TABLE 1: A fundamental difference between IVUS and OCT imaging.

	IVUS	*OCT*
Energy source	Ultrasound	Near-infrared light
Wavelength, μm	35–80	1.3
Resolution, μm	40–200 (axial), 200–300 (lateral)	15–20 (axial), 20–40 (lateral)
Maximum scan diameter, mm	15	7
Tissue penetration, mm	10	1–2.5
Blood clearing	Not required	Required
Advantages	More favorable imaging in larger vascular structures (e.g., left main)	Can measure and characterize calcium, differentiate between white and red thrombus **(Figs. 2A to D)**
Disadvantages	Inferior detection of stent malapposition and edge dissection	Cannot accurately assess residual plaque burden at stent edges

(IVUS: intravascular ultrasound; OCT: optical coherence tomography)

necrotic plaques are notorious for causing distal embolization during PCI and periprocedural myocardial infarction. Morphological predictors are attenuated plaque, plaque rupture, and thin-cap fibroatheroma. Representative images are shown in **Figures 3A and B**. In a large IVUS study, the incidence of a lipid-rich plaque was 43.8 and 27.9% in acute coronary syndrome (ACS) and stable coronary artery disease patients, respectively.[1] In this study, the adjusted odds ratio to predict post-PCI thrombolysis in myocardial infarction (TIMI) flow grade <3 was 5.9 (95% confidence interval: 2.4–14.5) and 6.6 (95% confidence interval: 1.4–32.1), respectively for ACS and stable coronary artery cases. In the presence of such a plaque, direct stenting and aggressive postdilatation should be avoided.

Angiography picks calcium in only 40% of the cases, while IVUS detects calcium in 73% of lesions. In general, angiographically detected calcium corresponds to more calcium (larger angle and length) by IVUS. Similar is the case with OCT and as it can penetrate calcium, it has the added advantage of measuring thickness and area for calcified plaque evaluation. Representative images of calcium in IVUS and OCT and the severity of calcium have been demonstrated in **Figures 4A to F**. Larger calcium angle and thickness are associated with poor stent expansion. The arc of calcium is classified as none or in quadrants. Calcium location is defined as superficial if present in the intimal luminal interface or deep if it is closer to the adventitia than the lumina. IVUS cannot penetrate calcium, so assessment is limited to calcium arc and length. As a proxy to direct measurement, IVUS calcium

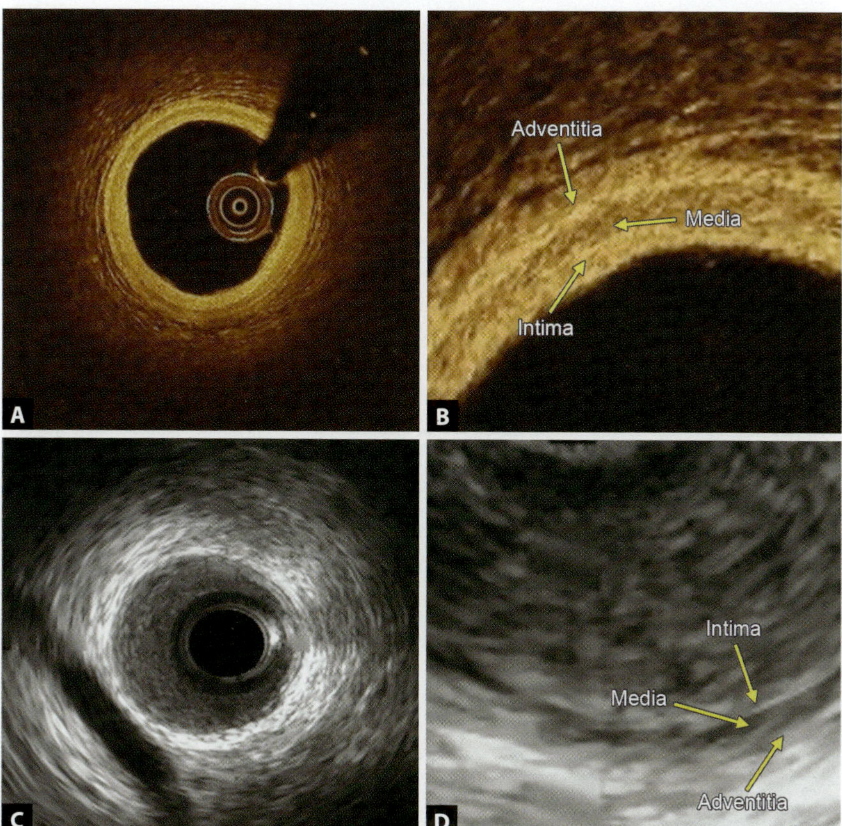

Figs. 1A to D: The appearance of a normal segment of a coronary artery in OCT (A) and IVUS (C). Zoomed-in OCT image showing vessel wall structure in a normal coronary segment (B). In OCT, intima appears as a thin signal-rich layer, media is a signal-poor layer, and adventitia is a heterogeneously appearing signal-rich layer. These layers are separated by signal-rich internal and external elastic lamina (B). In IVUS, the intima and adventitia appear as echogenic layers, while the media is echolucent (D). (IVUS: intravascular ultrasound; OCT: optical coherence tomography)

with a smooth surface and reverberations or irregular surfaces without reverberation indicates thinner calcium (OCT maximum calcium thickness <0.50 mm). On the other hand, IVUS calcium with an irregular surface without reverberations indicates thicker calcium (OCT calcium thickness >1 mm).[2] OCT can penetrate calcium to assess the thickness, area, and volume of the calcium. The presence of calcium of more than 180° arc, thickness of >0.5 mm, and length of >5 mm by OCT or circumferential extension of >180° by IVUS are predictors of poor stent expansion, smaller stent area, and greater stent eccentricity.[3] The above features should prompt consideration for the use of plaque modification techniques like rotational atherectomy, orbital atherectomy, intravascular lithotripsy or cutting and/or scoring balloons.

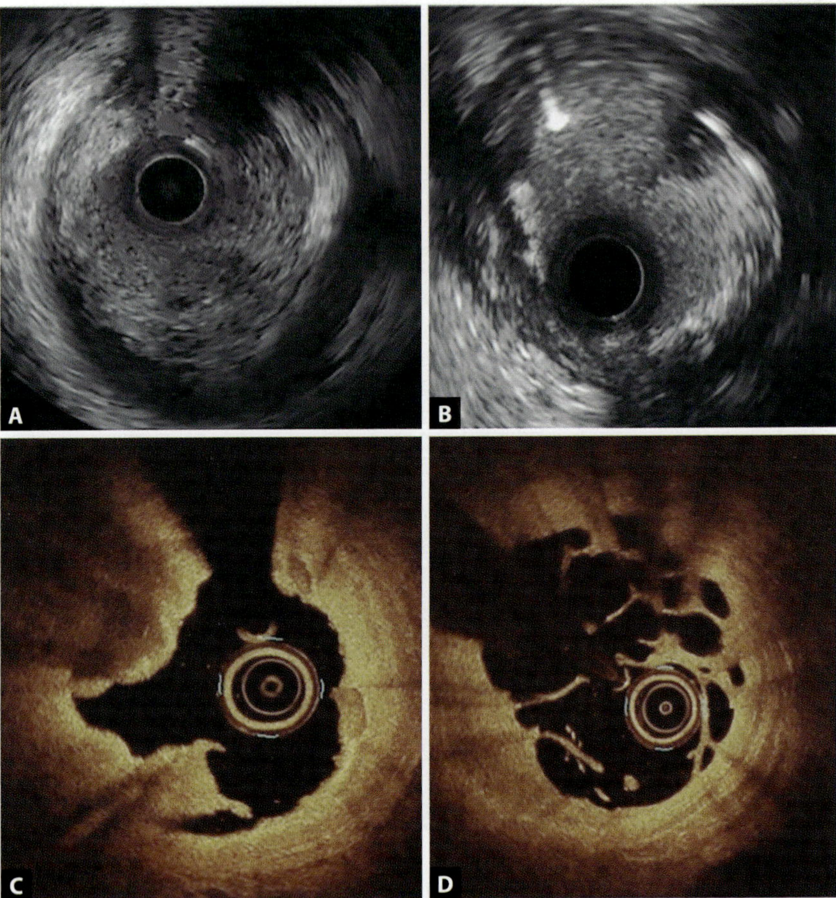

Figs. 2A to D: In IVUS, thrombus appears as a hypoechoic structure within the lumen of the vessel (A) or stent (B) with an acoustic shadow. In OCT, red thrombus appears as a signal-rich mass within the lumen with high backscattering at the leading edge with high attenuation beyond (C), while white thrombus appears as signal-rich mass with low attenuation (D). Figure D also showed multiple intraluminal channels suggestive of recanalized thrombus. (IVUS: intravascular ultrasound; OCT: optical coherence tomography)

Intravascular imaging helps in identifying the mechanism for in-stent restenosis (ISR)—stent underexpansion, neointimal hyperplasia, and neoatherosclerosis **(Figs. 5A to F)**. The approach to treating each of them is different.[4] Stent underexpansion needs adequate dilatation, which sometimes requires lithotripsy or laser therapy. Neointimal hyperplasia needs plaque modification followed by drug-eluting sent or drug-coated balloon angioplasty. Neoatherosclerosis needs to be treated as a de novo atherosclerotic lesion. The current guideline recommends IVUS/OCT imaging to detect stent-related mechanical problems leading to restenosis

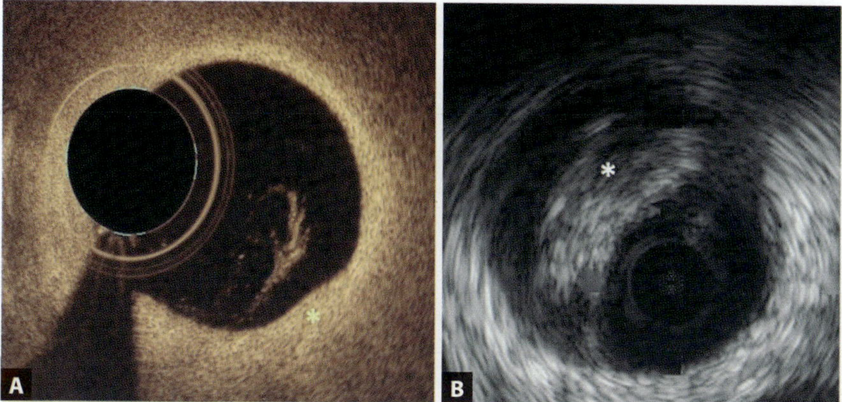

Figs. 3A and B: (A) The lipid core appears as signal-poor areas in the plaque with irregular border in OCT and (B) hypoechoic areas within the plaque in IVUS. Asterisks in (A) and (B) represent the lipid core. (IVUS: intravascular ultrasound; OCT: optical coherence tomography)

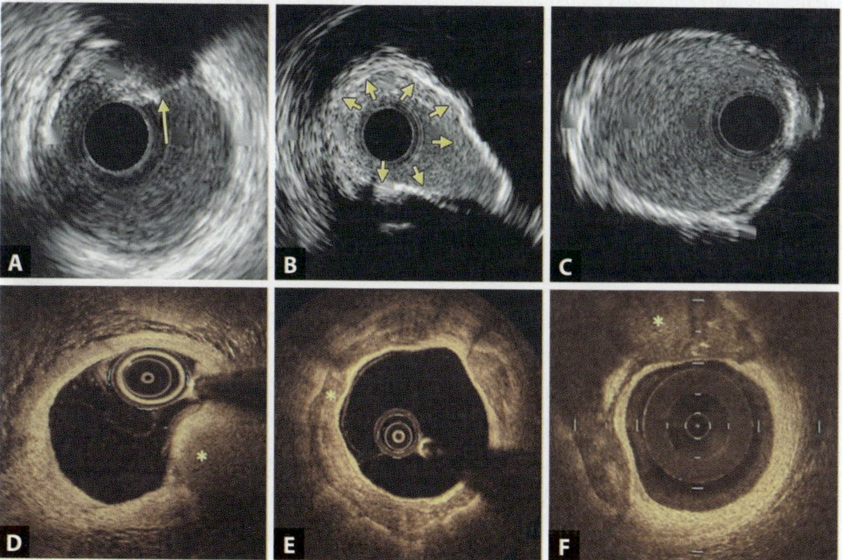

Figs. 4A to F: (A to C) IVUS and (D to F) OCT images of calcified segments of coronary arteries. In IVUS, calcium appears as a hyperechoic line with an acoustic shadow. In OCT, calcium appears as heterogeneous signal-poor regions with sharp borders. Figures A and D show a calcium nodule protruding into the lumen in IVUS and OCT images, respectively. Figure B shows a 270° calcium with the acoustic shadow, which makes the deeper assessment of the vessel impossible. Figure C shows a 360° calcium with acoustic shadow. Figure E shows superficial calcium and F shows deep calcium in OCT images. Arrows in A and B show the inner surface of calcium. Asterisks in D, E, and F represent the core of calcium. (IVUS: intravascular ultrasound; OCT: optical coherence tomography)

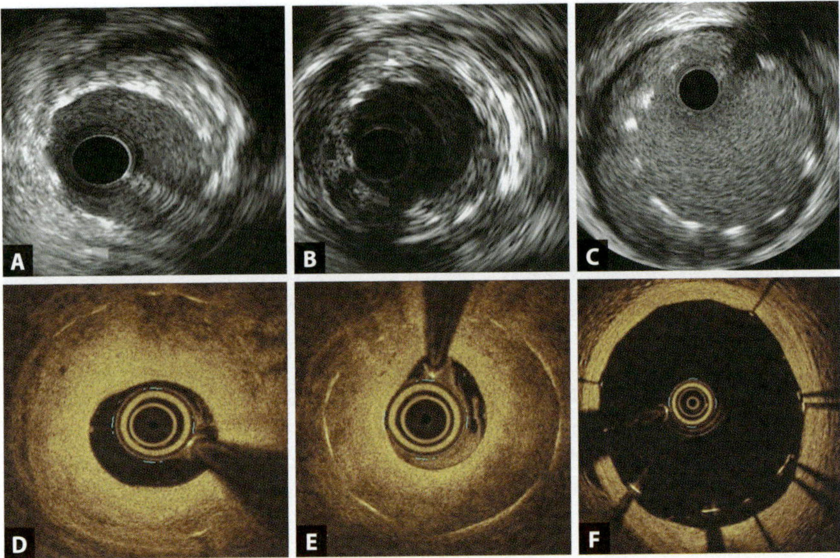

Figs. 5A to F: Intravascular imaging showing various major mechanisms responsible for in-stent restenoses such as (A) underexpanded stent, (B and D) neointimal hyperplasia, (C and F) malapposition, and (E) neoatherosclerosis.

(recommendation Class IIa, level of evidence C).[5] Other unusual lesions like spontaneous coronary artery dissections can also be detected by IVUS and OCT; however, one should be prudent.

Assessment of Lesion Significance

Fractional flow reserve (FFR) is the gold standard for assessment of lesion significance in non-left main vessels. The use of IVUS and OCT for this purpose is not accurate. However, IVUS derived MLA of <3.2 mm^2 correlates well with an FFR value of <0.8.[6] OCT-derived cut-offs are smaller. In the OMEF study, MLA of <2.0 mm^2 showed an excellent discriminative power to predict FFR of ≤0.80. An MLA of <3.1 mm^2 best predicted an FFR of ≤0.8 for proximal coronary segments.[6a] For left main coronary artery (LMCA) lesions, there is a better correlation between IVUS and FFR. An IVUS MLA of <6 mm^2 correlates well with an FFR value of <0.75 in the western population.[7] Smaller MLA cut-offs have been seen in Asian patients. Studies from Korea suggested that an IVUS MLA of 4.5–4.8 mm^2 correlate well with a positive FFR.[8] The cut-off MLA of >6 mm^2 has been used to defer LMCA revascularization. For LMCA lesions, there is a better correlation between IVUS and FFR. The cut-off MLA of >6 mm^2 has been used to defer LMCA revascularization. OCT has limitations in the assessment of LMCA especially the ostium due to the inability to acquire the bloodless field.

Determination of Stent Size

- *Intravascular ultrasound-guided stent size:* In the DES era, stent and post-stent adjunct balloon sizing are based on reference distal vessel lumen diameter or distal vessel external elastic lamina (EEL) diameter. The vessel EEL-based sizing is preferred when the vessel segment is disease-free or has a fibrotic plaque; wherein, the EEL can be identified reliably. Distal lumen reference-based sizing is the most straightforward approach which is followed by optimization of mid and proximal stent segments.[9] The lumen-based approach is used when there is plaque and identification of EEL is not feasible. The stent lengths are based on proximal and distal landing zones, which are ideally disease-free segments. However, if such a zone is unavailable then the plaque burden should be <50%.[10] Lipid-rich plaque and thin-cap fibroatheroma should be avoided at landing zones. A representative case of IVUS-guided stenting is shown in **Figures 6A to D**.
- *Optical coherence tomography-guided stent size:* The selection of stent size is based on lumen diameters or the smaller of the proximal or distal reference external elastic lamina diameter if >180° of its circumference was visible.[11] However, OCT often cannot identify the EEL at the lesion site.

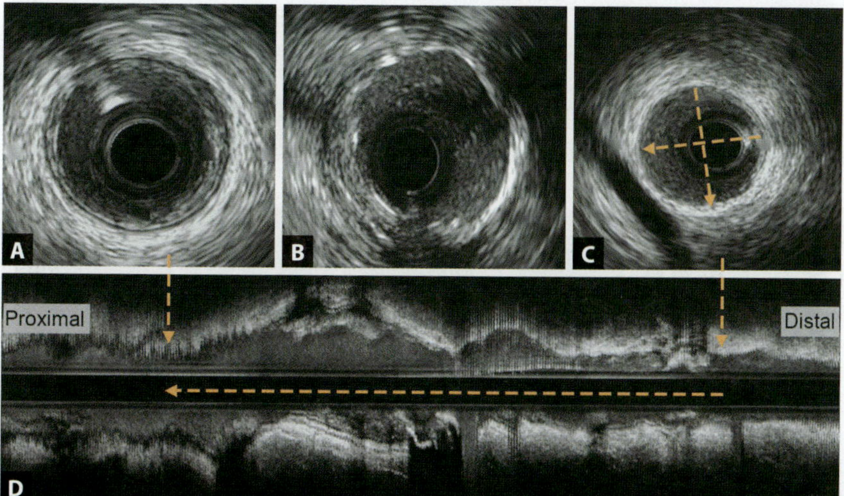

Figs. 6A to D: (A to C) IVUS images showing cross-sections at various levels of the coronary artery. Figures A and B are the selected segments for proximal and distal landing zones, respectively, as they are disease-free. The diameter of the stent is decided based on the distal reference vessel (C). Dotted line in C represent the coronary artery diameters. Figure D depicts the longitudinal section of coronary segment studied. Dotted line in D represents the distance between the proximal and distal landing zones (distance between A and C) based on which stent length is decided. (IVUS: intravascular ultrasound)

The ILLUMIEN III study thus introduced a novel method for choosing stent sizes. If the EEL was visible for >180°, then the stent size is based on the smaller of the proximal and distal vessel EEL diameter rounded down by 0.25 mm to the next stent diameter. If the EEL is not visible for >180° then stent size is based on 100% of the lumen diameter. The selection of the landing zone is the same as that with IVUS. A representative image for OCT-guided PCI is shown in **Figures 7A to E**. OCT can be used for coronary imaging except in the case of ostial left main disease (class of recommendation—2a, level of evidence—B).

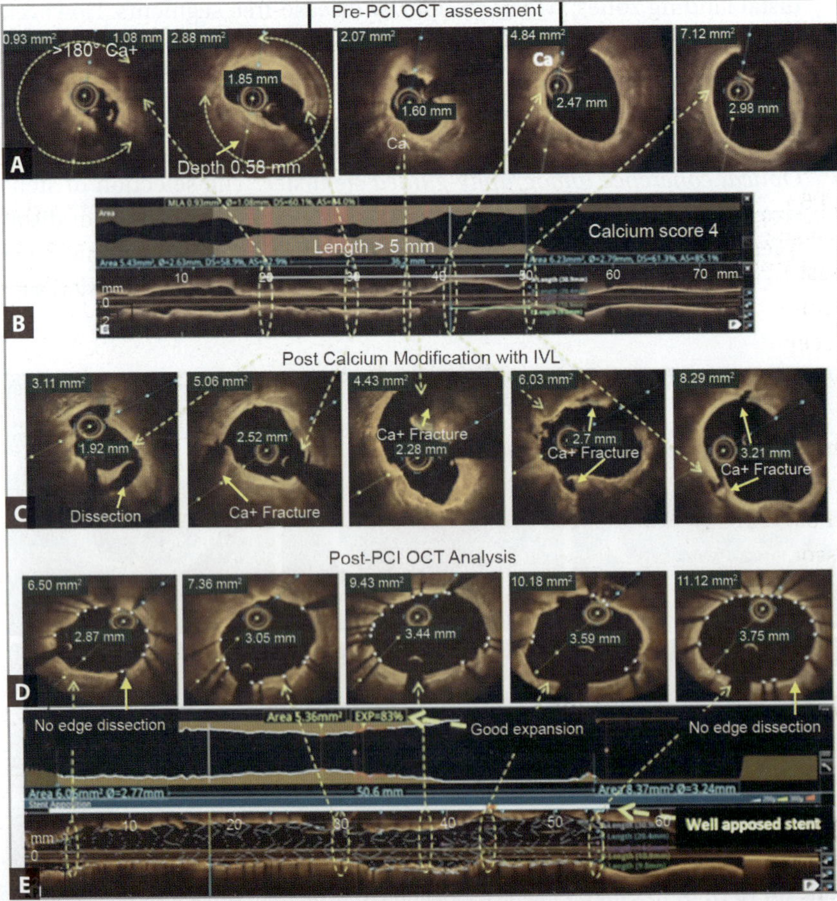

Figs. 7A to E: OCT-guided management of calcified left anterior descending (LAD). (A and B) Prepercutaneous coronary intervention (PCI) assessment showed a heavily calcified LAD with a calcium arc >180°, a calcium thickness of 0.58 mm, and a length of >5 mm resulting in a calcium score of 4; (C) Fractures in the calcium after modification with intravascular lithotripsy (IVL); (D and E) Post-PCI assessment showed 83% stent expansion, no edge dissection, and a well-apposed stent. (OCT: optical coherence tomography)

POSTPERCUTANEOUS CORONARY INTERVENTION IMAGING USES

Iterative imaging helps with the further steps of additional plaque modification, and optimal stenting—that is avoiding underexpansion and geographical miss and identifying complications and their management.

Optimal Stent Expansion

Postdilation is more frequently used following imaging, which leads to a larger minimal stent area compared to angiography alone. According to the current ESC expert consensus document, in non-LMCA, an absolute minimum stent area of >5.5 mm^2 or relative expansion minimum stent area by average reference lumen area of >80% is recommended.[12] The cut-offs for LMCA are 7 and 8 mm^2 in distal and proximal LMCA, respectively.

The minimum lumen area detected by OCT is smaller than IVUS. OCT detected MLA of >5.4 mm^2 was associated with an FFR of >0.9 and an MLA of <4.5 mm^2 was associated with a higher MACE.[13] In the ILLUMIEN III study, the stent segment was divided into proximal and distal halves, and on the post-PCI OCT, the MSA of each half was compared to the respective reference lumen area; >95% was considered optimal and >90% was considered acceptable stent expansion. A higher absolute stent expansion is associated with lower chances of stent failure.

Post-PCI MSA is the most consistent and strongest predictor of stent thrombosis and restenosis.[10,14,15] The larger the MSA, the lesser the chances for restenosis. Usually, the underexpansion is more severe and diffuse in-stent thrombosis compared to ISR. Prati et al. showed MSR <4.5 mm^2 was associated with MACE events (cardiac death, stent thrombosis, target lesion restenosis, and target vessel MI).[16]

Post-stent Implantation Complications

Geographical Miss and Edge Dissection

Longitudinal geographical miss (GM) is defined as an angiographically injured or diseased segment not covered by a stent, and axial GM a balloon/artery size ratio <0.9 or >1.3. In a study by Costa et al., GM occurred in 66.5% of patients; 47.6% had longitudinal GM, 35.2% had axial GM, and 16.5% had both. The overall rate of longitudinal geographical miss was 31.3% without much difference between the procedures done with and without OCT co-registration.[16] Thus, geographical miss is not infrequent even with intravascular imaging guidance of PCI. Geographical miss has been associated with restenosis and stent thrombosis. The presence of greater stent edge plaque burden, calcium or attenuated plaque or greater stent expansion at the stent edge is associated with edge dissections. An untreated

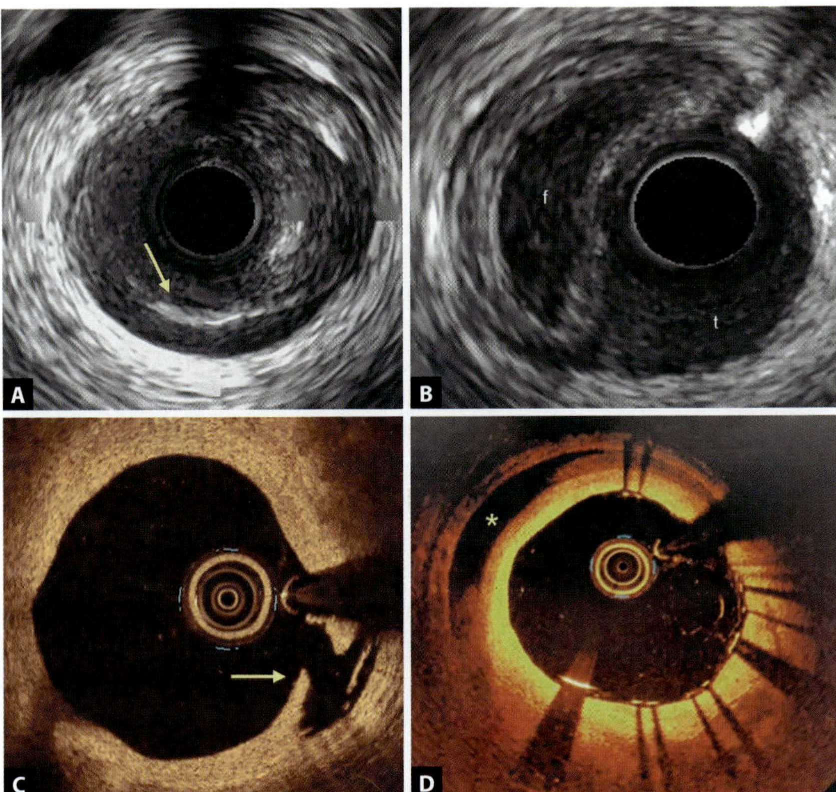

Figs. 8A to D: (A and C) Coronary dissection appears as a disruption in the continuity of the arterial wall with a flap. (B) Imaging can help to identify the true lumen (t), which is characterized by the presence of all three layers, that is, intima, media and adventitia, from the false lumen (f). (D) Intramural hematoma can be identified as an accumulation of blood within the media that may displace the internal elastic membrane inward and the external elastic membrane outward, with or without identifiable entry or exit points. Arrows in A and C point at the dissection flaps in IVUS and OCT, respectively. Asterisk in D represents the blood accumulated within the media of an intramural hematoma. (IVUS: intravascular ultrasound; OCT: optical coherence tomography)

edge dissection is associated with stent thrombosis and restenosis especially if the lumen area within the dissection is <5 mm^2 (by OCT), the dissection length is >3 mm, the residual distal edge dissection is >200 µm in width and the dissection flap radial extent is >60°.[17] Representative images of stent edge dissection are shown in **Figures 8A to D**. Stent edge dissection is more frequently picked up with OCT than IVUS.

Tissue Protrusion

Tissue protrusion was seen in up to 31% of patients with stable coronary artery disease and 69% of patients with ACS.[18,19] In ADAPT-DES and HORIZON-AMI studies, which used post-PCI IVUS in ACS patients, tissue protrusion was not associated with adverse events due to greater stent expansions. Large tissue protrusion leading to a small residual lumen area was associated with early stent thrombosis. However, in a post-PCI OCT study, irregular tissue protrusion due to lipid plaque or thrombus was associated with stent thrombosis.[20]

Acute Malapposition

It is defined as the inadequate contact of the outer stent surface with the outer wall. Acute malposition is detected by OCT twice as frequently compared with IVUS.[21,22] Causes are stent under deployment, resistant lesions at the landing zone or vessel spasm and underfilling of the vessel. Hence, NTG should be used to identify the true size of the vessel. In the various cross-sectional studies with OCT and IVUS, it was seen that more than half of them resolved in the 9-month follow-up.[23,24] Acute malapposition is especially important in the setting of a stent underexpansion. In the absence of stent underexpansion, malapposition was not associated with early or late adverse outcomes irrespective of length and thickness. The EAPCI recommends correcting extensive acute stent malapposition >0.4 mm with longitudinal extension >1 mm. Length of malapposition of >10 mm predisposes for very late stent thrombosis.[25]

OPTICAL COHERENCE TOMOGRAPHY VERSUS INTRAVASCULAR ULTRASOUND-GUIDED PERCUTANEOUS CORONARY INTERVENTION

Intravascular ultrasound-guided PCI leads to larger MSA as seen in the study by Habara et al. and the OPINION trial.[22,26] This is because IVUS-based stent sizing is based on EEL diameter leading to larger stent and balloon sizes. The visualization of EEL by OCT is limited. However, in the ILUMIEN III study, EEL visibility >180° was noted in up to 70% of the patients by the operator. In this study, the stent sizing was based on EEL diameter in the majority of the patients and the results were noninferior to IVUS. Based on trials like OPINION, ILUMIEN III, and iSIGHT,[21,22,27] OCT is noninferior to IVUS for stent expansion, and acute and long-term results. The OCTIVUS trial was a head-to-head trial concerning clinical outcomes powered for noninferiority.[28] It showed that OCT was noninferior to IVUS in clinical outcomes. The incidence of procedural complications was lower with OCT and the incidence of contrast-induced nephropathy was equal in both groups. The ILUMIEN IV trial investigated OCT-guided PCI against angiography-guided PCI in complex patients and lesions. Do positive guided PCI led to larger MSA, it did not reduce the 2-year rate of target vessel failure.

Both modalities are useful in detecting post-PCI complications; however, OCT provides better image quality, can better define calcium and differentiate between red and white thrombus.

OPTIMIZATION OF BIORESORBABLE SCAFFOLD

Due to some inherent properties of the bioresorbable scaffold (BRS), adequate lesion preparation, scaffold expansion, and prevention of malapposition are very critical during PCI. As BRSs are radiolucent, cine angiography is inadequate to assess these aspects and intravascular imaging is important. BRS underexpansion and malapposition is associated with target lesion failure. Malapposition at the time of implantation may hinder the process of incorporation of the scaffold in the vessel wall and become a nidus for thrombus during strut dismantling. Device failure should undergo investigation with intravascular imaging preferably with OCT. However, evidence supporting the usage of intravascular imaging for improving outcomes in BRSs is scanty.[29]

LEFT MAIN STENT STRATEGY

Preintervention assessment of left main coronary artery disease, direct imaging assessment of disease at the ostia of the left anterior descending, and left circumflex bifurcation lesions in the left main coronary artery help to select the appropriate stent strategy and predict side-branch occlusion—and stent optimization. This holds good for nonleft main coronary artery bifurcation lesions also.[30,31] Current guidelines recommend the use of IVUS for planning stenting of the left main lesion (class of recommendation—2a, level of evidence—B).[5]

CHRONIC TOTAL OCCLUSION LESIONS

Intravascular ultrasound has specific applications during chronic total occlusion (CTO) interventions. In the anterograde approach, the use of IVUS includes resolving proximal cap ambiguity, facilitating re-entry into the true lumen after subintimal wiring, and confirming the distal true lumen guidewire position before stenting. In the retrograde approach, IVUS (which is advanced on the anterograde guidewire) is useful in guiding the crossing of the retrograde guidewire from the false lumen into the true lumen, which can also be done by use of the reverse controlled anterograde-retrograde tracking technique.[25] IVUS guidance is associated with better CTO treatment outcomes. In a series of 31 cases, the use of IVUS led to the successful revascularization of all the previously failed CTO PCIs.[32] In a randomized setting, the guided procedure reduced 12 months MACE compared to angiography alone.[33]

IMAGING OF SAPHENOUS VENOUS GRAFTS

Saphenous venous graft vessels are larger than the coronary vessels making angiographic assessment difficult. Aggressive stent expansion is associated with periprocedural embolization of plaque material and myocardial necrosis, with no improvement of target vessel revascularization rates at 1 year.[21] Stent oversizing may also cause graft perforation. IVUS is reasonable for selecting appropriately sized stents. OCT can define the graft wall characteristics with greater accuracy and provide information about stent restenosis.

RECOMMENDATIONS

European Society of Cardiology Recommendations (2018)[34]

Intravascular ultrasound or OCT should be used in selected patients for stent optimization (IIa). IVUS should be considered to optimize the treatment of unprotected left main disease (IIa). In patients with stent failure, IVUS or OCT is reasonable to determine the mechanism of stent failure (IIa).

American Heart Association Recommendations (IIa)[5]

In patients undergoing stent implantation, IVUS can be useful for procedure guidance in cases of left main or complex lesions stenting to reduce ischemic events (IIa). In patients undergoing stent implantation, OCT is a reasonable alternative to IVUS for procedural guidance except for ostial left main disease (IIa). In patients with stent failure, IVUS or OCT is reasonable to determine the mechanism of stent failure (IIa). Intravascular imaging is recommended for lesion assessment of intermediate left main disease (IIa).

CONCLUSION

Both IVUS and OCT improve outcomes of PCI, particularly in complex lesions and stent failures. Each has its advantages and limitations. All interventionalists should familiarize themselves with both imaging modalities.

REFERENCES

1. Kimura S, Kakuta T, Yonetsu T, Suzuki A, Iesaka Y, Fujiwara H, et al. Clinical Significance of Echo Signal Attenuation on Intravascular Ultrasound in Patients With Coronary Artery Disease. Circ Cardiovasc Interv. 2009;2(5):444-54.
2. Wang X, Matsumura M, Mintz GS, Lee T, Zhang W, Cao Y, et al. In Vivo Calcium Detection by Comparing Optical Coherence Tomography, Intravascular Ultrasound, and Angiography. JACC Cardiovasc Imag. 2017;10(8):869-79.
3. Hoffmann R. Treatment of calcified coronary lesions with Palmaz-Schatz stents. An intravascular ultrasound study. Eur Heart J. 1998;19(8):1224-31.
4. Shlofmitz E, Torguson R, Zhang C, Craig PE, Mintz GS, Khalid N, et al. Impact of Intravascular Ultrasound on Outcomes Following PErcutaneous Coronary InterventioN in Complex Lesions (iOPEN Complex). Am Heart J. 2020;221:74-83.
5. Lawton JS, Tamis-Holland JE, Bangalore S, Bates ER, Beckie TM, Bischoff JM, et al. 2021 ACC/AHA/SCAI Guideline for Coronary Artery Revascularization. J Am Coll Cardiol. 2022;79(2):e21-129.

6. Ben-Dor I, Torguson R, Gaglia M, Gonzalez M, Maluenda G, Bui A, et al. Correlation between fractional flow reserve and intravascular ultrasound lumen area in intermediate coronary artery stenosis. EuroInterv. 2011;7(2):225-33.
6a. Vergallo R, Lombardi M, Kakuta T, Pawlowski T, Leone AM, Sardella G, et al. Optical Coherence Tomography Measures Predicting Fractional Flow Reserve: The OMEF Study. J Soc Cardiovasc Angiogr Interv. 2024;3(4):101288.
7. Jasti V, Ivan E, Yalamanchili V, Wongpraparut N, Leesar MA. Correlations Between Fractional Flow Reserve and Intravascular Ultrasound in Patients With an Ambiguous Left Main Coronary Artery Stenosis. Circulation. 2004;110(18):2831-6.
8. Park SJ, Ahn JM, Kang SJ, Yoon SH, Koo BK, Lee JY, et al. Intravascular Ultrasound-Derived Minimal Lumen Area Criteria for Functionally Significant Left Main Coronary Artery Stenosis. JACC Cardiovasc Interv. 2014;7(8):868-74.
9. Truesdell AG, Alasnag MA, Kaul P, Rab ST, Riley RF, Young MN, et al. Intravascular Imaging During Percutaneous Coronary Intervention. J Am Coll Cardiol. 2023;81(6):590-605.
10. Choi SY, Maehara A, Cristea E, Witzenbichler B, Guagliumi G, Brodie B, et al. Usefulness of Minimum Stent Cross Sectional Area as a Predictor of Angiographic Restenosis After Primary Percutaneous Coronary Intervention in Acute Myocardial Infarction (from the HORIZONS-AMI Trial IVUS Substudy). Am J Cardiol. 2012;109(4):455-60.
11. Mintz GS. Intravascular ultrasound and outcomes after drug-eluting stent implantation. Coron Artery Dis. 2017;28(4):346-52.
12. Hong MK. Intravascular ultrasound predictors of angiographic restenosis after sirolimus-eluting stent implantation. Eur Heart J. 2006;27(11):1305-10.
13. Meneveau N, Souteyrand G, Motreff P, Caussin C, Amabile N, Ohlmann P, et al. Optical Coherence Tomography to Optimize Results of Percutaneous Coronary Intervention in Patients with Non–ST-Elevation Acute Coronary Syndrome: Results of the Multicenter, Randomized DOCTORS Study (Does Optical Coherence Tomography Optimize Results of Stenting). Circulation. 2016;134(13):906-17.
14. Doi H, Maehara A, Mintz GS, Yu A, Wang H, Mandinov L, et al. Impact of Post-Intervention Minimal Stent Area on 9-Month Follow-Up Patency of Paclitaxel-Eluting Stents. JACC Cardiovasc Interv. 2009;2(12):1269-75.
15. Prati F, Romagnoli E, Burzotta F, Limbruno U, Gatto L, La Manna A, et al. Clinical Impact of OCT Findings During PCI. JACC Cardiovasc Imag. 2015;8(11):1297-305.
16. Costa MA, Angiolillo DJ, Tannenbaum M, Driesman M, Chu A, Patterson J, et al. Impact of Stent Deployment Procedural Factors on Long-Term Effectiveness and Safety of Sirolimus-Eluting Stents (Final Results of the Multicenter Prospective STLLR Trial). Am J Cardiol. 2008;101(12):1704-11.
17. Kobayashi N, Mintz GS, Witzenbichler B, Metzger DC, Rinaldi MJ, Duffy PL, et al. Prevalence, Features, and Prognostic Importance of Edge Dissection After Drug-Eluting Stent Implantation: An ADAPT-DES Intravascular Ultrasound Substudy. Circ Cardiovasc Interv. 2016;9(7):e003553.
18. Choi SY, Witzenbichler B, Maehara A, Lansky AJ, Guagliumi G, Brodie B, et al. Intravascular Ultrasound Findings of Early Stent Thrombosis After Primary Percutaneous Intervention in Acute Myocardial Infarction: A Harmonizing Outcomes with Revascularization and Stents in Acute Myocardial Infarction (HORIZONS-AMI) Substudy. Circ Cardiovasc Interv. 2011;4(3):239-47.

19. Qiu F, Mintz GS, Witzenbichler B, Metzger DC, Rinaldi MJ, Duffy PL, et al. Prevalence and Clinical Impact of Tissue Protrusion After Stent Implantation. JACC Cardiovasc Interv. 2016;9(14):1499-507.
20. Soeda T, Uemura S, Park SJ, Jang Y, Lee S, Cho JM, et al. Incidence and Clinical Significance of Poststent Optical Coherence Tomography Findings: One-Year Follow-Up Study From a Multicenter Registry. Circulation. 2015;132(11):1020-9.
21. Ali ZA, Maehara A, Généreux P, Shlofmitz RA, Fabbiocchi F, Nazif TM, et al. Optical coherence tomography compared with intravascular ultrasound and with angiography to guide coronary stent implantation (ILUMIEN III: OPTIMIZE PCI): a randomised controlled trial. Lancet. 2016;388(10060):2618-28.
22. Kubo T, Shinke T, Okamura T, Hibi K, Nakazawa G, Morino Y, et al. Optical frequency domain imaging vs. intravascular ultrasound in percutaneous coronary intervention (OPINION trial): one-year angiographic and clinical results. Eur Heart J. 2017;38(42):3139-47.
23. Im E, Kim BK, Ko YG, Shin DH, Kim JS, Choi D, et al. Incidences, Predictors, and Clinical Outcomes of Acute and Late Stent Malapposition Detected by Optical Coherence Tomography After Drug-Eluting Stent Implantation. Circ Cardiovasc Interv. 2014;7(1):88-96.
24. Prati F, Kodama T, Romagnoli E, Gatto L, Di Vito L, Ramazzotti V, et al. Suboptimal stent deployment is associated with subacute stent thrombosis: optical coherence tomography insights from a multicenter matched study. From the CLI Foundation investigators: the CLI-THRO study. Am Heart J. 2015;169(2):249-56.
25. Galassi AR, Sumitsuji S, Boukhris M, Brilakis ES, Di Mario C, Garbo R, et al. Utility of Intravascular Ultrasound in Percutaneous Revascularization of Chronic Total Occlusions. JACC Cardiovasc Interv. 2016;9(19):1979-91.
26. Habara M, Nasu K, Terashima M, Kaneda H, Yokota D, Ko E, et al. Impact of Frequency-Domain Optical Coherence Tomography Guidance for Optimal Coronary Stent Implantation in Comparison With Intravascular Ultrasound Guidance. Circ Cardiovasc Interv. 2012;5(2):193-201.
27. Chamié D, Costa JR, Damiani LP, Siqueira D, Braga S, Costa R, et al. Optical Coherence Tomography Versus Intravascular Ultrasound and Angiography to Guide Percutaneous Coronary Interventions: The iSIGHT Randomized Trial. Circ Cardiovasc Interv. 2021;14(3):e009452.
28. Kang DY, Ahn JM, Yun SC, Hur SH, Cho YK, Lee CH, et al. Optical Coherence Tomography-Guided or Intravascular Ultrasound-Guided Percutaneous Coronary Intervention: The OCTIVUS Randomized Clinical Trial. Circulation. 2023;148(16):1195-206.
29. Yamaji K, Ueki Y, Souteyrand G, Daemen J, Wiebe J, Nef H, et al. Mechanisms of very late bioresorbable scaffold thrombosis. J Am Coll Cardiol. 2017;70(19): 2330-44.
30. Zhang YJ, Pang S, Chen XY, Bourantas CV, Pan DR, Dong SJ, et al. Comparison of intravascular ultrasound guided versus angiography guided drug eluting stent implantation: A systematic review and meta-analysis. BMC Cardiovasc Disord. 2015;15(1):153.
31. Bavishi C, Sardar P, Chatterjee S, Khan AR, Shah A, Ather S, et al. Intravascular ultrasound-guided vs angiography-guided drug-eluting stent implantation in complex coronary lesions: meta-analysis of randomized trials. Am Heart J. 2017;185:26-34.

32. Park Y, Park HS, Jang GL, Lee DY, Lee H, Lee JH, et al. Intravascular ultrasound guided recanalization of stumpless chronic total occlusion. Int J Cardiol. 2011;148(2):174-8.
33. Kim BK, Shin DH, Hong MK, Park HS, Rha SW, Mintz GS, et al. Clinical Impact of Intravascular Ultrasound-Guided Chronic Total Occlusion Intervention With Zotarolimus-Eluting Versus Biolimus-Eluting Stent Implantation: Randomized Study. Circ Cardiovasc Interv. 2015;8(7):e002592.
34. Neumann FJ, Sousa-Uva M, Ahlsson A, Alfonso F, Banning AP, Benedetto U, et al. 2018 ESC/EACTS Guidelines on myocardial revascularization. Eur Heart J. 2019;40(2):87-165.

CHAPTER 10

Coronary Physiology in Contemporary Percutaneous Coronary Intervention: Practical Approach

Anil Dhall, Ayush Malhotra

INTRODUCTION

Demonstration of improvement of pressure and flow during the first angioplasty itself made us understand the importance of physiology **(Fig. 1)**.

For many years, most decision making in CAD (coronary artery disease) was dependent of anatomy and coronary angiography (CAG) continues to remain the gold standard for diagnosis and management. Two-dimensional silhouette image provided by CAG has well-recognized limitations, because both physician's visual assessment and quantitative coronary analysis have shown poor correlation with functional stenosis severity. CAG does not accurately represent the true complexity of coronary luminal morphology, and gives no indication of functional influence of luminal changes on coronary blood flow.[2]

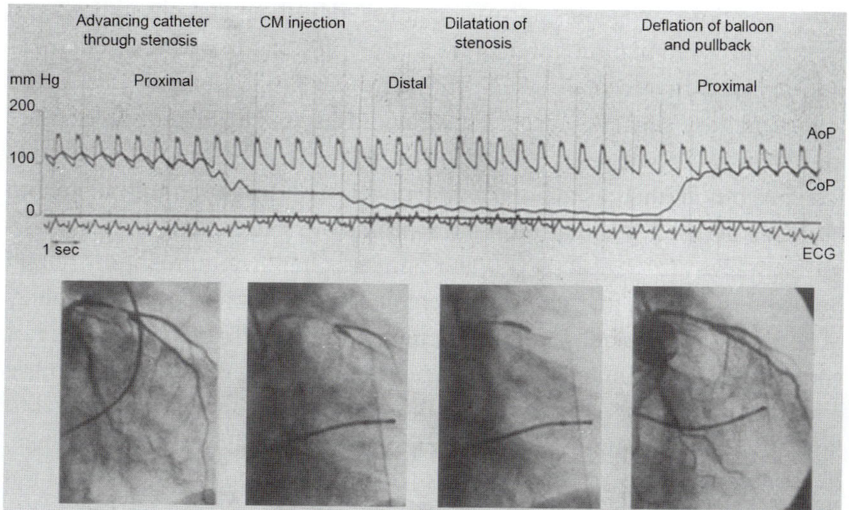

Fig. 1: First case of percutaneous coronary intervention. In 1979, coronary pressure across the stenosis before and after balloon angioplasty was recorded in the first case of coronary intervention. (AoP: aortic pressure; CM: contrast media; CoP: coronary pressure)

Source: Reproduced with permission from Grüntzig et al.[1]

PHYSIOLOGIC CONCEPTS

The two major fundamental questions in interventional cardiology while deciding for treatment of CAD is whether one should treat or not. How should one treat? Everything else is commentary. Treatment of CAD traditionally was based on presence of symptoms or demonstration of inducible ischemia coupled with angiographic anatomy and assessment of left ventricular function. Angiographic assessment held the key in decision making depending on the amount of myocardium subtended by the occluded or the diseased vessel.

The assessment was based on a angiographic lumenogram which has many challenges, because it is a two-dimensional plane assessment of a three-dimensional vessel which could have in its lumen conditions such as thrombosis, dissections, calcium and can be confounded by branch vessels. 95% of the coronary circulation is in the microcirculation, however, what is visible on a coronary angiogram is 5% of the coronary tree which is in the epicardium. The left coronary system perfuses during diastole and the right coronary system supplying the thin wall structures perfuses during both phases. We have postulated a three-compartment model where >0.5 millimeter diameter vessels are visible angiographically which are called epicardial vessels and between 0.5 and 0.1 millimeter diameter are prearterioles which are dependent on sympathetic innervation and endothelial dependent shear wall stress and the <0.1 mm arterioles are under autoregulation, myogenic control or controlled by the metabolic milieu.

Coronary circulation autoregulates itself and that is why revascularization decisions were made when the coronary flow reserve (CFR) or the autoregulatory capacity was exceeded and traditionally a 70% occlusion of bigger epicardial vessels or 50% occlusion of left main (LM) were traditionally taken as our guidelines. As we have evolved, we have learnt to understand our CAG better. We can also do intracoronary imaging using tools such as intravascular ultrasound (IVUS) and optical coherence tomography (OCT) but even these remain anatomical references and do not cover physiology of coronary circulation. The measurement of myocardial blood flow at rest contains only very limited diagnostic information; however, when we achieve a level of maximum vasodilatation, the pressure becomes proportional to flow. As we move from the autoregulation to a completely vasodilated state, the pressure gradient across stenosis is then related to the flow across the stenosis. Under normal conditions there is little, if any, resistance in the epicardial coronaries as most of the resistance is in the microvasculature. A concept of fractional flow reserve (FFR) was developed after we had experimented with Doppler pressure wires to actually see only a pullback gradient.

Principles that govern the association between pressure and flow in the coronary circulation form the basis, from which all clinically applicable coronary physiologic indices have developed. Small changes in microvascular resistance and/or distal coronary pressure alter myocardial blood flow, with microvascular vasodilation and increase in distal coronary end-diastolic pressure augmenting myocardial perfusion while microvascular vasoconstriction and/or decrease in distal coronary end-diastolic pressure have the opposite effect. Pathologic states that interfere with normal blood flow regulation adversely influence myocardial contraction. In diseased states, impaired myocardial blood flow occurs in response to microvascular dysfunction, changes in epicardial vessel resistance, or a combination of both. Several conditions interfere with normal vasodilator capacity of microcirculation, thus blunting the potential for maximally increasing coronary blood flow.

In order to achieve accurate FFR measurements, induction of maximal vasodilatation via declines in myocardial circulatory resistances is essential.[3] For the duration of pharmacologic induction of maximal hyperemia, there is minimal coronary resistance that remains constant, which results in an incremental-linear relationship between blood flow and perfusion pressure.[3,4] The ideal hyperemic stimulus must have a short onset until maximum hyperemia is attained, be easy to administer, have a duration long enough to facilitate pressure pullback recordings, have limited side effects, and be eliminated quickly.[5,6]

CORONARY FLOW RESERVE

Coronary flow reserve is the ratio of maximum blood flow during hyperemia in the coronary artery being interrogated to the resting blood flow of the same artery. It is predicated on the fact that functionally significant coronary stenosis will cause compensatory lower microcirculatory resistance and lead to blunting of further increases in blood flow during hyperemia. CFR provides assessment of both epicardial and microcirculatory status, within the territory of the coronary artery of interest. CFR is measured using temperature sensor wires by thermodilution or by Doppler wires. CFR correlates well with noninvasive myocardial perfusion studies. A CFR of <2 indicates impaired flow and predicts unfavorable outcomes. Correlation between CFR and FFR is modest. A discrepancy whereby normal CFR coincides with abnormal FFR or abnormal CFR coincides with normal FFR occurs in 30–40%.[7] Although CFR is a better prognostic indicator, FFR remains a better measurement, as it specifically assesses functional significance of epicardial lesions. Moreover, CFR is dependent on systemic hemodynamics and has less reproducibility as compared to FFR.[8]

Wide range of intracoronary physiological tools can follow every such domains. Although the entire coronary circulation is covered/tackled

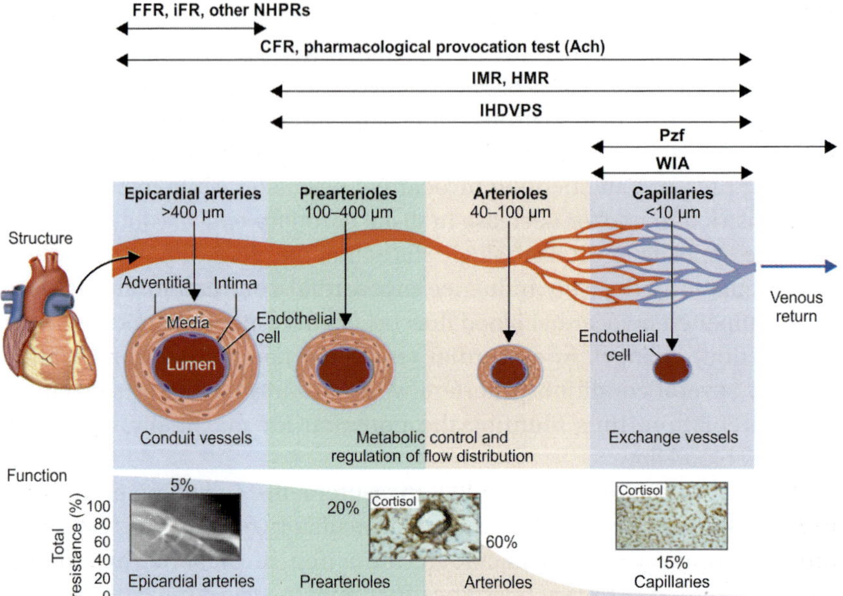

Fig. 2: Structural and functional components of coronary circulation.[9] (Ach: acetylcholine; CFR: coronary flow reserve; FFR: fractional flow reserve; HMR: hyperemic microvascular resistance; IHDVPS: instantaneous hyperemic diastolic velocity pressure slope; IMR: index of microvascular resistance; NHPR: nonhyperemic pressure ratio; Pzf: zero flow pressure; WIA: wave-intensity analysis)

by CFR **(Fig. 2)**, various other indexes have been evolved for estimating certain specific parameters of the heart circulation. Normally, the myocardial perfusion is controlled by appropriate regulation of the epicardial arteries, microcirculation, and myocardial bed.[9]

HYPEREMIC AND NONHYPEREMIC PRESSURE INDICES

Fractional flow reserve is the most widely used intracoronary tool to define flow-limiting epicardial stenoses, with randomized clinical trials and observational studies supporting deferral[10,11] or performance[10,12] of revascularization based on FFR values, predominately in patients with chronic coronary syndrome (CCS).

Coronary pressure-derived FFR is the current gold standard of care for the functional assessment of lesion severity in patients with intermediate grade stenosis (typically around 40–80% stenosis) without evidence of ischemia in noninvasive testing, or in those with multivessel disease.[13]

Fractional flow reserve is defined as the ratio of maximal blood flow in the presence of an epicardial stenosis. The mathematical derivation based on assumptions is shown below:

Derivation of Fractional Flow Reserve

$$FFR = \frac{\text{Maximum Myocardial Flow (Stenosis)}}{\text{Maximum Myocardial Flow (Normal)}}$$

$$\text{Myocardial Flow} = \frac{\Delta\ \text{Pressure}}{\text{Resistance}}$$

$$FFR = \frac{(Pd\text{–}Pv)/\cancel{\text{Resistance}}}{(Pa\text{–}Pv)/\cancel{\text{Resistance}}}$$

at maximal hyperemia

$$FFR = \frac{Pd\text{–}Pv}{Pa\text{–}Pv}$$

$$FFR = \frac{Pd}{Pa}$$

Under physiological conditions, Pv is either 0 or negligible compared to Pd or Pa, therefore, FFR can simply be derived from ratio of distal to proximal coronary pressure at maximal hyperemia, i.e., FFR = Pd/Pa. Where, Pa—proximal coronary pressure, Pd—distal coronary pressure, Pv—central venous pressure, on a maximal hyperemic myocardial blood flow in the absence of stenosis.[14]

Maximal hyperemia is the cornerstone of physiology used to assess epicardial vessel stenosis. Hyperemia is achieved by maximal vasodilation of resistance vessels, to increase the myocardial flow. Multiple agents can be used to cause hyperemia, such as adenosine, papaverine, dipyridamole, and nitroprusside **(Table 1)**.[15]

Fractional flow reserve is highly sensitive and specific functional index of epicardial stenosis.

- Fractional flow reserve is not influenced by hemodynamic parameters (pulse, BP, and contractility).[16]
- Fractional flow reserve is highly reproducible.[16]
- *Fractional flow reserve accounts for the influence of collateral vessels:* FFR value across a stenosis will account for physiological influence of collateral in both—(1) vessel that provides collaterals to another more severely stenosed artery (retrograde flow) and (2) the vessel which receives collaterals from another less severely stenosed artery (antegrade flow), thus accounting for functional influence of collaterals at maximal hyperemia.[17]
- Fractional flow reserve has high spatial resolution also. It reaches a per segment accuracy with a high spatial resolution of few millimeters, as compared to other tests which are per vessel accurate. This spatial resolution allows accurate identification of exact anatomic position of stenosis which is of clinical value in vessels with serial or ostial lesions.[17]

TABLE 1: Different vasodilators available for FFR measurement.

Vasodilators	*Comments*	*Side effects*
Adenosine (IV): 140 µg/kg/min	Intravenous line should be placed in a large, preferably central vein (femoral vein or a large antecubital vein)	• Decrease of blood pressure by 10–15% • Burning or angina-such as chest pain during infusion • Not to be used in patients with severe obstructive lung disease
Adenosine (IC): • 30–60 pg for the left coronary artery • 20–30 µg for the right coronary artery	• Does not require central venous cannulation • Only creates very short-lasting hyperemia that is insufficient to make a pressure pullback recording	Sometimes atrioventricular block seconds after injection in right coronary artery
Papaverine (IC): • 16–20 mg for the left coronary artery • 12–16 mg for the right coronary artery	• Alternative agent • Creating sufficiently long hyperemia (30–60 s) to make a pullback recording • Less used in the United States and Western Europe	• Transient QT prolongation • Very rarely, ventricular tachycardia or torsade de pointes
Nitroprusside (IC): • 0.6 µg/kg • 100 µg	• As effective as adenosine to induce maximal hyperemia but with a more sustained effect • Further studies are needed	The hypotensive effect does not result in any side effects
Regadenoson (IV): 400 µg for the peripheral infusion	• Effect may be identical to intravenous adenosine • Further studies are needed	• Chest discomfort, flushing and headache • Most events were brief and self-limiting

(FFR: fractional flow reserve)

Fractional flow reserve was validated initially by comparing it to invasive gold standard of absolute flow at three different pressure levels in 12 different stenosis and was found to have a linear relation. It was then subjected to clinical validation data in more than 24 studies, in more than 1,500 patients and a cut off value of 0.75 was arrived at.[18] A low FFR can be generated in two different ways either there could be severe flow-limiting stenosis or there is a gross increase in coronary flow which is not being able to be taken care of despite not having very severe stenosis. This was subjected to multiple different trials which that FFR-guided percutaneous coronary intervention (PCI) should be preferred management strategy in this group of patients.[19-23]

- DEFER showed that it was safe to defer PCI in lesions with an FFR >0.75.
- FAME-I showed that treating lesions with an FFR >0.80 with first-generation DES was harmful and that a deferred PCI strategy was safer and cost-saving.
- FAME-II showed that deferring PCI in lesions with an FFR <0.80 was harmful compared to optimal medical therapy.
- While more expensive at the beginning, the cost of this strategy decreased by 50% at 1 year.
- In addition, FAME-II confirmed the findings of DEFER.

Fractional flow reserve-based assessment strategy at the time of angiography results in reclassification of revascularization strategy, i.e., PCI, bypass surgery, or medical therapy. Among patients with intermediate grade stenosis, >40% were reclassified in their management strategy after FFR assessment.[21] Thus, the FFR's role in guiding revascularization in various situations is well established and implemented by various guidelines (2018 ESC/EACTS guidelines)[24] on international platforms.

PITFALLS IN CORONARY PRESSURE MEASUREMENTS

Although associated with potential drawbacks, intravenous administration enables achieving a more consistent hyperemic effect, which allows a pressure pull back during steady state hyperemia for the hemodynamic analysis of all abnormalities along the length of coronary artery.[25] In normal coronary arteries, expected FFR value is 1.0, meaning absence of obstacles to coronary flow in diseased coronary arteries. FFR value below 0.80 indicates hemodynamically significant stenosis, causing myocardial ischemia with an accuracy of 90%.[25] To date, FFR is the gold standard for detection of myocardial ischemia, because it is much more accurate in distinguishing functionally significant stenosis than noninvasive provocative tests, such as exercise electrocardiogram, myocardial perfusion scintigraphy, and stress echocardiography. FFR has class 1A recommendation by current guidelines.[21]

Calibration and Equalization

It should begin with calibration and equalization of both a pressure wire and a fluid-filled pressure monitoring system. If pressure waveforms look suspicious, pull back pressure wire to the guide catheter tip to verify equal pressures **(Fig. 3)**.

After equalization (when sensor at tip of guiding catheter): Wait for 20–30 seconds before advancing wire farther (gives time for small air bubbles to be flushed away from sensor cavity). If signal changes, re-equalization can be done by various methods such as flushing the guiding catheter, checking the height of the transducer, checking whether guidewire introducer needle has been removed or by manipulating pressure wire to ensure the sensors

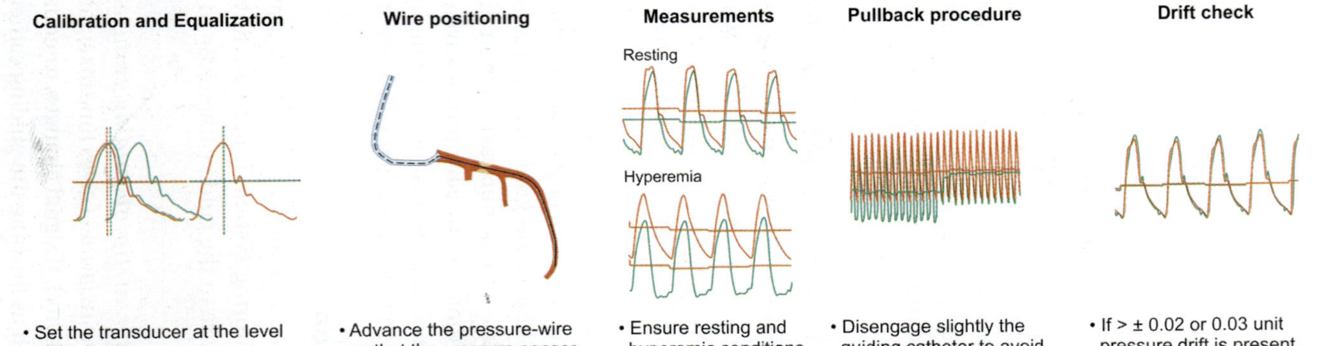

Fig. 3: Steps to perform FFR.[25] (FFR: fractional flow reserve)

not against the vessel wall. The cause of drift can range from having an air bubble at the sensor tip to high contrast concentration in catheter, due to temperature changes, loose connection, leak in guide connections, irregular rhythm or multiple ectopic beats, and improper zero.

- Flush the wire, then connect. Zeroing of the pressure sensor then takes place automatically. Catheter must be lying flat and not be moved.
- The wire is then advanced into the coronary artery until the pressure sensor is positioned precisely at the end of the guide catheter.
- Flush/pressure equalization between the wire and aortic pressure must then be performed.
- Prior to advancing the pressure wire, intracoronary nitroglycerin should be administered, in order to prevent spasm and minimize resistance in the epicardial vessels.
- The pressure sensor of the wire must be positioned directly distal to the lesion that is to be investigated.
- Presence of viscous contrast in the coronary artery can affect the pd/pa ratio and hence the system should be flushed with saline prior to measurement.
- One of the major drawbacks of this procedure includes signal drift (drift related the wire) which leads to false values of FFR. After a long procedure, differences may sometimes occur between aortic and distal pressures even if this difference does not correspond to a true pressure gradient.

Signal Drift (Figs. 4 and 5)

When the difference is due to drift, the two pressure tracings have exactly the same form. However, there will be a separation from the initially equal aortic catheter and coronary pressures (measured at the tip of the guiding) at the end of the procedure. After the FFR measurement, the coronary wire is pulled back into the guiding catheter, and Pd/Pa is recorded again. In the absence of any drift, Pd/Pa should be 1 or range of 0.97–1.03.[25]

There are instances when it is tedious to push the wire forward distally, it can be made viable by placing the pressure sensor at a distance of nearly

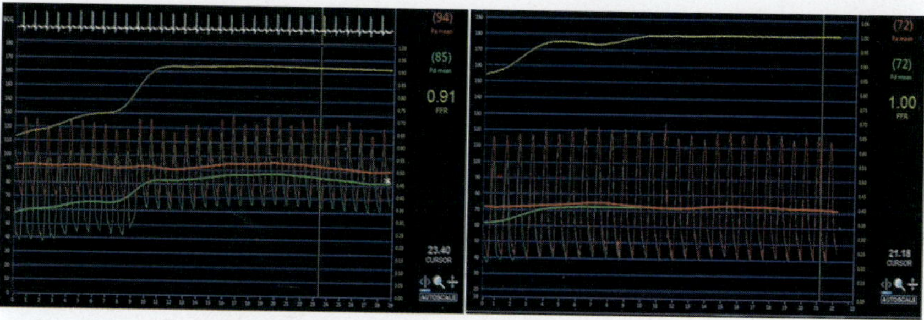

Fig. 4: Separation from the initially equal aortic and coronary pressures (measured at the tip of the guiding catheter) at the end of the procedure.

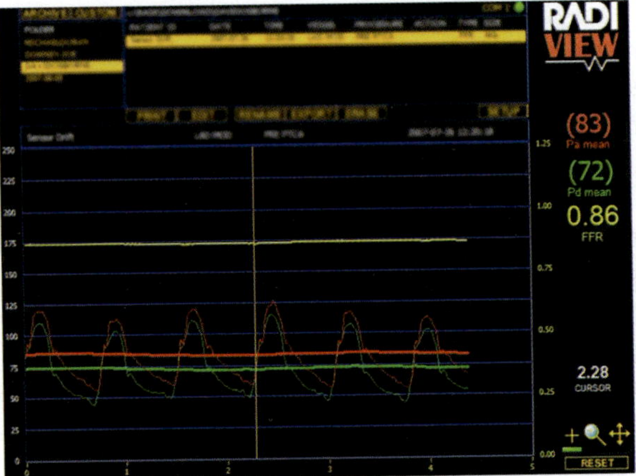

Fig. 5: Signal drift.

2–3 cm from target lesion thereby also preventing accordion effect and injury caused by the wire. Prior to the measurement of pressure, it is important to gently disengage the guiding catheter as it is required to avert pressure damping even when the case does not involve ostial lesion. Both aortic and distal coronary pressure waveforms need to be checked so that probable errors from contrast medium, aortic pressure damping, pressure drift, and whipping noise can be detected.

Drift related to aortic pressure/procedure:

- Changing height of aortic transducer
- Capillary forces in catheter (flushing with 5–10 mL of saline)
- Wedged guide catheter in ostium causing damping of aortic waveform
- Needle in Y-connector
- Catheter with side holes
- Aortic pressure damping due to some contrast injectors.

After the FFR measurement, the coronary wire is pulled back into the guiding catheter, and Pd/Pa is recorded again. In the absence of any drift, Pd/Pa should be 1 or range of 0.97–1.03.

NONHYPEREMIC PRESSURE RATIO

Nonhyperemic pressure ratios (NHPRs) are resting indices, which measure the Pd/Pa ratio during the diastolic phase when microvascular resistance is stable. In the cardiac cycle, represented in the **Figures 6A and B** show the period of a cardiac cycle in which NHPRs are calculated. Instantaneous wave-free ratio (iFR) is measured during the wave-free period (WFP) when the resistance is constant and minimal.

Nonhyperemic pressure ratio is increasingly utilized in clinical practice owing to a more favorable side effect profile, reduced cost and procedure

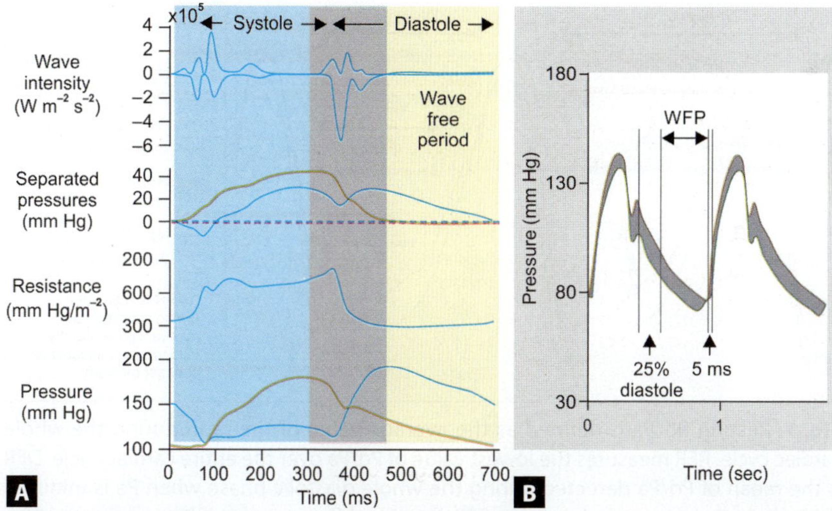

Figs. 6A and B: (A) Showing pressure waveforms and wave intensity during systole and diastole; (B) Showing diastolic wave-free period (WFP).
Sources: Davies et al. Circulation. 2006;113(14):1768-78. and Davies JE, et al. JACC. 2012;59:1392-402.

time, and ease of use compared with pharmacological hyperemia. This facilitates multiple intraprocedural measurements either in different vessels or at different stages of the PCI procedure. Guidance by iFR, a widely utilized NHPR, was noninferior to FFR guidance of revascularization for major adverse cardiac events (MACE) at 1 year[20,26] and 5-year follow-ups.[27]

Measurement of coronary pressure is done during a period where the microcirculatory resistance is constant. During that period, the measured pressure is proportional to the flow, similar to adenosine induced hyperemia. Resting ratio (Pd/Pa, iFR, rFR, etc.)—no adenosine, relies on adequate ECG/stable R-R cycle, reduces discomfort to patient, reduces time to set up/infuse hyperemic agent **(Fig. 7)**.

INSTANTANEOUS WAVE-FREE RATIO

The challenge of stable maximal hyperemia and use of coronary hyperemic agents was sought to be overcome by closer examination of the diastolic wave-free period wherein hyperemic agents were not needed and pressure difference was proportional to flow. This is measuring quaternary pressure during a period where microcirculatory resistance is constant and it mimics the constant microcircuit resistance induced by adenosine whereby measure pressure proportional to flow. iFR also, therefore, unmasked transcoronary pressure drop by increasing flow during diastole and has a 94% overall classification agreement with FFR.[28,29]

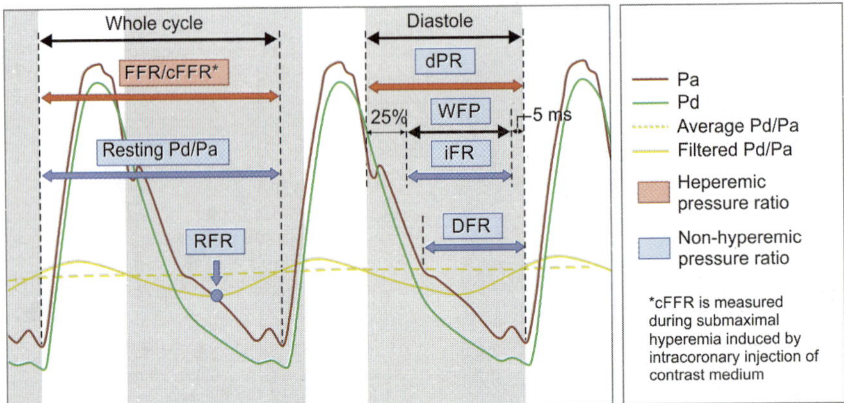

Fig. 7: Resting Pd/Pa is defined as the average value of the ratio during the whole cardiac cycle. RFR measures the lowest value of Pd/Pa over the entire cardiac cycle. DFR is the mean of Pd/Pa detected during the whole diastolic phase when Pa is minimal. (DFR: diastolic hyperemia-free ratio; FFR: fractional flow reserve; iFR: instant wave-free ratio; Pa: aortic pressure; Pd: distal pressure beyond the stenosis; RFR: resting full-cycle ratio; WFP: wave-free period)

This was validated in two large studies called "iFR-SWEDEHEART" and "DEFINE" which confirmed that IFR in most cases was as useful as FFR; however, the cut off for iFR was taken as 0.89 as compared to 0.80 for FFR.

Another advantage of iFR is its ability to individually assess lesions severity in the context of diffuse vessel disease, thus minimizing FFR limitations in the setting of serial coronary stenosis. This scan be used for automatic co-registration precision PCI and even pre-PCI prediction of benefits. By using co-registration of the iFR pullback trace and coronary angiogram, iFR is able to detect lesion-specific pressure drop along the whole length of the vessel and differentiate focal from diffuse coronary disease.[28,29] Thus allowing proper identification of which lesions should be treated if any, secondly accurately predicting to what extent coronary physiology will improve after PCI for each lesion and thirdly to confidently decide the number, length of lesion.

Besides, FFR, IFR and resting Pd/Pa, other physiological indices to assess coronary stenosis are given in **Table 2**. There are some gender differences among the physiological indices. The FFR is slightly higher in female. Similarly, other indices also show some variations according to the gender **(Table 3)**.

We continued the progress in coronary interventions and interventions were guided not only by our improved understanding of physiology but also imaging **(Tables 4 and 5)**. We did have some hiccups in our understanding of the physiology, when in the "FORZA" trial it was compared with OCT and 350 patients were randomized with angiographic intermediate lesions.

TABLE 2: Various physiologic indices.

Physiologic index	*Definition*	*Cut-off value*	*Features*
Fractional flow reserve (FFR)	Ratio of distal coronary pressure to aortic pressure in hyperemic status	<0.80	• Epicardial coronary artery specific index • Reflecting maximal flow limitation due to epicardial coronary artery disease • Extensive clinical data
Instantaneous wave-free ratio (iFR)	Ratio of distal coronary pressure to aortic pressure during the diastolic wave-free period in resting status	≤0.89	• Epicardial coronary artery specific index • No need of hyperemia • Noninferior outcome to FFR-guided revascularization
Resting full cycle ratio (RFR)	Lowest value of the ratio of distal coronary pressure to aortic pressure in resting status	= 0.89	• Epicardial coronary artery specific index • No need of hyperemia • High degree correlation and agreement with iFR
Diastolic pressure ratio (dPR)	Average ratio of distal coronary pressure to aortic pressure during the diastolic period in resting status	≤0.89	• Epicardial coronary artery specific index • No need of hyperemia • High degree correlation and agreement with iFR
Coronary flow reserve (CFR)	Ratio of hyperemic coronary flow and resting coronary flow	<2.0–2.5	• Reflects both epicardial coronary artery disease and microvascular dysfunction • Influenced by various factors, such as hemodynamics, conditions, or contractility • Enormous data regarding its prognostic value
Coronary flow capacity (CFC)	Combination of coronary flow reserve and coronary stress flow	CFR <1.74 and coronary stress flow <1.12 mL/min/g	• Reflects comprehensive coronary physiologic status • Less influenced by resting flow conditions
Index of microcirculatory resistance (IMR)	Distal coronary artery pressure multiplied by hyperemic mean transit time	>25 U	• Microcirculation-specific index • Proven prognostic value in many studies

Contd...

Contd…

Physiologic index	*Definition*	*Cut-off value*	*Features*
Hyperemic microvascular resistance (hMR)	Ratio of maximal coronary flow velocity to distal coronary artery pressure during hyperemia	>2.5 mm Hg/cm/s	• Microcirculation-specific index • Relatively few outcome data

TABLE 3: Gender comparison of various physiological assessment techniques.

FFR		*NHPR*	*CFR*
Women	• Relatively high FFR compared with men • More favorable outcomes in cases with deferral of PCI by FFR compared with men • Favorable outcomes compared to angiography-guided PCI strategy	• Similar rate of lesion significance compared with FFR • Similar event rate compared with FFR-guided PCI strategy	• Lower CFR compared with men • Higher resting flow compared with men • Low CFR is dissociated with poor outcome
Men	• Relatively low FFR compared with women • Favorable outcomes compared with angiography-guided PCI strategy	• Lower rate of lesion significance compared with FFR • Similar event rate compared with FFR-guided PCI	• Higher CFR compared with women • Lower resting flow compared with women • Low CFR is associated with poor outcome

(CFR: coronary flow reserve; FFR: fractional flow reserve; NHPR: nonhyperemic pressure ratio; PCI: percutaneous coronary intervention)

It was found that if you optimize the lesion with OCT plus angioplasty or with IVUS—assessing intermediate, non-LM lesions—the only downside is that it is associated with the implantation of more stents compared to physiology-guided interventions. Most operators came to the conclusion that if you want to be judicious about using intracoronary devices, use physiology in the assessment of LM disease. We also understood that lesion dimensions as well as plaque burden were actually important and hence, if the LM has an cross-sectional area of >6 mm^2 on intracoronary imaging assessment, it will have a negative FFR most likely and do not require intervention. If it is ≤4.5 mm^2, it is very likely to require intervention and the true use of FFR came between 4.5 and 6 mm^2, wherein it could actually determine what lesion should be

TABLE 4: Major randomized controlled trials using wire-based physiological assessment.

Study name		*Follow-up*	*Population*	*Comparison*	*Primary endpoint*	*Result*	*p value*
DEFER	325	15 years	Patients with de novo stenosis Deferral with FFR = 0.75 vs. (DS >50%)	Performed PCI with FFR ≥0.75	MI	2.2% vs. 10.0%	0.033
FAME	1,005	5 years	Patients with multivessel disease	FFR-guided vs. angiography—composite of death, MI, or guided PCI	Revascularization	28.0% vs. 31.0%	0.31
FAME II	888	5 years	With FFR 50.80	Patients with de novo stenosis FFR-guided PCI plus OMT vs. OMI alone	Composite of death, MI, or urgent revascularization	13.9% vs. 27.0%	<0.001
DANAMI-3-PRIMULTI	627	1 year	Patients with STEMI with 1 clinically significant stenosis in the noninfarct-related vessel	FFR-guided complete revascularization vs. no further invasive treatment (culprit only)	Composite of death, nonfatal 13.0% vs. MI, or ischemia-driven revascularization	22.0%	0.004
Compare-acute	885	1 year	Patients with STEMI with 21 clinically significant stenosis in the noninfarct-related vessel	FFR-guided complete revascularization vs. no further invasive treatment (culprit only)	Composite of death, nonfatal MI, revascularization, and cerebro-vascular events	7.8% vs. 20.5%	<0.001

Contd...

Contd...

Study name		*Follow-up*	*Population*	*Comparison*	*Primary endpoint*	*Result*	*p value*
iFR-SWEDEHEART	2,037	2 years	(DS 40–70%)	Patients with de novo stenosis FFR-guided vs. iFR-guided PCI	Composite of death, nonfatal MI, or unplanned revascularization	8.4% vs. 8.7%	0.93
DEFINE-FLAIR	2,492	2 years	(DS 40–70%)	Patients with de novo stenosis FFR-guided vs. iFR-guided PCI	Composite of death, nonfatal MI, or unplanned revascularization	10.5% vs. 11.8%	0.25

(DANAMI-3-PRIMULTI: Danish Study of Optimal Acute Treatment of Patients with ST-Elevation Myocardial Infarction-Primary PCI in Patients with ST-Elevation Myocardial Infarction and Multivessel Disease: Treatment of Culprit Lesion Only or Complete Revascularization; DEFINE-FLAIR: Functional Lesion Assessment of Intermediate Stenosis to Guide Revascularization; DS: diameter stenosis; FAME: Fractional Flow Reserve Versus Angiography for Multivessel Evaluation; FFR: fractional flow reserve; iFR: instantaneous wave-free ratio; iFR-SWEDEHEART: Evaluation of iFR versus FFR in Stable Angina or Acute Coronary Syndrome; MI: myocardial infarction: OMT: optimal medical therapy; PCI: percutaneous coronary intervention; STEMI: ST segment elevated myocardial infarction)[30,31]

TABLE 5: Advantages and disadvantages of physiology and intravascular imaging coregistration.

Coregistration technique	*Advantages*	*Disadvantages*
iFR	• A pressure drop can be visually depicted alongside the angiogram • Allows for prediction of post-PCI outcome and enables tailoring of PCI approach • Physiological data can be collected in single pullback	iFR coregistration technology is relatively new, more data is awaited on its clinical use and how it might influence clinical outcomes
IVUS	• Provides detail regarding the vessel wall and nature of the disease including its composition • No significant difference in fluoroscopy times versus OCT coregistration • Images can be acquired in single pullback • No need for blood clearance in vessel for image acquisition • Theoretical reduced risk of dissection propagation (due to lack of blood displacement) • Better placed to image left main, ostial lesions, chronic total occlusions	• Smaller evidence-base for use of IVUS coregistration • Requires some additional contrast injection for the coregistered images
OCT	• Multiple RCTs investigating use of OCT coregistration • Provides detail regarding the vessel wall and nature of the disease including its composition • No significant difference in fluoroscopy times versus IVUS coregistration • Images can be acquired in single pullback • Better placed to image in-stent restenosis, calcium, thrombi, ruptured, and erosive plaques	Limited utility in patients with impaired renal function (contrast injection)

(iFR: instantaneous wave-free ratio; IVUS: intravascular ultrasound; OCT: optical coherence tomography; PCI: percutaneous coronary intervention; RCT: randomized controlled trials)

intervened and what should not be intervened. Even at this time, despite our advances, we were not sure whether we could use the same physiology to confirm the judicious completion of an adequate PCI and, therefore, we came to certain guidelines as to an adequate PCI. We understood that we should deploy stents from normal segment to normal segment which means <50%

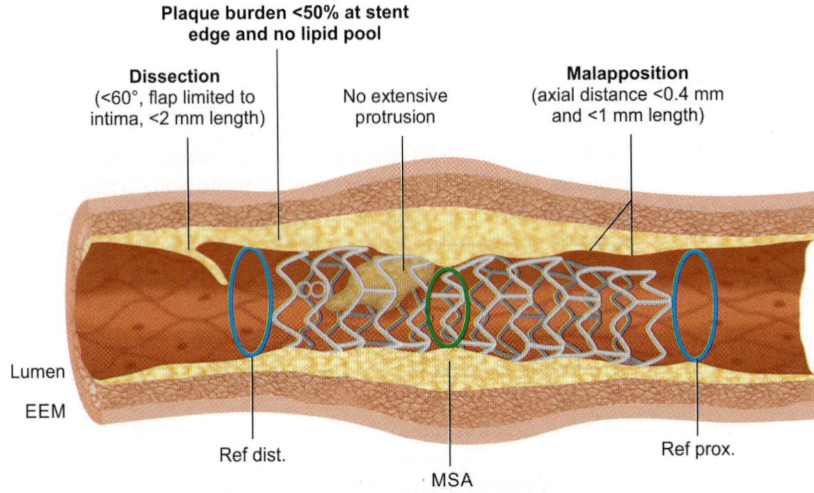

Fig. 8: Relation between reference proximal–distal end of lesion with stent apposition. (IVUS: intravascular ultrasound; MSA: minimal stent area; OCT: optical coherence tomography)

plaque burden. We also realize that by different trials we should achieve MLA of >5.5 mm^2 on IVUS or >4.5 mm^2 on OCT **(Fig. 8)**.

Physiology guidance is to decide not just whether to treat and where to treat. We can then use it to see what will be the individual impact or step up of iFR at any particular point and angiographic versus physiology mismatch will be avoided **(Fig. 9)**. Therefore, this is done when automatic storage instruction is possible, the machine has to be configured and it can be used after performing a PCI. It came as a matter of surprise when DEFINE PCI showed that 24% of patients after a seemingly optimal PCI continue to have a suboptimal FFR and this could be resolved in a large number of cases.

Because of problems that we have not visualized, the potential causes were diffuse diseases which were not angiographically apparent, geographical mismatch, inadequate coverage of lesion, stent under-/overexpansion or under size stents and serial stenosis. If you were to see that one in four patients with aFFR ≤0.90, 81% were thought to have residual ischemia which was focus and this could actually be used. Two-thirds of the stenosis approximately distal to the sent, one-third were inside the stent and if we see there is an opportunity for improvement because if we treat this then the residual lesion reduces from 24 to 5%. Therefore, today we have a role of FFR not just in pre-PCI physiologic assessment but also in post-PCI physiology assessment. To simplify further, we realize that we could also get similar results as hyperemic FFR with using just contrast, so contrast is a milder hyperemic agent.

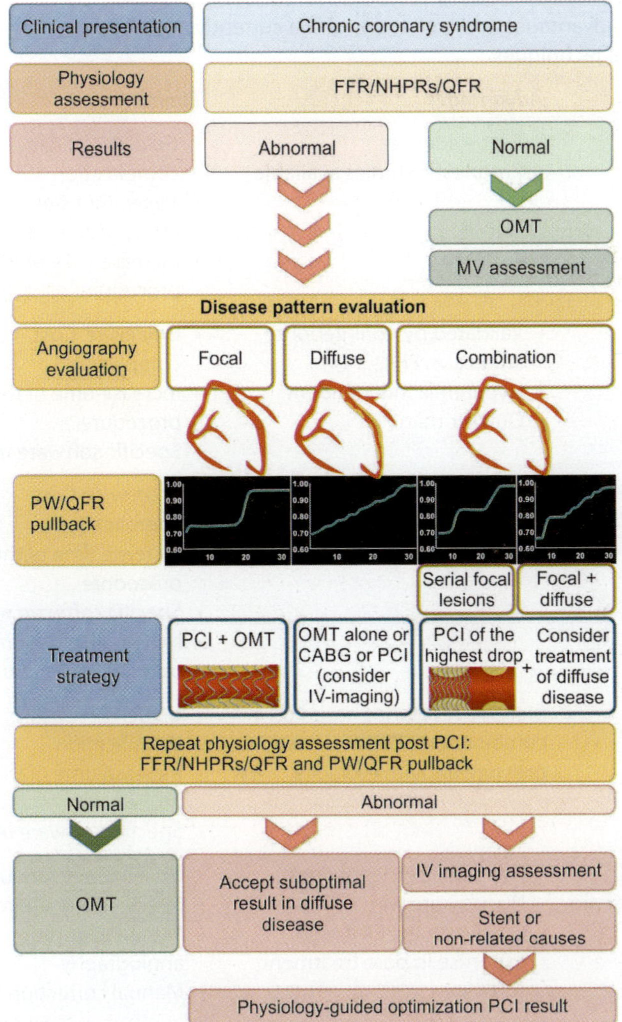

Fig. 9: Schematic clinical management of coronary disease based on physiological assessment. Normal values of pressure wire-based or angiography-based indices suggest investigating the microvascular function. Abnormal epicardial physiology means that an appropriate management should be planned based on a careful evaluation of atherosclerotic pattern. Post-PCI physiology assessment identifies residual ischemia with the need to optimize the suboptimal post-PCI physiology results. (CABG: coronary artery bypass graft; FFR: fractional flow reserve; IV: intravascular; MV: microvascular; NHPRs: nonhyperemic pressure ratios; OMT: optimal medical therapy; PCI: percutaneous coronary intervention; PW: pressure wire; QFR: quantitative flow ratio)

Though it has limitations because contrast hyperemia is too short for pull back tracing and there is not much evidence on contrast FFR **(Table 6)**. It looks too simple but there are technical challenges with 28% drifting, 18%

TABLE 6: Advantages and limitations of the currently available coronary physiology assessment techniques.

	Advantages	*Limitations*
FFR	• Best evidences • Prognostic studies available	• *Guidewire:* Cost, complication • *Hyperemia:* Cost and side effect of adenosine • Increase time of the procedure
iFR	• Validated by noninferiority studies vs. FFR • Hyperemia independent • Quicker than FFR	• *Guidewire:* Cost, complication • Increase time of the procedure • Specific software required
Other NHPR	• Hyperemia independent • Quicker than FFR	• *Guidewire:* Cost, complication • Increase time of the procedure • Specific software required • No evidence regarding outcome prediction
HSR	Stenosis resistance based on a combination of intracoronary pressure and flow velocity	• *Guidewire:* Cost, complication • Increase time of the procedure • Specific software required
QFR, CAAS VFFR, FFR angio system	• Hyperemia independent • No pressure wire • Quicker than FFR if high expertise in post-treatment software	• No evidence for outcomes • Specific software required • Precise acquisition of angiography • Manual correction by expert
FFR CT	• Noninvasive • Increase performance of CCTA	• Cost • Offline analysis
CFR	• Study all coronary tree • Prognostic performance	• Overall assessment (macro- and microcirculation) • *Variability:* Intrinsic + variable resting condition • *Guidewire:* Cost, complication • *Hyperemia:* Cost and side effect of adenosine. Increase time of the procedure

(CCTA: coronary computed tomography angiography; CFR: coronary flow reserve; FFR: fractional flow reserve; HSR: hyperemic stenosis resistance; iFR: instantaneous wave-free ratio; NHPR: nonhyperemic pressure ratio; QFR: quantitative flow ratio; vFFR: vessel fractional flow reserve)

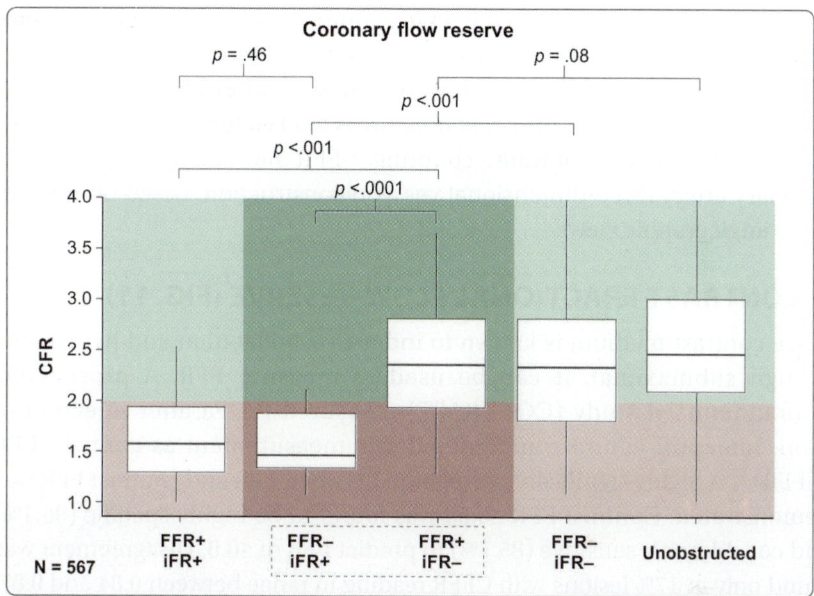

Fig. 10: CFR box plots separated by FFR/iFR discordant groups. Median denoted by horizontal black line. IQR denoted by box. Whiskers is the range of values. CFR >2 in green. CFR <2 in pink. CFR was significantly higher in the FFR1/iFR group versus the FFR/iFR1 group.[37] (CFR: coronary flow reserve; FFR: fractional flow reserve; iFR: instantaneous wave-free ratio)

guide damping, 5% interminability of which 23% there could be discrepancy between FFR and iFR. The myocardial mass subtended especially with regards to chronic total occlusion (CTO) and female gender is an issue and it is a continuous variable with an event rate not zero but above 0.8 because this is so how we resolve the FFR versus CFR discordance **(Fig. 10)**. Optimized PCI by using FFR is possible though, we have to really check that we are doing it correctly—to avoid drift and to finish with good result. It can be used with clinical and imaging background that will help in optimized completion. On even using CT angiogram for a completely virtual noninvasive FFR and quantitative flow ratio (QFR).

Quantitative flow ratio: The most validated angio-derived physiological index is quantitative flow ratio (QFR), which computes FFR from the ICA without the need for dedicated PW or hyperemic stimuli, sharing the same abnormality cut-off (0.80). QFR integrates the three-dimensional angiographic reconstruction of the vessel, derived from two angiographic projections with at least 25° of difference, and coronary flow is estimated from frame counting. QFR can be analyzed both online and offline, with a shorter analysis time than FFR (5.0 min vs. 7.0 min). QFR is efficient in precisely assessing the hemodynamic evaluation of coronary stenosis and produces great accuracy closest to the optimal value as compared to the FFR responses 84% sensitivity and 88% specificity.[32-36]

Another index similar to QFR which commands benefits but with a few disadvantages is vessel FFR. Instead of a full length coronary evaluation, vessel FFR permits only single lesion analysis and does not need a full-fledged evaluation. The aortic root pressure is tracked for determining hyper-dynamic flow instead of frame counting.[36] FFR allows a full left and right coronary artery three-dimensional vessel reconstruction, based on three or more angiographic views.

CONTRAST FRACTIONAL FLOW RESERVE (FIG. 11)

Since contrast medium is known to induce vasodilatation and hyperemia, though submaximal, it can be used to measure FFR. A prospective nonrandomized study (CONTRAST) measured Pd/Pa after injection of 6 mL Iomeprol contrast and coined this measurement as contrast FFR (CFFR).[38] A highly significant correlation between FFR and contrast FFR was demonstrated. Contrast FFR ≤0.83 was found to be highly specific (96.1%) and considerably sensitive (85.7%) to predict FFR of ≤0.8. Disagreement was found only in 17% lesions with CFFR reading in range between 0.84 and 0.87. Accuracy to predict FFR ≤0.8 was higher for contrast FFR, when compared to resting Pd/Pa or iFR. In a multicenter study involving 1,026 coronary stenosis, contrast FFR of ≤0.85 was found to have AUC of 0.89 in predicting an FFR value of ≤0.80.[39]

The results of these studies indicated that contrast FFR is feasible and has greater accuracy than iFR and resting Pd/Pa to predict functionally significant FFR. However, there are no randomized controlled international trials for CFFR, nor a consensus on amount of contrast required for FFR measurement and hyperemia induced by contrast is short lived.

- *Manual IC bolus of contrast:* Inject 6–10 mL of contrast[1,2]
- *Power injector IC bolus of contrast:* 10 mL at 4 mL/s, 300 psi[1,2]
  - Guide catheter should be disengaged from the ostium to avoid wedging phenomenon.
  - After any injection of contrast medium flushing of the guiding catheter with saline is recommended to avoid pressure damping due to contrast medium viscosity.
- *To document cFFR:*
  1. *Select recording:* Quick FFR
  2. Click on Rec
  3. Annotation → Contrast IC

CLINICAL CONFOUNDERS (FIG. 12)

Severe Aortic Stenosis

The dual impact of severe aortic valve stenosis and CAD is not only common, 25–50% of it also faces therapeutic and diagnostic challenges. Coronary

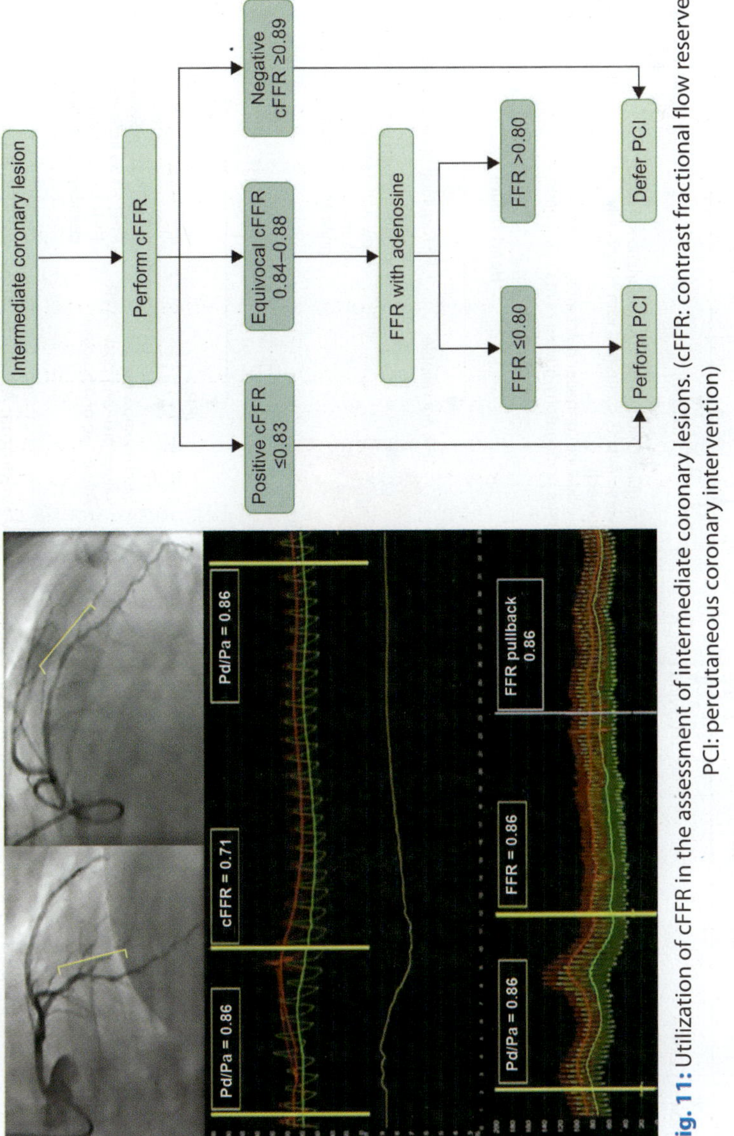

Fig. 11: Utilization of cFFR in the assessment of intermediate coronary lesions. (cFFR: contrast fractional flow reserve; PCI: percutaneous coronary intervention)

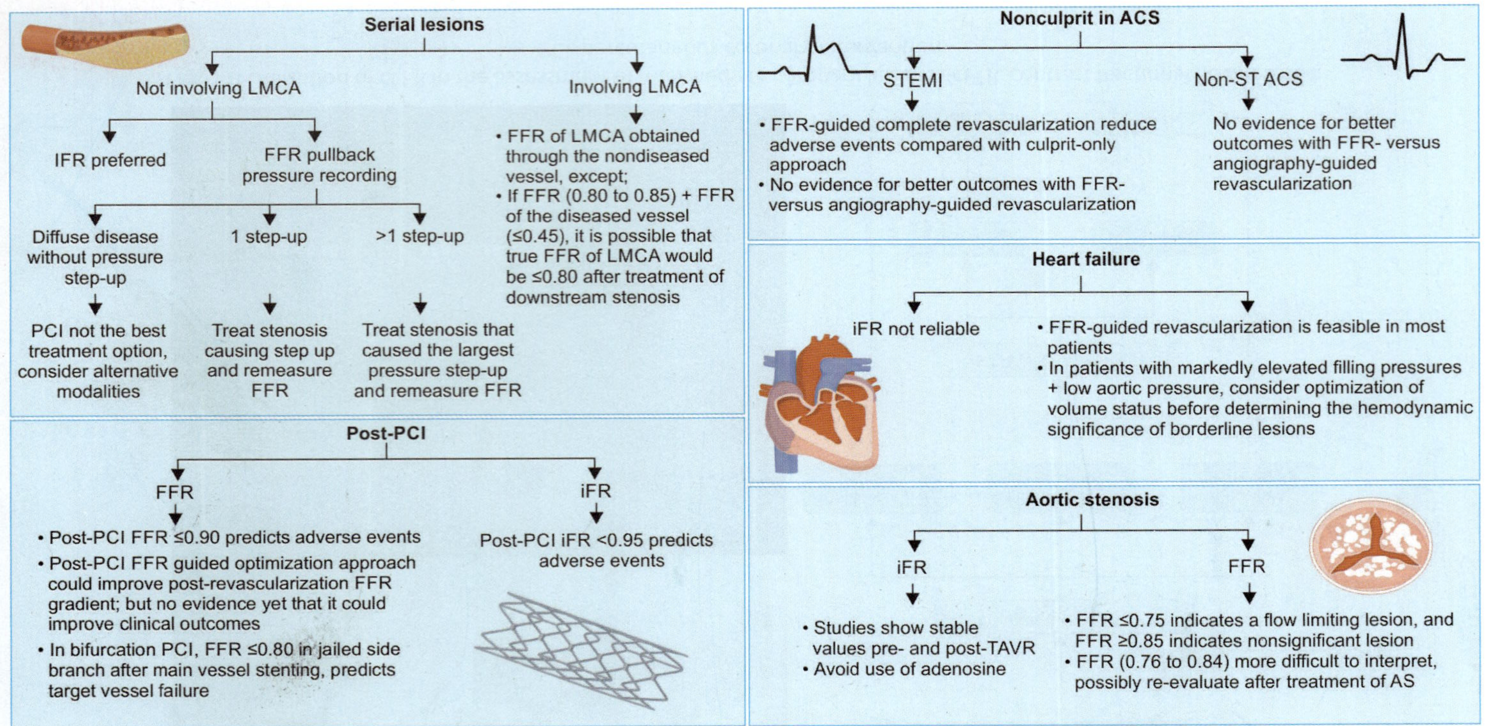

Fig. 12: Use of FFR/iFR in special patient subgroups. (ACS: acute coronary syndrome; AS: aortic stenosis; FFR: fractional flow reserve; iFR: instantaneous wave-free ratio; LMCA: left main coronary artery; PCI: percutaneous coronary intervention; STEMI: ST elevation myocardial infarction)

physiological estimations are the major assessing factors which decide the choice of revascularization prior to SAVR (surgical aortic valve replacement) or TAVR (transcatheter aortic valve replacement). The hemodynamics involving aortic stenosis increases left ventricular systolic and diastolic pressures along with diastolic impairment. Just as in case of patients with heart failure and severe AS result in rise in venous pressures and elevated left ventricular end-diastolic pressures (LVEDPs) thereby directly effecting the coronary pressures and flow which in turn also impact physiological indices. However, post TAVR, a sudden drop in afterload and regression of LV hypertrophy takes place accompanied by decreased resting flow and increased aortic pressures.[43] Resting physiological indices have to meet disadvantages for patients with pronounced AS as they may not withstand vasodilator difficulties. Among the premier studies, coronary physiological evaluations have shown improvement in CFR within 12 months follow-up after TAVR and also leading to instant reduction in afterload and improved microvascular function.[44]

Conclusively, following indications are observed: Prior to TAVR, usually the NHPR is not normal whereas FFR shows false normalcy. Post TAVR, NHPR exhibits varied ranges and FFR goes down (Pa goes up). Although any alteration in the decision for pre TAVR is almost negligible (treatment of post TAVR is only <10% of the lesions). After 6–12 months follow-up, NHPR may rise appreciably posing higher reclassification (~30%). For normal baseline (FFR >0.85), FFR is stable but might decline at 0.75–0.85.[45-48] Overall, determining functionally significant coronary lesions might be challenging among patients with severe AS. Changes in coronary blood flow and microvascular resistance might be attributed to the valvular disorder and epicardial coronary disease among patients with AS, a statement particularly relevant among patients with borderline physiological testing results. Studies suggest that iFR may be a better tool given the more stable results shown in pre- and post-TAVR patients, and the ability to avoid use of adenosine. In the use of FFR, a value ≤0.75 definitely indicates a flow-limiting lesion, and FFR ≥0.85 a physiologically nonsignificant lesion. FFR values in between those values can be more difficult to interpret. There is smaller risk for a specific lesion to go beyond ischemic threshold during FFR evaluations, which also ensures that in contrast to the sole angiography guidance, FFR pathway has fewer events of MACE despite the variations around TAVR.[47] An enhanced rate of defection in majority of the lesions (78.2%) was established during >0.80 FFR preservation suggesting that post TAVR even slight change in FFR is usually not clinically significant and the decision of not electing revascularization proves to be safe. The pre-TAVR values and its comparison to the post-TAVR data suggested wider differences in nonhyperemic pressure ratio (NHPR) for coronary lesions thereby indicting that FFR is more reliable.

Atrial Fibrillation

Atrial fibrillation (AF) is most common arrhythmia associated with CAD. Rapid ventricular rates (RVRs) are observed in AF patients due to increased myocardial oxygen demand and a state of pseudo-hyperemic which could worsen baseline Pd/Pa documentation iFR evaluations.[49] Although baseline values also get affected in non-RVR states and with those patients whose microvascular system is dysfunctional.[50] The verification is exhibited by iFR and FFR values which are assessed for the severity of coronary artery stenosis in routine studies. Both NHPRs including iFR get affected by resting (nonhyperemic) heart rate and blood pressure leading to 2.5–4.4 times enhanced variations as compared to FFR variance.[51] Reliable and reproducible FFR measurements are obtained for AF patients in comparison to iFR evaluations in AF. Overall, these indications suggest that there is first a coronary blood flow during diastole which later substantially drops at systole,[16] which remains consistent whatever the heart rate, whereas the span of diastole relies on heart rate affecting significantly NHPR as compared to FFR.

Left Main Coronary Artery Disease and Multiple Lesions

The LM assessment gets affected by the dysfunction of left anterior descending coronary artery (LAD) and the severity of the disease by FFR is evaluated during the LAD of pressure-sensor wire,[52,53] which should be placed in stenosis free artery as recommended. However, the flow of blood passing through LM is governed by the outflow within branch vessels (here it includes both the LAD and LCx—left circumflex artery), the FFR value could get affected even if one vessel is diseased and the other vessel hosts the pressure sensor. An animal model was proposed by Fearon et al.[54] in which an artificial stenosis was developed through balloon inflation PCI patients in the LAD, LCx, or both for comparing the real versus actual FFR as studied in 25 patients with 91 sample evaluation **(Figs. 13A and B)**. The true FFR found from left main coronary artery (LMCA) was observed to be low as compared to the apparent FFR.

Owing to the crosstalk phenomenon, the physiological studies of serial stenosis still pose problematic as serial stenosis greatly impacts the vessel hemodynamic more so at the time of maximal hyperemia **(Figs. 14 and 15)**. The proximal lesion gradient shows faulty results due to false Pd value, the reduction in flow from proximal stenosis misleads to the higher value indicators of the distal lesion.[41] Hyperemic PW pullback assists in identifying the larger pressure drop segment which needs to be first stented, although it tends to also overevaluate the severity of the lesion and thereby treating the nonstenotic segment. Reportedly, NHPR and NHPR-pullback are not significantly affected because autoregulation targets stable and resting coronary flow thereby averting crosstalk stenosis. If there is concomitant LM

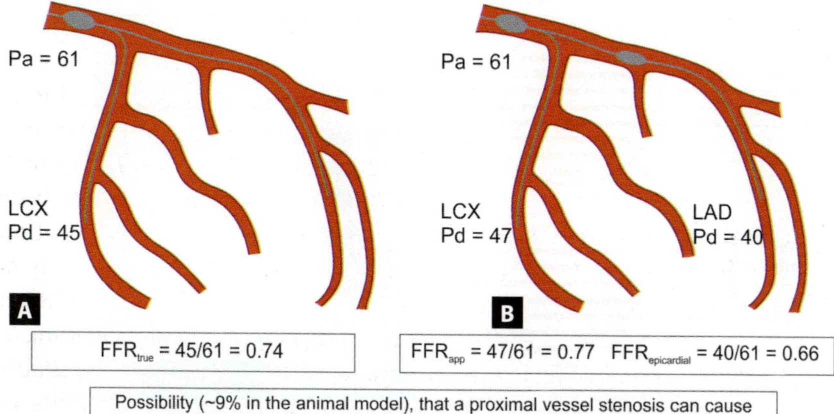

Figs. 13A and B: Effect of downstream lesion in FFR assessment of left main. (FFR: fractional flow reserve; LM: left main)

coupled with LAD or LCx disease, placing the distal PW in a major obstructed branch is a promising approach so that there is a separate identification of the drop in pressure due to the LM disease (proximal stenosis) **(Fig. 16)**.[42]

In case of intermediate grade LM disease, assessment using pressure-derived FFR is more challenging due to the requirement for disengagement of guiding catheter and inability to administer intracoronary adenosine. Some observational data exist to support the use of FFR, to decide if revascularization should be deferred or performed.[22] In a study, which included 230 patients with intermediate grade LMS stenosis, only 23% showed FFR of <0.80, who therefore underwent bypass surgery and rest with FFR of >0.80 were deferred treatment. However, clinical outcomes at 5 years were similar in both groups.[23]

Serial coronary lesions influence the FFR estimations and for every lesion, iFR pullback gives more accurate hemodynamic evaluations signifying the importance of each coronary lesion in series versus FFR evaluation more often during comparison of focal with the lesions with diffused disease present in series although clinical outcomes are still not confirmed during interventions of such lesions relying on iFR changes.[20,55]

Left Ventricular Hypertrophy

There is no direct influence of left ventricular hypertrophy (LVH) on FFR as determined after investigations also no notable changes are observed with absence or presence of LVH.[56] Corollary studies of the DANAMI-3-PRIMULTI along with cardiac magnetic resonance have indicated that LVH has probably no interaction with the direct relation of diameter stenosis to FFR.[57] Also clinically due to LVH there was no advantage of FFR-guided revasculariza-tion in comparison to angiographic revascularization. The clinical outcomes

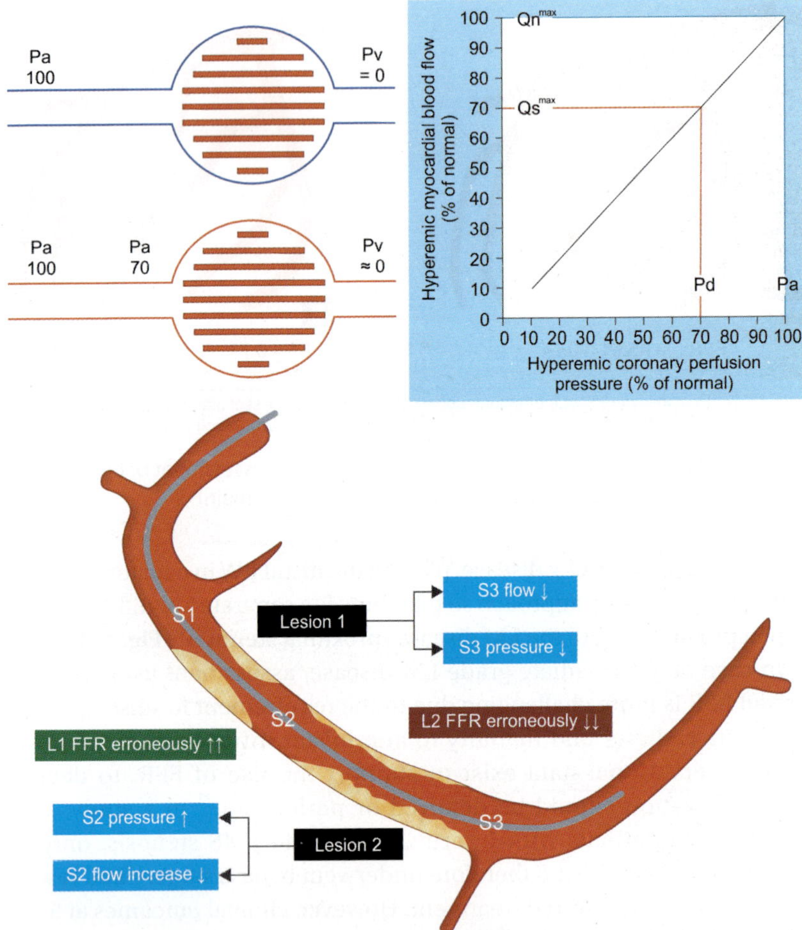

Fig. 14: *Multiple stenoses:* The crosstalk phenomenon. Coronary flow physiology is affected by the complex interplay between serial stenoses. The proximal lesion (1) reduces flow and pressure leading to an increase gradient across the distal lesion and FFR reduction (severity overestimation). Conversely the distal lesion might increase the interlesion pressure (S2) reducing the pressure gradient across the proximal one, thus leading to FFR increase (severity underestimation). (FFR: fractional flow reserve; Pa: aortic pressure; Pd: distal pressure; Pv: venous pressure; Qn: hypothetical maximal myocardial flow without stenosis; Qs: maximal myocardial flow in the presence of stenosis).

indicate a direct relationship of LVH with microvascular dysfunction and reduced coronary flow. The combined effect microvascular dysfunction, high degree of myocardium, and the hemodynamic impacts behind LVH pose a complex challenge in maintaining simple hyperemic Pd/Pa ratio for FFR. It is quite likely that, in case of LVH patients, the declining effect of FFR impacting the myocardial territory of the vessel facing stenosis is eventually

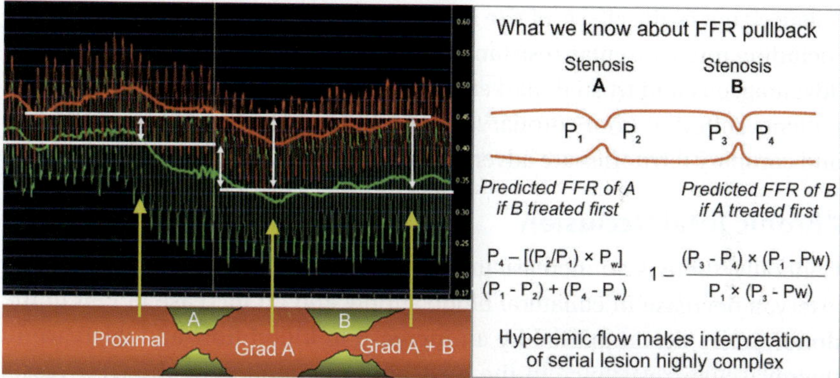

$$\frac{P_4 - [(P_2/P_1) \times P_w]}{(P_1 - P_2) + (P_4 - P_w)} \qquad 1 - \frac{(P_3 - P_4) \times (P_1 - Pw)}{P_1 \times (P_3 - Pw)}$$

Fig. 15: Showing FFR pullback interpretation of serial lesions.[26,54] (FFR: fractional flow reserve)

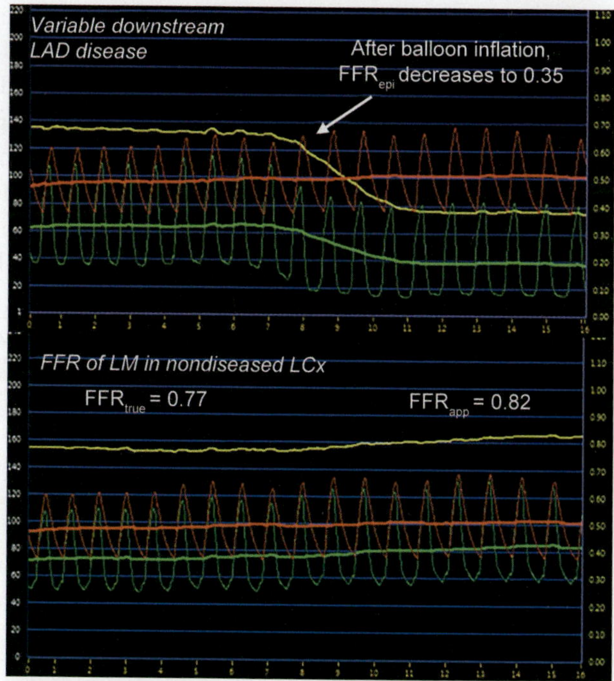

Fig. 16: Case example of LM-FFR by use of simultaneous coronary pressure recordings during the creation of variable downstream stenosis using balloon inflation. (Top panel) The coronary pressure is recorded from the LAD pressure wire before and after balloon inflation within a newly placed LAD stent (the green line is distal coronary pressure, the red line is aortic pressure, and the yellow line is FFR value). (Bottom panel) The coronary pressure is recorded simultaneously from the LCx pressure wire (FFR_{true} and FFR_{app}) before and after inflation of the balloon in the LAD, ultimately leading to complete occlusion (the green line is distal coronary pressure, the red line is aortic pressure, and the yellow line is the FFR value).[26,54] (FFR: fractional flow reserve; LAD: left anterior descending; LCx: left circumflex artery; LM: left main)

balanced out by the effects of rise in FFR which occurs with enhanced LVEDP including microvascular resistance. Conclusively, FFR appears to be more advantageous and trusted marker having hemodynamic importance among patients suffering from coronary lesions, LVH even when large myocardial and coronary territories are adverse.

Chronic Total Occlusion

Generally, there is an increase in FFR in the chronic total occlusion (CTO) artery, a decrease in collateral blood supply and an increase in FFR in the donor artery accompanied by an increase in blood flow and decrease in microvascular resistance in the myocardium supplied by the CTO vessel **(Table 7)**.

Myocardial Bridge

As the left coronary artery perfuses in diastole, physiologic evaluation of myocardial bridge (MB) is a conceptual challenge. In view of objective evidence of ischemia in the presence of MB, we strongly recommend the use of intracoronary hemodynamic evaluation of MB by FFR. Several reports have shown reduced FFR associated with myocardial bridging and its normalization with successful coronary stenting. Two local hemodynamic features specific to MB, so-called "overshooting" and "sucking" effects, occurred in a number of patients during dobutamine provocation **(Figs. 17A to F)**.

TABLE 7: Utilization of coronary physiology in various complex coronary lesions.

Complex clinical scenarios	*FFR/NHPR*	*Key points*	*Outcome studies?*
Bifurcation lesions	FFR/NHPR	Deceptive angio, difficult access	Yes
Ostial, LM	FFR	IV adeno for ostial, LM. LM+LAD use FFR >0.6. IVUS for <0.6	Yes
Diffuse/serial disease	Pullback pressure	ΔP hyperemia/rest w co-registration	No
CABG[40]	FFR	MVD not need CABG of all vessels. SVG biology trumps physiology but assessment correct	Yes
STEMI/NSTEMI	FFR/NHPR, IMR	Primulti and Danami say yes to nonculprit if <0.8. IMR >40 u worse outcomes	Yes
CTO	FFR	Δmyoc bed and collateral flow indices	Yes
TAVR	FFR/NHPR	CBF increases after TAVR, FFR decreases	No

(CABG: coronary artery bypass graft; FFR: fractional flow reserve; NSTEMI: non-ST-elevation myocardial infarction; STEMI: ST elevation myocardial infarction)

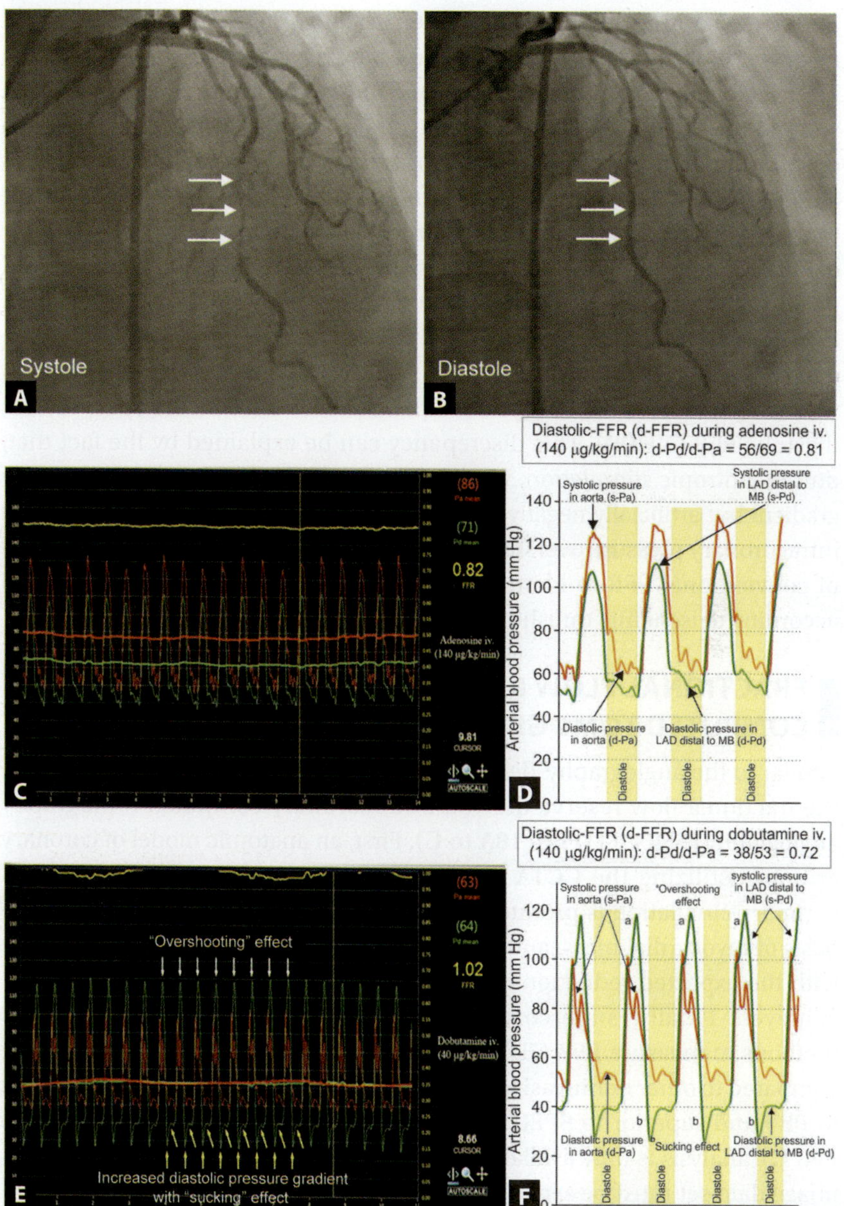

Figs. 17A to F: *Example of MB invasive functional assessment with schematic graphics.* Coronary angiography revealed MB in the medial segment of left anterior descending (LAD) artery with systolic compression (A) and diastolic decompression (B) of intramyocardial segment ("milking effect"). Conventional-FFR and diastolic-FFR (d-FFR) measurements during adenosine (C and D), and peak dobutamine infusion (E and F). (d-Pa: aortic blood pressure waveform during diastole; d-Pd: distal intracoronary pressure waveform during diastole; FFR: fractional flow reserve; MB: myocardial bridging; Pa (red line): aortic blood pressure waveform during the whole cardiac cycle; Pd (green line): distal intracoronary pressure waveform during the whole cardiac cycle)[78]

The "overshooting" effect existed when systolic pressure gradient reached negative value, meaning that the average intracoronary pressure distal to the MB overshooted the average aortic blood pressure during systole. It has been studied that d-FFR (diastolic FFR) during inotropic stimulation with high doses of dobutamine, in comparison to vasodilation with adenosine, provides a more reliable assessment of functional significance of MB correspondent to stress-induced myocardial ischemia. The optimal cut-off of ≤0.76 for d-FFR at peak dobutamine dose has the best sensitivity, specificity, and positive and negative predictive value for discriminating the MB in relation to exercise stress-induced myocardial ischemia. It has been shown that the decrease systolic pressure across the MB during dobutamine provocation was a major determinant of the discrepancies between conventional FFR and diastolic FFR (NHPR). This discrepancy can be explained by the fact that, during inotropic stimulation, MB produces an increase of diastolic pressure gradient but artificially negative systolic pressure gradient secondary to distal intracoronary pressure overshooting. This is the main reason for the inability of conventional FFR to identify patients with functionally significant MB according to ischemic threshold ≤0.80.[76,77]

FRACTIONAL FLOW RESERVE DERIVED FROM COMPUTED TOMOGRAPHY

Similar to the angiography-derived FFR, several steps are required to obtain the fractional flow reserve derived from coronary computed tomography angiography (FFR CT) **(Figs. 18A to C)**. First, an anatomic model of coronary arteries ustilizing the CCTA data is done. Then a physiologic model of coronary circulation is produced. Resting coronary flow is modeled on the basis of myocardial mass, and maximal hyperemia is modeled in agreement with the expected reduction in resistance if adenosine injection would be achieved. Finally, supercomputers use computational fluid dynamics methods to measure FFR CT.[58-60] The diagnostic performance is interesting compared to other noninvasive tests. The PACIFIC trial showed it comparable to PET and superior to SPECT. The weakness remains an off-line analysis. FFR CT analysis is only available at a central laboratory in California. CCTA image data set must be sent to postprocessing which still takes 1–4 hours. In addition to the cost of process, the performance also depends strongly on the quality of the image. Severe calcification, motion artifact, and stenting decrease the quality of analysis. For example, in PACIFIC trial, analyzability of FFR CT was only 75% at the patient level.[61] FFR CT is a feasible and safe with a significantly lower rate of nonobstructive coronary artery disease (NOCAD) at ICA. At 1-year follow-up, the FFR CT strategy appeared lower cost than the ICA strategy with an equivalent cardiac event rate and the same level of quality of life.[62,63] The SYNTAX III trial, in patients with LM or 3-vessel CAD,

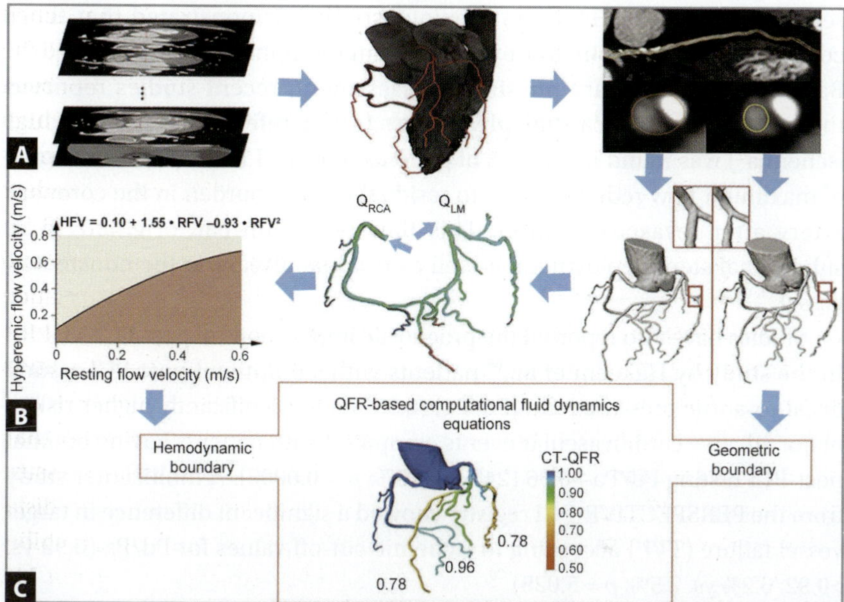

Figs. 18A to C: Computed tomography-derived quantitative flow ratio. The framework of CT-QFR computation includes: (A) Lumen contour and coronary tree automatic reconstruction and CT-QFR computation; (B) Patient-specific virtual hyperemic flow estimation; (C) QFR computational fluid dynamics equations. (CT: computed tomography; HFV: hyperemic flow velocity; LM: left main; QFR: quantitative flow ratio; RCA: right coronary artery; RFV: resting flow velocity)
Adapted with permission from Li et al.
Source: Li Z, Zhang J, Xu L et al. Diagnostic Accuracy of a Fast Computational Approach to Derive Fractional Flow Reserve From Coronary CT Angiography. JACC Cardiovasc Imaging. 2020 Jan;13(1 Pt 1):172-175.

showed that CCTA analysis made the same revascularization decision as ICA analysis, and that the use of FFR CT changed the decision in 7% of cases.[64] In FORECAST trial, use of FFR CT reduced ICA, and did not differ significantly from control group in cost or clinical outcomes.[65] However, control group had mainly CCTA (63%) as the initial test. Studies with adequate statistical power to compare the performance of FFR CT with other noninvasive tests in the management of chronic coronary syndrome are expected.

POST-PERCUTANEOUS CORONARY INTERVENTION FRACTIONAL FLOW RESERVE

Post-angiographically successful PCI does not necessarily result in functionally optimized PCI. Low post-PCI physiologic indexes predict worse outcomes. Post-PCI physiologic assessment enables optimization of PCI results and improves outcome. The success of PCI is generally assessed by CAG, despite its well-accepted limitations in defining stenosis severity before PCI. However, previous studies demonstrated that there could be residual ischemia even after angiographically successful PCI. Based on intracoronary physiology assessment, recent studies reported that suboptimal epicardial physiology (often referred to as "residual ischemia") was found in 10–36% of patients. Post PCI FFR shows the degree of maximum flow reduction due to residual disease burden in the coronary artery after revascularization. This flow reduction can originate from suboptimal stent deployment as well as residual disease in the nonstented vessel.[66-68]

Studies have also reported the prognostic implications of post-PCI NHPRs. In the study by Hakeem et al.,[69] patients with suboptimal post-PCI resting distal-to-aortic pressure ratio (Pd/Pa) (0.96) had a significantly higher risk of major adverse cardiovascular events compared with patients having optimal post-PCI resting Pd/Pa >0.96 (24% vs. 15%; $p = 0.0006$). A multicenter study from the PERSPECTIVE-PCI registry showed a significant difference in target vessel failure (TVF) according to ischemic cut-off values for Pd/Pa (0.92 vs. >0.92; 6.2% vs. 2.5%; $p = 5.029$).[70]

The DEFINE PCI (Physiological Assessment of Coronary Stenosis after PCI) has given results for epicardial residual ischemia post-angiography PCI, reported as iFR < 0.89 occurring in 24% trials of patients.[71] 81.6% of patients with suboptimal post-PCI iFR had focal residual disease. Post-PCI FFR in patients with complex CAD is predictive of adverse cardiac events at 1 year. On a vessel level, low post-PCI FFR was associated with a significantly higher rate of TVF, as well as cardiac death alone.

Regardless of stent type used, low post-PCI FFR values have consistently been associated with worse clinical outcomes. In a patient-level meta-analysis, post-PCI FFR showed an inverse relationship with subsequent events [hazard ratio (HR): 0.86, 95% confidence interval (CI): 0.80–0.93; $p < 0.001$).[72] One of the limitations is that the optimal cut-off values for the post-PCI FFR varied among the studies, although they were slightly lower among the studies using second-generation drug-eluting stent (DES) (0.84–0.90) compared with earlier reports with bare-metal stent or mainly first-generation DES. The heterogeneity of the optimal cut-off values of post-PCI FFR stems from the fact that the values were set to predict subsequent clinical events that would be affected by study population, event rates, and the definition of clinical events of each study, whereas the optimal cut-off value of pre-PCI FFR was determined to identify the presence of ischemia using noninvasive stress tests.[73] Also, the optimal cut-off value of post-PCI FFR could be lower in the left anterior descending (LAD) artery than non-LAD,[74] because the LAD generally supplies a larger subtended myocardium, which is one of the key determinants of hyperemic coronary flow and consequently FFR.[75]

The FFR SEARCH study main findings of our study are the following: (1) poststenting FFR is safe, feasible, and can be easily performed when using a rapid exchange microcatheter maintaining wire access. (2) Impaired coronary physiology expressed by FFR <0.90 was common (37.8% of patients). (3) Post-PCI FFR <0.90 was not associated with an increase in overall MACE, but on a vessel level analysis, resulted into a higher rate of TVRs and a trend toward higher rate of ST during a follow-up of 2 years. The FFR cutoff <0.90 was derived from a post hoc analysis of the FAME Trials and was supported by a large meta-analysis, however, never tested in a prospective fashion. Using this threshold, more than one-third of the final results judged as acceptable by angiography were categorized as suboptimal, highlighting its clinical relevance. Hence, post-PCI physiological assessment may play a more important role for evaluation and localization of residual disease outside the stented segment rather than for stent optimization, for which intracoronary imaging is the established method. Many studies and post hoc analyses of RCTs have established that post-PCI FFR value is an independent predictor of long-term clinical outcomes.[69] Previous trials have demonstrated that "higher is better," although the best cut-off value of post-PCI FFR varied from 0.86 to 0.96 for the prediction of clinical events.[68,69] Post-PCI FFR was an independent predictor of TVF (target vessel failure) as well as of the composite of cardiac death and MI in patient undergoing FFR-guided DES implantation.

CONCLUSION

For decisions on epicardial revascularization and findings in coronary microcirculation, the evaluation of coronary physiology has emerged as a dependable tool for managing patients successfully **(Fig. 19 and Flowchart 1)**. Despite multiple evidences supporting the use of FFR in numerous clinical scenarios, FFR remains significantly underutilized. With further adoption of appropriate use criteria for PCI, coronary physiology evaluation via FFR would be expected to continue to rise in PCI. Coronary physiology assessment helps the management, improve the prognosis and quality of life of patients with CAD. Ongoing clinical trials will help in improving patient selection for FFR by providing more insight into the use of FFR in specific subgroups of patients, including those with aortic stenosis, ACS, and pre- to post-PCI evaluation. On the basis of availability of coronary physiological indexes and its ranges, it is possible to plan and conduct personalized treatment and acquire greater precision.

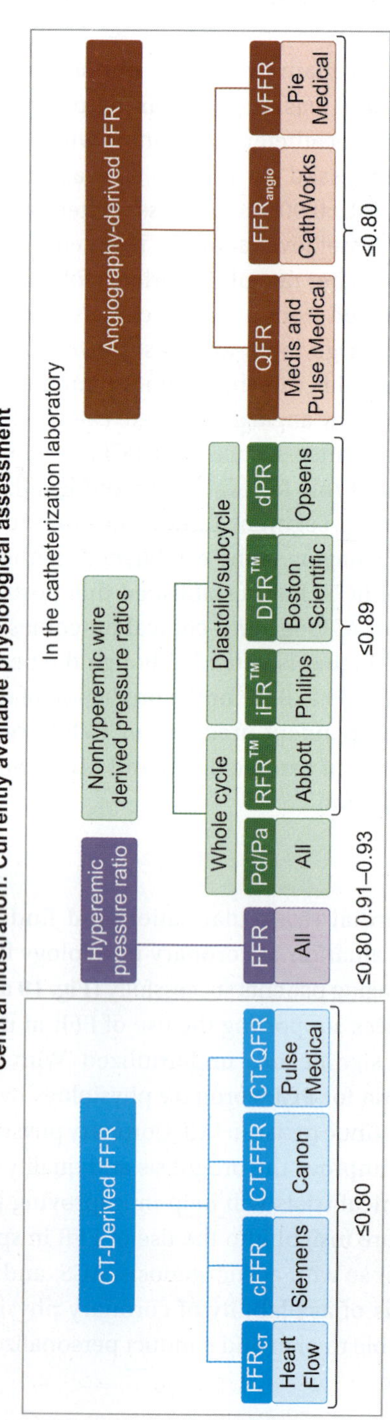

Fig. 19: Presently available techniques for physiologic assessment.[30]
Source: Kogame N et al. JACC Cardiovasc Interv. 2020;13(14):1617-38.

Flowchart 1: Proposed algorithm for post-PCI optimization.[69]

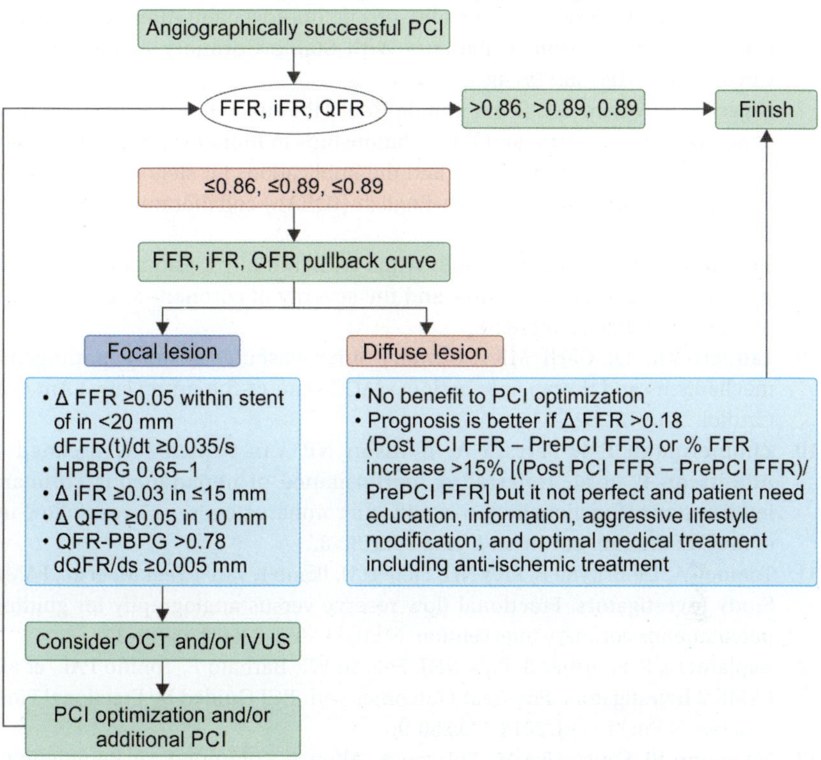

(FFR: fractional flow reserve; iFR: instantaneous wave-free ratio; PCI: percutaneous coronary intervention; QFR: quantitative flow ratio)

REFERENCES

1. Grüntzig AR, Senning A, Siegenthaler WE. Nonoperative dilatation of coronary-artery stenosis: percutaneous transluminal coronary angioplasty. N Engl J Med. 1979;301:61-8.
2. Serruys PW, Di Mario C, Meneveau N, de Jaegere P, Strikwerda S, de Feyter PJ, et al. Intracoronary pressure and flow velocity with sensor-tip guidewires: a new methodologic approach for assessment of coronary hemodynamics before and after coronary interventions. Am J Cardiol. 1993;71:41D-53D.
3. Sandhu PS, Kaul U. Fractional flow reserve: How to interpret in different situations. In: Sethi R, Khanna NN, Kumar JS (Eds). NIC Companion Book of Interventional Cardiology, 1st edition. New Delhi: Jaypee Brothers Medial Publisher; 2017. pp. 30-41.
4. Beltrame JF, Crea F, Kaski JC, Ogawa H, Ong P, Sechtem U, et al. International standardization of diagnostic criteria for vasospastic angina. Eur Heart J. 2017;38:2565-8.
5. Toth GG, Johnson NP, Jeremias A, Pellicano M, Vranckx P, Fearon WF, et al. Standardization of fractional flow reserve measurements. J Am Coll Cardiol. 2016;68(7):742-53.

6. Nishi T, Piroth Z, De Bruyne B, Jagic N, Möbius-Winkler S, Kobayashi Y, et al. Fractional Flow Reserve and Quality-of-Life Improvement After Percutaneous Coronary Intervention in Patients With Stable Coronary Artery Disease. Circulation. 2018;138:1797-804.
7. Nijjer SS, de Waard GA, Sen S, van de Hoef TP, Petraco R, Echavarría-Pinto M, et al. Coronary pressure and flow relationships in humans: phasic analysis of normal and pathological vessels and the implications for stenosis assessment: a report from the Iberian-Dutch-English (IDEAL) collaborators. Eur Heart J. 2016;37:2069-80.
8. Uren NG, Melin JA, De Bruyne B, Wijns W, Baudhuin T, Camici PG. Relation between myocardial blood flow and the severity of coronary-artery stenosis. N Engl J Med. 1994;330:1782-8.
9. Taqueti VR, Di Carli MF. Coronary microvascular disease pathogenic mechanisms and therapeutic options: JACC state-of-the-art review. J Am Coll Cardiol. 2018;72:2625-41.
10. Zimmermann FM, Ferrara A, Johnson NP, van Nunen LX, Escaned J, Albertsson P, et al. Deferral vs. performance of percutaneous coronary intervention of functionally non-significant coronary stenosis: 15-year follow-up of the DEFER trial. Eur Heart J. 2015;36:3182-8.
11. Tonino PA, De Bruyne B, Pijls NH, Siebert U, Ikeno F, van' t Veer M, et al.; FAME Study Investigators. Fractional flow reserve versus angiography for guiding percutaneous coronary intervention. N Engl J Med. 2009;360:213-24.
12. Xaplanteris P, Fournier S, Pijls NHJ, Fearon WF, Barbato E, Tonino PAL, et al.; FAME 2 Investigators. Five-Year Outcomes with PCI Guided by Fractional Flow Reserve. N Engl J Med. 2018;379:250-9.
13. Neumann FJ, Sousa-Uva M, Ahlsson A, Alfonso F, Banning AP, Benedetto U, et al. The Task Force on myocardial revascularization of the European Society of Cardiology (ESC) and European Association for Cardio-Thoracic Surgery (EACTS) Guidelines on myocardial revascularization. Eur Heart J. 2019;40:87-165.
14. Pijls NH, Van Gelder B, Van der Voort P, Peels K, Bracke FA, Bonnier HJ, et al. Fractional flow reserve. A useful index to evaluate the influence of an epicardial coronary stenosis an myocardial blood flow. Circulation. 1955;92:3183-93.
15. De Bruyne B, Pijls NH, Barbato E, Bartunek J, Bech JW, Wijns W, et al. Intracoronary and intravenous adenosine 5'-triphosphate, adenosine, papaverine, and contrast medium to assess fractional flow reserve in humans. Circulation. 2003;107:1877-83.
16. De Bruyne B, Bartunek J, Sys SU, Pijls NH, Heyndrickx GR, Wijns W. Simultaneous coronary pressure and flow velocity measurements in humans: feasibility, reproducibility, and hemodynamic dependence of coronary flow velocity reserve, hyperemic flow versus slope index, and fractional flow reserve. Circulation. 1996;94:1842-9.
17. Melikian N, Cuisset T, Hamilos M, De Bruyne B. Fractional flow reserve - the influence of the collateral circulation. Int J Cardiol. 2009;132:109-10.
18. Pijls NHJ, Fearon WF, Tonino PAL, Siebert U, Ikeno F, Bornschein B, et al. Fractional flow reserve versus angiography for guiding percutaneous coronary intervention in patients with multivessel coronary artery disease: 2-year follow-up of the FAME (Fractional Flow Reserve Versus Angiography for Multivessel Evaluation) study. J Am Coll Cardiol. 2010;56(3):177-84.

19. Fearon WF, Pijls NH, Tonino PA, Siebert U, Ikeno F, Bornschein B, et al.; FAME study investigators. Fractional flow reserve versus angiography for guiding percutaneous coronary intervention in patients with multivessel coronary artery disease: 2 year follow up of the FAME study. J Am Coll Cardiol. 2010;56: 177-84.
20. Davies JE, Sen S, Dehbi HM, AL-Lamee R, Petraco R, Nijjer SS, et al. Use of the instantaneous wave free ratio or fractional flow reserve in PCI. N Eng J Med. 2017;376:1824-34.
21. Van Belle E, Rioufol G, Pouillot C, Cuisset T, Bougrini K, Teiger E, et al. Out come impact of coronary revaslularisation strategy reclassification with fractional flow reserve at time of diagnostic angiography. Insights from a large French multicenter Fractional flow reserve registry. Circulation. 2014;129:173-85.
22. Mallidi J, Atreya AR, Cook J, Garb J, Jeremias A, Klein LW, et al. Long-term outcomes following fractional flow reserve-guided treatment of angiographically ambiguous left main coronary artery disease. A meta-analysis of prospective Cohort studies. Catheter Cardiovasc Interv. 2015;86:12-8.
23. Hamilos M, Muller O, Cuisset T, Ntalianis A, Chlouverakis G, Sarno G, et al. Long-term clinical outcome after fractional flow reserve-guided treatment in patients with agiographically equivocal left main coronary artery stenosis. Circulation. 2009;120:1505-12.
24. De Bruyne B, Pijls NH, Kalesan B, Barbato E, Tonino PA, Piroth Z, et al.; FAME 2 trial Investigators. Fractional flow reserve guided PCI versus medical therapy in stable coronary artery disease. N Engl J Med. 2021;367:991-1001.
25. Koo B, Lee J, Hwang D. Park S, Shiono Y, Yonetsu T, et al. Practical Application of Coronary Physiologic Assessment: Asia-Pacific Expert Consensus Document: Part 1. JACC Asia. 2023;3(5):689-706.
26. Götberg M, Christiansen EH, Gudmundsdottir IJ, Sandhall L, Danielewicz M, Jakobsen L, et al.; iFR-SWEDEHEART Investigators. Instantaneous Wave-free Ratio versus Fractional Flow Reserve to Guide PCI. N Engl J Med. 2017;376: 1813-23.
27. Götberg M, Berntorp K, Rylance R, Christiansen EH, Yndigegn T, Gudmundsdottir IJ, et al. 5-Year outcomes of PCI guided by measurement of instantaneous wave-free ratio versus fractional flow reserve. J Am Coll Cardiol. 2022;79:965-74.
28. Fearon WF, Nishi T, De Bruyne B, Boothroyd DB, Barbato E, Tonino P, et al.; FAME-2 Trial Investigators. Clinical outcomes and cost-effectiveness of fractional flow reserve-guided percutaneous coronary intervention in patients with stable coronary artery disease: Three-year follow-up of the FAME-2 trial. Circulation. 2018;137:480-7.
29. Gotberg M, Cook CM, Sen S, Nijjer S, Escaned J, Davies JE. The evolving future of instantaneous wave-free ratio and fractional flow reserve. J Am Coll Cardiol. 2017;70(11):1379-402.
30. Kogame N, Ono M, Kawashima H, Tomaniak M, Hara H, Leipsic J, et al. The impact of coronary physiology on contemporary clinical decision making. JACC Cardiovasc Interv. 2020;13(14):1617-38.
31. Collet C, Miyazaki Y, Ryan N, Asano T, Tenekecioglu E, Sonck J, et al. Fractional flow reserve derived from computed tomographic angiography in patients with multivessel CAD. J Am Coll Cardiol. 2018;71(24):2756-69.

32. Kern MJ, Samady H. Current concepts of integrated coronary physiology in the catheterization laboratory. J Am Coll Cardiol. 2010;55(3):173-85.
33. Tu S, Westra J, Yang J, von Birgelen C, Ferrara A, Pellicano M, et al.; FAVOR Pilot Trial Study Group. Diagnostic Accuracy of Fast Computational Approaches to Derive Fractional Flow Reserve From Diagnostic Coronary Angiography: The International Multicenter FAVOR Pilot Study. JACC Cardiovasc Interv. 2016;9:2024-35.
34. Westra J, Andersen BK, Campo G, Matsuo H, Koltowski L, Eftekhari A, et al. Diagnostic Performance of In-Procedure Angiography-Derived Quantitative Flow Reserve Compared to Pressure-Derived Fractional Flow Reserve: The FAVOR II Europe-Japan Study. J Am Heart Assoc. 2018;7:e009603.
35. Xu B, Tu S, Qiao S, Qu X, Chen Y, Yang J, et al. Diagnostic accuracy of angiography-based quantitative flow ratio measurements for online assessment of coronary stenosis. J Am Coll Cardiol. 2017;70:3077-387.
36. Collet C, Onuma Y, Sonck J, Asano T, Vandeloo B, Kornowski R, et al. Diagnostic performance of angiography-derived fractional flow reserve: a systematic review and Bayesian meta-analysis. Eur Heart J. 2018;39:3314-21.
37. Cook CM, Jeremias A, Petraco R, Sen S, Nijjer S, Shun-Shin MJ, et al. Fractional flow reserve/instantaneous wave-free ratio discordance in angiographically intermediate coronary stenoses: an analysis using Doppler-derived coronary flow measurements. JACC Cardiovasc Interv. 2017;10(24):2514-24.
38. Leone AM, Scalone G, De Maria GL, Tagliaferro F, Gardi A, Clemente F, et al. Efficacy of contrast medium induced Pd/Pa ratio in predicting functional significance of intermediate coronary artery stenosis assessed by fractional flow reserve: insights from the RINASCI study. EuroIntervention. 2015;11(4):421-7.
39. Leone AM, Martin-Reyes R, Baptista SB, Amabile N, Raposo L, Franco Pelaez JA, et al. The multi-center evaluation of the accuracy of the contrast medium induced Pd/Pa ratio in predicting FFR (MOMENTO-FFR) study. EuroIntervention. 2016;12(6):708-15.
40. Pellicano M, De Bruyne B, Toth GG, Casselman F, Wijns W, Barbato E. Fractional flow reserve to guide and to assess coronary artery bypass grafting. Eur Heart J. 2017;38:1959-68.
41. Nijjer SS, Sen S, Petraco R, Mayet J, Francis DP, Davies JE. The Instantaneous wave-Free Ratio (iFR) pullback: a novel innovation using baseline physiology to optimise coronary angioplasty in tandem lesions. Cardiovasc Revasc Med. 2015;16:167-71.
42. Modi BN, De Silva K, Rajani R, Curzen N, Perera D. Physiology-Guided Management of Serial Coronary Artery Disease A Review. JAMA Cardiol. 2018;3:432-8.
43. Camuglia AC, Syed J, Garg P, Kiaii B, Chu MW, Jones PM, et al. Invasively assessed coronary flow dynamics improved following relief of aortic stenosis with transcatheter aortic valve implantation. J Am Coll Cardiol. 2014;63(17):1808-9.
44. Wiegerinck EM, van de Hoef TP, Rolandi MC, Yong Z, van Kesteren F, Koch KT, et al. Impact of aortic valve stenosis on coronary hemodynamics and instantaneous effect of transcatheter aortic valve implantation. Circ Cardiovasc Interv. 2015;8(8):e002443.
45. Pesarini G, Scarsini R, Zivelonghi C, Piccoli A, Gambaro A, Gottin L, et al. Functional assessment of coronary artery disease in patients undergoing

transcatheter aortic valve implantation: influence of pressure overload on the evaluation of lesions severity. Circ Cardiovasc Interv. 2016;9:e004088.

46. Scarsini R, Lunardi M, Venturi G, Pighi M, Tavella D, Pesarini G, et al. Long-term variations of FFR and iFR after transcatheter aortic valve implantation. Int J Cardiol. 2020;317:37-41.
47. Lunardi M, Scarsini R, Venturi G, Pesarini G, Pighi M, Gratta A, et al. Physiological versus angiographic guidance for myocardial revascularization in patients undergoing transcatheter aortic valve implantation. J Am Heart Assoc. 2019;8:e012618.
48. Sabbah M, Joshi FR, Minkkinen M, Holmvang L, Tilsted HH, Pedersen F, et al. Long-term changes in invasive physiological pressure indices of stenosis severity following transcatheter aortic valve implantation. Circ Cardiovasc Interv. 2022;15:e011331.
49. Range FT, Schafers M, Acil T, Schäfers KP, Kies P, Paul M, et al. Impaired myocardial perfusion and perfusion reserve associated with increased coronary resistance in persistent atrial fibrillation. Eur Heart J. 2007;28(18):2223-30.
50. Kochiadakis GE, Skalidis EI, Kalebubas MD, Igoumenidis NE, Chrysostomakis SI, Kanoupakis EM, et al. Effect of acute atrial fibrillation on phasic coronary blood flow pattern and flow reserve in humans. Eur Heart J. 2002;23(9):734-41.
51. Berry C, Veer MV, Witt N, Kala P, Bocek O, Pyxaras SA, et al. VERIFY (VERification of instantaneous wave-free ratio and fractional flow reserve for the assessment of coronary artery stenosis severity in everyday practice): a multicenter study in consecutive patients. J Am Coll Cardiol. 2013;61(13):1421-7.
52. De Bruyne B, Pijls NH, Heyndrickx GR, Hodeige D, Kirkeeide R, Gould KL. Pressure-derived fractional flow reserve to assess serial epicardial stenoses: theoretical basis and animal validation. Circulation. 2000;101(15):1840-7.
53. Pijls NH, de Bruyne B, Bech GJ, Liistro F, Heyndrickx GR, Bonnier HJ, et al. Coronary pressure measurement to assess the hemodynamic significance of serial stenoses within one coronary artery: validation in humans. Circulation. 2000;02(19):2371-7.
54. Fearon WF, Yong AS, Lenders G, Toth GG, Dao C, Daniels DV, et al. The impact of downstream coronary stenosis on fractional flow reserve assessment of intermediate left main coronary artery disease: human validation. JACC Cardiovasc Interv. 2015;8(3):398-403.
55. De Bruyne B, Pijls NH, Heyndrickx GR, Hodeige D, Kirkeeide R, Gould KL. Pressure-derived fractional flow reserve to assess serial epicardial stenoses: theoretical basis and animal validation. Circulation. 2000;101(15):1840-7.
56. Chhatriwalla AK, Ragosta M, Powers ER, Sarembock IJ, Gimple LW, Fischer JJ, et al. High left ventricular mass index does not limit the utility of fractional flow reserve for the physiologic assessment of lesion severity. J Invasive Cardiol. 2006;18(11):544-9.
57. Sabbah M, Nepper-Christensen L, Lonborg J, Helqvist S, Køber L, Høfsten DE, et al. Fractional flow reserve-guided PCI in patients with and without left ventricular hypertrophy: a DANAMI-3-PRIMULTI substudy. EuroIntervention. 2020;16(7):584-90.
58. Koo BK, Erglis A, Doh JH, Daniels DV, Jegere S, Kim HS, et al. Diagnosis of ischemia-causing coronary stenoses by noninvasive fractional flow reserve computed from coronary computed tomographic angiograms. Results from the prospective multicenter DISCOVER-FLOW (Diagnosis of Ischemia-Causing

Stenoses Obtained via Noninvasive Fractional Flow Reserve) study. J Am Coll Cardiol. 2011;58:1989-97.

59. Min JK, Leipsic J, Pencina MJ, Berman DS, Koo BK, van Mieghem C, et al. Diagnostic accuracy of fractional flow reserve from anatomic CT angiography. J Am Med Assoc. 2012;308:1237-45.
60. Nørgaard BL, Leipsic J, Gaur S, Seneviratne S, Ko BS, Ito H, et al. Diagnostic performance of noninvasive fractional flow reserve derived from coronary computed tomography angiography in suspected coronary artery disease: the NXT trial (Analysis of Coronary Blood Flow Using CT Angiography: next Steps). J Am Coll Cardiol. 2014;63:1145-55.
61. Driessen RS, Danad I, Stuijfzand WJ, Raijmakers PG, Schumacher SP, van Diemen PA, et al. Comparison of coronary computed tomography angiography, fractional flow reserve, and perfusion imaging for ischemia diagnosis. J Am Coll Cardiol. 2019;73:161-73.
62. Douglas PS, Pontone G, Hlatky MA, Patel MR, Norgaard BL, Byrne RA, et al. Clinical outcomes of fractional flow reserve by computed tomographic angiography-guided diagnostic strategies vs. usual care in patients with suspected coronary artery disease: the prospective longitudinal trial of FFR (CT): outcome and resource impacts study. Europ Heart J. 2015;36:3359-67.
63. Douglas PS, De Bruyne B, Pontone G, Patel MR, Norgaard BL, Byrne RA, et al. 1-Year Outcomes of FFRCT-Guided Care in Patients with Suspected Coronary Disease: The PLATFORM Study. J Am Coll Cardiol. 2016;68:435-45.
64. Collet C, Onuma Y, Andreini D, Sonck J, Pompilio G, Mushtaq S, et al. Coronary computed tomography angiography for heart team decision-making in multivessel coronary artery disease. Eur Heart J. 2018;39:3689-98.
65. Curzen N, Nicholas Z, Stuart B, Wilding S, Hill K, Shambrook J, et al. Fractional flow reserve derived from computed tomography coronary angiography in the assessment and management of stable chest pain: the FORECAST randomized trial. Eur Heart J. 2021;42:3844-52.
66. Biscaglia S, Uretsky B, Barbato E, Collet C, Onuma Y, Jeremias A, et al. Invasive coronary physiology after stent implantation: another step toward precision medicine. JACC Cardiovasc Interv. 2021;14:237-46.
67. Lee JM, Lee SH, Shin D, Choi KH, van de Hoef TP, Kim HK, et al. Physiology-based revascularization: a new approach to plan and optimize percutaneous coronary intervention. JACC Asia. 2021;1:14-36.
68. Collet C, Sonck J, Vandeloo B, Mizukami T, Roosens B, Lochy S, et al. Measurement of hyperemic pullback pressure gradients to characterize patterns of coronary atherosclerosis. J Am Coll Cardiol. 2019;74:1772-84.
69. Hakeem A, Ghosh B, Shah K, Agarwal S, Kasula S, Hacioglu Y, et al. Incremental prognostic value of post-intervention Pd/Pa in patients undergoing ischemia-driven percutaneous coronary intervention. JACC Cardiovasc Interv. 2019; 12:2002-14.
70. Shin D, Lee SH, Lee JM, Choi KH, Hwang D, Lee HJ, et al. Prognostic implications of post-intervention resting Pd/Pa and fractional flow reserve in patients with stent implantation. JACC Cardiovasc Interv. 2020;13:1920-33.
71. Caullery B, Riou L, Barone-Rochette G. Coronary Angiography Upgraded by Imaging Post-Processing: Present and Future Directions. Diagnostics. 2023;13:1978.

72. Johnson NP, Toth GG, Lai D, Zhu H, Açar G, Agostoni P, et al. Prognostic value of fractional flow reserve: linking physiologic severity to clinical outcomes. J Am Coll Cardiol. 2014;64:1641-54.
73. Pijls NH, De Bruyne B, Peels K, Van Der Voort PH, Bonnier HJ, Bartunek J Koolen JJ, et al. Measurement of fractional flow reserve to assess the functional severity of coronary-artery stenoses. N Engl J Med. 1996;334:1703-8.
74. Hwang D, Lee JM, Lee HJ, Kim SH, Nam CW, Hahn JY, et al. Influence of target vessel on prognostic relevance of fractional flow reserve after coronary stenting. EuroIntervention. 2019;15:457-64.
75. Leone AM, De Caterina AR, Basile E, Gardi A, Laezza D, Mazzari MA, et al. Influence of the amount of myocardium subtended by a stenosis on fractional flow reserve. Circ Cardiovasc Interv. 2013;6:29-36.
76. Klues HG, Schwarz ER, vom Dahl J, Reffelmann T, Hl R, Potthast K, et al. Disturbed intracoronary hemodynamics in myocardial bridging: early normalization by intracoronary stent placement. Circulation. 1997;96:2905-13.
77. Escaned J, Cortés J, Flores A, Goicolea J, Alfonso F, Hernández R, et al. Importance of diastolic fractional flow reserve and dobutamine challenge in physiologic assessment of myocardial bridging. J Am Coll Cardiol. 2003;42:226-33.
78. Aleksandric SB, Djordjevic-Dikic AD, Dobric MR, Giga VL, Soldatovic IA, Vukcevic V, et al. Functional assessment of myocardial bridging with conventional and diastolic fractional flow reserve: vasodilator versus inotropic provocation. J Am Heart Assoc. 2021;10(13):e020597.

CHAPTER 11

Balloon Uncrossable Lesions: Technical Approach

AV Ganesh Kumar

INTRODUCTION

Balloon uncrossable lesions are typically encountered in long calcific lesions, chronic total occlusions, in-stent restenosis, and side branch access in bifurcation lesions. Very occasionally they might be encountered in patients with acute coronary syndromes, it might also happen that a lesion which was earlier negotiable with a balloon is subsequently found to be uncrossable. This chapter will help you to understand the tips and tricks of negotiating such a lesion and achieve a successful revascularization.

It is very important that prior to labeling a lesion as uncrossable, it is preferable to confirm that the wire is placed in the distal true lumen as use of adjunctive devices and aggressive manipulation will increase the chances of perforation and complications.

MECHANISMS TO ACHIEVE SUCCESSFUL CROSSING (FLOWCHART 1)

- Increase the support
- Balloon-mediated atheromodification
- Plaque modification devices

Flowchart 1: Step-wise approach to noncrossable lesions.

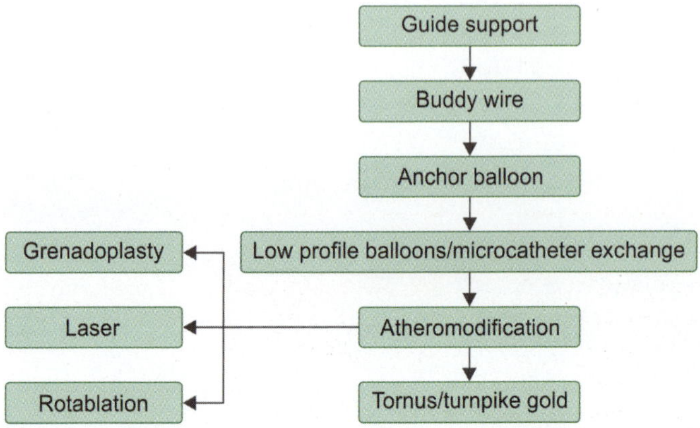

Guide support
↓
Buddy wire
↓
Anchor balloon
↓
Low profile balloons/microcatheter exchange
↓
Atheromodification → Grenadoplasty / Laser / Rotablation
↓
Tornus/turnpike gold

Increase the Support

Passive Support

Innate guide design with back up support against opposite aortic wall provides coaxial guide alignment and avoids the need for active guide manipulation. Selection of guide catheters should be based on cuspal depth, orientation of coronary ostia, and the length of engaging vessel (LMCA/PROXIMAL RCA); it is also preferable to anticipate placement of longer vascular sheath as it will overcome peripheral tortuosity and provide good guide stability. We also prefer to base our guide selection on the diagnostic coronary angiogram catheter sizes and catheter orientation in the coronary ostia. In the authors experience, **Table 1** can be a good basis for guide selection.

Most of the time, it is difficult to change the guide after wire crossing, hence prior appropriate guide selection is useful.

Active Support

- *Anchoring:* Balloon anchoring increases guide support, side branch anchor (Conus for RCA, Diagonal for LAD) with a small balloon is the most feasible initial option as it can allow better tracking of plaque modification devices. Sometimes patient might develop chest pain or rarely perforation can occur because of size mismatch and trauma leading to perforation. Hence, sizing should preferably be 1:1 sizing avoiding balloon slippage and vessel trauma. Distal anchoring can also be performed by going subintimal, reaching the distal true lumen and inflating the balloon leading to pinning of the primary guidewire; sometimes, a stent can also be used as to jail the secondary wire called as buddy wire stent anchor[1] increasing the guide support a leading to enhanced trackability.[1]
- *Wire support:* Presence of additional wires (buddy wire) provides both active and passive support with better guide alignment and enhanced trackability, usually this should be the initial choice in noncrossable lesions. Wire support can be enhanced by exchanging the primary wire with extra support wires which have stiffer shafts, Grand Slam (Asahi Intec) and Sion-ES Wire (Asahi Intec) are the two most commonly used support guidewires in our practice. Using of such wires will remove proximal tortuosity and further enhance guide support.

TABLE 1: Basis for guide selection.

Left main coronary artery	*Right coronary artery*
• *PB (ASAHI INTEC), EBU (MEDTRONIC):* Normal anterior orientation and superior orientation • *Amplatz:* Posterior orientation	• *Horizontal orientation:* Judkins right • *Superior orientation:* Amplatz/Hockey stick • *Inferior orientation:* Multipurpose, Judkins right

Deep wire crossing is a technique in which a polymer jacketed wire is placed via the septal perforators deep into the ventricle through arterioluminal communications, Khelimskii et al.[2] reported a 3.2% incidence of in-hospital major adverse cardiac events with this technique. Retrograde trapping of antegrade wire can sometimes be useful in retrograde CTO cases to enhance support.

- *Guide catheter extensions (GCE):* They are one of the mainstay in managing technically challenging and uncrossable lesions. Guide catheter extensions help to remove proximal tortuosity, enhance guide alignment, deliver devices in calcified and tortuous vessels and they are also helpful in anomalous coronary artery origins and chronic total occlusions, GuideLiner V3 Catheter (Teleflex, USA), Guidezilla II Guide Extension Catheter (Boston Scientific, USA), and Guideplus Catheter (Nipro Corp, Japan) are the most commonly used GCE in India. They do not require removal of Y connector as compared to Heartrail II Guiding Catheter (Terumo, Japan) and Proxis System (St Jude Medical, USA). Delivery of the catheter extensions to the target site can be accomplished with a compliant balloon inflated at nominal pressures just proximal to target lesion or via the inch worming technique (intermittent inflation and deflation of a small balloon positioned halfway in and half out the guide catheter extension, with advancement of the guide catheter extension when the balloon is being simultaneously deflated).

  Coaxial anchoring of guide catheter extensions can be performed via a balloon inflation by a second guide catheter stabilizing the extension.[1]

  Complications associated with use of guide catheter extensions include air embolism, vessel dissection, and sometimes stent deformation, hence periodic back flush is needed and forceful injections and maneuvering need to be avoided. Chandra S et al.[3] have provided a detailed account on guide catheters and its role in interventional cardiology.

Balloon-mediated Atheromodification

Lower the Better

A lower profile balloon like the mini Trek (Abbott Vascular) and Apex push (Boston scientific) with a single marker can significantly enhance the chances of crossability; the profile of a balloon is maximum at the site of marker and hence if we are able to negotiate the marker into the proximal cap, a high pressure inflation will usually alter the proximal cap and will subsequently allow a different balloon to cross the lesion. Often, serial dilation with gradually increasing diameters will be required to successfully negotiate the lesion or it might also happen sometimes that a previously balloon crossable lesion becomes noncrossable after balloon dilation as the disruption of calcium alters the intraluminal geometry leading to luminal encroachment and making it uncrossable and we might have to use atheroablative devices like rotablation for such cases.

TABLE 2: Low-profile balloons.

	Tip entry profile	*Crossing profile*
NIC Nano Hydro (0.85 mm) (SIS Medical)	0.016″	0.0195″
NIC 1.1 Hydro (SIS Medical)	0.016″	0.0205″
Ikazuchi Zero 1.0 (Kaneka Medical)	0.016″	0.023″
Mini Trek 1.2 (Abbott v)	0.018″	0.026″
Alveo HP 0.75 (Brosmed com)	0.0156″	0.0203″

Grenadoplasty

It is most commonly used technique in which a small low-profile balloon **(Table 2)** is advanced as far as possible into the proximal cap and inflated at high pressures till it ruptures (intentionally). This balloon rupture creates a contrast jet that modifies the plaque leading to successful crossing with a new balloon. In our experience, we have been using the low-profile ALVEO-HP noncompliant balloons which can be inflated at high pressures and enhances the success rate, the approximate success rate is around 50% for grenadoplasty as reported by Voo et al. with a small risk of staining and perforation with this technique.

Wire Cutting Technique

This is a combination of balloon and wire-mediated atheromodification, in which two wires are made to cross the lesion, balloon is advanced over the first guidewire and deeply wedged into the lesion as far as possible, the second guidewire is then withdrawn keeping the balloon inflated leading to cutting and modification of proximal cap. Success rate of this technique is approximately 60%.[4] A modification of the same is seesaw wire cutting technique where two balloons are serially inflated and deflated at the proximal cap leading to a cutting effect with the pinned wire.[1]

Plaque Modification Devices

Laser

Excimer laser coronary atherectomy (ELCA) is very effective for treatment of balloon uncrossable lesions. The mechanism of action of laser is photothermal, photochemical, and photomechanical disruption of resistant plaque,[5] subsequent cutting balloon dilations will lead to enhanced luminal area. ELCA offers advantages in terms of simplicity of use, fast learning curve, and higher technical success rate, and its ability to be compatible with any 0.014 inch guidewire gives it an added advantage over other atheroablative devices. The photoacoustic effect created by laser leads to fracture in calcium and subsequent dilation of lesions. ELCA should always be performed after flushing out the contrast and under continuous saline infusion, while presence of contrast will lead to large bubble formation and increases risk of perforation. The authors have been using ELCA as first choice in noncrossable lesions after primary attempts are unsuccessful, but the availability of this modality in India is only in a very few centers.

Atherectomy

Use of rotational and orbital atherectomy can greatly facilitate crossing of such lesion, the biggest hurdle faced is the exchange with the Rotawire which will require microcatheter advancement to the distal lumen to exchange to Rotawire and frequently a microcatheter is not able to cross the lesion. Hence, advancing the microcatheter as deep as possible into the lesion and then exchanging with a Rotawire can done followed by rotablation. A lowest profile microcatheter called as Mogul (Nipro Japan) can cross the uncrossable lesions for Rotawire exchange. This catheter is under pending regulators approval in India and is likely to be available soon for the end users. Newer atherectomy guidewires, such as the Viperwire Advance flex tip (CSI Inc., St Paul), with improved handling characteristics can facilitate atherectomy of balloon uncrossable lesions.

Microcatheters

Dedicated plaque modification microcatheters such as the Tornus (Asahi Intecc) and the Turnpike Gold (Teleflex) are sometimes quite helpful in balloon uncrossable lesions. They have to be rotated (spinning 18–20 times) with a gentle push through the lesion and should be allowed to counter clock after each cycle of clockwise spinning (to release the tension and prevent uncoiling of these braided catheter). The Tornus microcatheter should be advanced using counter-clockwise rotation and withdrawn using clockwise rotation. The Turnpike Gold microcatheter is advanced by turning clockwise and withdrawn by turning counter-clockwise. Once the lesion is crossed, it can be exchanged with a Rotawire for further atheromodification or it can be removed and exchanged with a low-profile balloon to dilate the lesion.[1] The use of microcatheters has declined with the advent of newer low-profile balloons and usage of LASER; microcatheters like FINECROSS (Terumo Inc) and CORSAIR (Terumo Inc) are not plaque modifying but sometimes screwing and unscrewing motion (fine cross should never be rotated, only corsair pro) can lead to negotiating such a lesion and exchange with a high support wire can enhance balloon trackability. Mogul microcatheter launched by Nipro recently has been found to be quite helpful in providing backup support and crossing resistant lesions.

Combinations of plaque modification devices:

- *Combined use of rotational atherectomy and excimer LASER (RASER angioplasty):* LASER which allows sufficient plaque modification that allows microcatheter advancement and exchange with a Rotawire followed by calcium debulking with rotational atherectomy which will allow subsequent balloon expansion and optimal stent expansion.

- *ELCA-Tripsy:* Plaque modification by LASER followed by shockwave intravascular lithotripsy (Shockwave Medical Inc.) can also be used for optimal lesion preparation.

CONCLUSION

In the authors experience, a combination of the above techniques is usually required to negotiate such lesion. First of all, balloon uncrossable lesions should be anticipated by the operator and a 7Fr or 8Fr guide catheter with good back-up support should be selected for engagement. Changing the guide catheter may not be possible or cumbersome after crossing the lesion with guidewire. Then the use of low crossing profile balloons followed by use of anchor balloons and finally a guide extension (at time GE can be used upfront) should be tried first before committing to plaque modification devices. These lesions are usually calcific in nature and the true extent and disease burden should be complimented by intravascular imaging so that appropriate devices can be used.

Use of adjunctive devices will increase the procedural time and increase the risk of thrombosis, hence ACT (activated clotting time) monitoring should be periodically performed (every half hour in our practice); subintimal techniques like the external crush and the subintimal distal anchor technique are preferably to be avoided as the chances of complications are quite high and the success reports are quite few and anecdotal.

Catheterization laboratories where chronic total occlusions are performed routinely by CTO operators will frequently encounter such lesions and hence it is very pertinent that these laboratories should be well equipped with the relevant adjunctive therapeutics for uncrossable lesions.

REFERENCES

1. Elrayes MM, Xenogiannis I, Nikolakopoulos I, Vemmou E, Wollmuth J, Abi Rafeh N, et al. An algorithmic approach to balloon-uncrossable coronary lesions. Catheter Cardiovasc Interv. 2021;97(6):E817-25.
2. Khelimskii D, Badoyan A, Krestyaninov O. The deep-wire crossing technique: a novel method for treating balloon-uncrossable lesions. J Invasive Cardiol. 2019;31(12):E362-8.
3. Chandra S, Tiwari A, Chaudhary G, Yadav R. Guide catheter extension systems: Hype or a need? Indian Heart J. 2021;73(5):535-8.
4. Hu XQ, Tang L, Zhou SH, Fang ZF, Shen XQ. A novel approach to facilitating balloon crossing chronic total occlusions: the "wire-cutting" technique. J Interv Cardiol. 2012;25(3):297-303.
5. McQuillan C, Jackson MWP, Brilakis ES, Egred M. Uncrossable and undilatable lesions-A practical approach to optimizing outcomes in PCI. Catheter Cardiovasc Interv. 2021;97(1):121-6.

CHAPTER 12

Ectatic Coronaries with Heavy Thrombus Burden in Primary Percutaneous Coronary Intervention: Approach

Ajith R Bhagawat

INTRODUCTION

Coronary artery ectasia (CAE) is defined as localized or diffuse dilatation of the coronary artery up to 1.5 times the contiguous diameter of healthy (normal) segment of the vessel. It is differentiated from coronary artery aneurysm (CAA) by width to length ratio of the dilated coronary segment (CAE: >1.5 times and width:length <1; CAA: >1.5 times and width:length >1). An anatomical classification of CAE was proposed by Markis et al., dividing into four phenotypes according to its extension in the coronary tree: Type I—diffuse ectasia of two or three vessels; type II—diffuse ectasia in one vessel and focal dilatation in another vessel; type III—diffuse ectasia of one vessel only and focal aneurysm as type III and IV, respectively.[1]

EPIDEMIOLOGY AND RISK FACTORS

The reported prevalence of 1.2–4.9% among patients undergoing coronary angiography. CAE can be due to both congenital and acquired causes. While it is known that CAE is often a sequelae of childhood Kawasaki's disease, atherosclerosis accounts for approximately half of the cases in adults. Other 20–30% cases of CAE are caused by congenital anomalies. Only 10–20% of cases of CAE have been reported resulting from inflammatory or connective tissue diseases.[2]

Several reports showed a gender predominance with a high prevalence of CAE in men. Hypertension, smoking, dyslipidemia, familial hypercholesterolemia, and cocaine abuse reported a higher risk. Nevertheless, in contrast with coronary artery disease (CAD), CAE has an inverse association with diabetes mellitus due to negative remodeling of the artery wall, the impairment of compensatory vessel enlargement. Right coronary artery (RCA) is the most frequently involved, followed by left anterior descending (LAD), left circumflex (LCx), and less frequently left main (LM).

CLINICAL FEATURES AND MANAGEMENT

The clinical manifestations of CAE are heterogeneous, ranging from occasionally recognized during coronary angiography or computed tomography (CT) to different possible scenarios like acute coronary syndrome (ACS), effort angina, exercise-induced ischemia, microvascular dysfunction, compression of adjacent cardiac or noncardiac structures and rarely rupture with acute cardiac tamponade.

The gold standard for the diagnostic assessment of CAE remains coronary angiography: The typical angiographical features are delayed antegrade contrast filling, segmental back flow, and local deposition of dye in the dilated coronary segment, all of them able to depict the severe flow disturbances of CAE.[3] Coronary imaging [such as intravascular ultrasound (IVUS) and optical coherence tomography (OCT)] is useful to better assess vessel wall architecture and to distinguish between aneurysm and complex plaques angiographically. This is crucial for prognostic stratification and therapeutic guidance, due to the high risk of ACS associated with the presence of an ulcerated or ruptured atherosclerotic plaque. Moreover, IVUS might be helpful to precisely estimate the minimal lumen area and the percentage of the stenosis, to evaluate the thrombotic and calcific burden of the lesion, and to guide stent sizing and implantation when percutaneous coronary intervention (PCI) is planned. Compared to IVUS, OCT has greater axial and spatial resolution that might be helpful in CAE to assess atherosclerotic plaque features, thrombus burden, and mechanisms of PCI failure. However, its application in large vessel is limited by the low penetration depth, with loss of image definition as the distance of the anatomical structures from the lens increases.

Other technologies such as CT and MRI can provide important information on CAE anatomical features, such as shape, maximum diameter, and presence of concomitant stenosis, avoiding the pitfalls of coronary angiography. Furthermore, CT allows a three-dimensional reconstruction of the coronary tree that might clarify anatomical and functional relations with other adjacent structures (i.e., fistulous communications with cardiac or noncardiac chambers). Beside this, transthoracic and transesophageal echocardiography have a role for long-term follow-up in adulthood of patients with history of Kawasaki disease.

Coronary artery ectasia can present as acute coronary syndrome with or without any underlying atherosclerotic plaque rupture and can advance into acute myocardial infarction (AMI). Clinical observations have demonstrated that thrombosis, embolization, and rupture of the involved segments are the leading causes of AMI and sudden death in patients with CAE. It complicates primary percutaneous coronary intervention (PPCI) because of the high thrombus burden that can cause distal embolization leading to no-reflow. Hence, the success of PPCI in CAE is suboptimal due to organized thrombus, slow flow during the procedure, and floating stent struts causing recurrent vessel closure in the ectatic segments.

Coronary angiography is commonly used for quantification of the thrombus burden and defined as the presence of a filling defect with reduced contrast density or haziness. Most widely used Thrombolysis in Myocardial

Infarction (TIMI) scale relies on the relative estimated size of the thrombus and of the affected vessel, using a score ranging from grade 0 (no thrombus) to grade 5 (very large thrombus with complete occlusion).

Current guidelines recommend primary PCI as the preferred treatment option in ST-elevation myocardial infarction (STEMI) patients.[4] Compared to thrombolysis, primary PCI is more effectively obtain patency of the infarct-related artery (IRA), resulting in smaller infarcts, less number of acute and long-term adverse events, including recurrent MI and death. Management of lesions with a large thrombus burden during primary PCI is still challenging. Several pharmacological and mechanical approaches have been suggested in reducing thrombus burden.

PHARMACOLOGICAL THERAPY

Dual Antiplatelet Therapy

Early administration of dual antiplatelet therapy (DAPT) decreases thrombus burden and improves clinical outcome. Aspirin in a loading dose of 150–300 mg orally inhibits thromboxane A2-mediated platelet inhibition. Onset starts within 30–60 minutes and lasted up to lifespan of platelets. A potent P2Y12 inhibitor (prasugrel 60 mg or ticagrelor 180 mg or clopidogrel 600 mg) must be used for more aggressive platelet aggregation. Prasugrel and ticagrelor have a more rapid onset of action, greater potency, and are superior to clopidogrel in clinical outcomes. An intravenous P2Y12 agent (e.g., cangrelor) may also be considered in patients not pretreated with oral P2Y12 receptor inhibitors at the time of PCI or in those who are intubated or unable to have oral agents.

Glycoprotein IIb/IIIa Inhibitors

Glycoprotein IIb/IIIa inhibitors (GPIs) (abciximab, tirofiban, and eptifibatide) are more potent inhibitor of platelet aggregation by competing with von Willebrand factor (vWF) and fibrinogen for GPIIb/IIIa receptor binding. GPIs have been found to be effective in dissolving angiographically proven thrombus and in restoring TIMI flow. Abciximab is the most used in clinical experience in the setting of STEMI undergoing primary PCI, although high bleeding rates remain a concern.

Based on available data, recent guidelines state that routine use of upstream GPIs in STEMI patients undergoing PPCI is not recommended and should be considered only for bailout therapy if there is evidence of large thrombus burden, slow or no-reflow or a thrombotic complication, or could be administered upstream only in high-risk patients undergoing transfer for primary PCI.

Intracoronary GP IIb/IIIa intracoronary administration of abciximab in the infarct-related artery has theoretical advantage over IV route that it can provide higher local concentration, resulting in a higher receptor occupancy leading to higher rate of thrombus resolution. Some small studies have shown benefits of intracoronary bolus administration of abciximab but these results have not been confirmed in large-scale clinical trial. However, in the absence of conclusive evidence, the role of intracoronary bolus of GPIs still needs to be established by large randomized trials.

Anticoagulants

Effective anticoagulation is needed during primary PCI to inhibit the coagulation cascade and progression of thrombus. Anticoagulant options for primary PCI include UFH (unfractionated heparin), enoxaparin, and bivalirudin. Based on large body of experience, the routine use of UFH during primary PCI is primary recommendation. A meta-analysis involving 23 PCI trials (30,966 patients, 33% primary PCI) demonstrated superiority of enoxaparin over UFH in reducing mortality and bleeding outcomes, particularly in patients undergoing primary PCI. Bivalirudin should be considered in patients at high bleeding risk and heparin-induced thrombocytopenia.

Vasodilators

Several vasodilators have been used intracoronary during primary PCI in large thrombus burden to decrease risk of distal embolization and no-reflow.

- *Nitroglycerin:* Nitroglycerin is an endothelium-dependent coronary vasodilator acting by releasing nitric oxide, which subsequently activates cyclic GMP leading to reduction in intracellular calcium resulting in smooth muscle relaxation. Nitroglycerin may be useful when there is associated spasm of epicardial coronary artery. It has been shown to cause coronary artery dilation with doses as little as 5 mg. The use in moderate doses (50–200 mg) produces maximal or nearly maximal dilation, while larger doses (>450 mg) result in no further dilation.
- *Nitroprusside:* Nitroprusside is an endothelial-independent direct donor of nitric oxide. It produces more balanced arterial and venous dilation thus effectively dilating both the epicardial coronary arteries and the small resistance arterioles. Intracoronary nitroprusside has been shown to be a safe and effective therapy for no-reflow during primary PCI in the setting of intracoronary thrombi. Doses of 50–100 mg bolus can be used intracoronary and repeated as needed.
- *Adenosine:* Adenosine is an endogenous purine nucleoside with a very short half-life (5–10 s). It is primarily a vasodilator of small coronary resistance arterioles, with no effect on the large epicardial arteries. It has been shown to decrease slow flow/no-reflow, during primary PCI in presence of intracoronary thrombi. Intracoronary bolus doses of 30–60 μg

have a lower incidence of flushing, headache, and dyspnea compared to IV dose. Contraindications are high-grade AV block or sick sinus syndrome or active or severe bronchospastic lung disease.

- *Calcium channel blockers:* Intracoronary nicardipine (200 mg) is more potent and prolonged microvascular dilation with minimal negative chronotropic and inotropic effects as compared to IC verapamil (200 mg) and diltiazem (1 mg). It has been shown to be safe and effective for the reversal of no-reflow during interventions of native and saphenous vein graft (SVG) lesions.
- *Intracoronary thrombolysis:* Intracoronary delivery of thrombolytic agent results in higher concentration of thrombolytics at the site of thrombus and more effective thrombolysis. Small studies of local delivery of fibrinolytics as an adjunct to primary PCI demonstrated promising results in STEMI patients with a large thrombus burden and failed manual aspiration and showed reduced thrombus burden and improved myocardial reperfusion without any major bleeding. Intracoronary bolus of urokinase (200,000 U) and low-dose intracoronary alteplase (10 mg or 20 mg) are used in various trials. At present, there is no sufficient data for intracoronary use of fibrinolytics. There are currently two ongoing Phase III trials to evaluate intracoronary low-dose alteplase, the Adjunctive Low-dose tPA in Primary PCI for STEMI (STRIVE) trial and tenecteplase, the Restoring Microcirculatory Perfusion in STEMI (RESTORE-MI) trial which may further address the issue.
- *Percutaneous devices:* At present, two types of devices are available—thrombectomy devices and embolic protection devices. Thrombectomy devices aim at reducing thrombus burden, while embolic protection devices aim at capturing the debris liberated during PCI.
- *Thrombectomy devices:* Thrombectomy devices are broadly divided into two groups—manual and mechanical.
- *Manual thrombus aspiration:* Current generation devices have low crossing profile, hydrophilic coating, flexibility, and tapered distal tip. Catheter system is advanced over the guidewire and distal end of catheter system is placed proximal to the thrombus and proximal end is attached to a suction device. With the continued suction, the catheter is advanced distally through the thrombus to allow complete retrieval of the thrombus. Most commonly used manual devices in clinical practice are Export AP (Medtronic). Although this is not routinely recommended during primary PCI, selective and bailout aspiration thrombectomy is reasonable in patients with large residual thrombus burden after opening the vessel with a guidewire or a balloon.
- *Mechanical thrombectomy devices:* The most commonly used mechanical thrombectomy device is the AngioJet rheolytic thrombectomy (RT) catheter. AngioJet uses high velocity saline jets, which leads to dissolution

of thrombus and creates a strong suction of approximately 600 mm Hg at the catheter tip, which produces Venturi effect leading to suction of the thrombus. Based on available literature, it may be concluded that the AngioJet is beneficial in patients with large thrombus burden but not in minimal thrombus. A major concern for this rheolytic thrombectomy is hemolytic anemia with prolonged use. Therefore, total device time use should be limited to 10 minutes. Hemolysis induces the release of adenosine, which can precipitate bradyarrhythmias, hence placement of a temporary pacing wire is recommended, especially when performing thrombectomy in the right coronary artery. Recently, "Penumbra" was introduced as a totally automated mechanical thrombus aspiration device. Although it is primarily recommended for thrombus aspiration from large cerebral vessel in acute stroke, it is increasingly used in coronary system as well.

X-sizer Thrombectomy System

The power-sourced X-sizer thrombectomy catheter (ev3, Minneapolis, MN, USA) is considered one of the most user-friendly mechanical thrombectomy devices. It consists of a helical cutter enclosed within a protective housing, attached to a dual-bore catheter shaft containing guidewire and vacuum extraction lumens. Activation of the handheld controller rotates the helical cutter at 2,100 rpm, which entraps and macerates the thrombus, and extracts it into a vacuum collection bottle.

Excimer Laser Coronary Atherectomy

The CVX-300 cardiovascular laser excimer system (Spectranetics) is the only coronary laser-emitting device currently approved by the US-FDA. It uses Xenon chloride (XeCl) as the active medium and generates pulses of short wavelength, high-energy ultraviolet (UV) light having a wavelength of 308 nm. Laser-generated acoustic shock waves can separate thrombus from the vessel wall, dissolve clot, and vaporize procoagulant mediators. Laser also has an inhibitory effect on platelet aggregation leading to "stunned platelet phenomenon".[5]

Embolic Protection Devices

Embolic protection devices (EPDs) have been developed to decrease distal embolization during SVG interventions and carotid artery stenting. While there is evidence to support embolic protection devices in SVG interventions, these have not been replicated in the setting of STEMI. EPDs can be divided into three distinct types based on their mechanism of operation: distal occlusion aspiration devices (e.g., PurcuSurge Guardewire, TriActive), distal filters (e.g., filterwire EZ, SpiderRX), and proximal occlusion aspiration devices (e.g., Proxis).[6]

Stenting Strategy

Direct Stenting

A direct stenting strategy reduces the incidence of distal embolization by minimal manipulation and trapping the thrombus behind the stent. There are some disadvantages of direct stenting including, underestimation of the true vessel size, failure to cross in tortuous or calcified lesions, inadequate stent expansion and late stent malapposition, that may increase the risk of restenosis or stent thrombosis. Direct stenting with or without thrombus aspiration might be applied safely in selected patients with AMI with low thrombus grade.

Covered Stent

Covered stents are made up of bare metal stent (BMS) platform covered with a fine mesh that can trap the thrombus and prevent distal embolization. Two types of coronary stents have been evaluated in randomized trials: MGuard (InspireMD) and STENTYS (STENTYS SA). Similar associated lesions like aneurysmal lesions can be effectively achieved with a covered stent.

Deferred Stenting

Deferred strategy may potentially limit the risk of distal coronary embolization in the presence of high thrombus burden. It allows 24–48 hours of intense antithrombotic therapy, including prolonged intravenous GPIIb/IIIa inhibition and heparin anticoagulation. Subsequent angiography frequently shows reduced thrombus burden and PCI may be performed with a significantly lower risk of distal embolization.

Follow-up

The optimal antithrombotic therapy is debated and included DAPT, anticoagulation, or combination of them. An aggressive antithrombotic for first 6 weeks (anticoagulation + DAPT) with INR target between 2.5 and 3 followed by anticoagulation and single antiplatelet therapy appears a reasonable strategy; however, it needs individualized approach.

CONCLUSION

PCI in ectatic coronaries with heavy thrombus burden may lead to no-reflow. It also leads to difficulty in stent sizing which frequently results in stent malapposition. Appropriate use of adjunct devices may help in procedural success and potent antiplatelet therapy improves the clinical outcomes.

REFERENCES

1. Markis JE, Joffe CD, Cohn PF, Feen DJ, Herman MV, Gorlin R. Clinical significance of coronary arterial ectasia. Am J Cardiol. 1976;37(2):217-22.
2. Ozgur Ulas Ozcan, Sadi Gulec. Coronary artery ectasia. cor et vasa 55 (2013) e242–e247.
3. Akram Kawsara, Iván J Núñez Gil, Fahad Alqahtani et al. Management of Coronary Artery Aneurysms. Am Coll Cardiol Intv 2018;11:1211–23.
4. Sunil V Rao, Michelle L O'Donoghue, Marc Ruel, et al. 2025 ACC/AHA/ACEP/NAEMSP/SCAI Guideline for the Management of Patients With Acute Coronary Syndromes: A Report of the American College of Cardiology/American Heart Association Joint Committee on Clinical Practice Guidelines. J Am Coll Cardiol. 2025:S0735-1097(24)10424-X.
5. Hiruma T, Tanaka T, Nanasato M, Isobe M. Excimer laser coronary atherectomy for acute myocardial infarction with coronary artery ectasia and massive thrombosis. AsiaIntervention. 2023;9(2):152-3.
6. Bangalore S, Bhatt DL. Embolic protection devices. Circulation. 2014; 129(17):e470-6.

CHAPTER 13

Approach to Percutaneous Coronary Intervention in Calcified Lesions

Sarita Rao, Roshan Rao, Abhishek Rathore, Achukatla Kumar

INTRODUCTION

Ischemic heart disease (IHD) stands as the primary cause of fatalities and health burden in the adult population of India. With an alarming mortality rate of 109.23 deaths per 100,000 individuals, IHD led to approximately 1.5 million deaths in the country.[1] Coronary artery calcification (CAC) is most common in patients diagnosed with coronary artery disease (CAD).[2] Despite significant progress in interventional procedures, patients with moderate-to-severe CAC face a less favorable prognosis following percutaneous coronary intervention (PCI) compared to those without calcifications.[2-4]

The prevalence of CAC rises with age, particularly in men and individuals diagnosed with stable angina or diabetes.[5] CAC serves as a standalone indicator of advanced CAD, and the extent of calcification is closely associated with the likelihood of cardiac events in the future.[6] As the population ages, there is a growing number of old patients with several comorbidities, deemed unsuitable or elevated-risk candidates for coronary artery bypass surgery (CABG), who are now being directed toward PCI for cases involving intricate coronary anatomy.[7,8]

In angiographic investigations, substantial coronary calcification has been noted in around 20–30% of PCI patients.[9] There has been a notable rise in the frequency of PCIs conducted in significantly calcified CAD patients. This increase is influenced, at least in part, by the ongoing clinical need for enhancing life expectancy and the regular implementation of revascularization procedures in the older population.[4]

PATHOPHYSIOLOGY OF CORONARY CALCIFICATION

Calcification was observed in both the intimal and medial layers of coronary arteries. Intimal calcification poses the risk of significant luminal obstruction, potentially leading to downstream ischemia. On the other hand, calcification localized in the media and periadventitia primarily results in diminished vascular compliance.[3] The process of arterial calcification is complex, involving the apoptosis of macrophages within the lipid core and the transformation of vascular smooth muscle cells into an osteoblast phenotype.

This transformation leads to the formation of sheets or nodules of calcium, and fractures in these calcified structures can result in their breakthrough, forming nodules.[10] Compared to lipid plaques,[11] calcified plaques exhibit reduced compliance, presenting various technical challenges during PCI, such as difficulties in device delivery, equipment damage or entrapment, stent underexpansion, and complications like coronary rupture.

CLINICAL IMPLICATIONS OF CORONARY CALCIFICATION

Coronary artery calcification is universal in all patients with documented CAD. While not all plaques manifest calcification, a notable association exists between the burden of coronary calcium and the presence of atherosclerosis. Initially considered a result of age-related degeneration, CAC is now acknowledged to be intricately linked with CAD.

Encountering moderate-to-severe calcification occurs in approximately one-third of coronary lesions, often linked to increased lesion complexity involving coronary bifurcations and chronic total occlusions. The prevalence of such calcification is expected to rise with factors such as advancing age, chronic kidney disease (CKD), and diabetes.[9,12,13] Patients with severely calcified coronary lesions experience higher overall mortality, poorer outcomes irrespective of clinical presentation, and are less likely to undergo complete revascularization.[4,14,15] Managing heavily calcified lesions poses challenges, including difficulties in dilation, a heightened risk of coronary dissection and perforation, stent delivery failure, stent under expansion, malposition, polymer disruption, and impaired drug delivery with drug-eluting stents (DES).[3,4,9,16,17] These challenges contribute to elevated rates of target lesion failure, restenosis, stent thrombosis, myocardial infarction, and increased mortality.

Lesions characterized by high calcium content (LHCC) among these features represent a formidable challenge, exerting a substantial adverse impact on both the immediate and prolonged outcomes of PCI.

TECHNICAL CHALLENGES IN PERCUTANEOUS CORONARY INTERVENTION FOR CALCIFIED LESIONS

The presence of CAC poses notable challenges due to distinct technical considerations of the procedure and the complexity of the patient population. Calcifications impose constraints on the effectiveness of both balloon angioplasty and the successful delivery and expansion of stents. Additionally, patients with calcified lesions are often older and exhibit a higher prevalence of comorbidities, including renal dysfunction, anemia, and a history of prior CABG.[3,17-19] Studies have underscored that calcifications independently elevate the risk of stent failure and subsequent ischemic events, serving as an independent predictor of major adverse cardiac events (MACE), including death, following PCI.[4,9,20,21] The emergence of newer generation DES, engineered to be less thrombogenic, has demonstrated superiority over earlier DES and bare-metal stents (BMS) in the management of calcified lesions.[18,22]

Coronary calcification has been linked to unfavorable postintervention outcomes, potentially attributable to suboptimal stent expansion. In a comprehensive analysis involving 6,855 participants from two significant randomized controlled trials (RCTs), ACUITY and HORIZONS-AMI, there was a robust association between moderate-to-severe coronary calcification and adverse events, including ischemic target lesion revascularization and stent thrombosis at 1 year.[9] An additional combined analysis covering seven clinical trials of DES, encompassing 6,296 participants, identified complex coronary calcification as the sole predictor of unfavorable outcomes post-intervention, encompassing overall mortality.[4] The recent MACE trial, involving 350 participants across 33 sites, underscored the association of severe calcification with lower lesion and procedural success rates, alongside elevated overall adverse events at 1 year.[23,24]

IMAGING MODALITIES FOR CORONARY CALCIFICATION

Although computer tomography scanning is routinely employed in elective scenarios, emergency cardiac patients undergoing coronary angiography are the initial cohort in which LHCC is typically detected. The precision of coronary angiography in recognizing elevated calcium levels is suboptimal, particularly in in-stent restenosis. Advanced intravascular imaging techniques not only improve LHCC detection but also facilitate a thorough evaluation of calcium burden, distribution, and eccentricity. Optical coherence tomography (OCT) and intravascular ultrasound (IVUS) stand out as the two primary modalities for intravascular imaging **(Figs. 1A and B)**.

A clinical OCT-based scoring system has been incorporated into practice, offering a straightforward assessment of calcific plaque volume and the potential risk of stent underexpansion and adverse outcomes.[25] The scoring system assigns scores based on specific criteria: A maximum calcium arc angle exceeding 180° receives a score of 2, a maximum calcium thickness surpassing 0.5 mm earns a score of 1, and a calcium length exceeding 5 mm also receives a score of 1. A recommendation for calcium modification before stenting is made if the total score is greater than 2 out of 4, as all these parameters have demonstrated independent predictive value for stent underexpansion. Recently, a scoring system based on IVUS was instituted **(Flowchart 1)**.[26,27]

CALCIUM MODIFICATION DEVICES

Procedures for treating vascular problems involve various devices. Those without a balloon include rotational atherectomy (RA) (Rotablator), orbital

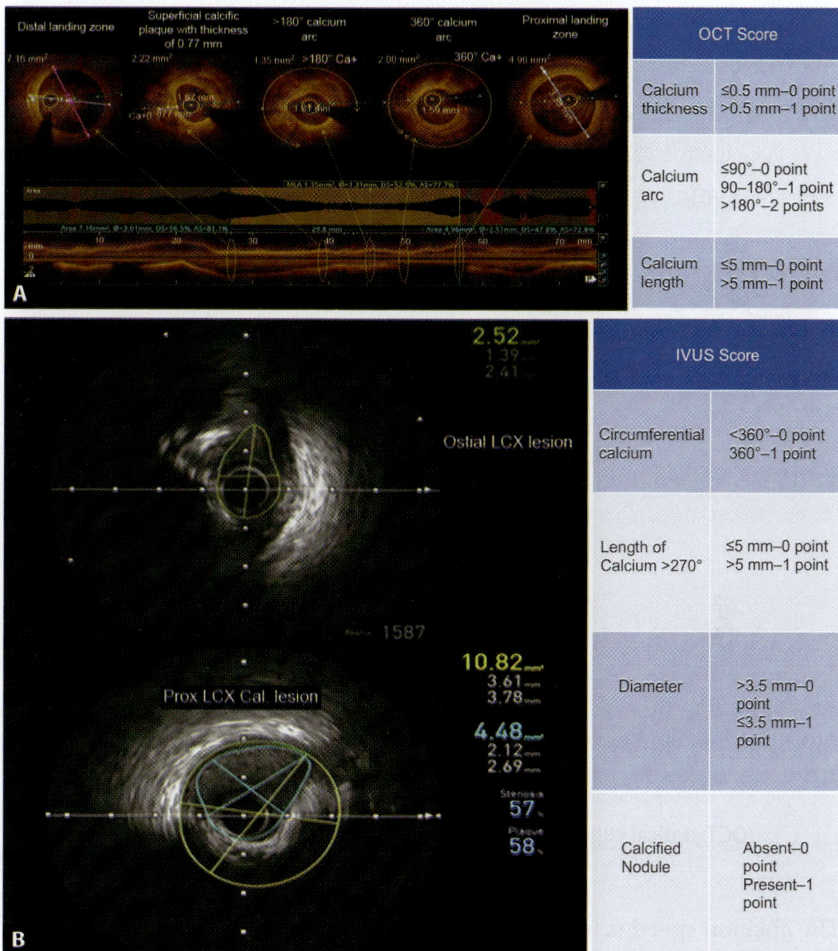

OCT Score	
Calcium thickness	≤0.5 mm–0 point >0.5 mm–1 point
Calcium arc	≤90°–0 point 90–180°–1 point >180°–2 points
Calcium length	≤5 mm–0 point >5 mm–1 point

IVUS Score	
Circumferential calcium	<360°–0 point 360°–1 point
Length of Calcium >270°	≤5 mm–0 point >5 mm–1 point
Diameter	>3.5 mm–0 point ≤3.5 mm–1 point
Calcified Nodule	Absent–0 point Present–1 point

Figs. 1A and B: OCT and IVUS imaging modalities. (Cal: calcific; IVUS: intravascular ultrasound; LCX: left circumflex coronary artery; OCT: optical coherence tomography)

atherectomy (OA) (Diamondback 360), and RA combined with an excimer laser (CVX-300 Excimer Laser System). Alternatively, procedures using devices with a balloon include cutting balloons (WOLVERINE), scoring balloons like AngioSculpt, Scoreflex, and NSE Alpha, as well as the ultra-high pressure noncompliant balloon OPN and the coronary lithoplasty device (CL) by Shockwave Medical. However, their widespread use is limited by complications, technical difficulties, operator expertise, and healthcare resource utilization.

Rotational Atherectomy

Rotational atherectomy continues to be the predominant atherectomy device globally for calcified lesions.[28] The Burr size from 1.25 to 2 is available.

Flowchart 1: Imaging modalities, calcium scoring system, and device selection.

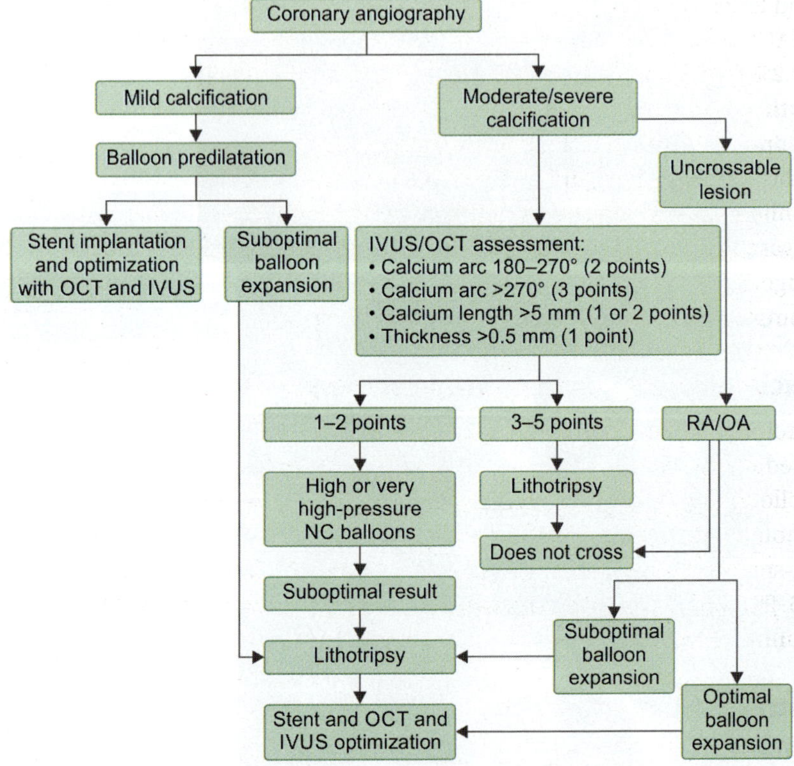

(**OCT:** optical coherence tomography; IVUS: intravascular ultrasound)

The ablation speed is from 120,000 to 220,000 rpm. Burr does unidirectional cutting and ablation. It is extremely useful to modify luminal intimal calcium.

The ROTAXUS trial, the pioneering RCT exploring routine RA before paclitaxel-eluting stent implantation in calcified CAD, involved 240 participants with severely calcified lesions.[29] At the 2-year follow-up, no differences were observed in death, target lesion revascularization, and MI among those with or without RA.[30] Recent equipment advancements include the RotaPro™ system with a digital speedometer and a more maneuverable RotaWire Drive™ for enhanced procedural efficiency.

Orbital Atherectomy

Orbital atherectomy was initially developed in 2007 for peripheral intervention, received FDA approval in 2013 for coronary intervention. This technique operates through the rapid, continual elliptical rotation of the crown, leading to a rise in orbital diameter. It has a bidirectional orbiting crown with differential sanding technology. It enables modification of both luminal intimal and deep calcium.

The ORBIT I trial enrolled 50 participants with calcified CAD for the safety and feasibility of OA.[31] Achieving procedural success in 94% of cases, adverse MACE events were recorded in 12.1% at the 6-month and increased to 21.2% for 5 years.[32] The subsequent ORBIT II trial, involving 443 participants with complex calcified lesions, met both primary safety and efficacy endpoints. Rates of in-hospital MI, target vessel revascularization, or cardiac mortality were low, and at 3 years, cumulative MACE events were 23.5%.[33] While no significance was noted in various outcomes, higher target vessel revascularization rates were observed in the group with ≥95% stenosis. The ongoing ECLIPSE study targets to register approximately 2,000 participants, comparing OA with conventional balloon angioplasty.[34]

Excimer Laser Coronary Atherectomy

Excimer laser coronary atherectomy (ELCA), introduced to human medical procedures in 1988, originally emerged as a viable substitute for balloon angioplasty in addressing intricate coronary lesions.[35,36] It delivers photoablation via a catheter for tissue breakdown. ELCA, primarily used for in-stent restenosis, demonstrated success in the ELLEMENT registry, where 96.4% of patients with underexpanded stents showed improvement in the luminal area.[37]

Intravascular Lithotripsy

Intravascular lithotripsy (IVL) draws on the lithotripsy principle applied in managing calculi for over 30 years. Its introduction to coronary intervention took place in 2015. It used balloon-based sonic emitters for the breakdown of calcium. It has excellent results in modifying deep as well as superficial calcium selectively with literally no injury to soft tissue.

The Disrupt CAD I trial, a prospective study, evaluated lithoplasty in 60 participants with severely calcified atherosclerotic plaques.[38] Stent delivery was successful in all patients, and at 6 months, the MACE rate was 8.3%. The subsequent Disrupt CAD II trial involved 120 participants and identified calcium fractures in 78.7% of lesions after lithoplasty.[39] Disrupt CAD III, designed for regulatory approval, enrolled 431 participants and reported a success rate of 92.4%.[40] At 30 days, 92.2% of participants were free from MACE. The OCT sub-study revealed calcium fractures in 67.4% of lesions.[40]

Specialized Angioplasty Balloons

Before atherectomy devices emerged, these balloons traditionally constituted the primary approach for prestenting treatment in calcified lesions. There are microblades mounted to ablate calcium. Recent retrospective data have not shown significant differences in outcomes in comparing cutting balloon angioplasty to alternative calcium-modifying approaches like RA and conventional balloon angioplasty.[41-43] Improved results were observed with a combination of RA and scoring balloons.

CONCLUSION

Healthcare professionals have long acknowledged that certain characteristics of coronary artery lesions contribute to the complexity of interventions. The presence of complex lesions is linked to unfavorable cardiovascular outcomes and an increased risk of subsequent ischemic events. The introduction of novel devices in recent years has significantly broadened the range of tools available for addressing heavily calcified lesions. The challenge lies in the operator's ability to acquaint themselves with the strengths and limitations of each device, enabling the adoption of the most suitable, individualized approach for the specific target lesion. The emergence of new percutaneous techniques, coupled with high-resolution intracoronary imaging, has opened up opportunities to tackle the treatment of heavily calcified lesions, which are known to pose a high risk of periprocedural complications.

REFERENCES

1. Institute for Health Metrics and Evaluation (IHME). Findings from the global burden of disease study 2019. Seattle, WA: IHME; 2021.
2. Genereux P, Redfors B, Witzenbichler B, Arsenault MP, Weisz G, Stuckey TD, et al. Two-year outcomes after percutaneous coronary intervention of calcified lesions with drug-eluting stents. Int J Cardiol. 2017;231:61-7.
3. Madhavan MV, Tarigopula M, Mintz GS, Maehara A, Stone GW, Genereux P. Coronary artery calcification: pathogenesis and prognostic implications. J Am Coll Cardiol. 2014;63:1703-14.
4. Bourantas CV, Zhang YJ, Garg S, Iqbal J, Valgimigli M, Windecker S, et al. Prognostic implications of coronary calcification in patients with obstructive coronary artery disease treated by percutaneous coronary intervention: a patient-level pooled analysis of 7 contemporary stent trials. Heart. 2014;100:1158-64.
5. Mori H, Torii S, Kutyna M, Sakamoto A, Finn AV, Virmani R. Coronary artery calcification and its progression: what does it really mean? JACC Cardiovasc Imaging. 2018;11:127-42.
6. Yano Y, O'Donnell CJ, Kuller L, Kavousi M, Erbel R, Ning H, et al. Association of coronary artery calcium score vs age with cardiovascular risk in older adults: an analysis of pooled population-based studies. JAMA Cardiol. 2017;2:986-94.
7. Barbato E, Carrie D, Dardas P, Fajadet J, Gaul G, Haude M, et al. European Expert consensus on rotational atherectomy. EuroIntervention. 2015;11:30-6.
8. Sharma SK, Tomey MI, Teirstein PS, Kini AS, Reitman AB, Lee AC, et al. North American expert review of rotational atherectomy. Circ Cardiovasc Interv. 2019;12:e007448.
9. Généreux P, Madhavan MV, Mintz GS, Maehara A, Palmerini T, Lasalle L, et al. Ischemic outcomes after coronary intervention of calcified vessels in acute coronary syndromes. Pooled analysis from the HORIZONS-AMI (Harmonizing Outcomes With Revascularization and Stents in Acute Myocardial Infarction)

and ACUITY (Acute Catheterization and Urgent Intervention Triage Strategy) trials. J Am Coll Cardiol. 2014;63:1845-54.

10. Akers EJ, Nicholls SJ, Di Bartolo BA. Plaque calcification: do lipoproteins have a role? Arterioscler Thromb Vasc Biol. 2019;39:1902-10.
11. Virmani R, Burke AP, Farb A, Kolodgie FD. Pathology of the vulnerable plaque. J Am Coll Cardiol. 2006;47:C13-8.
12. Andrews J, Psaltis PJ, Bartolo BAD, Nicholls SJ, Puri R. Coronary arterial calcification: a review of mechanisms, promoters and imaging. Trends Cardiovasc Med. 2018;28:491-501.
13. Kassimis G, Raina T, Kontogiannis N, Patri G, Abramik J, Zaphiriou A, et al. How should we treat heavily calcified coronary artery disease in contemporary practice? From atherectomy to intravascular lithotripsy. Cardiovasc Revasc Med. 2019;20:1172-83.
14. Huisman J, Van Der Heijden LC, Kok MM, Danse PW, Jessurun GA, Stoel MG, et al. Impact of severe lesion calcification on clinical outcome of patients with stable angina, treated with newer generation permanent polymercoated drug-eluting stents: a patient-level pooled analysis from TWENTE and DUTCH PEERS (TWENTE II). Am Heart J. 2016;175:121-9.
15. Huisman J, van der Heijden LC, Kok MM, Louwerenburg HW, Danse PW, Jessurun GAJ, et al. Two-year outcome after treatment of severely calcified lesions with newer generation drug-eluting stents in acute coronary syndromes. J Cardiol. 2017;69:660-5.
16. Moussa I, Ellis SG, Jones M, Kereiakes DJ, McMartin D, Rutherford B, et al. Impact of coronary culprit lesion calcium in patients undergoing paclitaxel-eluting stent implantation (a TAXUS-IV Sub Study). Am J Cardiol. 2005;96;1242-7.
17. Kuriyama N, Kobayashi Y, Yamaguchi M, Shibata Y. Usefulness of rotational atherectomy in preventing polymer damage of everolimus-eluting stent in calcified coronary artery. JACC Cardiovasc Interv. 2011;4:588-9.
18. Guedeney P, Claessen BE, Mehran R, Mintz GS, Liu M, Sorrentino S, et al. Coronary Calcification and Long-Term Outcomes According to Drug-Eluting Stent Generation. JACC Cardiovasc Interv. 2020;13:1417-28.
19. Copeland-Halperin RS, Baber U, Aquino M, Rajamanickam A, Roy S, Hasan C, et al. Prevalence, correlates, and impact of coronary calcification on adverse events following PCI with newer-generation DES: Findings from a large multiethnic registry. Catheter Cardiovasc Interv. 2018;91:859-66.
20. Mosseri M, Satler LF, Pichard AD, Waksman R. Impact of vessel calcification on outcomes after coronary stenting. Cardiovasc Revasc Med. 2005;6:147-53.
21. Wang FF, Han JL, He R, Zeng XZ, Zhang FC, Guo LJ, et al. Prognostic value of coronary artery calcium score in patients with stable angina pectoris after percutaneous coronary intervention. J Geriatr Cardiol. 2014;11:113-19.
22. Lange RA, Hillis LD. Second-Generation Drug-Eluting Coronary Stents. N Engl J Med. 2010;362:1728-30.
23. Sharma SK, Bolduan RW, Patel MR, Martinsen BJ, Azemi T, Giugliano G, et al. Impact of calcification on percutaneous coronary intervention: MACE-trial 1-year results. Catheter Cardiovasc Interv. 2019;94:187-94.
24. Beohar N, Kaltenbach LA, Wojdyla D, Pineda AM, Rao SV, Stone GW, et al. Trends in usage and clinical outcomes of coronary atherectomy: a report from the National Cardiovascular Data Registry CathPCI Registry. Circ Cardiovasc Interv. 2020;13:e008239.

25. Fujino A, Mintz GS, Matsumura M, Lee T, Kim SY, Hoshino M, et al. A new optical coherence tomography-based calcium scoring system to predict stent underexpansion. EuroIntervention. 2018;13:e2182-9.
26. Zhang M, Matsumura M, Usui E, Noguchi M, Fujimura T, Fall KN, et al. Intravascular ultrasound-derived calcium score to predict stent expansion in severely calcified lesions. Circ Cardiovasc Interv. 2021;14:e010296.
27. Jadhav KP, Kavalipatu KNR, Kuchulakanti PK, Reddy RP, Athuluri R, Prakash G, et al. Coronary Artery Calcification: From Cell to Stent—A Review. Indian J Clin Cardiol. 2021;2(2):97-109.
28. Fourrier JL, Bertrand ME, Auth DC, Lablanche JM, Gommeaux A, Brunetaud JM. Percutaneous coronary rotational angioplasty in humans: preliminary report. J Am Coll Cardiol. 1989;14:1278-82.
29. Abdel-Wahab M, Richardt G, Joachim Büttner H, Toelg R, Geist V, Meinertz T, et al. High-speed rotational atherectomy before paclitaxel-eluting stent implantation in complex calcified coronary lesions: the randomized ROTAXUS (Rotational Atherectomy Prior to Taxus Stent Treatment for Complex Native Coronary Artery Disease) trial. JACC Cardiovasc Interv. 2013;6:10-9.
30. de Waha S, Allali A, Büttner HJ, Toelg R, Geist V, Neumann FJ, et al. Rotational atherectomy before paclitaxel-eluting stent implantation in complex calcified coronary lesions: two-year clinical outcome of the randomized ROTAXUS trial. Catheter Cardiovasc Interv. 2016;87:691-700.
31. Parikh K, Chandra P, Choksi N, Khanna P, Chambers J. Safety and feasibility of orbital atherectomy for the treatment of calcified coronary lesions: the ORBIT I trial. Catheter Cardiovasc Interv. 2013;81:1134-9.
32. Bhatt P, Parikh P, Patel A, Chag M, Chandarana A, Parikh R, et al. Long-term safety and performance of the orbital atherectomy system for treating calcified coronary artery lesions: 5-year follow-up in the ORBIT I trial. Cardiovasc Revasc Med. 2015;16:213-6.
33. Lee M, Généreux P, Shlofmitz R, Phillipson D, Anose BM, Martinsen BJ, et al. Orbital atherectomy for treating de novo, severely calcified coronary lesions: 3-year results of the pivotal ORBIT II trial. Cardiovasc Revasc Med. 2017;18:261-4.
34. Généreux P, Kirtane AJ, Kandzari DE, Armstrong EJ, Krucoff MW, Redfors B, et al. Randomized evaluation of vessel preparation with orbital atherectomy prior to drug-eluting stent implantation in severely calcified coronary artery lesions: design and rationale of the ECLIPSE trial. Am Heart J. 2022;249:1-11.
35. Litvack F, Grundfest W, Eigler N, Tsoi D, Goldenberg T, Laudenslager J, et al. Percutaneous excimer laser coronary angioplasty. Lancet. 1989;334:102-3.
36. Appelman YE, Piek JJ, Strikwerda S, Tijssen JG, de Feyter PJ, David GK, et al. Randomised trial of excimer laser angioplasty versus balloon angioplasty for treatment of obstructive coronary artery disease. Lancet. 1996;347:79-84.
37. Lee T, Shlofmitz RA, Song L, Tsiamtsiouris T, Pappas T, Madrid A, et al. The effectiveness of excimer laser angioplasty to treat coronary in-stent restenosis with peri-stent calcium as assessed by optical coherence tomography. EuroIntervention. 2019;15:e279-88.
38. Brinton TJ, Ali ZA, Hill JM, Meredith IT, Maehara A, Illindala U, et al. Feasibility of shockwave coronary intravascular lithotripsy for the treatment of calcified coronary stenoses. Circulation. 2019;139:834-6.
39. Ali ZA, Nef H, Escaned J, Werner N, Banning AP, Hill JM, et al. Safety and effectiveness of coronary intravascular lithotripsy for treatment of severely

calcified coronary stenoses: the Disrupt CAD II study. Circ Cardiovasc Interv. 2019;12:e008434.

40. Hill JM, Kereiakes DJ, Shlofmitz RA, Klein AJ, Riley RF, Price MJ, et al. Intravascular lithotripsy for treatment of severely calcified coronary artery disease. J Am Coll Cardiol. 2020;76:2635-46.
41. Mauri L, Bonan R, Weiner BH, Legrand V, Bassand JP, Popma JJ, et al. Cutting balloon angioplasty for the prevention of restenosis: results of the Cutting Balloon Global Randomized Trial. Am J Cardiol. 2002;90:1079-83.
42. Tian W, Mahmoudi M, Lhermusier T, Kiramijyan S, Ota H, Chen F, et al. Comparison of rotational atherectomy, plain old balloon angioplasty, and cutting-balloon angioplasty prior to drug-eluting stent implantation for the treatment of heavily calcified coronary lesions. J Invasive Cardiol. 2015;27:387-91.
43. Redfors B, Maehara A, Witzenbichler B, Weisz G, Stuckey TD, Henry TD, et al. Outcomes after successful percutaneous coronary intervention of calcified lesions using rotational atherectomy, cutting-balloon angioplasty, or balloon only angioplasty before drug-eluting stent implantation. J Invasive Cardiol. 2017;29:378-86.

CHAPTER

14

Rotational and Orbital Atherectomy: Basics and Technique

Sridhar Kasturi

INTRODUCTION

Calcified coronary arteries are more often observed in patients with advanced age, diabetes mellitus, coronary artery bypass graft (CABG), and chronic kidney disease (CKD), and moreover percutaneous coronary intervention (PCI) of this subset of patients associated with increased plaque burden, complex interventional procedures, postprocedural stent fracture, improper expansion, malapposition, dissections with intramural hematoma (IMH), and perforation leading to increased acute and long-term complications particularly if adequate plaque modification is not done with appropriate plaque modification devices prior to implanting drug-eluting stents (DES). Additionally, these patients are prone for stent dislodgments, prolonged procedural time causing more exposure to radiation, and delayed endothelialization of stent struts during follow-up. As per the results of ADAPT–DES, all-comers DES registry, study population of 8,582 patients showed evidence of moderate-to-severe calcification in about 30.8% of NSTEMI-ACS and STEMI PCI patients. HORIZON-AMI and ACUITY-AMI CORONARY CALCIUM results showed increased cardiac death, all-cause death, myocardial infarction (MI), target lesion revascularization (TLR), and major adverse cardiac event (MACE) as the severity of calcium increases, and, moreover, it showed significant increase in the MACE rate in patients with calcium versus those without calcium at 1-year follow-up.[1] PCI of calcific coronaries is associated with high-vascular access related complications due to advanced age, requirement of bigger sheaths and catheters, and more frequently associated with calcification of peripheral access site vessels. However, major bleeding complications related access site can be reduced by opting to radial site with slender sheath and intravascular ultrasound (IVUS)-guided femoral puncture.

ASSESSMENT OF CALCIUM SEVERITY, ANGIO VERSUS INTRAVASCULAR IMAGING

Angio shows moderate calcium as moderate dense radiopacities noted during cardiac cycle before contrast injection while severe calcium seen as a dense radiopacities on both sides of the vessel wall (tram track) without cardiac motion before contrast injection. Although angiography has high specificity in detecting calcium but its role is limited in the assessment of depth, circumferential extent, and exact length of the calcific plaque which are essential components of plaque modifications of PCI procedure.[2] Before planning PCI, it would be essential to interpret angio images with careful assessment of calcium severity for any need for plaque modification especially when angio suggestive of moderate-to-severe calcification. PCI with intravascular imaging guides in assessing distribution of plaque and severity of plaque burden in terms of thickness, circumferential distribution, length, and calcium expansion index for precise planning of plaque modification strategies. Coronary angiography underestimates the severity of coronary calcium, and moreover grating sensation with difficulty while passing ballon, dog-boning or inadequate balloon expansion on angio necessitates intravascular imaging assessment of severity of calcium which will be useful in guiding plaque modification and optimization of DES implantation. The inability to cross a severely calcified vessel with an IVUS or optical coherence tomography (OCT) catheter often necessitates upfront plaque modification devices and in some instances these procedures may need guide extension catheters with guide support to facilitate placement of imaging catheters, balloons, plaque modification devices and stents and additionally this may be needed even after adequate plaque modification in some cases **(Fig. 1)**. IVUS scores over OCT in patients with severe LV dysfunction, CKD, ostial lesions of left main (LM), large caliber/aneurysmal vessels, and unstable hemodynamic status. As the IVUS identifies only the leading edge of calcific plaque with poor penetration of calcific plaque which is a limitation for measuring thickness of thick calcific plaque, not useful to detect deep calcium and that is situated underneath the superficial calcium, and similarly it has limitations in detecting microcalcifications/spotty

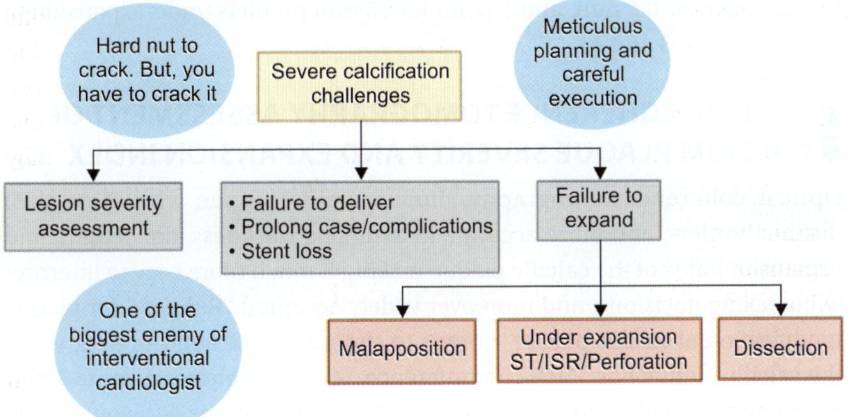

Fig. 1: Assessment of calcium severity. (ISR: in-stent restenosis; ST: stent thrombosis)

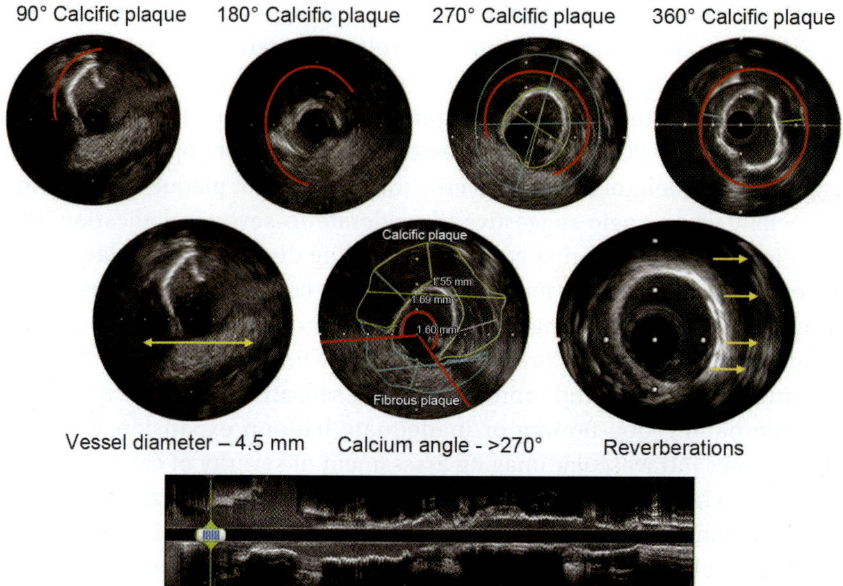

Fig. 2: Calcium index score by intravascular ultrasound.

calcification and when calcium is situated beneath the large necrotic core. Even in some cases, dense fibrotic plaques may reflect IVUS waves mimicking calcific plaque, therefore operator should be wise enough to consider all these facts while interpreting IVUS images during PCI procedure.

As per the IVUS imaging, calcium score of 2 or more than 2 points predicts underexpansion of the stent—2 points for Arc >270 degrees, length >5 mm, 1 point each for calcified nodule (CN), smaller vessel diameter (<3.5 mm) and reverberations <90 degrees **(Fig. 2)**.

A calcific lesion with a score of 4—2 points for Ca Arc >180 degrees, 1 point for Ca thickness 0.5 mm, and 1 point for >5 mm predicts underexpansion of the stent **(Figs. 3 and 4)**.

OPTICAL COHERENCE TOMOGRAPHY ASSESSMENT OF CALCIUM PLAQUE SEVERITY AND EXPANSION INDEX

Optical coherence tomography shows calcific plaque with clear well distinct borders, and more accurate in assessing thickness, arc, length, and expansion index of the calcific plaque making it much more easy to interpret while taking decisions, and moreover widely accepted "Rule of 5 for plaque modification of calcific plaque" criteria to choose modification strategy when the calcific plaque has >50% circumference, >0.5 mm thickness, and >5 mm length of the calcific plaque is a user friendly general rule for decision making as suggested by Fujino et al.,[3] which recommends atherectomy if calcium

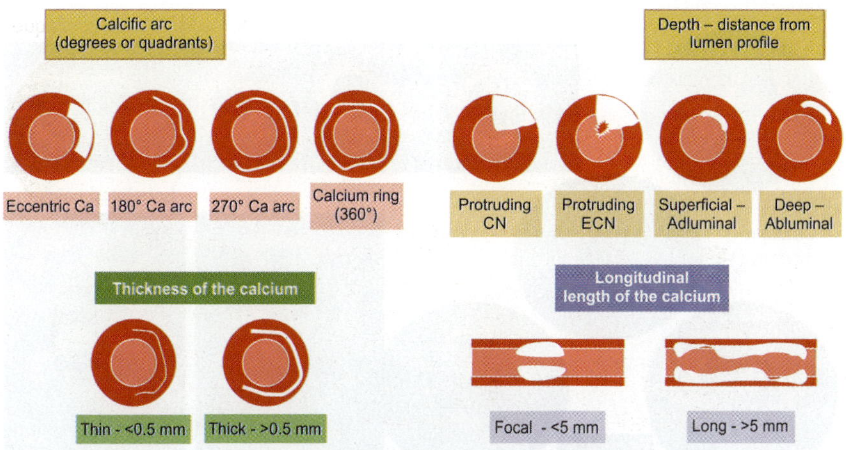

Fig. 3: Intravascular imaging assessment of the calcium.

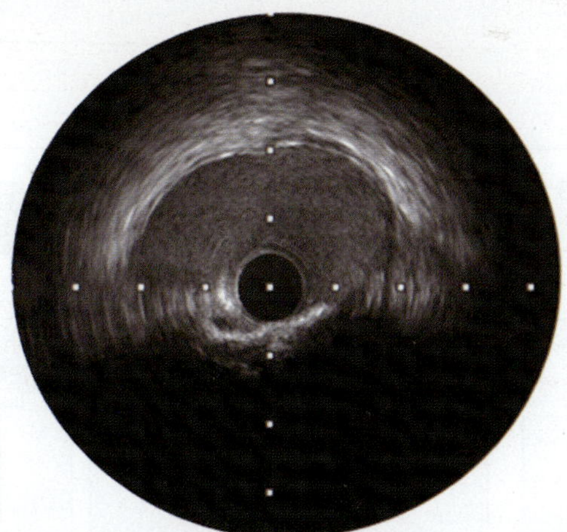

Fig. 4: Calcium nodule.

thickness >0.5 mm (1 point), calcified vessel length >5 mm (1 point), calcified angle >180° (2 points), score of 4 predicts underexpansion without calcium modification, and furthermore OCT can predict plaque fracture if plaque thickness is <0.54 mm, and Arc <221°. OCT can identify plaque modification indicators better than any other imaging modality such as: (1) A reduction in calcium plaque volume, (2) fractures/cuts/dissections, and (3) gain in the mean luminal area **(Figs. 5 and 6)**.

Recent edition of OCT with Ultreon Software helps in the automatic detection of vessel size and quantification of calcium by using artificial intelligence. Additionally, use stent boost to get adequate stent expansion in multiple planes wherever IVI is not feasible or affordable. CN contributes to 5–7% of ACS due to acute coronary thrombosis, and it is associated with

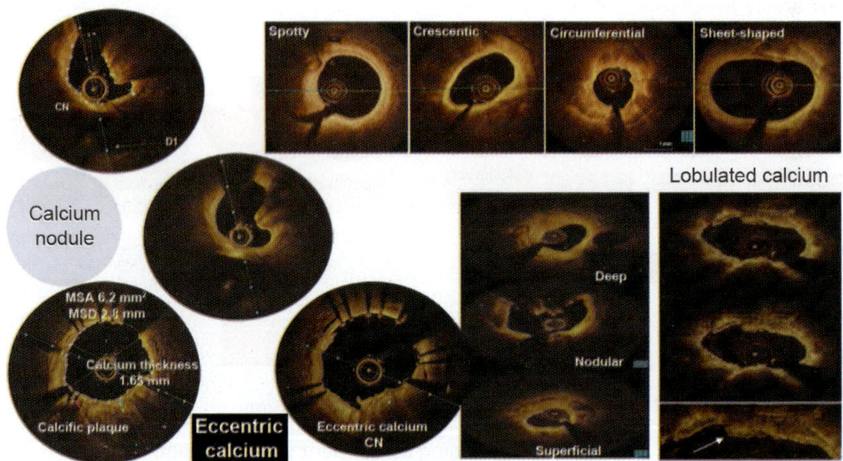

Fig. 5: Assessment of calcium by optical coherence tomography.

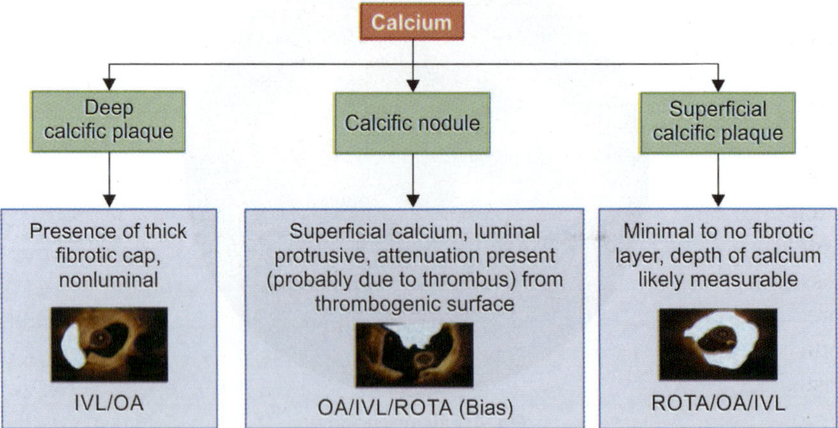

Fig. 6: Tips and tricks in assessing the calcium for any need of plaque modification. (IVL: intravascular lithotripsy; OA: orbital atherectomy)

worse acute and long-term outcomes following PCI. OCT is very useful in differentiating two main morphologies of calcium nodules: (1) Eruptive CN—has irregular surface appearance, associated with disruption of the intimal fibrous cap with superimposed thrombus; and (2) Protruding CN—multiple or single nodule of calcium protrusion into the lumen.[4] Eruptive CN is associated with better stent expansion but associated with high recurrence rate and increased MACE compared to protruding CN which is more resistant and frequently associated with underexpansion. CN is commonly seen in the proximal mid-right coronary artery (RCA), proximal LAD, proximal LCx, and LM which is seen as bright protruding shadow of leading border with broad dark shadow beneath it. PCI of CN lesions is associated with more event rate and difficult to treat, despite using plaque modification devices, and sometimes it requires combination of plaque modification device to get adequate stent expansion. However, it is associated with high recurrence rate and requires regular follow-up to manage it appropriately. IVUS catheter position close to CN or eccentric calcium suggests effectiveness of Rota for adequate plaque modification in that position and if position of catheter is adjacent to the side of the vessel wall, away from calcific plaque, use large size burr, adjust the wire related bias by pulling or pushing guidewire and exchanging Rota floppy with Rota extra support to have adequate contact of burr with calcific plaque for effective modification or else it may not ablate properly **(Fig. 7)**.

Noncompliant (NC) balloons: These are useful for mild-to-moderate calcific lesions, and more effective and safer compared to semicompliant balloons because of uniform dilatation even at higher inflation pressures. These are associated with high rate of perforations, dissections with IMH, and balloon rupture in severely calcified lesions, especially in eccentric/calcific nodule lesions. Cutting balloons are useful to prepare proximal segments, ostial lesions, straight coronary segments without tortuosity or acute bends, and for further plaque modification following intravascular lithotripsy (IVL) **(Fig. 8)**, rotational atherectomy (RA), or orbital atherectomy (OA). Scoring ballons are useful in similar lesions but they are more deliverable, hence, useful to prepare even distal lesions and tortuous lesions. In contrast to regular NC balloons, scoring and cutting ballons produce more controlled dissections, less tissue injury, less inflammation, and more gain in luminal area. High pressure OPN NC balloon (super-NC Balloon) is a twin-layered balloon with minimal increase of diameter at burst pressure 35 atm (maximal pressure tested up to 45 atm) and is suitable to tackle crossable undilatable calcified lesions (avoid eccentric calcific or CN lesions to avoid perforation) and

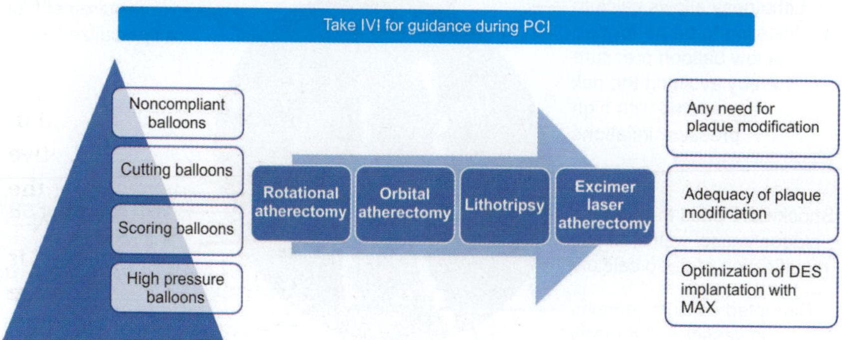

Fig. 7: What to choose and when to use plaque modification device in PCI calcific lesions. (DES: drug-eluting stents; IVI: intravascular imaging; PCI: percutaneous coronary intervention)

underexpanded stents. However, it has high profile with poor capability to cross very tight lesions compared to regular NC balloons.

MERITS AND DEMERITS OF BALLOON-BASED PLAQUE MODIFICATION

Intravascular Lithotripsy

Intravascular lithotripsy is a 12-mm long balloon catheter with three emitters inside the balloon between two radiopaque markers, its profile smaller than other modifying balloons, and slightly larger profile than a noncompliant balloon because of the integration of EHL emitters into the shaft and is available in 7 sizes ranging from 2.5 to 4.0 mm **(Figs. 9 and 10)**.

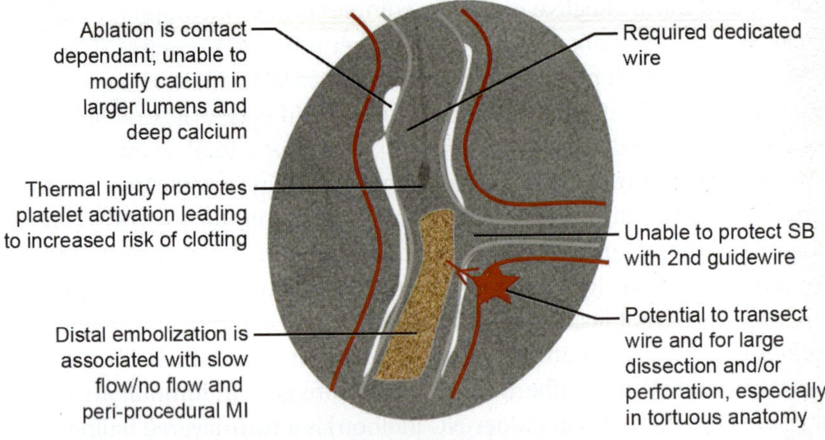

Fig. 8: Rota for plaque modification.

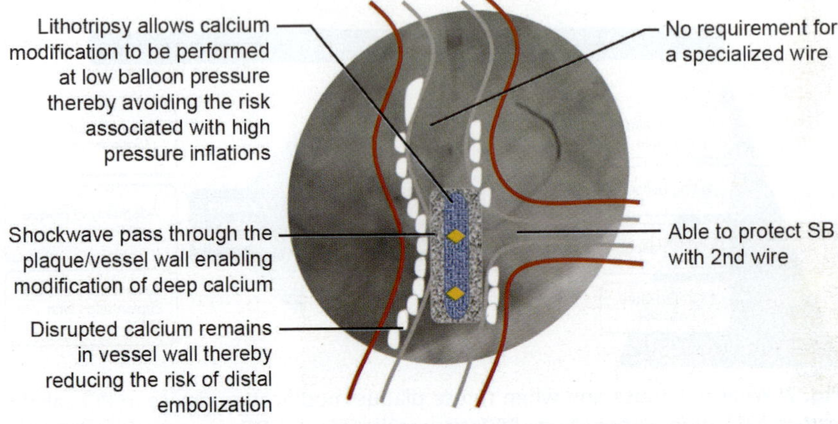

Fig. 9: Intravascular lithotripsy for plaque modification.

Crossing profile and flexibility influences trackability of the device, a longer shaft length allows the placement of device to treat more distally located lesions, and larger IVL balloons are available to meet the size of proximal vessels including left main coronary artery to get effective plaque modification. IVL modifies calcified plaques by delivering an electrical discharge at the emitters vaporizes the fluid generating a series of circumferential ultrashort pulses of high-intensity acoustic energy, which, by virtue of its compressive and decompressive components, results in effective circumferential modification of both superficial and deep calcium. In contrast to both RA and OA, which generate nanoparticles that may embolize distally and impair

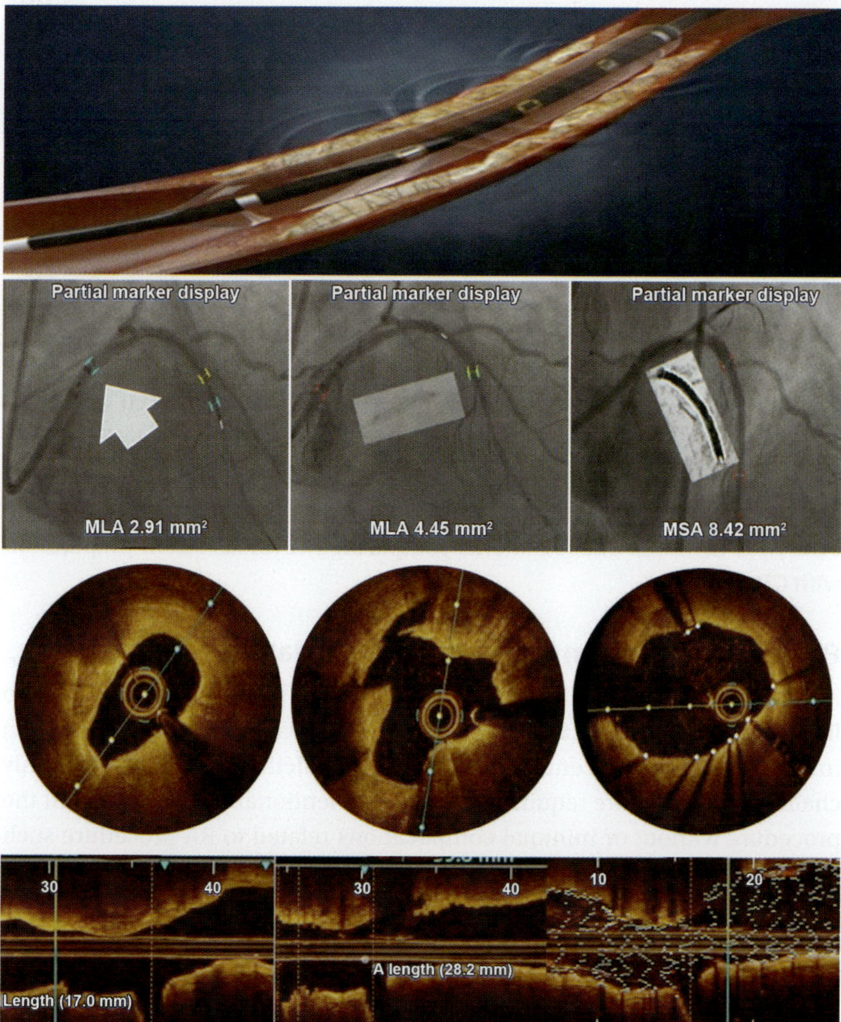

Fig. 10: Intravascular lithotripsy-induced calcium fractures after plaque modification for optimal stent expansion. (MLA: mean luminal area; MSA: mean stent area)

microcirculatory function, larger calcium fragments generated by lithotripsy remain in situ with virtually no debris production, avoid the trauma produced by blades and burrs and their related risk. IVL has potential advantage over the ROTA particularly in high-risk bifurcation lesions with high prediction for SB closure, patients with severe LV dysfunction and clinical probability of high risk of slow flow, no flow, and dissection. IVL has ability to fracture a calcified plaque outside an underexpanded stent, and lesions resistant to other balloon-based strategies therefore allow appropriate stent expansion and apposition. IVL is also effective for plaque modification of large vessels (use 3.5-mm and 4-mm diameter IVL) and bifurcation lesions owing to the maintenance of SB wire during modification. The OCT studies showed calcium fracture as the predominant mechanism of action of IVL, the number of fractures was proportional to the magnitude of calcification. Calcium fracture was identified in 78.7% of CAC plaques, with multiple fractures in more than half of the lesions **(Fig. 11)**.

Recent evidence from the Disrupt CAD I and Disrupt CAD II trials demonstrated very low rates of coronary periprocedural complications (rates of in-hospital myocardial infarction were 5.0% in Disrupt CAD I and 5.8% in Disrupt CAD II), with no unresolved complex dissections (types D to F), perforations, abrupt closures, and slow- or no-reflow events.[5] The pivotal Disrupt CAD III trial demonstrated no perforations, abrupt closures, or no-reflow events following IVL alone despite treatment of more complex lesions than were treated in the Disrupt CAD I and Disrupt CAD II studies.

The ROTAXUS trail of RA versus Balloon preparation of calcific lesions of 240 patients showed no benefit of primary outcome late lumen loss but higher procedural success, and similar results were noticed even in recent PREPARE-CAL trail of 200 patients comparing RA versus lesion preparation with CB or SC.

Plaque Modification Strategies with Ablation

Although it has been available for over 3 decades, it is used less often due to limited number of skillful operators and nonavailability of this facility even in many tertiary care centers. RA of severely calcified coronaries is highly challenging procedure requiring special interventional skills to carry out the procedure without or minimal complications related to RA procedure such as perforation, burr entrapment or burr stall, SB loss, and slow flow or no flow phenomenon.[6] Developing special skills to operate, choosing suitable lesions with meticulous planning, and execution of procedure with image guidance and adjunctive devices are the essential elements for the achievement of successful procedure.

Rotational atherectomy device consists of diamonds coated burr, advancer, and console, and the device has a burr at the tip, requires guide

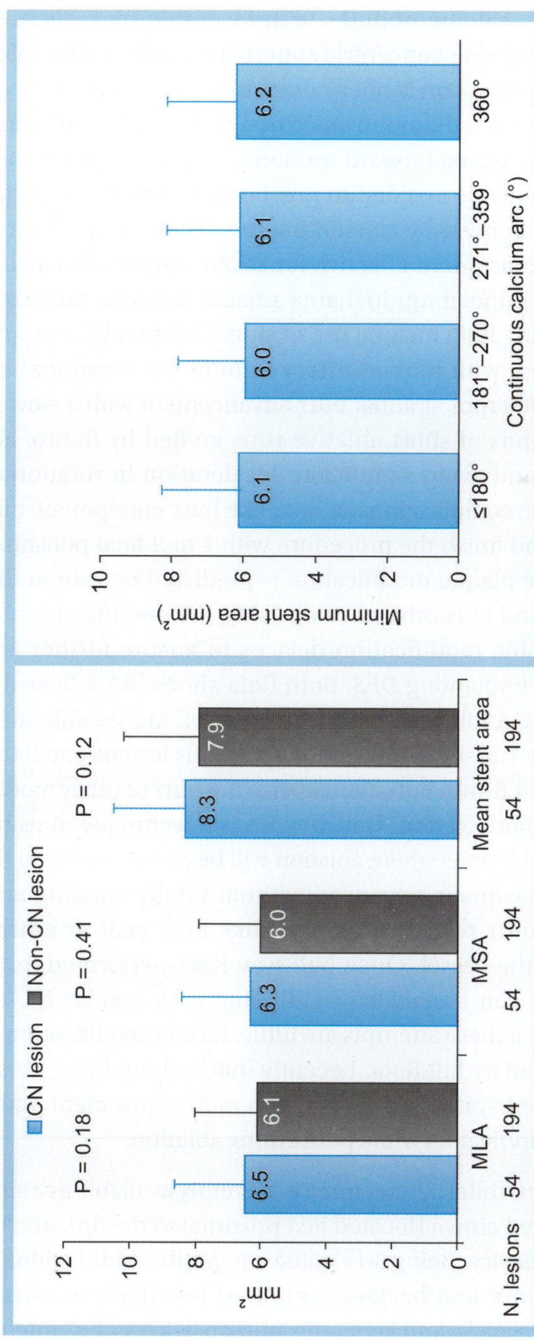

Fig. 11: IVL—impact of calcium eccentricity on the safety and effectiveness of coronary intravascular lithotripsy pooled analysis from the DISRUPT CAD studies—IVL-induced calcium fractures proportional to the magnitude of coronary artery calcium including eccentric and CN leading to consistent improvements in stent expansion and luminal gain in both eccentric and concentric calcified coronary lesions. (CN: calcified nodule; IVL: intravascular lithotripsy)

catheter according to the burr size such as 6F (1.25–1.5 mm), 7F (1.75 mm), 8F (2.25–2.38 mm), 10F (2.5 mm). It is very useful for undilatable or balloon uncrossable lesions, calcific nodules with favorable bias, serial or long calcified lesions containing concentric superficial calcium, and bifurcation lesions in which SB protection is not a concern. It has a nickel-plated bullet-shaped burr coated with diamond microscopic crystals with centripetal forward cutting only during forward motion. Additional guidewires in the main vessel or SB must be avoided to prevent wire cutting or perforation. Rota results are influenced by calcific plaque eccentricity, luminal area, burr size, and wire bias, more effective for severe superficial calcium with calcific arc >270° and mean luminal area smaller than the burr size. Basic principles of operating Rota include use of single 1.5-mm burr (appropriate in >90% of the cases) with burr-to-artery ratio of 0.6, rotational speed of about 140,000–180,000 rpm, gradual burr advancement with a slow pecking motion, 15–20 seconds of short ablative runs guided by fluoro, acoustic, and tactile inputs, and avoid significant deceleration in rotational speed >5,000 rpm to reduce complications of Rota like burr entrapment/burr stall/ burr detachment, and finish the procedure with 1 or 2 final polishing runs.[7] Evidence of effective plaque modification is predicted by gain in the MLA, fractures, fissures, and cuts otherwise upsizing the modification device or opt for other available modification devices to ensure further adequate modification before implanting DES. Both Rota-shock (RA followed by IVL) and Orbital-Tripsy (OA followed by IVL) are useful and feasible in severely calcified vessels. Use 1.25-mm burr for long tortuous lesions and if unable to cross the lesion with 1.5-mm burr, then upsize the burr or other modification devices for further modification. Half-way RA is a technique of using RA to ablate long angulated lesions where ablation will be carried out until the point of acute angle or maximally advanced without totally crossing angulated curves to prevent burr-related problems, like burr stall or entrapment, and perforation of the vessel. Once half-way Rota performed, remaining uncrossed segment can be tackled by dilating with regular NC or other devices like IVL, and if these attempts are futile, further modification of distal segment can be opted by full Rota. Recently induced modified Rotapro is a user-friendly resigned system which is much more convenient and easy to setup with warning indicators while performing ablation.

Orbital atherectomy: Orbital atherectomy is currently available as a single 1.25 eccentrically mounted crown (located just proximal to the tip), and easier to setup modification device. Being 6-Fr guide compatible bidirectional cutting device (during forward and backward motion) less likely to cause crown entrapment or crown stall), and generates microparticles of <2 microns with forward flow during ablation, and less heat generation contributes to less proneness for distal embolization and slow/no flow. OA has the advantage of more ablation capability with increase in the crown speed thus provides more effective ablation of long lesions with concomitant superficial and deep calcium. Orbital motion of OA should be carried out with 1:1 slow motion at 1 mm/s without keeping any tension on the crown, and its orbital motion reduces the limitation of wire bias; therefore, it is more effective for ablation of eccentric and calcium nodules compared to Rota ablation **(Fig. 12 and Box 1)**.

Generally, OA ablation should be carried out with 80,000 rpm speed and restricting 120, 000 rpm speed to only large vessels with straight segment, but high-speed ablation using 120,000 rpm speed should be avoided in vessels with high tortuosity, severe angulation, and <3-mm diameter to reduce risk of vessel perforation. Higher speed with slow coronal movement in a uniform motion at the speed of about 1–3 mm/s within the target vessel produces greater degree of plaque modification. To sum up, OA is more useful for ablating large vessels, lesions with severe superficial calcium, eccentric calcium or CN, and crossable aorto-ostial lesions with reverse cutting **(Figs. 13 and 14)**.[8]

ORBIT 1 study showed 98% device success rate in 94% of patients, and moreover dissections without any sequelae were noticed in 12% of patients, and none showed slow flow/no flow. Similar device success (98.6%) and procedural success (91.4%) rates were observed in ORBIT 11 study with evidence of severe dissections in 2.3% of patients. ORBIT 1 and ORBIT 2 trials have established safety, feasibility, and effectiveness of OA for the modification of severely calcified lesions. Coronary perforation is a major complication of OA which is observed in 0.7–2% of patients; however, it can be reduced by avoiding OA of highly tortuous coronary lesions. OA produces

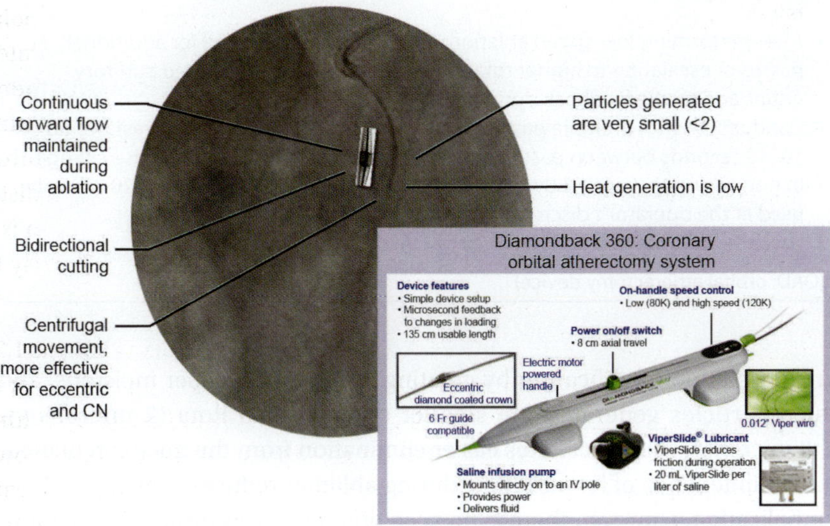

Fig. 12: Orbital atherectomy for plaque modification. (CN: calcified nodule)

BOX 1: Technical tips to perform orbital atherectomy.

- Before starting orbital atherectomy (OA), check for crown motion and speed by using advancer knob and speed controls on the back side of electric handle including glide switch mode, keep saline glide pump on, and check for proper application and relief of the break.
- Advance the OAD crown approximate 3–5 mm proximal to the lesion, unlock control knob and relieve any tension on the crown with backward movement of advancer knob.
- It is advisable to activate glide mode for rapid and smooth advancement of the crown in the guide catheter and deactivate glide switch once the crown reaches the target site.
- It is essential to maintain 1:1 motion between the crown and advancer knob. If loss of 1:1 motion occurs, slowly retract the crown and reengage the lesion with slow forward movement.
- Slow and steady advancement of the crown at 1 mm/s traverse rate results in better luminal gain as compared to 10 mm/s traverse rate in the same number of passes.
- Avoid pecking or forceful motion of the crown which may result in forward movement faster than 10 mm/s leading to increase in the complication rate.
- As the device has forward and backward cutting capability, it is essential to maintain the slow and gentle movement of the crown while ablating in either direction.
- Each pass should be carried out with 10–15 seconds run time with an interval of 10–15 seconds, and maximum run time should not exceed 30 seconds and the device will give a reminder beep at the end of preset run time, allowing time to decide where to rest the device between runs. A single run should not exceed 30 seconds and the total treatment time should not exceed 5 minutes.
- Carry out multiple number of passes of OA until there is no resistance or no change in noise or pitch while advancing the crown.
- It is essential to avoid high-speed ablation (120 k) in tortuous lesions, severe angulations, and vessels smaller than 3.0 mm in diameter to reduce complication rate.
- After performing low-speed ablation, decision about the need for additional passes or escalation to higher rotational speed can be taken based auditory, visual, and tactile feedback during ablation.
- Conduct OA with multiple passes of 10–15 seconds duration with a rest period of 10–15 seconds between passes until there is no resistance and no noise change.
- In non-tortuous vessels 3.0 mm or larger, high-speed ablation using 120 k may be used at the operator's discretion.
- Lock the control knob and remove the OAD.

(OAD: orbital atherectomy device)

greater plaque modification by creating longer and deeper incisions, and microparticles generated are smaller compared to Rota (2 microns vs. 5-8 microns) which facilitates easier elimination from the microcirculation, and maintenance of forward flow during ablation reduces chances of distal embolization. However, there is no such difference was observed in clinical studies. In vast majority of cases, OA can be performed using radial approach,

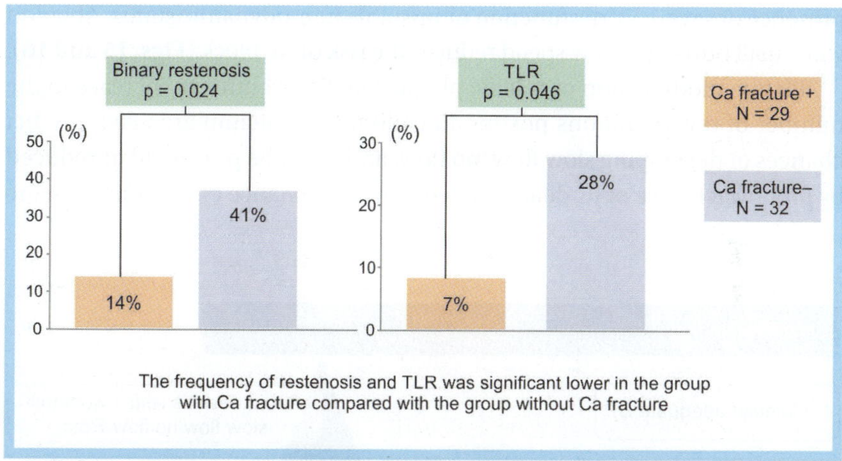

Fig. 13: Restenosis and TLR at 10-month follow-up in calcified lesions. (TLR: target lesion revascularization)

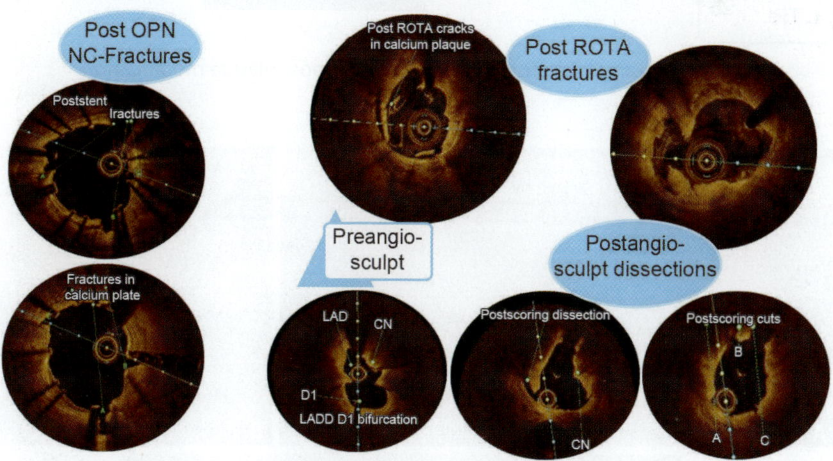

Fig. 14: Post plaque modification evidence of fractures indicates favorable outcomes.

hence it can reduce significant number of access site related complications and shortens the duration of hospitalization.

Bradyarrhythmias: Prophylactic temporary pacemaker implantation (TPI) to tackle AV blocks and complete heart block (CHB), preferably with balloon tip to reduce the risk of perforation, is recommended when patients are undergoing plaque modification with RA or OA of severely calcified Dominant RCA or LCX, severe MVD with LM, and last remaining vessel, especially in the presence of severe LV dysfunction or unstable hemodynamic status. Ablation with small burrs and slow speed reduces the risk of AV block **(Figs. 15 and 16)**.

Plaque modification of calcific plaque length >24 mm, an increase in the number of reverberations postmodification, and calcium arc >300° predict chances of developing slow flow/no flow, and it can be prevented or reduced by prophylactic use of IC dilators, adequate maintenance of systemic pressure

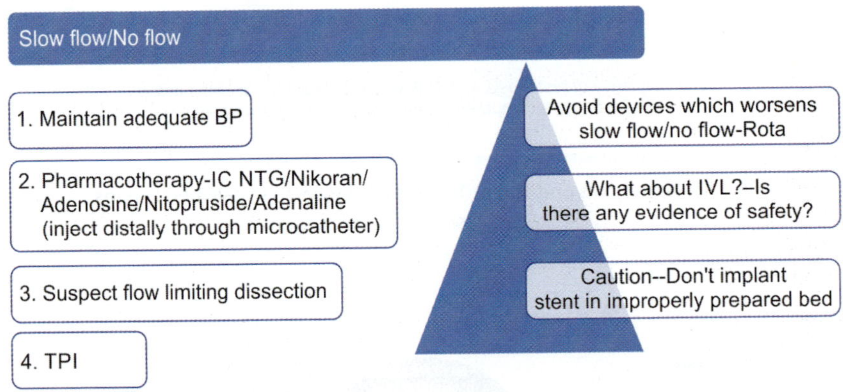

Fig. 15: Tips and tricks for slow flow/no flow-post plaque modification.

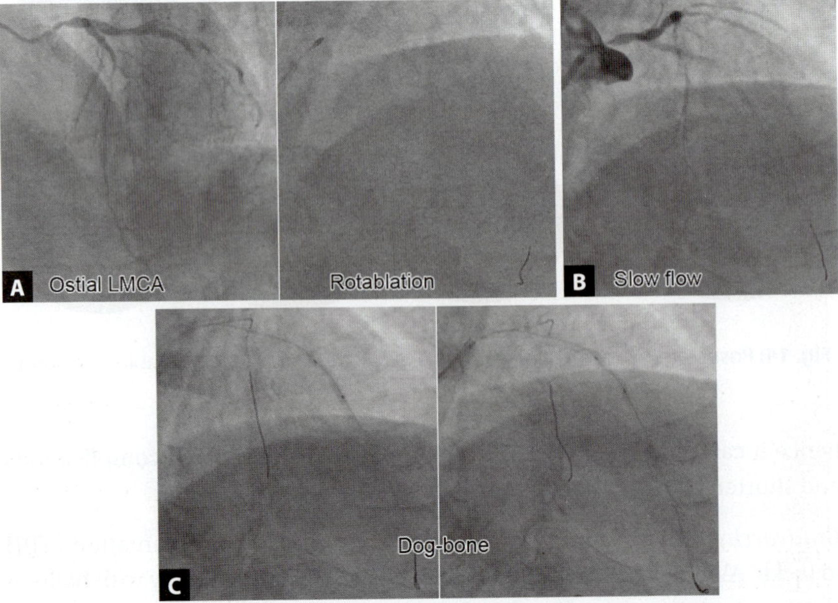

Figs. 16A to C: A case example of slow flow post ROTA status. (A) Rotablation of ostium of LMCA; (B) slow-flow after Rota of LM and LAD; (C) Rota for unexpandable lesion—Dogbone effect. (LAD: left anterior descending; LMCA: left main coronary artery)

with inotropes, and maintaining ACT more than 250 seconds. Furthermore, it can be reduced by avoiding ablation with big burrs, high-speed ablation, long runs of ablation and limiting ablation runs with more than 5,000 rpm deceleration **(Table 1)**.

After plaque modification, repeat intravascular imaging should be repeated to see the adequate plaque by evidence of fractures or cuts and increase in the mean luminal gain, and if OCT/IVUS images shows no evidence of fractures, and thickness of calcific plaque >0.5 mm, it suggests

TABLE 1: Difference between rotational and orbital atherectomy.

	Rotational atherectomy	*Orbital atherectomy*
Device	Rotablator	Diamondback 360
Available sizes	1.25, 1.5, 1.75, 2.0, 2.25, 2.38, and 2.5	1.25 mm
Guide catheter compatibility	<1.75 mm burrs: 6 Fr guide	6 Fr guide
Guidewire	0.009" floppy or extra-support rotawire	0.012"/0.014" VIPERWIRE advanced coronary guidewire
Flush solution	• Rotaglide infusion under a pressure bag • *Alternative:* Heparin, nitroglycerin, and verapamil in normal saline	ViperSlide, standard infusion rate
Mechanism of actions	• Rotational • Diamond-tipped burr spins concentrically on the wire • Atheroablation via differential cutting • Particle size (5–10 µm)	• Orbital • Eccentrically mounted diamond coated crown uses centrifugal force • Atheroablation via differential sanding • Particle size (<2 µm)
Technical features	• Front-cutting unidirectional burr • *Speed:* 140,000–180,000 rpm, avoid deceleration >5,000 rpm • Burr movement with pecking motion/short ablative runs (<25 s)	• Diamond coated crown, bidirectional • *Speed:* 80,000–120,000 rpm, larger ablative arc with higher speed • Continuous slow forward and backward crown movement
Cons: • Learning curve • Perforation • Slow/no-reflow • Burr entrapment	 • Long • Moderate • Moderate • Moderate	 • Short • Low • Low • Crown entrapment unlikely

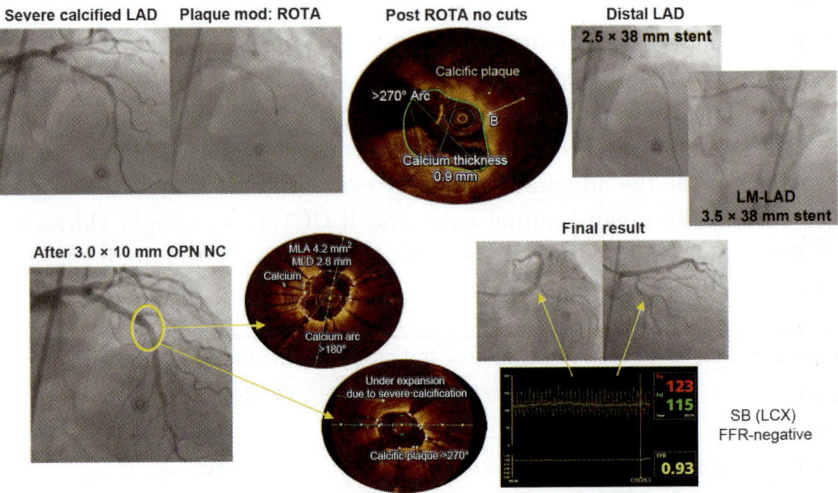

Fig. 17: Post-Rota OCT assessment of plaque modification: Inadequate plaque modification (thickness of calcium >0.5 mm and no fractures) underexpansion of the stent was managed with high pressure balloon dilatations using OPN NC balloon at 40–45 atm inflations. (NC: noncompliant; OCT: optical coherence tomography)

inadequate plaque modification, and further modification strategies should be planned like upsizing Rota burr/increasing the speed of the OA crown/ opting for other devices (IVL/OPN NC/CB/scoring balloons), followed by repeat run of IVI to confirm adequate modification prior to implanting DES. Most of these patients require additional supportive devices like guide extension catheters to facilitate imaging catheters, balloons, and stents to cross severely calcified tortuous segments and distal lesions, and helpful in preventing extension of IMH, help in expediting the procedure, and furthermore, it assists in performing balloon trapping to exchange wires, microcatheters, and balloons **(Fig. 17)**.

Aortoostial lesions: These are prone for higher rate of vessel recoiling, in-stent restenosis (ISR), and target lesion failure and repeat revascularization. It is also necessary to do the plaque modification of aortoostial lesions with proper coaxial position of guide catheter, otherwise it may lead to risk of Rota wire breakage, and furthermore substituting extra support Rota wire with Rota floppy gives some more support and avoids kinking of wire at ostial site. OA can be used when it is crossable and ablation can be done with backward motion with good coaxial position of guide. IVL is also useful for ostial lesions by applying 3.5-mm/4-mm diameter balloons depending upon LM size, and care should be taken in placing IVL with just 1–2 mm proximal end of IVL balloon extension into the aorta in order to avoid wastage of IVL pulses and for effective modification of ostium. During IVL therapy, it is preferable to give short duration of pulses that is 5 pulses instead of 10 pulses for prevention of profound hypotension-related deleterious side effects as a result of total occlusion of left main coronary artery (LMCA) with IVL balloon, especially in patents with left dominant system or totally occluded RCA with unstable hemodynamic status.

TREATMENT ALGORITHM FOR A CALCIFIED LESION EMPLOYING INTRACORONARY IMAGING (FLOWCHART 1)

Rotational atherectomy or LASER is considered when an imaging catheter or small profile balloon cannot pass the calcified lesion (balloon uncrossable lesions). Lesion modification by atherectomy or IVL or Laser devices is considered when intracoronary imaging findings indicate criteria with risk of stent underexpansion, such as calcium arc (>180°), thickness (>500 μm), or insufficient lesion expansion (remaining indication) by balloons including NC balloon, OPN balloon, and scoring devices. Once the lesion is pretreated with balloon or plaque modification devices, imaging should be performed to confirm the success of lesion preparation by detecting the presence of fracture and dissection and gain in mean luminal area. DES implantation

Flowchart 1: Treatment algorithm for a calcified lesion employing intracoronary imaging.

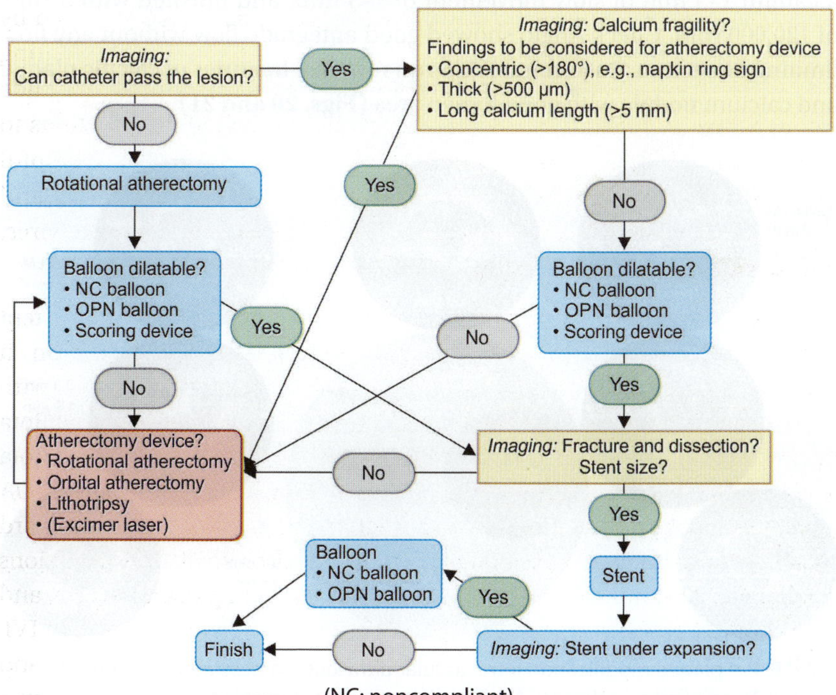

(NC: noncompliant)

should be carried out after selecting appropriately sized stent based on intravascular imaging, then poststent optimization must be done by identifying and rectifying any significant malapposition, expansion, and medial edge dissection to improve acute and long-term outcomes.

Case 1: Plaque modification with orbital atherectomy of LM bifurcation (T-tap technique) under IVUS guidance.
A 61-year-old male, known hypertensive, diabetic, CKD, and anemia, underwent PCI (2010) with stenting of LAD (3 × 30 mm endeavor resolute stent) and OM (2.5 × 23 mm mini vision stent), presented with chest heaviness associated with SOB. Diagnosed as ACS—unstable angina, 2D ECHO—good LV function, EF—60%. *Investigations:* Hb—8.6 g/dL, serum Cr—1.4 mg/dL, eGFR—56 mL/min, RBS—197 mg/dL.

CAG-DVD with ostial LCx 90% stenosis and mid-RCA 90% stenosis
The LMCA engaged through 7 Fr, right radial access, EBU 3.5-7 Fr guiding catheter, check Angio was taken, lesion was crossed with 0.014" run through wire, and predilated with 2.0 × 10 mm balloon at 10-12 atm. Prestenting IVUS run was taken from LCx to LM which show calcific nodules at ostial LCx with severe superficial calcium of distal LM and proximal LCx **(Figs. 18 and 19)**.

Orbital atherectomy was performed after exchanging viper wire with work horse wire over the corsair microcatheter. OA was carried out using 1.25-mm crown at 80,000 rpm speed, 5 runs with forward and backward cutting with a careful 1-3 mm of slow movement of 1-3 mm, and finished with 2 runs of 120,000 rpm. Check Angio showed good antegrade flow without any flow limiting dissection. Postorbital IVUS run revealed fractures of calcific plaque and calcium nodule with good lumen area **(Figs. 20 and 21)**.

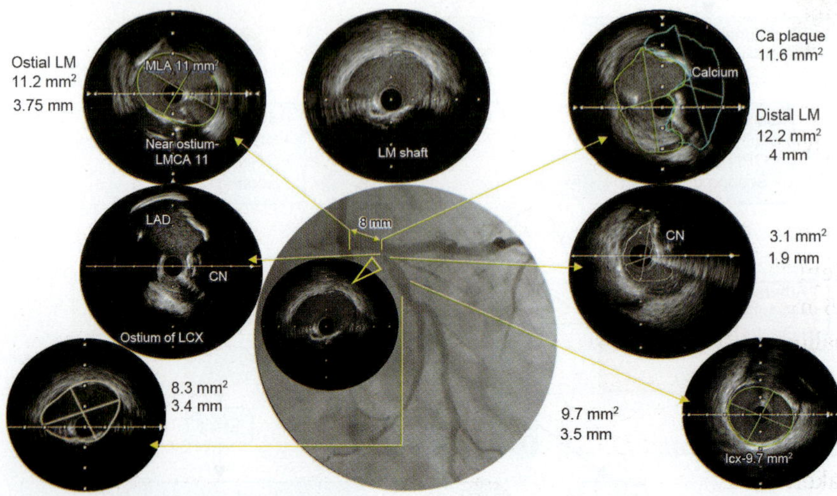

Fig. 18: Pre plaque modification intravascular ultrasound assessment of left main (LM)-LCX. (CN: calcified nodule; LMCA: left main coronary artery; MLA: mean luminal area)

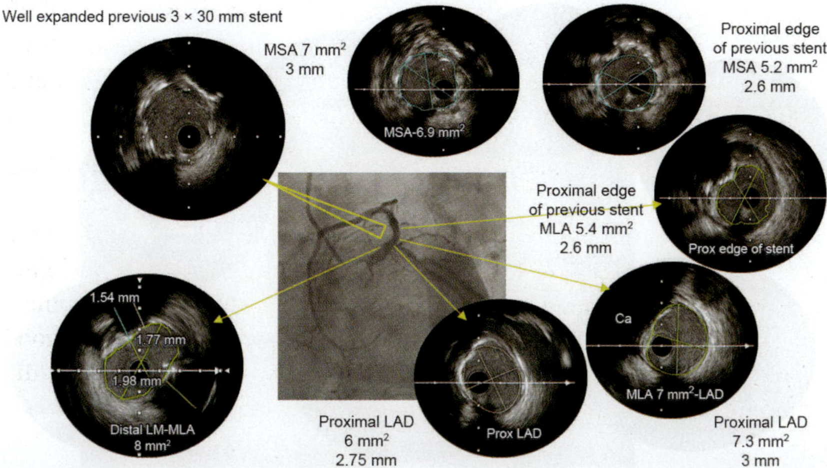

Fig. 19: Pre-plaque modification intravascular ultrasound assessment of left main (LM)-LAD. (LAD: left anterior descending; MLA: mean luminal area; MSA: mean stent area)

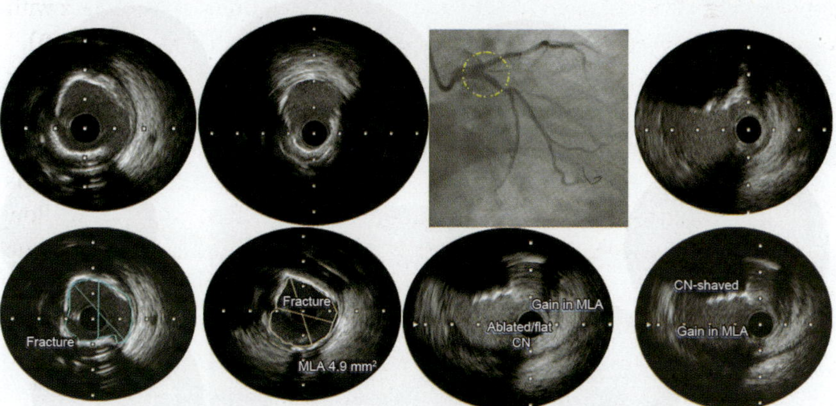

Fig. 20: Post-plaque modification with OA under IVUS. (CN: calcified nodule; IVUS: intravascular ultrasound; MLA: mean luminal area; OA: orbital atherectomy)

Subsequently, stenting of LM to LCx was done with 4.0 × 15-mm stent deployed at 12 atm, stented portion of LCx was post dilatated with 3.5 × 15-mm NC Trek balloon, and POT of LM was done with 5 × 6 mm POT PTCA balloon. IVUS run of LAD was taken which showed good gain in the luminal area with mild ISR at proximal LAD struts of previous stent, recrossed wire in LAD and kissing balloon dilatation done with 3.5 × 15 mm NC Trek balloon in LCx, 3.0 × 15 mm NC Trek balloon in LAD at 16 atms. Post-kissing IVUS run taken in LAD and LCx showed good luminal area with well-expanded stent in LCx, POT 5.0 × 6 mm NC balloon at distal LM at 14–16 atm. IVUS run in LAD run shows ostioproximal LAD intramural hematoma **(Fig. 22)**.

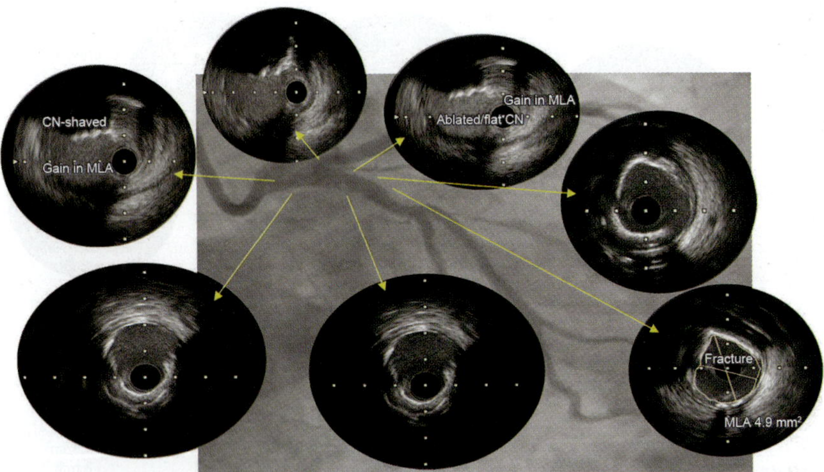

Fig. 21: Post-orbital intravascular ultrasound run revealed fractures of calcific plaque and calcium nodule with good lumen area. (MLA: mean luminal area)

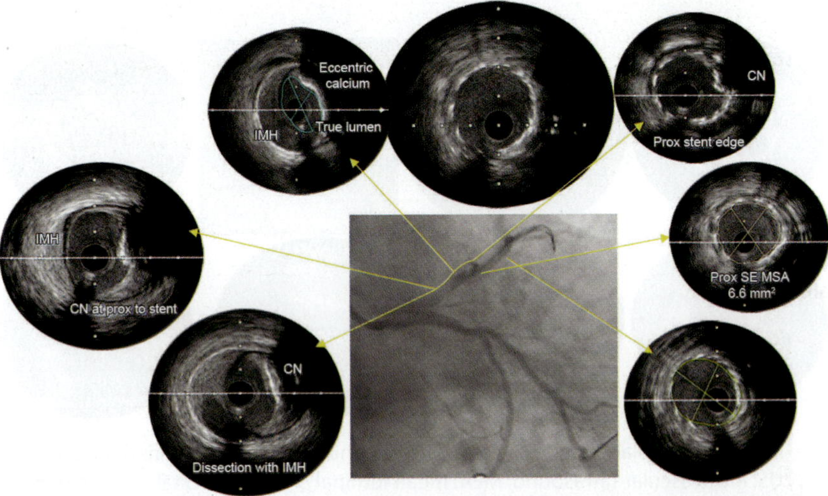

Fig. 22: Intravascular ultrasound run of LAD to left main showed ostioproximal LAD intramural hematoma. (CN: calcified nodule; LAD: left anterior descending; MSA: mean stent area)

Rewiring of both LAD and LCx over with crossed dual lumen catheter, Sion blue wire placed in LAD, and BMW wire placed in LCx. Balloon unable to cross in LAD and LCx. Guide plus guideliner used for support 3.5 × 15 mm balloon in LCx passed, stent unable to cross in LAD. 3 × 15 mm balloon crossed with guide liner support in LAD and dilated at 12 to 14 atm. Resolute Onyx 3.5 × 15 mm stent deployed from LMCA–LAD at 12 atm for 10 seconds and kissing balloon dilatation done with 3.5 × 15 mm NC Trek balloon in LCx, 3.0 × 15 mm NC Trek balloon in LAD at 18 atms, postdilation with 3.5 × 15 mm

NC Trek balloon at proximal LAD stent at 10–12 atm. Poststenting IVUS run taken in LAD and LCx suggestive of well-opposed stent with no evidence of edge dissection, no evidence of intramural hematoma. The final result was good with TIMI III flow with no complications **(Figs. 23 and 24)**.

Clinical History

A 75-year-old female, known HTN, CAD-S/P PTCA + DES to LCx IRA 2013 presented with complaint of SOB II with upper backache for the past

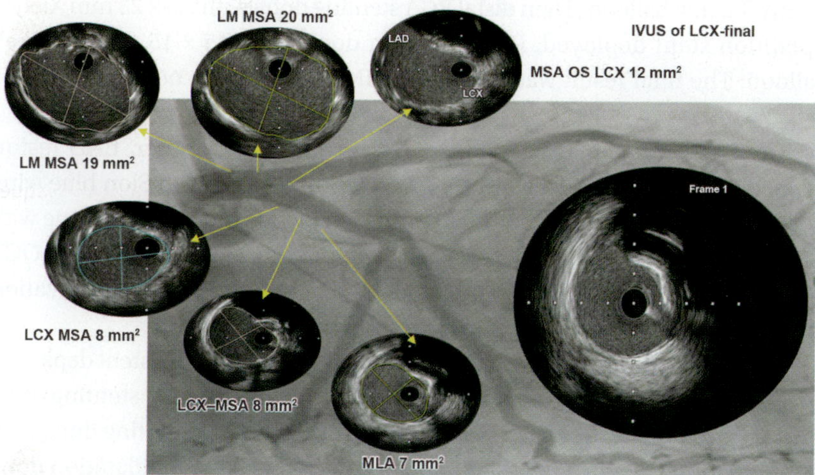

Fig. 23: Poststenting IVUS of LCX-LM showing well apposed and expanded stent struts. (IVUS: intravascular ultrasound; LM: left main; OS: oculus sinister; MLA: mean luminal area; MSA: mean stent area)

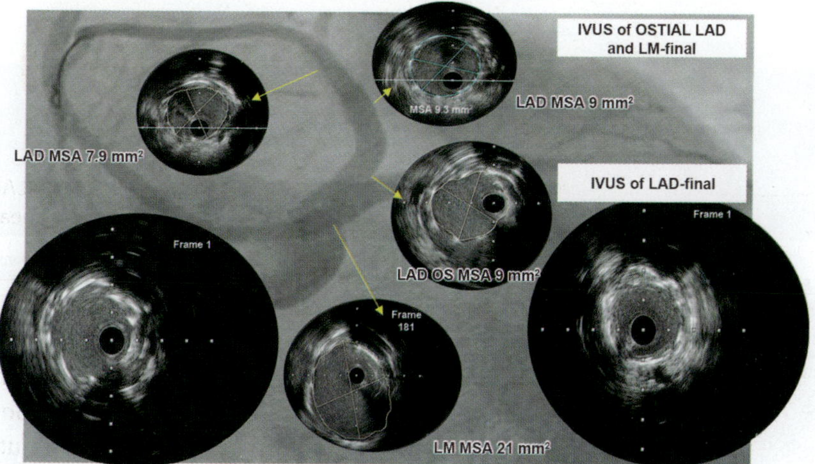

Fig. 24: Poststenting IVUS of LAD-LM showing well apposed and expanded stent struts. (IVUS: intravascular ultrasound; LAD: left anterior descending; LM: left main; OS: oculus sinister; MLA: mean luminal area; MSA: mean stent area)

2–3 months. ECG—left bundle branch block (LBBB), 2D Echo—severe LV dysfunction.

CAG: LMCA: Calcified distal 70%, LAD: Ostioproximal 95% calcific lesion, followed by 70% tubular lesion, LCx: Mid 40% ISR, distal 40% lesion and RCA: Proximal to mid mild ISR. Distal ISR 80% stenosis after stent. Advice: CABG/image-guided ROTA/IVL multivessel PCI.

Right coronary artery engaged with JR 3.5–7-Fr guiding catheter, RCA lesion crossed with 0.014" run through wire. Predilatation done with 2.0 × 10 mm Tazuna balloon. Then distal RCA stenting done with 3.5 × 23 mm Xience Xpedition stent deployed. Postdilatation done with 3.5 × 15 mm NC Trek balloon. The final result was good with TIMI III flow with no complications **(Fig. 25)**.

The LMCA engaged with EBU 3.5–7-Fr guiding catheter, LAD lesion crossed with 0.014" run through wire. LCx lesion crossed with Sion blue wire. Rota done with 1.5-mm burr at 1.6 L rpm. Then plaque modification done with 3.0 × 15 mm IVL balloon and 5 cycle given in proximal LAD. Prestenting OCT was done which showed LM to proximal LAD tight stenosis with calcification and fibro calcification lesion in mid LAD **(Fig. 26)**.

Mid LAD stenting done with 2.75 × 38 mm Xience Xpedition stent deployed. Postdilatation done with 3.0 × 15 mm balloon. Then LM–LAD stenting done with 3.0 × 26 mm Resolute Onyx stent deployed. Then LCx stenting done with 2.75 × 26 mm Resolute Onyx stent deployed. Kissing balloon dilatation done in LAD and LCx **(Fig. 25)**. Poststenting OCT was done which showed well-expanded stent struts with no edge dissection. The final result was good with TIMI III flow with no complications **(Figs. 27 to 30)**.

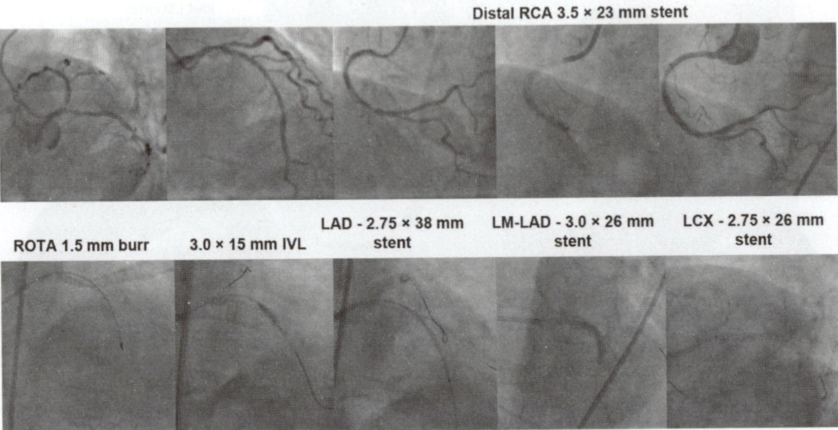

Fig. 25: Angioplasty of RCA, plaque modification of LAD with ROTA followed by IVL and stenting of LM. LAD & LCX. (IVL: intravascular lithotripsy; LAD: left anterior descending; LM: left main; RCA: right coronary artery)

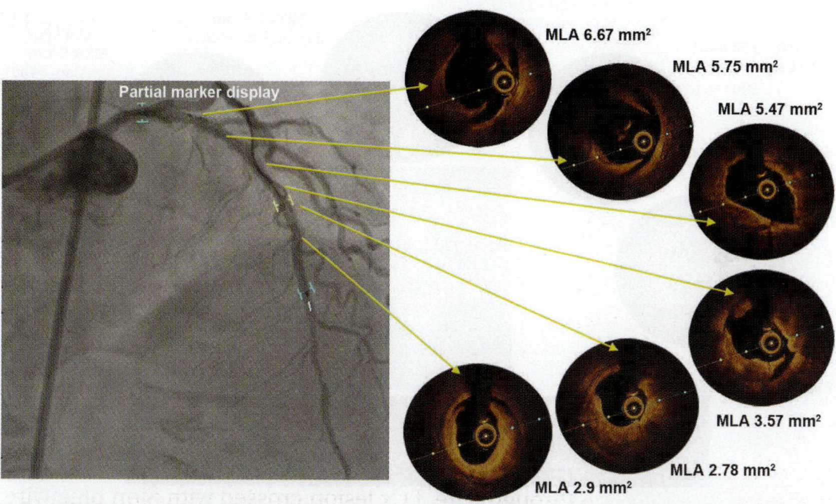

Fig. 26: Prestenting optical coherence tomography showing severe calcified lesion.

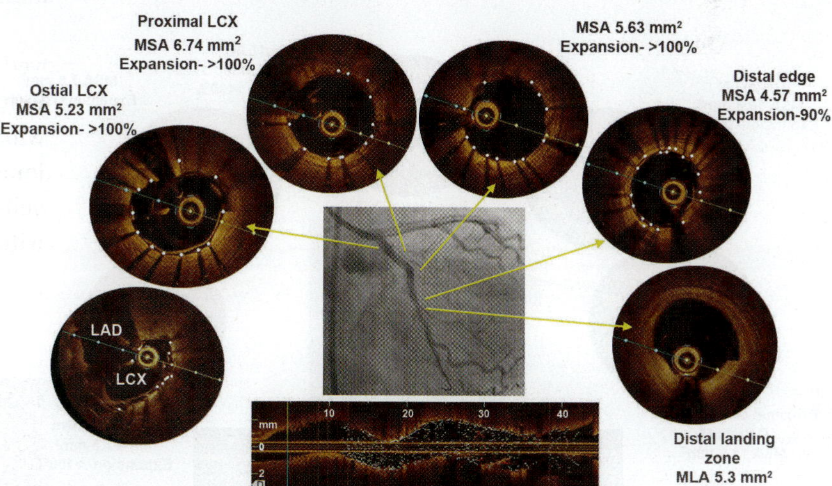

Fig. 27: Poststenting optical coherence tomography of LCX showing well expanded and apposed stent struts.

CONTRAST-INDUCED NEPHROPATHY

Patients who are undergoing PCI for severely calcified coronaries are at risk of contrast-induced nephropathy (CIN) which contributes to additional risk to the already existing high-risk status associated with these complex interventional procedures, therefore, it is essential to evaluate these subsets of patients to screen carefully for preventing or further worsening of renal dysfunction. CIN can be prevented by adequate hydration during

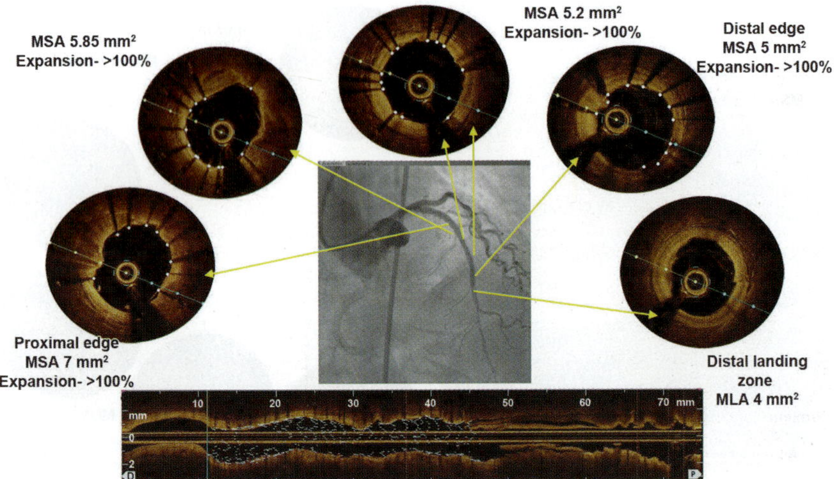

Fig. 28: Poststenting optical coherence tomography of mid LAD showing well expanded and apposed stent struts.

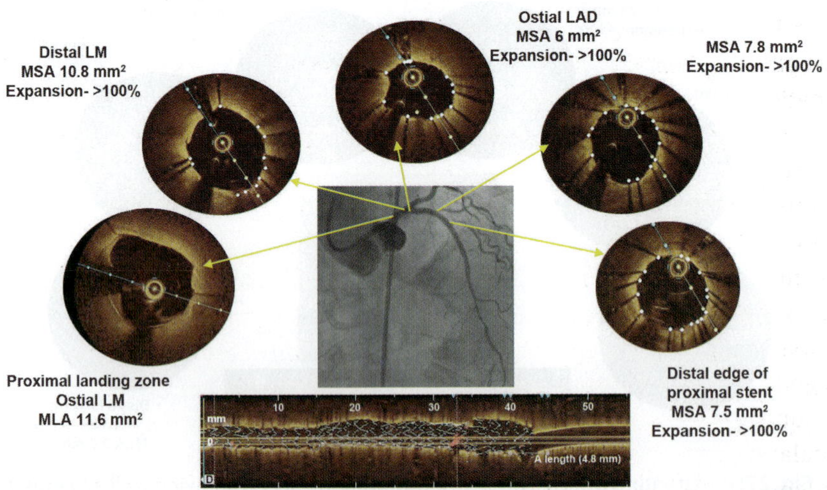

Fig. 29: Poststenting optical coherence tomography of LM-LAD showing well expanded and apposed stent struts.

periprocedure period with isotonic saline, usage of low osmolar or isoosmolar contrast agents, minimizing contrast dose. Whenever possible plan for implementing IVUS-guided low contrast or Zero-contrast PCI to reduce the risk of CIN, and not to delay dialysis management for patients who develop significant renal dysfunction with acidosis and low urine output to improve survival rate with low morbidity.

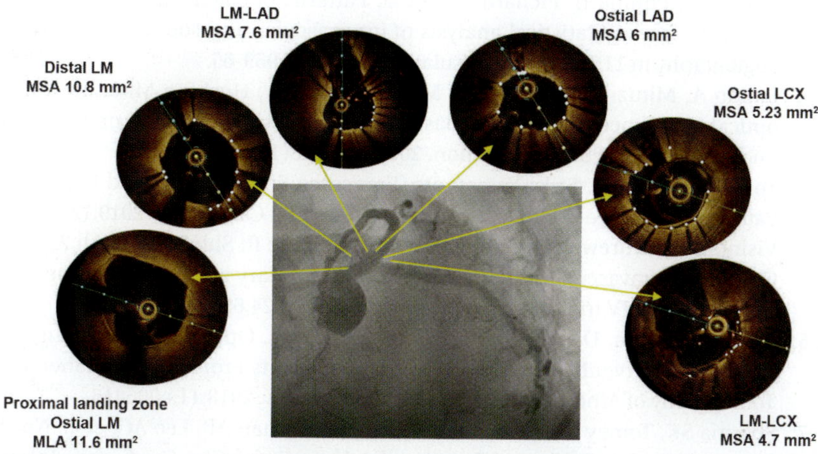

Fig. 30: Poststenting optical coherence tomography of LM bifurcation showing well expanded and apposed stent struts.

CONCLUSION

Pre-PCI intravascular imaging assessment of plaque morphology, lesion length, circumferential distribution, and expansion index is helpful in guiding meticulous lesion preparation, especially in diffuse, severe calcific lesions by using appropriate debulking devices. After lesion preparation, confirm adequate plaque modification with IVUS/OCT otherwise upsize the device or use additional adjunctive devices for further modification. Precise sizing of the stent and selection proper selection of landing zones with normal or minimal plaque burden are mandatory to get the best results. Finally, DES implantation should be optimized by looking for any malapposition, expansion, medial edge dissection, and needs to be rectified if they are significant. Avoid mismatch with reference vessel as oversizing leads to more frequent MACE; and undersizing leads to more frequent under expansion malapposition and scaffold thrombosis. It is strongly recommended to do adequate poststent dilation with appropriately sized NC high-pressure balloons to achieve good stent apposition and expansion without leaving any significant medial edge dissection.

REFERENCES

1. Généreux P, Madhavan MV, Mintz GS, et al. Ischemic outcomes after coronary intervention of calcified vessels in acute coronary syndromes. Pooled analysis from the HORIZONS-AMI (Harmonizing Outcomes With Revascularization and Stents in Acute Myocardial Infarction) and ACUITY (Acute Catheterization and Urgent Intervention Triage Strategy) TRIALS. J Am Coll Cardiol 2014; 63:1845-54.

2. Mintz GS, Popma JJ, Pichard AD, et al. Patterns of calcification in coronary artery disease. A statistical analysis of intravascular ultrasound and coronary angiography in 1155 lesions. Circulation. 1995;91:1959-65.
3. Fujino A, Mintz GS, Matsumura M, Lee T, Kim SY, Hoshino M, et al. A new optical coherence tomography-based calcium scoring system to predict stent underexpansion. EuroIntervention. 2018 Apr 6;13(18):e2182-e2189.
4. Tomoyo Sugiyama, Erika Yamamoto, Francesco Fracassi. Calcified Plaques in Patients With Acute Coronary Syndromes. J Am Coll Cardiol Intv 2019;12:531-40.
5. Visinoni ZM, Jurewitz DL, Kereiakes DJ, Shlofmitz R, Shlofmitz E, Ali Z, et al. Coronary intravascular lithotripsy for severe coronary artery calcification: The Disrupt CAD I-IV trials. Cardiovasc Revasc Med. 2024;65:81-7.
6. Emile Mehanna, Dawn Abbott, Hiram G. Bezerra. Optimizing Percutaneous Coronary Intervention in Calcified Lesions Insights From Optical Coherence Tomography of Atherectomy. Circ Cardiovasc Interv. 2018;11:e006813.
7. Sharma SK, Tomey MI, Teirstein PS, Kini AS, Reitman AB, Lee AC, et al. North American Expert Review of Rotational Atherectomy. Circ Cardiovasc Interv. 2019;12(5):e007448.
8. Shlofmitz E, Shlofmitz R, Lee MS. Orbital Atherectomy: A Comprehensive Review. Interv Cardiol Clin. 2019;8(2):161-71.

CHAPTER 15

Rotational Atherectomy: Complications Prevention and Management

Deepak Davidson

INTRODUCTION

Rotablation is an awesome technology that is used in the management of angioplasty of calcified coronary lesions. This device, which I consider as the best innovation in the field of coronary angioplasty, was introduced by David Auth in 1988. This is a masculine device and is useful for managing difficult coronary interventions. However, rotablation is not without complications and has a steep learning curve so that this challenging procedure can be made simpler and free of complications. Thus, patients with calcified or difficult coronary lesions can be benefited mostly with this particular procedure. In this chapter, I shall take you through the potential complications that can happen during rotablation, how to prevent it, and manage these complications, in case an unfortunate event occurs.

AIR EMBOLISM

Air embolism is a rare complication that can happen during rotablation.

How does it happen?

The drive shaft and its sheath is 4.3 F in size and when it is used inside a 6F guide catheter, it occupies the entire lumen of the 6F guide catheter. Thus, you have only a small space between the guide catheter and the drive shaft sheath. So, inadvertently while pushing the drive shaft through the guide catheter into the coronary artery, air bubbles can be formed inside the guide catheter (especially in case of the 6F guide catheter) due to venturi effect. During contrast injection, these air bubbles can be pushed into the coronary arteries leading on to air embolism.

How can it we prevented?

- *Use of large-bore guide catheter:* It is always safe to use 7F guide catheter, so that you have a reasonable space between the guide catheter and the drive shaft, so that air bubble formation due to venturi effect can be prevented.
- *Having a good bad bleed:* If you are using a small guide catheter like 6F guide catheter, before injecting contrast into the coronary is always good to have a good bad bleed so that when you have a good bad bleed whatever

small bubbles are there inside the guide catheter can be removed and while injecting contrast, air embolism can be prevented.

Management of air embolism:
Inadvertently, if air bubbles are pushed into the coronaries, it can lead to myocardial infarction (MI), hypotension, etc.

- Immediately start 100% oxygen.
- Patient is likely to have hypotension so manage hypotension with fluids, vasopressors. If there is hemodynamic collapse, you might need to intubate the patient. Call for an anesthetist's help and then arrange for mechanical circulatory support device.
- *Mechanical circulatory support device:* In case the patient does not respond to other resuscitative measures, one might have to resort to mechanical circulatory support devices.
- Intracoronary adrenaline could be of use in these situations so that you can achieve good flow in the distal vasculature.
- Aspirating with aspiration catheters is also useful to remove the air bubbles from inside the coronaries.

SLOW FLOW WITH ANGINA AND MYOCARDIAL INFRACTION

During rotablation, up to 15% of patients can have slow flow inside the coronaries leading on to angina and myocardial infraction.

Why does this happen?
During aggressive rotablation, one can have micro particles going down the coronaries and this can clog the small distal blood vessels and capillaries, and this can lead to slow flow during rotablation.[1]

How can it be prevented?

- During difficult rotablation, it is always good to have a good blood pressure so that the flow is well augmented during the procedure.
- Shorter duration of burr run (15 seconds) rather than going to 30 seconds of burring is always safer to prevent slow flow, especially in heavily calcified coronaries, patients with acute coronary syndrome or LV disfunction. 10–15 seconds would be safer option compared to longer burr runs.
- To have a good breathing space of a coronaries between the burring for 10–15 seconds. Wait for at least a minute in sick patients or with LV disfunction before you start off with the next run.
- Smaller burr size could reduce the incidence of distal embolization. When you have a patient with LV disfunction or when you have a patient with heavy calcification, it is always safe to start off with 1.25 mm burr. Step up burr approach would be safer option rather than starting off

with a bigger burr size. If a larger burr is used initially, one might have to hit hard against the lesion rather than pecking, and this hitting hard against the lesion can lead on to deceleration which in turn leads to distal embolization and slow flow.

- Reduce rotational burr speed rather than going up 200,000 rpm. Lower burr speeds (140–160 rpm) could reduce the chances of distal embolization.
- Minimizing decelerations during rotablation that is always try to do peck rather than hitting hard against lesion. (Which can lead on to increase particulate matter going down the vessel leading on to slow flow.)
- *Use of flushing cocktail*: You need to have a good flush during the procedure, a good flushing cocktail can wash away the micro particles and prevent clogging of the capillaries. Nicorandil in flush is found to be beneficial to prevent slow flow.

Management of slow flow:

Slow flow is a rare thing to happen, however, it can even lead to hypotension and death.

How do we prevent slow flow?

Steps to deal with slow flow:

- Long lesions >15 mm are associated with higher incidents of slow flow.
- Heavily calcified lesions can lead on to slow flow significantly.
- Tortuous vessels
- Highly eccentric lesion
- Reduce left ventricular function with high left ventricular end-diastolic pressure (LVEDP) all these situations one could have slow flow.

Prevention of slow flow:

- Pretreatment preparation:
  - Dual antiplatelet preloading
  - Calcium channel bloggers 2 days prior to the procedure can reduce the incidence.
  - Discontinue beta-blockers 2 days prior to procedures.
  - If possible, reduce BP-lowering medications so that you have a good blood pressure during the procedure.
  - Adequate hydration to maintain a good blood pressure.
  - Adequate blood pressure is required to compensate for the liberal use of vasodilators.
  - Always try to maintain an act of above 300.
  - Temporary pacemaker to be inserted if rotablation is done for right coronary artery or a dominant circumflex artery, left main procedure, ostial left anterior descending (LAD) lesion or with larger bur size with 2 mm or more.

- *During procedure:*
  - Try to avoid high speed rotablation (low speed is associated with less incidence of distal embolization and slow flow)
  - Avoid deceleration of >3,000, never drop the rotational atherectomy speed to >5,000 rpm.
  - Try to begin with smaller burr size.
  - Always maintain a burr artery 0.6.

Burr approach to prevent chance of distal embolization:

- Long lesions can be divided into segments and treat separately limiting run to shorter intervals <15 seconds also.
- Intracoronary nitroglycerin before each Rota run
- Never allow the burr to remain in one location while rotating.

How to treat slow flow?
Maintain a good blood pressure with mechanical circulatory support or with vasopressors.

- IC medications can reverse slow flow.
- 100–200 μg up to 4 doses
- Adenosine 24 μg up to 4 doses
- 100 μg maximum of 1,000 μg nitroprusside
- Adrenaline, 50–200 μg. All these medications could be given intracoronary through microcatheter so that slow flow could be managed.

BRADYCARDIA AND ATRIOVENTRICULAR BLOCK

Bradycardia and atrioventricular (AV) block can happen during slow flow or during right coronary rotablation.[2]

How do we prevent this?
Measures could be very similar to prevention of slow flow.

How do we manage bradycardia in case it happens during rotablation?

- Have temporary pacemaker inserted prior to rotablation of the right coronary artery could prevent bradycardia and AV block.
- IV aminophylline

GUIDE WIRE TIP DETACHMENT

Why does this happen?
The radiopaque part of the Rota wire is 0.014 inch and rest of Rota wire is 0.009 inch. If the burr travels distally and if it reaches the most distal portion till radiopaque marker, the burr can detach radiopaque tip from the Rota wire and this distal radiopaque part of the wire can embolize distally.

How do we prevent this?
Make sure that during the burring, the burr should not be advanced to the distal end of the guidewire.

How do we manage if the guidewire detachment occurs?

- Attempt removal with a loop snare
- Stent implantation in the site of detachment so that you can plaster the detached wire between the stent at the vessel wall.

VESSEL PERFORATION

Vessel perforation in rotablation is rare but a serious complication of rotablation.[3]

How can it be prevented?

- Using small burr size reduces the chances of vessel perforation, especially when you have an eccentric lesion or tortuous or angulated segment. So, it is always safe to start off with smaller burr size in these situations.
- Reduce the Rota speed in tortuous segments. Tortuous segments are the notorious areas for vessel perforation, because of guidewire.

If you have perforation, how do you manage that?

- Prolonged balloon inflation
- Covered stent implantation
- Cardiac surgery

STUCK BURR

Why does it happen?

Burr has two halves. Distal part is covered with diamond crumbs and proximal part is smooth. Only the distal part can ablate a lesion and the smooth part cannot. So, while pulling back, it can get trapped. While moving forward, the burr is aligned to the outer curve of the vessel and while pulling out, its aligned to the inner curve.[4] So, while moving out, it can get trapped in an eccentric lesion. Factors associated with stuck burr are described in **Table 1**.

TABLE 1: Triggering factors.

Anatomical	*Technical*
Long	Bigger burr
Angulated lesions	High Rota speed
Eccentric lesions	Speed dropping >5,000 rpm
Spasm	Pushing than pecking
Stent ablation	Malalignment of guide at RCA ostium
RCA ostium	

(RCA: right coronary artery)

How does it happens?

- At high speeds, a small burr can slip across the lesion without burring. Ledge of calcium behind burr causes "Kokeshi" (Japanese doll) effect.
- While pushing vigorously (without pecking) a large burr against long, angulated, tortuous, and calcified lesion, speed may decrease and burr could stop and get stuck.
- Burr can jump and get entrapped, if it is activated near a proximal lesion, without relieving the tension on the drive shaft.

What to do if the burr gets stuck inside the coronary artery?

- Pray hard
- Surgical help
- Percutaneous removal

How do we percutaneously remove the stuck burr?

- Apply manual traction with on-dynaglide or off-dynaglide rotation (burp foot pedal while pulling the burr)
    - Advance the burr, increase rotation speed and pull back.

What are the issues while pulling the stuck burr?

- Proximal vessel can get dissected due to guide getting sucked in.
- Brutal force can lead to fracture of burr shaft.

In order to prevent the guide catheter from getting sucked into the coronary, disengage the guide catheter and keep a 0.014 wire in aorta, to prevent the guide from getting deep in the vessel **(Fig. 1)**.

- Deep intubation of guide catheter and pull the burr.

    If burr gets stuck in proximal RCA, deep intubation of guide can release the burr.

- Dilate a balloon by the side of burr and pull the burr.

    Make a crack between vessel and burr. Wire should be a coated wire to cross heavily calcified vessel. At times just having a wire by the side can facilitate removal of burr by buddy effect. Rarely, stiffer wires like Gaia, Conquest pro might be needed.

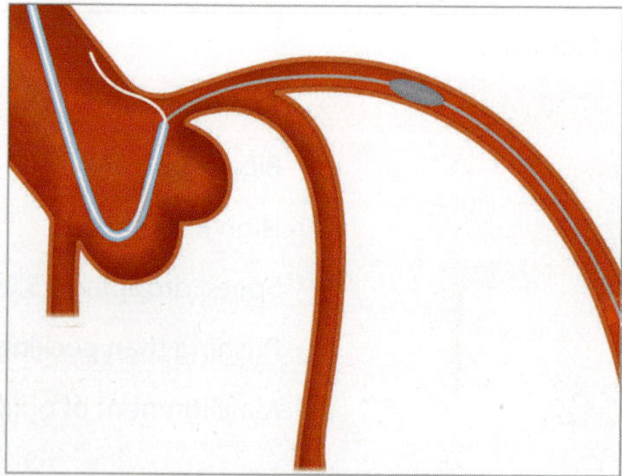

Fig. 1: A guidewire is kept in aorta to prevent the deep intubation of catheter into the coronary.

TABLE 1: Types of lasers available categorized by differences in wavelength.

Laser type	*Wavelength (nm)*	*Absorption depth (mm)*	*Mechanism*
XeCl (excimer)	308	0.05	Protein–lipids
Nd:YAG	1,060	2.0	Protein–water
	1,320	1.25	Water
Dye	480	0.5	Protein
Argon	488	0.5	Protein
HO:YAG	2,060	0.3	Water

(HO:YAG: holmium: yttrium-aluminum-garnet; Nd:YAG: neodymium-doped yttrium aluminum garnet; XeCl: xenon chloride)

Mechanism of Action of Laser

Three distinct mechanisms are involved in tissue ablation with excimer laser: (1) photochemical, (2) photothermal, and (3) photomechanical. Carbon-carbon bonds in the intravascular material are broken once the UV laser light is absorbed by the tissue (photochemical). As a result, the temperature of intracellular water increases, causing cellular rupture and generates a vapor bubble at the catheter tip (photothermal). The obstructive intravascular material is disrupted by the expansion and implosion of these vapor bubbles (photomechanical). The disrupted fragments are <10 µm in diameter, and are absorbed by the reticuloendothelial system avoiding any microvascular obstruction. Common terminologies used while performing excimer laser coronary atherectomy (ELCA) are fluence and rate.

The threshold energy required for the penetration of UV light into tissue and the creation of a steam bubble is called "fluence" (*range:* 30–80 mJ/mm^2). It has direct relationship on size of the bubble with higher fluence, larger bubble. The number of pulses emitted during a 1-second period is the "pulse repetition rate" (jack hammer effect) which is simply referred as "rate".

Equipment

The CVX-300 cardiovascular laser excimer system (Spectranetics; **Fig. 2**) uses Xenon chloride (XeCl) as the active medium. The light emitted has a wavelength of 308 nm (in the UVB spectrum) with a tissue penetration depth between 30 µm. It is the only coronary laser-emitting device currently approved by the US Food and Drug Administration (FDA).

Coronary catheters are available in four diameters (0.9, 1.4, 1.7, and 2.0 mm). Those most commonly used have a concentric array of laser fibers at the tip **(Fig. 3)**.

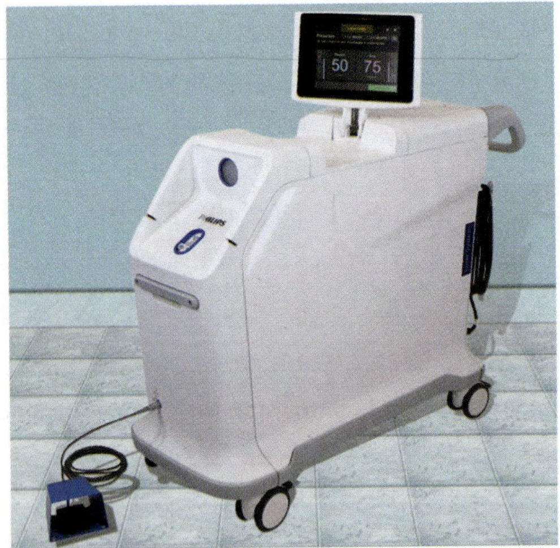

Fig. 2: CVX-300 excimer laser system.

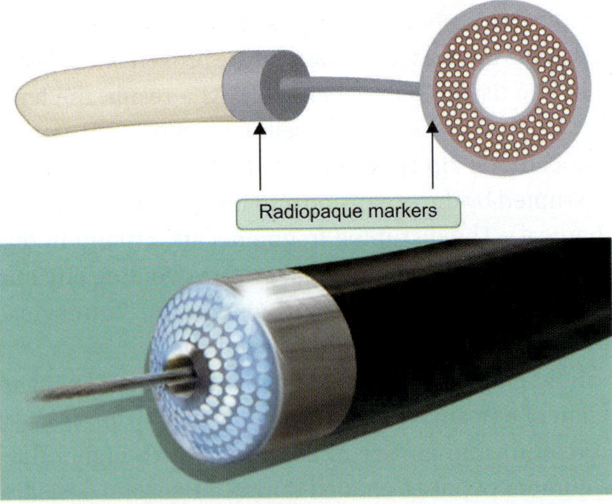

Fig. 3: Catheter tip with concentric array of fibers.

Procedural Technique and Tips

Prior to performing laser atherectomy, it is essential to observe certain safety measures. All persons inside the catheterization laboratory, including the patient, must wear protective spectacles to minimize the risk of retinal exposure to the UV light. All windows should be covered and doors locked. Following this safety checklist, the laser unit is warmed up and the selected catheter is connected and calibrated prior to being introduced into the body. Even when the catheter is in vivo, all staff in the vicinity should wear eye protection in case the catheter housing breaks, which could release UV light.

TABLE 2: Various ELCA catheters available with differentiating features.

	0.9 mm X-80	*1.4 mm*	*1.7 mm*	*2.0 mm*	*0.9 mm X-80 OTW*
Model number	110–004	114–009	117–016	120–009	110–002
Guidewire compatibility (in)	0.014	0.014	0.014	0.014	0.014
Guide catheter compatibility (F)	6	6/7	7	8	6
Minimum vessel diameter (mm)	2.0	2.2	2.5	3.0	2.0
Max tip outer diameter (in)	0.038	0.057	0.069	0.080	0.038
Max shaft outer diameter (in)	0.049	0.062	0.072	0.084	0.049
Working length (cm)	130	130	130	130	130
Fluence (mJ/mm^2)	30–80	30–60	30–60	30–60	30–80
Repetition rate (Hz)	25–80	25–40	25–40	25–40	25–80
Laser on/off time (seconds)	10/5	5/10	5/10	5/10	10/5

(ELCA: excimer laser coronary atherectomy)

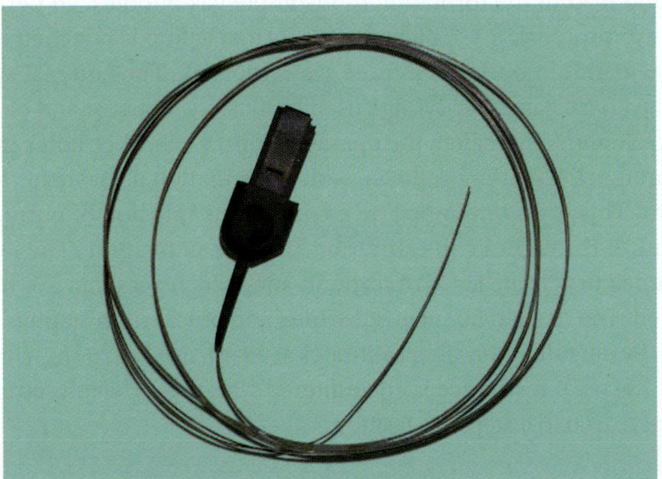

Fig. 4: 0.9-mm rapid exchange (RX) catheter.

The ELCA catheters are currently available in four diameters (0.9 mm, 1.4 mm, 1.7 mm, and 2.0 mm), and are of two types based on the arrangement of fiberoptic fibers within the catheter **(Fig. 4 and Table 2)**. They can either be concentric around the guidewire lumen or eccentrically localized toward one hemisphere. General concepts to consider when choosing a catheter are: (1) Its size should not exceed two-thirds the diameter of the target vessel, and (2) it should be able to deliver the intensity of energy needed to treat the target lesion based on the lesion's severity and consistency. Most commonly, the 0.9-mm catheter is used. Catheters can be conventional over-the-wire or newer rapid-exchange/monorail catheters. Monorail catheters are currently being utilized more commonly, given their advantages of better tip control and axial force transmission.

The proximal catheter end is then attached to the laser unit and its distal end calibrated. Calibration is an automated process, which is achieved by pointing the catheter tip towards the energy detector on the main laser unit and activating the laser. ELCA catheters are advanced on a short monorail segment compatible with any standard 0.014-inch guidewire. Care should be taken to select a guiding catheter that provides adequate support and that remains coaxial during lasing. In situations where the guiding catheter is not co-axial, guide extension catheters such as Guidezilla, Guideliner, Guideplus II, Telescope can be used. Once the system is turned on, the excimer laser generator requires around 5 minutes of start-up time.

A saline flush protocol is then employed before initiation of lasing. The concept behind this step is that both blood and contrast media consist of macromolecules, including proteins, that can absorb the bulk of the laser energy and lead to the formation of insoluble gas bubbles. To perform the saline flush protocol, a 1-L bag of 0.9% normal saline is attached to one of the triple manifold ports via a three-way stopcock. The contrast syringe is replaced with a clean 20-cc syringe used for flushing contrast and blood from the entire system. Thereafter, the operator infuses a 5–10-cc bolus of normal saline through the guiding catheter, with the initiation of lasing immediately afterward. This is accompanied by a continuous infusion of normal saline at 1–3 mL/s throughout the duration of laser activation. The system is programmed to activate for 5–10 seconds, after which goes into a 5–10 second rest period. The desired fluence, pulse rate, and pulse width settings are then selected. By default, the system calibrates at 45 mJ/mm^2 at 25 Hz, with a pulse width of 135 ns. If resistance is encountered with these default settings, they can be increased in a stepwise fashion.

The Five S's of Laser Success[6]

1. *Selecting the right patient:* Multiple morphology lesions (thrombus, calcium, and neointimal hyperplasia)
2. *Sizing:* Laser catheter diameter should not exceed two-thirds of the reference vessel diameter. Tighter the lesion, smaller the catheter. 0.9-mm catheter is most commonly used for uncrossable/undilatable lesions.

3. *Settings:* Fluence and pulse rate varying from 60/40 to 80/80. The 0.9-mm catheter permits 5 seconds activation and 10 seconds rest whereas the 0.9 mm × 80 catheter provides 10 seconds activation and 5 seconds rest, reflecting its use in more complex lesions. An audible alarm sounds at the end of the rest period to signal when to commence the next laser train.
4. *Saline:* Essential to remove contrast from the photoablation location. Flush is given at 1–2 mL/s. Application of laser in blood or contrast media is rarely performed in certain specific situations—such as treatment of an underexpanded stent—and should only be undertaken by experienced laser percutaneous coronary intervention (PCI) operators.[7]
5. *Speed:* The pulses of laser energy are delivered as the catheter is slowly (0.5 mm/s) advanced through the lesion, allowing adequate absorption and ablation. If the catheter is advanced too rapidly, the tissue does not have time to absorb the light energy and ablation will be suboptimal. Retrograde lasing can be performed on completion of antegrade lasing, particularly in severe lesions when there is anterograde resistance.

Clinical Indications

Acute Coronary Syndrome and Myocardial Infarction

Few reports with use of ELCA in intracoronary thrombus management providing excellent outcomes have been published in the recent years.[8,9] Considering the potential of ELCA for effective thrombus removal,[10] promotion of fibrinolysis,[11] platelet-stunning effects,[12] and concomitant plaque debulking,[13] It may be a beneficial tool in managing massive intracoronary thrombus in acute coronary syndrome (ACS) presentations. However, clinical data supporting the use of ELCA in AMI remains limited **(Fig. 5)**.

The Cohort of Acute Revascularization of Myocardial infarction with Excimer Laser (CARMEL) multicenter registry[14] is the largest study till date available that enrolled 151 acute myocardial infarction (AMI) patients, of which 65% had large thrombus burden in the culprit artery. Following ELCA, Thrombolysis in Myocardial Infarction (TIMI) flow grade was significantly increased (1.2–2.8), with an associated reduction in angiographic stenosis (83–52%). There was a low rate (8.6%) of major adverse coronary events (MACE). The maximal effect was observed in arteries with a large angiographic thrombus burden.

Uncrossable/Undilatable Lesions

When a lesion cannot be crossed with a low-profile device, or when the balloon inadequately expands with dilatation, ELCA may be applied, with a high success rate in such uncrossable or undilatable stenoses. The success rate may not be the same in lesions with significant calcification (calcified 79% vs. noncalcified 96%; $p < 0.05$).[15,16]

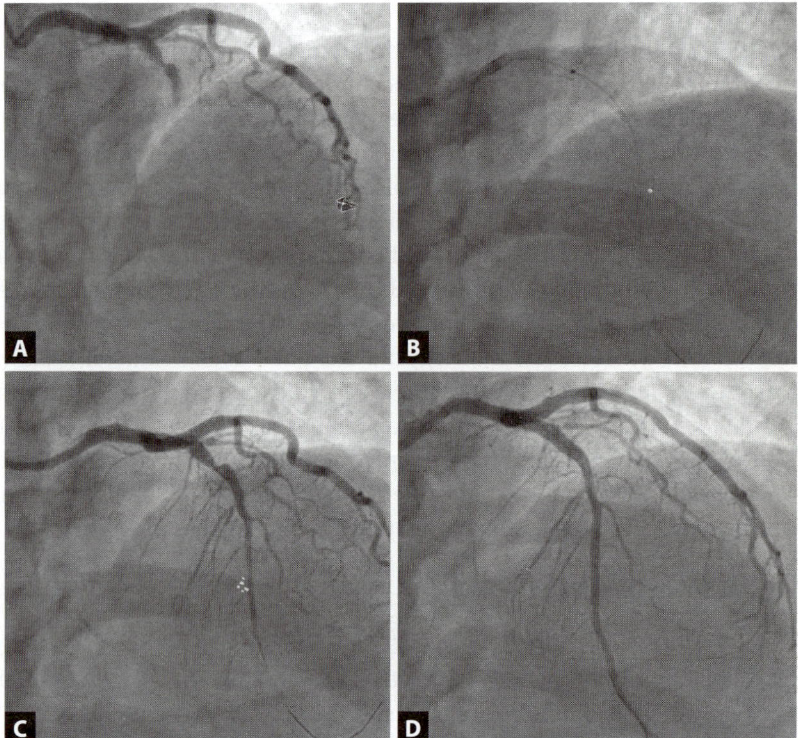

Figs. 5A to D: The use of ELCA in intracoronary thrombus. A 45-year-old man who underwent left anterior descending artery (LAD) stenting in 2011 now presented with anterior ST elevation MI with a thrombotically occluded LAD (A). ELCA was performed using 0.9-mm 6-F compatible catheter (B); 3,000 pulses were delivered over 10 trains with dramatic improvement in thrombus burden and obstructive stenosis (C). Case was completed with overlapping drug-eluting stent with excellent final angiographic result (D). (ELCA: excimer laser coronary atherectomy; MI: myocardial infarction).

In heavily calcified coronary lesions, the default technique for most of the PCI operators remains rotational atherectomy (RA), even among proficient ELCA users **(Fig. 6)**.

Chronic Total Occlusions

Despite attaining the distal wire position in chronic total occlusion (CTO), when the devices are unable to cross the proximal cap, ELCA can be considered. It may offer additional benefit as its ablative effect is transmitted through the lesion architecture, potentially weakening bonds between the constituent components of the CTO. A success rate of 86–90% for ELCA in CTO cases has been reported.[7,17,18]

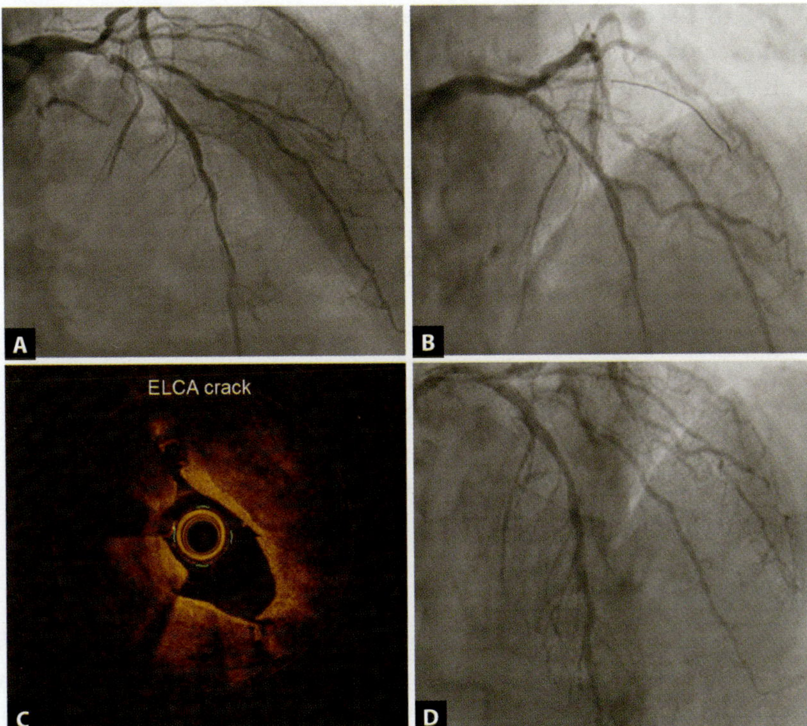

Figs. 6A to D: ELCA in calcium modification. A 64-year-old man, diabetic, chronic kidney disease, presented with chronic coronary syndrome. Left anterior descending artery (LAD) showed severe calcific disease and diseased good sized diagonal (A). Good angiographic luminal gain with TIMI III flow noted after lasing (B). Imaging with OCT showed intimal cracks after ELCA (C). Final angiographic result after drug-eluting stent (D). (ELCA: excimer laser coronary atherectomy).

Stent Underexpansion

Stent underexpansion is one of the risk factors for stent thrombosis. Rotational atherectomy (RA) risks metal fragment embolization and burr stalling. Despite maximal pressure balloon dilatation, ELCA remains the only technique to modify the underlying resistant atheroma by delivering energy to the abluminal stent surface without disrupting the stent architecture.[19,20] ELCA modifies the plaque behind the stent, which weakens the overall resistance, thus enabling subsequent complete stent expansion.[21-23] Within a stented environment, "contrast-milieu" lasing appears to be safe, facilitating high-pressure balloon stent expansion.[21-24]

In-stent Restenosis

In a study by Mehran et al., examination of 107 restenotic lesions in 98 patients showed that lesions treated with ELCA had greater intravascular ultrasound

(IVUS) cross-sectional area and luminal gain with more intimal hyperplasia ablation compared with balloon angioplasty alone.[25]

In a study by Rawlins J et al., where optical coherence tomography (OCT) was performed after ELCA for restenosis, its noted that laser therapy ablates both the luminal and abluminal atherosclerotic material.[26] This indicates that if the mechanism of restenosis is in part stent underexpansion, ELCA increases the likelihood of achieving greater stent expansion and more durable longer-term outcomes **(Fig. 7)**.

Saphenous Vein Grafts

Excimer laser coronary atherectomy is a safer alternative, allowing predictable debulking during SVG-PCI.[27,28] However, OCT images post-SVG ELCA showed that there are friable fragments that could embolize and cause no-reflow.[26] Therefore, when using ELCA for SVG-PCI, it is advisable to stent on a DPD system to prevent no-reflow.[26]

Contraindications

There are no absolute contraindications for the use of ELCA. Relative contraindications include acute angulation (>45°), coronary dissection, unprotected left main coronary artery. ELCA is also not recommended for heavy calcium and/or artery with the diameter of less than the catheter profile of 0.9 mm.

Complications

With the optimization of laser catheters and the introduction of safety techniques such as the saline infusion protocol, the incidence of previously seen serious complications such as flow-limiting dissections and vessel perforations has significantly decreased. Other measures used to prevent dissections include avoiding excessive force or over-sizing the laser catheter and starting from a low energy and increasing that slowly. If a flow-limiting dissection develops, the laser part of the procedure should be discontinued, and the dissection should be treated with balloon angioplasty and stent placement. Complications of ELCA are similar to those encountered during routine PCI. Specific issues may arise from interruption of the saline flush or contamination with contrast, which can generate excessive heat and increase the risk of vascular perforation.

ADVANCES AND FUTURE SCOPE

The use of ELCA has regained its momentum due to improved safety and performance with new, more-advanced catheters and the use of saline medium to deliver energy. Work is being performed toward development of

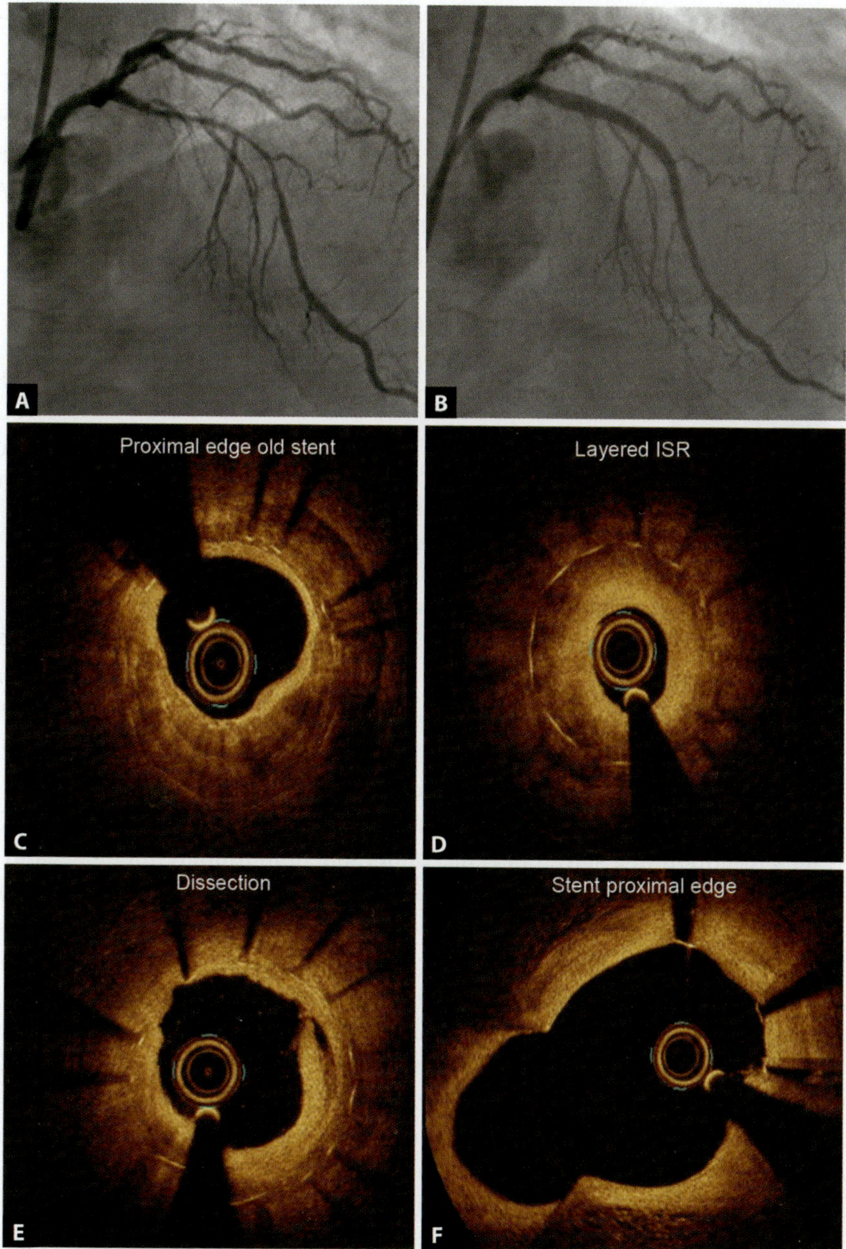

Figs. 7A to F: ELCA in in-stent restenosis. A 76-year-old man who underwent left anterior descending artery (LAD) stenting in 2009 now presented with chronic coronary syndrome with a severe in-stent restenosis (ISR) of LAD stent (A). Imaging with OCT showed neointimal hyperplasia with minimal lumen area (MLA) <2 mm^2 (C and D); ELCA was performed using 0.9-mm 6F compatible catheter; post-ELCA and balloon dilatation image (E). Case was completed with overlapping drug-eluting stent with excellent final angiographic and imaging result (B and F). (ELCA: excimer laser coronary atherectomy; OCT: optical coherence tomography).

laser catheters that can be used to ablate through heavily calcified plaques. This will be a significant advance, as laser is currently not very effective in heavily calcified lesions.

Laser use for underexpanded stents is a new approach for managing these difficult and clinically important cases. There have been reports of ELCA use in peri-stent calcium which is also promising. The use of laser with contrast in resistant lesions may also gain momentum, but should remain restricted to experienced laser users and to limited situations. In addition, saline flush should remain the standard practice.

Laser has also been used to modify and penetrate a resistant proximal CTO cap, which is important given advances in CTO-PCI. The combined use of laser and rotablation (RASER-PCI) is a useful approach for a subset of highly resistant and heavily calcified lesions.

In the era of moving toward stentless strategy, particularly in young patients after an ACS event with thrombotic lesion of the coronary arteries without significant luminal narrowing, ELCA laser can be considered for treating the thrombotic occlusion followed by drug-eluting balloon (DEB) usage is being considered by few operators. This technique, however, needs to be studied in large scale to identify if this is considered a safe option for young patients.

CONCLUSION

Excimer laser debulks and modifies the tissue with its photochemical, photothermal, and photokinetic properties without causing significant injury. After a disappointing start, ELCA has undergone important refinements and advancements that have earned it a renewed place in treating complex and resistant coronary lesions.

Excimer laser coronary atherectomy is a useful tool in the catheterization laboratory for treating lesions that are uncrossable or undilatable, a subset that is increasing with the aging population that we treat on a daily basis. ELCA is also helpful in cases where a stent was deployed but remains underexpanded, with accumulating evidence of its efficacy in this situation.

In addition, laser is increasingly used for CTO-PCI to facilitate the modification of the proximal CTO cap, to allow penetration with a wire and the completion of the procedure. Laser has been used in certain circumstances and by experienced operators in a contrast medium (rather than saline medium) to increase its effectiveness and allow the successful completion of complex PCI cases.

In comparison with rotablation, ELCA has the advantage of working with a normal 0.014″ PCI guidewire and in the presence of a second buddy wire (while rotablation cannot be done with 2 wires), which is frequently used in difficult lesions.

Overall, ELCA is an important tool in the interventionalists' armamentarium that, when used appropriately, allows the completion of difficult and demanding cases with successful outcomes, and therefore benefits our patients.

REFERENCES

1. Choy DSJ. History and state-of-the-art of lasers in cardiovascular disease. Laser Med Surg News Adv. 1988;6(3):34-8.
2. Cook SI, Eigler NL, Shefer A, Goldenberg T, Forrester JS, Litvack F. Percutaneous excimer laser coronary angioplasty of lesions not ideal for balloon angioplasty. Circulation. 1991;84:632-3.
3. Koster R, Kahler J, Brockhoff C, Münzel T, Meinertz T. Laser coronary angioplasty: history, present and future. Am J Cardiovasc Drugs. 2002;2:197-207.
4. Bittl JA, Sanborn TA, Tcheng JE. Clinical success, complications and restenosis rates with excimer laser coronary angioplasty. Am J Cardiol. 1992;70:1553-9.
5. Geschwind HJ, Dubois-Rande JL, Zelinsky R, Morelle JF, Boussignac G. Percutaneous coronary mid-infrared laser angioplasty. Am Heart J. 1991; 122:552-8.
6. Egred M, Brikalis ES. Excimer Laser Coronary Angioplasty (ELCA): Fundamentals, Mechanism of Action, and Clinical Applications. J Invasive Cardiol. 2020;32(2):E27-E35.
7. Topaz O. Laser for total occlusion recanalization. In: Waksman R, Saito S (Eds). Chronic Total Occlusions: A Guide to Recanalization. Hoboken, NJ: Wiley-Blackwell; 2009.
8. Rawlins J, Sambu N, O'Kane P. Strategies for the management of massive intra-coronary thrombus in acute myocardial infarction. Heart. 2013;99:510.
9. Whittaker A, Rawlins J, O'Kane P. Contemporary therapy of intracoronary thrombus: laser and bioresorbable scaffold. Cardiovasc Interv Ther. 2015;30:277-8.
10. Dahm JB, Topaz O, Woenckhaus C, Staudt A, Möx B, Hummel A, et al. Laser-facilitated thrombectomy: a new therapeutic option for treatment of thrombus-laden coronary lesions. Cath Cardiovasc Intervent. 2002;56:365-72.
11. Topaz O, Minisi AJ, Morris C, Mohanty PK, Carr Jr ME. Photoacoustic fibrinolysis: pulsed-wave, mid-infrared laser-clot interaction. J Thromb Thrombolysis. 1996;3:209-14.
12. Topaz O, Minisi AJ, Bernardo NL, McPherson RA, Martin E, Carr SL, et al. Alterations of platelet aggregation kinetics with ultraviolet laser emission: the "stunned platelet" phenomenon. Thromb Haemost. 2001;86:1087-93.
13. Topaz O, Bernardo NL, Shah R, McQueen RH, Desai P, Janin Y, et al. Effectiveness of excimer laser coronary angioplasty in acute myocardial infarction or in unstable angina pectoris. Am J Cardiol. 2001;87:849-55.
14. Topaz O, Ebersole D, Das T, Alderman EL, Madyoon H, Vora K, et al. Excimer laser angioplasty in acute myocardial infarction (the CARMEL multicenter study). Am J Cardiol. 2004;93:694-701.
15. Bittl JA. Clinical results with excimer laser coronary angioplasty. Semin Intervent Cardiol. 1996;1:129-34.

16. Bilodeau L, Fretz EB, Taeymans Y, Koolen J, Taylor K, Hilton DJ. Novel use of a high energy excimer laser catheter for calcified and complex coronary artery lesions. Cath Cardiovasc Interv. 2004;62:155-61.
17. Fernandez JP, Hobson AR, McKenzie D, Shah N, Sinha MK, Wells TA, et al. Beyond the balloon: excimer coronary laser atherectomy used alone or in combination with rotational atherectomy in the treatment of chronic total occlusions, non-crossable and non-expansible coronary lesions. EuroIntervention. 2013;9:243-50.
18. Holmes DR Jr, Forrester JS, Litvack F, Reeder GS, Leon MB, Rothbaum DA, et al. Chronic total obstructions and short-term outcome: the excimer laser angioplasty registry experience. Mayo Clin Proc. 1993;68:5-10.
19. Papaioannou T, Yadegar D, Vari S, Shehada R, Grundfest WS. Excimer laser (308 nm) recanalisation of in-stent restenosis: thermal considerations. Lasers Med Sci. 2001;16:90-100.
20. Burris N, Lippincott RA, Elfe A, Tcheng JE, O'Shea JC, Reiser C. Effects of 308 nanometer excimer laser energy on 316 L stainless-steel stents: implications for laser atherectomy of in-stent restenosis. J Invasive Cardiol. 2000;12:555-9.
21. Sunew J, Chandwaney RH, Stein DW, Meyers S, Davidson CJ. Excimer laser facilitated percutaneous coronary intervention of a nondilatable coronary stent. Cath Cardiovasc Intervent. 2001;53:513-7.
22. Fernandez JP, Hobson AR, Mckenzie DB, Talwar S, O'Kane PD. How should I treat severe calcific coronary artery disease? EuroIntervention. 2011;7:400-7.
23. Lam SC, Bertog S, Sievert H. Excimer laser in management of underexpansion of a newly deployed coronary stent. Catheter Cardiovasc Interv. 2014;83:E64-8.
24. Egred M. A novel approach for under-expanded stent: excimer laser in contrast medium. J Invasive Cardiol. 2012;24:E161-3.
25. Mehran R, Mintz GS, Satler LF, Pichard AD, Kent KM, Bucher TA, et al. Treatment of in-stent restenosis with excimer laser coronary angioplasty: mechanisms and results compared with PTCA alone. Circulation. 1997;96:2183-9.
26. Rawlins J, Talwar S, Green M, O'Kane P. Optical coherence tomography following percutaneous coronary intervention with excimer laser coronary atherectomy. Cardiovasc Revasc Med. 2014;15:29-34.
27. Giugliano GR, Falcone MW, Mego D, Ebersole D, Jenkins S, Das T, et al. A prospective multicenter registry of laser therapy for degenerated saphenous vein graft stenosis: the COronary graft Results following Atherectomy with Laser (CORAL) trial. Cardiovasc Revasc Med. 2012;13:84-9.
28. Ebersole D, Dahm JB, Das T, Madyoon H, Vora K, Baker J, et al. Excimer laser revascularization of saphenous vein grafts in acute myocardial infarction. J Invasive Cardiol. 2004;16:177-80.

CHAPTER 17

Treatment Strategy for Left Main Coronary Artery and Non-left Main Coronary Artery Bifurcation

Madhu Sreedharan

INTRODUCTION

Coronary bifurcations are common, accounting for up to 20% of all percutaneous coronary intervention (PCI)[1] and are associated with worse procedural and long-term outcomes. Bifurcations are composed of a proximal main vessel (PMV) that divides into two smaller branches, namely distal main vessel (DMV) and a side branch (SB) **(Fig. 1)**. The septum dividing the branches is called the carina. Endothelium at the carina is subject to high shear stress and so is relatively protected from atherosclerosis. The opposing lateral wall experiences low shear stress resulting in plaque formation. Thus, the carina is relatively free of disease while the plaque burden is typically opposite to the carina.[2]

SPECIAL CHARACTERISTICS OF BIFURCATION PERCUTANEOUS CORONARY INTERVENTION

Bifurcation lesions may occur at any branch point—but is most often seen in the left main coronary artery (LMCA) and the left anterior descending artery (LAD). The most important factor involved in treatment of the bifurcation is the preservation of the side branch. A significant side branch is one which you do not want to lose. Often it is the length of the side branch (side branch >73 mm supplies >10% of fractional myocardial mass) that is more important than the diameter.[3] Only 20% of non-left main SB supplies >10% of the myocardial mass.

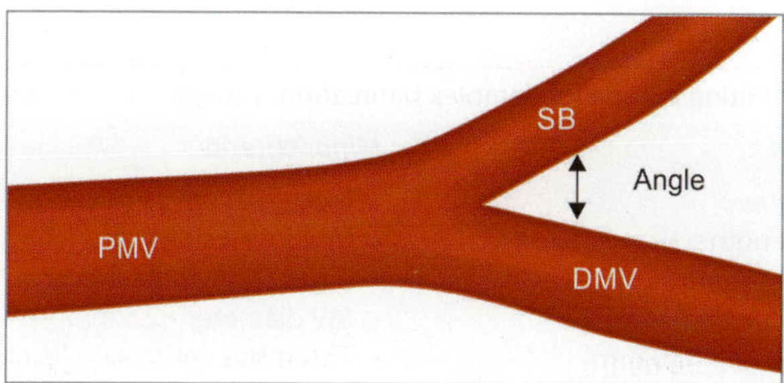

Fig. 1: Bifurcation anatomy. (PMV: proximal main vessel; DMV: distal main vessel; SB: side branch; Angle: bifurcation angle; carina is the septum between DMV and SB)

Medina classification is the most widely used to define bifurcation anatomy. A score of 1 is given to PMV, DMV, or SB having >50% stenosis.[4] Lesions involving both MV and SB (Medina Classification 1, 0, 1, 1, 1, 1, 0, 1, 1) have higher all-cause mortality and major adverse cardiac events (MACE) at 36 months.[5]

Calcification and bifurcation angles are other features which affect the outcomes in bifurcation PCI but not included in the Medina Classification. Calcification is more frequently seen in bifurcation. Rotablation is associated with less side branch compromise as compared to scoring or cutting balloons. Intravascular lithotripsy (IVL) offers a wire-based solution for calcific bifurcation lesions.

Bifurcation angle affects the outcome and the technique to be used. A 90° angle facilitates T stent while a more acute angle will result in T and protrude (TAP). A wide angle results in poor outcome with Culotte stent due to stent deformation and may be better dealt with DK Crush. In wide angles, crush or culotte techniques have been associated with higher MACE and angina while outcomes are unaffected with single stents.[6] Both very narrow and very wide angles increase likelihood of a poor outcome. A widely angulated side branch at high risk of compromise is best secured with a stent at the outset.

Coronary arteries follow the Murray's Law where the PMV diameter^3 = DMV diameter^3 + SB diameter^3. This has been simplified by the Finet's rule for maintaining the fractal geometry of the bifurcation which states that PMV diameter = (DMV d + SB d) × 0.678.[7]

BIFURCATION STRATEGIES

There are different ways by which a bifurcation lesion can be treated. It can be using a single stent primarily with a second stent if needed (provisional strategy) or electively using 2 stents (2 stent strategy). Most bifurcations can be treated with a provisional strategy (PS) while complex disease often requires a 2 stent strategy from the outset. DEFINITION criteria is one of the most useful ones to electively choose a 2 stent strategy **(Table 1)**.[8]

TABLE 1: Definition criteria for complex bifurcation: 1 major + any 2 minor criteria.

Major criteria	*Minor criteria*
LMCA bifurcation: • SB lesion length >10 mm • SB diameter stenosis >70% *Non-LMCA bifurcation:* • SB lesion length >10 mm • SB diameter stenosis >90%	• Mod—severe calcification • Multiple lesions • Bifurcation angle <45 or >70 • MV diameter <2.5 mm • Thrombus containing lesion • MV lesion length >25 mm

(LMCA: left main coronary artery; MV: main vessel; SB: side branch)

PROVISIONAL STRATEGY

Provisional is a layered strategy using a single stent with the option of using a second stent if needed. Both branches are wired and the main vessel is predilated for adequate lesion preparation. Routine SB dilatation is not recommended by the European Bifurcation Club (EBC) due to potential for SB dissection. However, critically narrowed SB may be dilated to prevent acute closure with stent deployment. Stent should be sized according to the DMV to prevent edge dissection and carinal shift into the SB. This would result in malapposition of the stent in the PMV as per the Murray's law. The proximal stent has to be expanded to overcome this with a POT (proximal optimization technique) **(Fig. 2)**. This is done with a short noncompliant balloon with the distal marker of the balloon at the carina and the proximal marker within the stent. A well done POT would optimize the proximal stent—preventing abluminal passage of the wire while trying to recross into SB and open the struts of the stent into the SB, scaffolding its ostium.

Following POT, a decision has to be made regarding treatment of the side branch. If the flow is good with no dissection/pinching of the side branch,

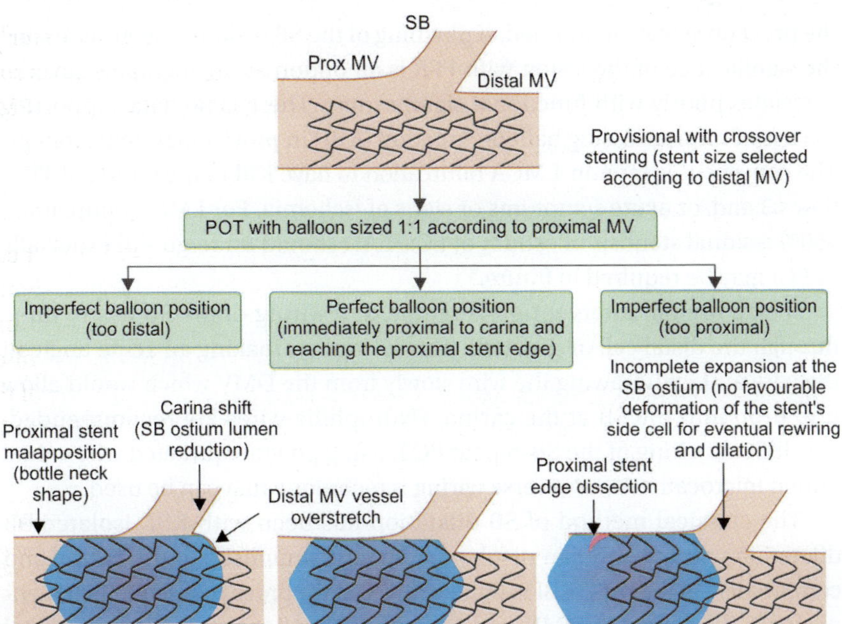

Fig. 2: Ideal way of doing a POT. (POT: proximal optimization technique; SB: side branch)

Source: Burzotta F, Lassen JF, Lefèvre T, Banning AP, Chatzizisis YS, Johnson TW, et al. Reproduced from the Percutaneous coronary intervention for bifurcation coronary lesions: the 15th consensus document from the European Bifurcation Club. EuroIntervention. 2021;16:1307-17.

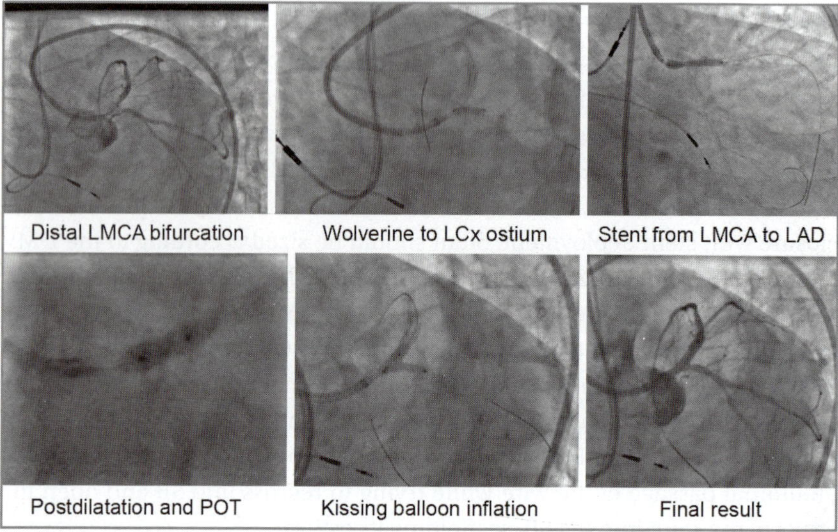

Fig. 3: Provisional strategy with KBI. (KBI: kissing balloon inflation; LAD: left anterior descending; LCx: left circumflex; LMCA: left main coronary artery; POT: proximal optimization technique)

the procedure may be stopped. If pinching of the SB ostium is seen, assessing the significance of the lesion with FFR is an option as angiographic severity correlates poorly with functional significance.[9] There is no data supporting the use of routine kissing balloon inflation (KBI) in provisional stent strategy. The consensus is for non-LMCA bifurcation to have KBI in the setting of TIMI flow <3 and/or acute symptoms or signs of ischemia. For LMCA bifurcation, >50% residual stenosis of ostium of LCx/LAD should undergo KBI especially as PCI may be required in future.[5]

If side branch intervention is requited, rewiring of the SB has to done through the distal cell of the stent. This is done by making an acute angle in the wire and withdrawing the wire slowly from the DMV which would allow it to drop into the SB at the carina. Hydrophilic wires are recommended. For difficult wiring of the SB-repeat POT, using polymer jacketed wires, dual lumen microcatheter, or reverse wiring is technique that can be used.

The classical method of SB dilatation has been with KBI. Isolated SB dilatation without KBI can displace stent struts opposite to the carina and compromise MV stent.[10] KBI is done with a 2 stage process of sequential high-pressure dilatation of DMV and SB with NC balloons sized to the distal vessel to ensure full expansion followed by a lower pressure simultaneous inflation to centralize the neocarina **(Fig. 3)**. The balloons should be deflated simultaneously. KBI restores FFR of SB to >0.75 in 92% of patients with FFR <0.75 following MV stenting.[9] KBI may result in MV stent distortion. Short balloons to reduce length of balloon overlap in the PMV and a final POT to

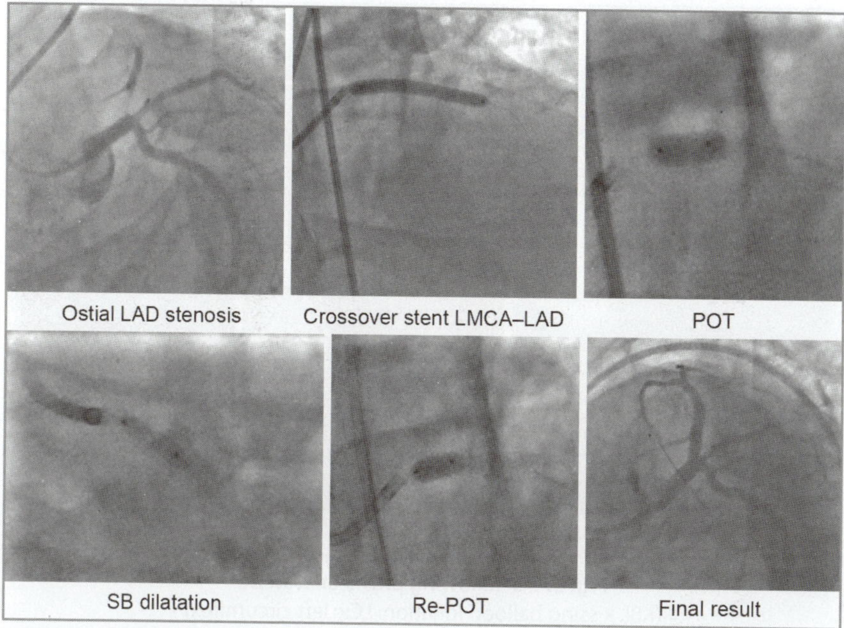

Fig. 4: Provisional strategy with POT–SB–POT. (LAD: left anterior descending; LMCA: left main coronary artery; POT: proximal optimization technique; SB: side branch)

remold the proximal segment of the stent are measures that can be taken to prevent this. This re-POT balloon should be placed proximal to the carina.

A strategy of POT → SB only dilatation → re-POT has been proposed to overcome the limitation of KBI **(Fig. 4)**.[11] This is highly dependent on optimal POT placement and distal wire crossing. The final POT balloon should cover the SB ostium to address malapposition induced by SB dilatation.

The SB wire should be jailed till the POT and re-wiring of the SB. Deploying MV stent with a jailed SB wire has not reduced SB occlusion, but it has been associated with increased flow recovery.[12] The jailed SB wire acts by creating a favorable change in the bifurcation geometry, serves as a marker of SB origin and finally if not able to re-wire, provides a track for a low profile balloon to be passed and dilated for flow restoration. Jailed wire may get trapped and fracture. Length of the wire jailed should be minimized to avoid this. If wire entrapment does occur with resistance felt on pulling back the wire, excessive pull on the wire should be avoided. Microcatheter or a low-profile balloon advanced over the jailed wire can help unentangle it. Jailed balloon or jailed microcatheter can also be used to protect patency of the SB.[13]

If there is persistent SB TIMI flow <3, extensive dissection or hemodynamic compromise following KBI, SB stenting should be undertaken. If SB stenting is needed, the options recommended are T, TAP, or culotte stenting **(Fig. 5)**. In the EBC trials comparing PS versus dual stenting strategy, the incidence of SB stenting was <20%.[14]

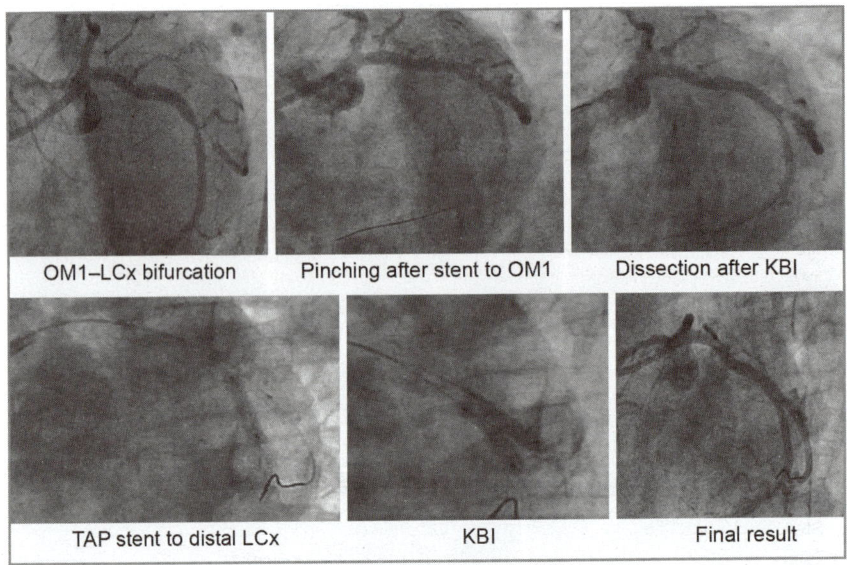

Fig. 5: TAP following provisional stent.
(KBI: kissing balloon inflation; LCx: left circumflex)

TWO STENT STRATEGIES

There are various stent strategies described of which the ones which have most data are the DK Crush and the Culotte stenting. If side branch access is not difficult, the MV should be stented first followed by T, TAP, or culotte. If the SB access is difficult, it should be stented first followed by DK Crush or reverse culotte.

DK CRUSH Stent (Fig. 6)

This was first described by Chen et al., in 2005 as a modification of the original crush technique.[15] In the original crush technique, rewiring the SB for KBI was often not successful due to 2 layers of stent across the SB ostium. Further balloon expansion was often inadequate. In the DK Crush modification, SB optimization by double kiss was described with success of KBI in 100%.

In this modification, both branches are wired and predilated for adequate lesion preparation. Stent is advanced to the SB and a balloon sized to the DMV is positioned in MV distally. SB stent is deployed with a 2-mm protrusion into the MV. Stent in SB is further optimized by high pressure dilatation of the stent delivery balloon after withdrawing it slightly. After removing the wire and balloon in the SB, the part of the stent in the MV is crushed with the balloon kept previously in the MV. A further dilatation with a balloon sized to the PMV to crush the stent fully—particularly in LMCA is recommended. If the stent is not completely crushed, the wire may go between the 2 layers

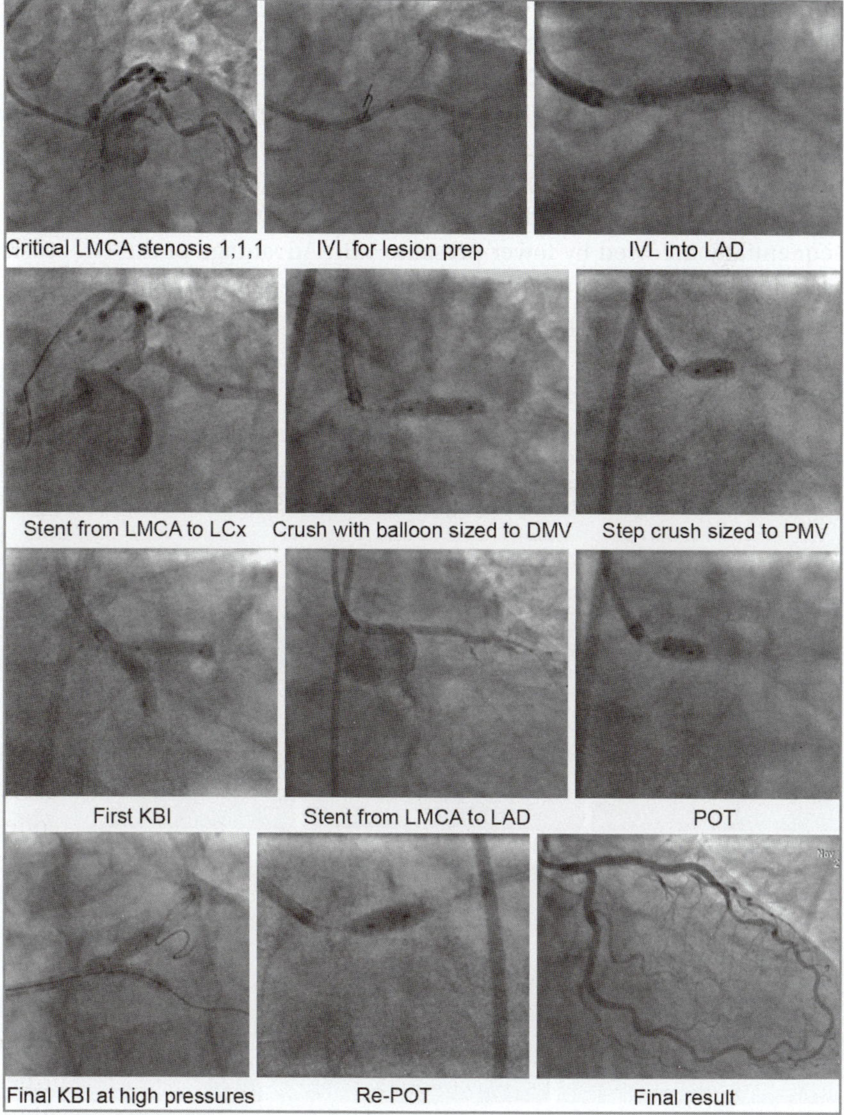

Fig. 6: Steps of DK CRUSH stent. (DMV: distal main vessel; IVL: intravascular lithotripsy; KBI: kissing balloon inflation; LAD: left anterior descending; LCx: left circumflex; LMCA: left main coronary artery; PMV: proximal main vessel; POT: proximal optimization technique)

of the incompletely crushed stent while trying to rewire the SB subsequently and this may result in opening of the stent struts into the MV. This can lead to a catastrophic situation preventing any device being taken down into the MV.

Following complete crushing of the stent, SB has to be rewired through the proximal or mid strut (unlike provisional stenting when rewiring has to be through the distal strut). Trying to cross via the distal strut may result in the wire going between the vessel wall and the crushed stent at the ostium of the SB resulting in a stent free space at the ostium leading to restenosis. Following wiring, the first KBI is done which opens up the SB ostium and deflects the neocarina away from MV lumen. The wire in the SB is taken out and the MV is stented—sized to the DMV. Following this POT is done, SB rewired followed by final KBI and a re-POT.

Balloon dilatations are done with short NC balloons at high pressures sequentially followed by lower pressure KBI. Advantage of the DK crush technique includes maintenance of the MV wire position throughout the procedure and ability to perform it using a 6F guide catheter transradially.

Culotte Stent (Fig. 7)

Chevalier et al., described Culotte stenting to ensure complete coverage of the bifurcation in 1998.[16] Bifurcation lesions with DMV and SB of similar sizes without a large bifurcation angle are the best subset for this technique.

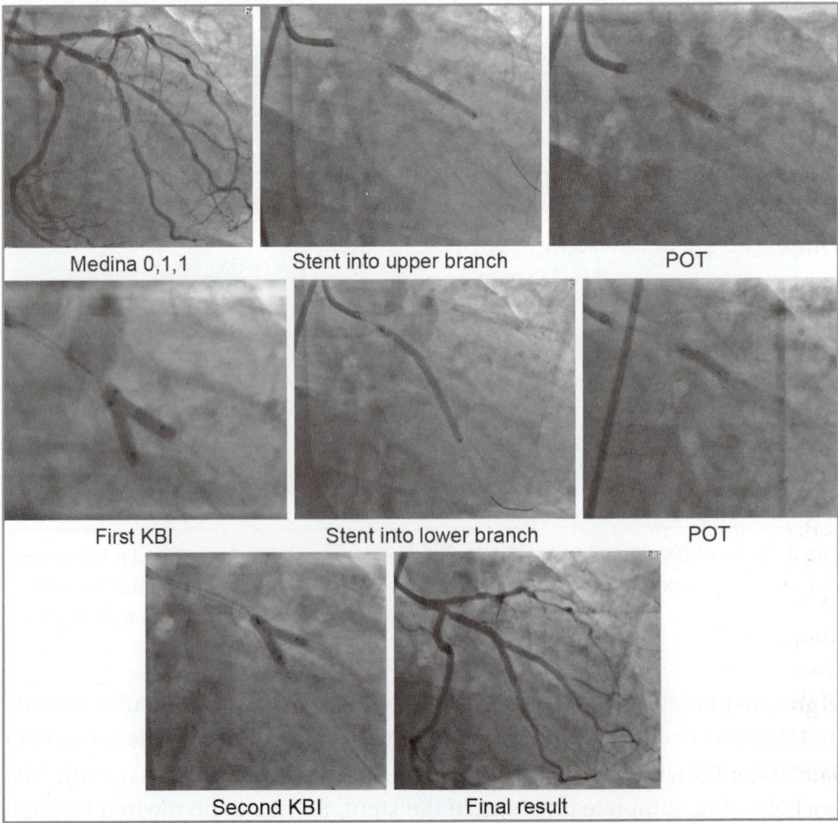

Fig. 7: Steps of DK culotte stent. (KBI: kissing balloon inflation; POT: proximal optimization technique)

In this, both branches are wired followed by dilatation and stenting of the MV (or the most angulated branch). Enough PMV coverage for POT is mandatory. POT is followed by wiring of the SB through the distal strut and dilatation of the SB. SB stent is delivered with protrusion into the PMV. POT is again done followed by wiring of the DMV through the distal strut. KBI is done followed by re-POT.

Several modifications of the culotte have evolved. Mini culotte refers to minimal protrusion of the second stent into PMV to minimize the length of the double stent layer. DK Culotte refers to KBI after the first rewiring. This reduces neocarina, degree of stent malapposition, and SB ostial stenosis.[17]

TRIALS OF BIFURCATION STRATEGIES (TABLES 2 AND 3)

The trials of non-LMCA bifurcation showed equipoise between provisional stent as compared to routine 2 stent techniques. The initial trials with first-generation DES was associated with increased periprocedural myocardial infarction (MI) and long-term mortality at 5 years which are not seen in the later trials EBC two and Nordic Baltic IV using second-generation DES. Complex bifurcations, however, had better outcomes with a 2 stent strategy—predominantly using DK crush technique, driven by lower rates of target vessel MI (TVMI) and target lesion revascularization (TLR) in the DEFINITION II trial.[18] This leads toward individualized therapy for each patient depending on the complexity of the lesion.

Several trials have addressed LMCA bifurcation lesions. DK CRUSH III compared DK Crush with Culotte stenting in distal LMCA bifurcation. Culotte stent was associated with higher MACE at 1 year and at 3 years driven by increased MI and TVR. Definite ST was also higher in the Culotte arm. Those with a bifurcation angle >70% and complex lesions as per the DEFINITION criteria had worse outcomes.

DK CRUSH V compared PS to DK Crush. Rate of SB stenting was high at 47% in the PS group reflecting the higher severity of disease. TLF at 12 months and at 3 years were higher in the PS group driven by higher rates of TVMI, TLR, and stent thrombosis.

In the EBC Main comparing PS with systematic 2 stent strategies, the incidence of MACE at 12 months was similar between both PS and 2 stent groups with no difference in individual end points. However, SB lesion length was only 7 mm and requirement of SB stenting was needed in only 22% of the PS group unlike in DK CRUSH V.

Though appearing to be discordant, the trial results are complimentary. Data shows that for most bifurcation lesions, a provisional strategy would provide good results. However, for the more complex lesions, as shown by the DEFINITION criteria, a systematic 2 stent strategy may be better. DK Crush provides the best long-term results in this subset. However, it is a complex

TABLE 2: All bifurcations: PS versus 2 stent RCTs.

	NORDIC	*BBK*	*CACTUS*	*BBC One*	*EBC Two*	*Nordic Baltic*	*Lin*	*DK Crush II*
Number	413	202	350	500	200	450	108	370
PS								
SB pre-dilatation	NS	NS	90.8%	NS	NS	64.2%	NS	36.8%
KBI	32%	100%	90.2%	26%	94%	36.1%	94.4%	79.5%
SB Stent	4.3%	19%	31%	3%	16%	3.7%	16.7%	28.6%
2 Stent								
Crush Var	Cr 50%	–	Cr 100%	Cr 68%	–	Mini 21%	DK 65%	DK 100%
Culotte	21%	–	–	30%	100%	66%	25%	–
Other	29%	T 100%	–	–	–	13%	10%	–
SB stented	95.1%	98.2%	100%	98%	97%	96.5%	94.4%	100%
FKBI	74%	100%	92.1%	72% Cr 89% Cu	96%	91.%	90.7%	100%
Follow-up	5 years	5 years	6 months	9 months	12 months	2 years	8 months	5 years
PS vs. 2 stent	15.8 vs. 21.8%	22.8 vs. 22.9%	15.8 vs. 15.8%	8 vs. 15.2%	7.7 vs. 10.3%	12.9 vs. 8.4%	38.9 vs. 11.1%	23.8 vs. 15.7%
P value	0.15	0.91	0.95	0.009 peri-procedural MI	0.53	0.12	<0.01 TLR	0.05 TLR

(KBI: kissing balloon inflation; MI: myocardial infarction; PS: provisional stent; RCT: randomized controlled trial; SB: side branch; TLR: target lesion revascularization)

TABLE 3: LMCA bifurcation RCT PS versus 2 stents.

	DK crush V	*EBC main*
Number	482	467
PS SB Predilatation KBI SB stented	 NS 78.9% 47.1%	 49% 89% 22%
2 stent SB stented DK Crush Culotte T/TAP FKBI	 100% 100% 99.6%	 94% 5% 53% 33% 93%
MACE definition	Cardiac death, target vessel MI, or clinically driven TLR	All-cause death, MI, or TLR
PS vs. 2 Stents	10.7 vs. 5% @ 12 months 16.9 vs. 8% @ 3 years	14. vs. 17.7%
P value	0.02 (12 months) ↓TVMI (ST) 0.005 (3 years) ↓TVMI and TLR	0.34

(KBI: kissing balloon inflation; LMCA: left main coronary artery; MACE: major adverse cardiac event; MI: myocardial infarction; SB: side branch; TLR: target lesion revascularization; TVMI: target vessel myocardial infarction)

procedure involving multiple steps and the results of the DK crush trials were at the hands of extremely experienced operators performing >300 PCIs/year for 5 years including at least 20 LMCA PCIs/year.

IMAGING IN BIFURCATION LESIONS

Intravascular imaging-guided PCI is associated with better outcomes particularly in complex subsets. In the OCTOBER trial, optical coherence tomography (OCT) guidance was compared to angiography-guided PCI in complex bifurcation in 1,201 patients. OCT was designed to achieve three aims:

1. *Optimal lesion coverage:* Less than 30% stenosis within 5 mm of stent edge with no lipid plaque or plaque rupture. No edge dissection visible on angiography
2. *Optimal stent expansion:* Residual diameter stenosis less than 10%. Less than 50% stenosis of the ostium of SB when stent was implanted in the MV only
3. Absence of stent malapposition or accidentally crushed or distorted stents.

The guiding principles of OCT were: (1) Predilatation of the lesions, (2) OCT for assessing the morphology, length, and diameter (MLD) of the lesion, (3) stent implantation and high pressure postdilatation with NC balloon followed by rewiring of the SB, (4) OCT evaluation for stent expansion and apposition, exclusion of geographical miss, evaluation of wire position in recrossing into the SB and ruling out abluminal rewiring of PMV, (5) sequential balloon inflation followed by simultaneous KBI, (6) final OCT of all segments for stent expansion, apposition and assessment of SB ostium. OCT was done (A) after predilatation, (B) after each rewiring, (C) final result of all stented segments. OCT was associated with a lower incidence of MACE at 2 years.[19]

CONCLUSION

Bifurcation PCI is complex and the loss of a significant SB is associated with poor outcomes. An individualized approach taking into consideration the lesion complexity and the skill of the operator should decide the strategy. The difference between the techniques may be less important that the meticulous application of the steps involved. Intravascular imaging should be mandatory in doing complex bifurcation subsets particularly those involving left main coronary artery for getting optimum long-term results.

REFERENCES

1. Lassen JF, Holm NR, Banning A, Burzotta F, Lefèvre T, Chieffo A, et al. Percutaneous coronary intervention for coronary bifurcation disease: 11th consensus document from the European Bifurcation Club. EuroIntervention. 2016;12(1):38-46.
2. Cheng C, Tempel D, van Haperen R, van der Baan A, Grosveld F, Daemen MJ, et al. Atherosclerotic lesion size and vulnerability are determined by patterns of fluid shear stress. Circulation. 2006;113(23):2744-53.
3. Kim HY, Doh JH, Lim HS, Nam CW, Shin ES, Koo BK, et al. Identification of Coronary artery side branch supplying myocardial mass that may benefit from revascularization. JACC Cardiovasc Interv. 2017;10(6):571-81.
4. Medina A, Suárez de Lezo J, Pan M. A New Classification of coronary bifurcation lesions. Rev Esp Cardiol Engl Ed. 2006;59(2):183.
5. Hildick-Smith D, Arunothayaraj S, Stankovic G, Chen SL. Percutaneous coronary intervention of bifurcation lesions. EuroIntervention. 2022;18(4):e273-91.
6. Collins N, Seidelin PH, Daly P, Ivanov J, Barolet A, Mackie K, et al. Long-term outcomes after percutaneous coronary intervention of bifurcation narrowings. Am J Cardiol. 2008;102(4):404-10.
7. Finet G, Gilard M, Perrenot B, Rioufol G, Motreff P, Gavit L, et al. Fractal geometry of arterial coronary bifurcations: a quantitative coronary angiography and intravascular ultrasound analysis. EuroIntervention. 2008;3(4):490-8.
8. Chen SL. DEFINITION criteria for left main bifurcation stenting – from clinical need to a formula. AsiaIntervention. 2023;9(1):20.
9. Koo BK, Park KW, Kang HJ, Cho YS, Chung WY, Youn TJ, et al. Physiological evaluation of the provisional side-branch intervention strategy for bifurcation lesions using fractional flow reserve. Eur Heart J. 2008;29(6):726–32.

10. Ormiston JA, Webster MWI, Jack SE, Ruygrok PN, Stewart JT, Scott D, et al. Drug-eluting stents for coronary bifurcations: bench testing of provisional side-branch strategies. Catheter Cardiovasc Interv. 2006;67(1):49-55.
11. Derimay F, Finet G, Souteyrand G, Maillard L, Aminian A, Lattuca B, et al. Benefit of a new provisional stenting strategy, the re-proximal optimisation technique: the rePOT clinical study. EuroIntervention. 2018;14(3):e325-32.
12. Hahn JY, Chun WJ, Kim JH, Song YB, Oh JH, Koo BK, et al. Predictors and outcomes of side branch occlusion after main vessel stenting in coronary bifurcation lesions: results from the COBIS II Registry (COronary BIfurcation Stenting). J Am Coll Cardiol. 2013;62(18):1654-9.
13. Dou K, Zhang D, Pan H, Guo N, Li L, Li Y, et al. Active SB-P vs. Conventional Approach to the Protection of High-risk Side Branches: The CIT-RESOLVE Trial. Cardiovasc Interv. 2020;13(9):1112-22.
14. Hildick-Smith D, Egred M, Banning A, Brunel P, Ferenc M, Hovasse T, et al. The European bifurcation club Left Main Coronary Stent study: a randomized comparison of stepwise provisional vs. systematic dual stenting strategies (EBC MAIN). Eur Heart J. 2021;42(37):3829-39.
15. Chen SL, Ye F, Zhang JJ, Zhu ZS, Lin S, Shan SJ, et al. DK crush technique: modified treatment of bifurcation lesions in coronary artery. Chin Med J (Engl). 2005;118(20):1746-50.
16. Chevalier B, Glatt B, Royer T, Guyon P. Placement of coronary stents in bifurcation lesions by the "culotte" technique. Am J Cardiol. 1998;82(8):943-9.
17. Hu F, Tu S, Cai W, Jiang Z, Zheng H, Xiao L, et al. Double kissing mini-culotte versus mini-culotte stenting: insights from micro-computed tomographic imaging of bench testing. EuroIntervention. 2019;15(5):465-72.
18. Zhang JJ, Ye F, Xu K, Kan J, Tao L, Santoso T, et al. Multicentre, randomized comparison of two-stent and provisional stenting techniques in patients with complex coronary bifurcation lesions: the DEFINITION II trial. Eur Heart J. 2020;41(27):2523-36.
19. Holm NR, Andreasen LN, Neghabat O, Laanmets P, Kumsars I, Bennett J, et al. OCT or Angiography Guidance for PCI in Complex Bifurcation Lesions. N Engl J Med. 2023;389(16):1477-87.

CHAPTER 18

Side Branch Crossing and Recrossing in Bifurcation: Troubleshooting Techniques

Dibya Kumar Baruah

INTRODUCTION

Coronary bifurcation lesions comprise approximately 20% of all percutaneous coronary interventions (PCI) performed.[1,2] Coronary bifurcation stenting (CBS) is associated with increased risk of stent thrombosis, in-stent restenosis, and major adverse cardiovascular events.[3] Given the extensive prevalence of bifurcation lesions, understanding the bifurcation anatomy and physiology, various techniques of bifurcation stenting are of paramount importance for effective performance during PCI. The most common and easily understandable classification of bifurcation lesion is the Medina classification[4] **(Fig. 1)**. This is a 3-digit binary code which defines a bifurcation by the presence of disease proximal and distal to the bifurcation in the main vessel (MV) and presence/absence of disease in the SB. Another classification based on carinal and take off angles proposed by Nomura T et al. is more practical and useful to understand the bifurcation anatomy[5] **(Fig. 2)**. Majority of bifurcation lesions can be treated with provisional stent technique (single stent strategy), and two stent strategy is determined by the complexity

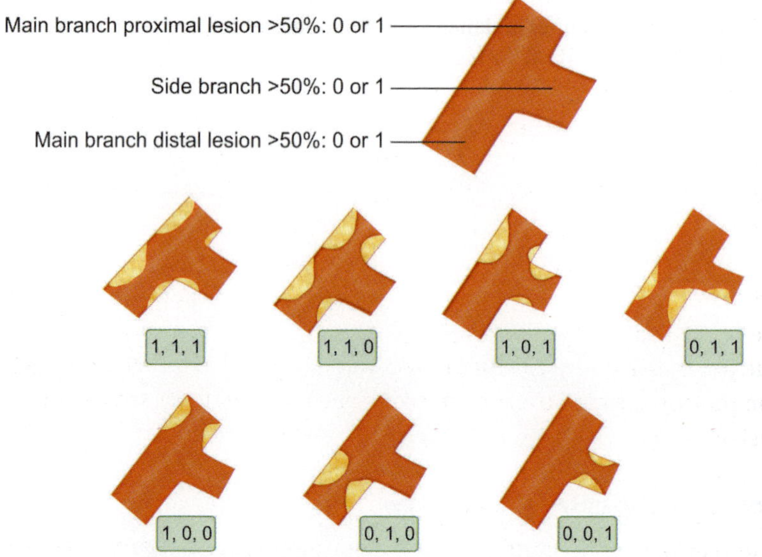

Fig. 1: Medina classification of bifurcation lesion.

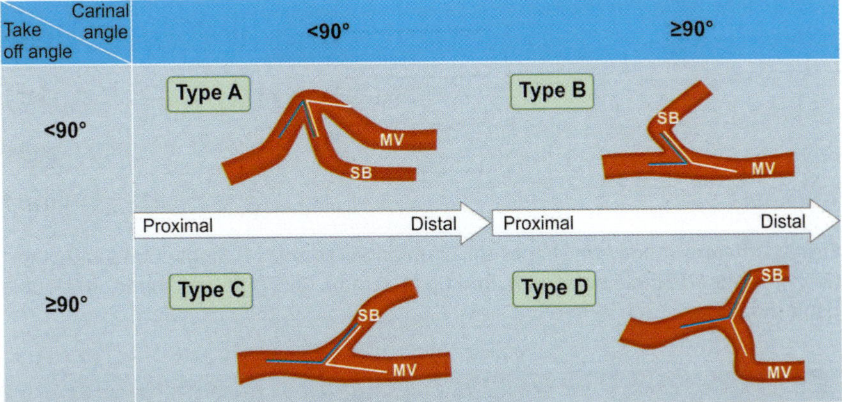

Fig. 2: Four types of bifurcation according to the take off and carinal angles. (MV: main vessel; SB: side branch)

of the lesion as defined by the DEFINITION trial.[6] It defines complex lesions as Medina 1,1,1/1,1,0 with major criteria of left main (LM) side branch (SB) >70% stenosis or non-LM SB >90% stenosis, SB >2.5 mm, and SB lesion length >10 mm with two minor criteria: moderate to severe calcification, multiple lesions, bifurcation angle <45, MV diameter <2.5 mm, thrombus, and MV lesion length >25 mm. Safe placement of appropriately selected guidewire in the MV and subsequent access to the SB is the first crucial step in CBS.

SIDE BRANCH WIRING

General Tips and Tricks for Noncomplex Side Branch Access

Wiring of the noncomplex side branch without acute angulation is usually obtained by majority of interventional cardiologists without any difficulties, however, in presence of acute angulation, it is not an easy walk for which different maneuvers are required. First step is appropriate selection of guidewire and preparation of the guidewire tip to desired shape. Based on the angulation, diseased severity and the size of the MV, four types of guidewire shapes can be used to cross the side branch: a single bend with short (2–3 mm) tip, a single bend with a long (4–6 mm) tip, a single wide bend and a double bend shape[7] **(Fig. 3)**. Usual practice of bifurcation stenting is to wire the more difficult branch first **(Figs. 4A to I)**. This will prevent wire twisting due to excessive torquing of the second guidewire while sailing through the complexities around the previously placed wire and makes subsequent steps easier.

Complex Side Branch Access

Complexities of the bifurcation are determined mostly by the plaque distribution, severity of the degree of stenosis in the MV or SB, and the angulation

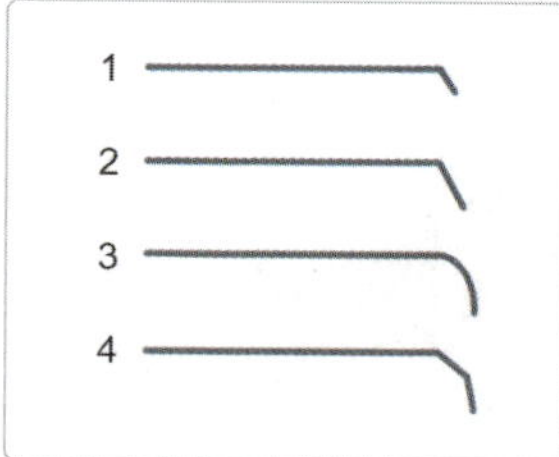

Fig. 3: Different guidewire shapes for bifurcation lesions: (1) Single bend with short (2–3 mm) tip. (2) Single bend with long tip (4–6 mm). (3) Single wide bend. (4) Double bend shape.

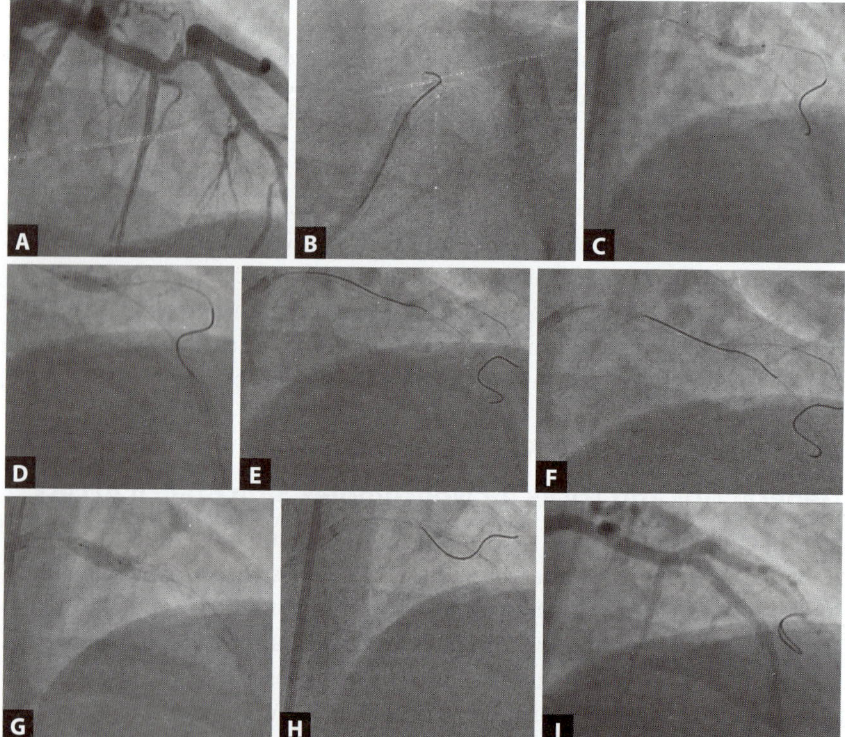

Figs. 4A to I: *Case example*: A 58-year-old man presented with anterior NSTEMI. Angiogram showed a complex bifurcation lesion with difficult side branch angle (A) treated with Culotte bifurcation stenting. Here a wide bend guidewire tip was used (B) for easy side branch access; (C) Side branch stenting; (D) POT; (E and F) Distal strut crossing to MV; (G) Re-POT after 2nd stent in LAD; (H) Distal strut crossing to side branch stent; (I) Final result. (NSTEMI: non-ST-elevation myocardial infarction; POT: proximal optimization technique)

of the SB take off. The task of crossing a complex bifurcation requires a great degree of skills and experiences. One should also know the predictors of SB occlusion that is seen more commonly during complex CBS.[3,8,9]

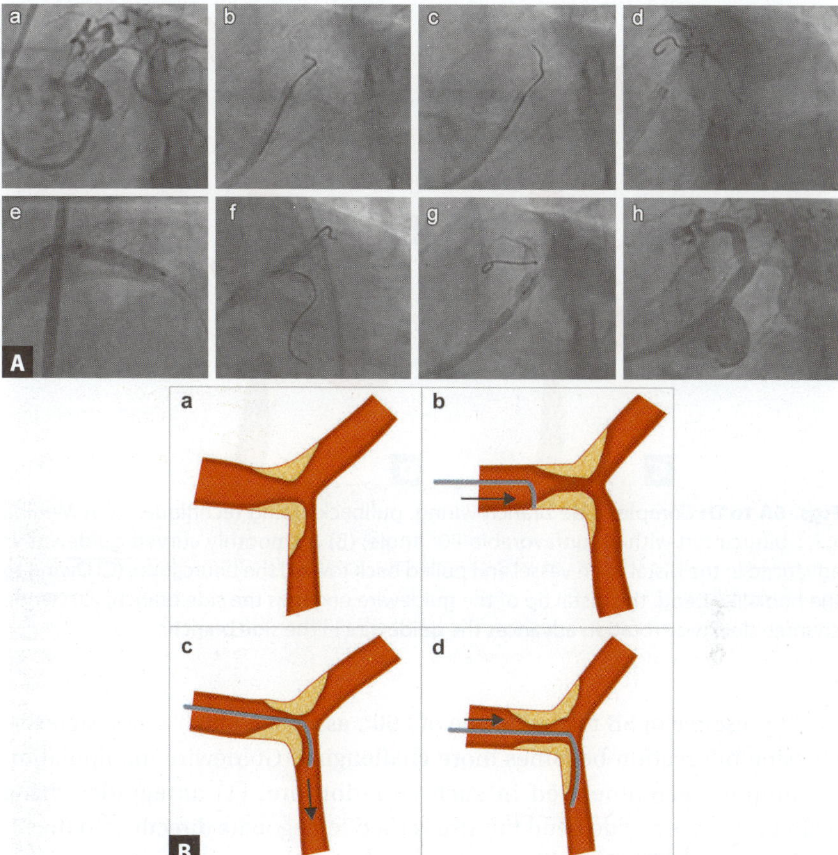

Figs. 5A and B: (A) *Case example:* A 68-year-old man presented with ACS. Coronary angiogram: (a) Widely angulated LM bifurcation Medina 0,1,1, treated with Mini crush two stent strategy, (b) Wide guidewire double curve tip to cross the MV, (c) Double curve is more obvious, (d) SB stenting, (e) MV stenting, (f) Kissing dilatation, (g) POT, and (h) Final result; (B) *Complex side branch wiring:* Antegrade wiring technique: (a) A Medina 1,1,1 bifurcation with an unfavorable 90° angle, (b) A guidewire that has been gently curved proximally to its J tip is advanced toward the bifurcation, (c) Owing to its second bend, the guidewire engages the side branch effectively, (d) Gentle turning counter-clockwise advances the guidewire in the side branch. (ACS: acute coronary syndrome; LM: left main; MV: main vessel; POT: proximal optimization technique; SB: side branch).

There are various techniques of side branch access in complex bifurcation. First step is the appropriate selection of guidewires (work horse, hydrophilic, or stiff) and preparation of the necessary curvature of the wire tip according to the angulation as well as size of the MV. In a situation of wide-angle bifurcation, especially in left main disease, a widely curve guidewire tip is helpful to cross the bifurcation either to the MV or to the SB **(Figs. 5A and B)**.

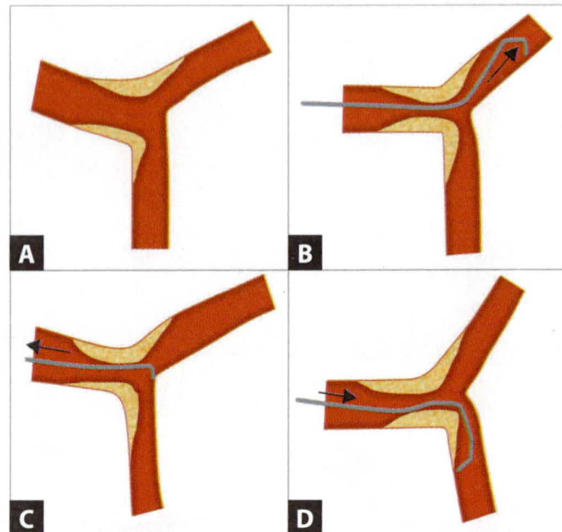

Figs. 6A to D: Complex side branch wiring: pullback wiring technique. (A) A Medina 1,1,1 bifurcation with an unfavorable 90° angle; (B) A smoothly curved guidewire is advanced in the distal main vessel and pulled back toward the bifurcation; (C) Owing to the hook-like bend, the distal tip of the guidewire engages the side branch; (D) Gentle counter-clockwise rotation advances the guidewire in the side branch.

In presence of SB take off angle of ≥90°, associated high-grade stenosis, crossing bifurcation becomes more challenging. Guidewire manipulation techniques recommended in such situation are: (1) antegrade wiring technique: here a wide bend tip wire is tried to negotiate directly into the SB from proximal MV, (2) pullback wiring technique consisting of the crossing the SB by retrieving the wire from the MV placed distal to the bifurcation **(Figs. 6A to D)**. With more acute carinal angulation (Type B, **Fig. 2**), same technique becomes the "reverse wire" technique (RWT).[10]

REVERSE WIRE TECHNIQUE FOR ACUTELY ANGULATED SIDE BRANCH

Angulated side branch is more challenging to wire. As a first step, one should make an appropriate guidewire shape by changing the tip, and second is necessary escalation of wires while trying to cross the most difficult branch first, and looking for different wire properties that may facilitate wiring. However, this technique may not be successful always to access an acutely angulated SB. To combat this situation, catheter-directed techniques can be applied. Different designs are available and can be of great help during CBS.[11,12] Commonly used catheters are angulated catheters [e.g., Super Cross (Teleflex)], deflectable catheters [e.g., Venture catheter (St. Jude Medical, St. Paul, MN, USA)], and double-lumen catheters [e.g., Twin-Pass (Teleflex)]. Balloon angioplasty or atherectomy of the main branch to modify the SB angle

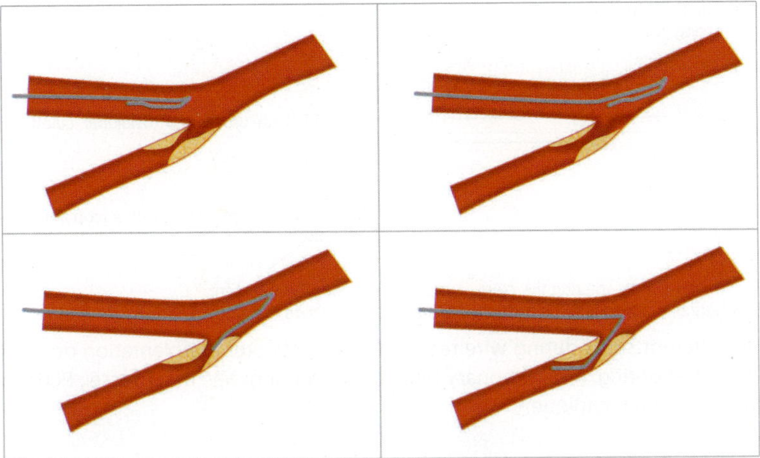

Fig. 7: Reverse wire technique.

for easy access is the last resort, but at the expense of risk of dissection and acute SB occlusion.[13] Even after all these efforts and application of different techniques, success does not come in all cases. In this challenging situation, "reverse wire technique (RWT)" becomes most useful guidewire technique. First described by Kawasaki et al. in 2008, original RWT uses a guidewire with a hairpin curve, which is delivered beyond the bifurcation zone 11. Subsequent gentle pullback and torquing allows reverse wiring of the side branch with the J-tip and subsequent advancement by doing anticlockwise torque **(Fig. 7)**. Useful modifications of this technique have been done by several authors including double lumen catheter facilitated RWT.[14-16]

WIRE RECROSSING AFTER MV STENTING: HOW TO MAKE IT A SUCCESS?

After implantation of the MV stent in provisional stenting or SB stenting in two stent strategy, the most important step toward a successful procedure is the recrossing of stent cell, which again requires specific skills and experiences. It can be a challenging task based on the technique applied, presence of the complexities of plaques (e.g., calcification), severity of stenosis, and angulation of the side branch, etc. Success can vary from patient to patient with the use of same strategy based on the presence or absence of the above factors.

Few important steps during recrossing the MV stent should be kept in mind, such as keeping the SB wire in place till successful recrossing, adequate POT of the MV stent, and based on the bifurcation strategy, careful selection of distal cell or proximal cell for crossing **(Fig. 8)**. Coronary imaging, especially optical coherence tomography (OCT), can guide to choose the right cell crossing in certain situation.[17] In a tip of the month (TOTM) of

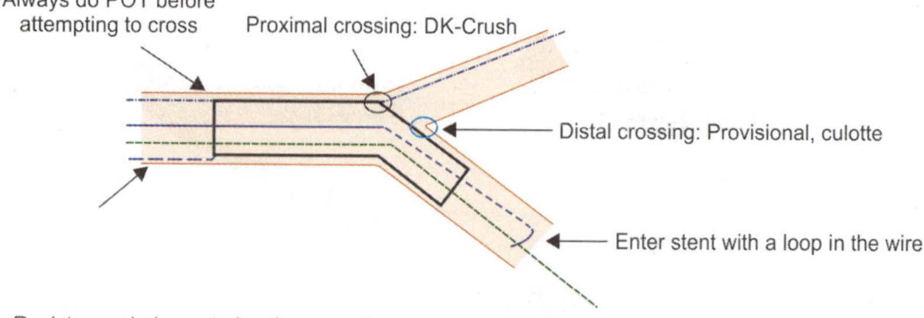

Fig. 8: Different steps during wire recrossing after MV stent implantation during CBS and troubleshooting. (CBS: coronary bifurcation stenting; MV: main vessel; POT: proximal optimization technique)

bifurcation stenting, Tamara M Atkinson has mentioned the following steps for a successful recrossing of stent during CBS:[18]

- Maintain the jailed wire until successful rewiring is performed with a separate wire.
- Common reason associated with rewiring failure is underexpanded stent in the MV preventing the wire to reach the SB ostium. That is why, always perform POT on the MV with a distal balloon tip marker positioned at the level of the carina before rewiring.[19]
- Minimize the passage of wire behind the MV stent by utilizing one or more of the following:
  - Use a J configuration of the wire tip while entering the MV stent
  - Use a dual-lumen microcatheter
  - Pull back the MV wire to wire the SB
- Shape the wire with a long tip (4–6 mm) and a wide or double bend. If one shape fails, reshape the tip or consider changing to a stiffer, hydrophilic, or graded transition wire.
- Use the pullback technique, where the wire is advanced past the carina and then pulled back to catch the proximal (DK-crush) or distal strut[20,21] (provisional or culotte) **(Figs. 4E and H)**.
- Use a dual lumen angled or steerable microcatheter to direct the wire into the SB.
- Inflate the balloon in the distal MV to direct the wire into the SB (balloon block and support technique).[22]
- Use a different angiographic view.

Presence of proximal tortuosity and acutely angulated SB produces difficulties in recrossing the stent. In such situation, microcatheter can ease the negotiation of guidewire through the tortuosity and Venture catheter can make possible to enter the side branch.[23-25] Real difficulties during CBS arise when multiple attempts with different wires fail to recross a major side branch with compromise flow. This can be managed with advancement of a small balloon over the jailed SB wire under the MV stent and dilate the SB ostium. This will allow SB reflow and also helps to recross the SB to finish with final kissing balloon dilatation and final POT of the MV stent.

CONCLUSION

Careful assessment and understanding the complexities of the lesion in the index patient is essential to adapt the right bifurcation strategy. Appropriate guidewire selection and preparation of suitable wire tip shape based on the vessel size and angulation is crucial in crossing and recrossing during bifurcation stenting. In challenging situation adaption of advance techniques can help in troubleshooting of wire crossing strategy during CBS.

REFERENCES

1. Lassen JF, Holm NR, Stankovic G, Lefevre T, Chieffo A, Hildick-Smith D, et al. Percutaneous coronary intervention for coronary bifurcation disease: consensus from the first 10 years of the European Bifurcation Club meetings. EuroIntervention. 2014;10(5):545-60.
2. Louvard Y, Thomas M, Dzavik V, Hildick-Smith D, Galassi AR, Pan M, et al. Classification of coronary artery bifurcation lesions and treatments: time for a consensus! Catheter Cardiovasc Interv. 2008;71(2):175-83.
3. Nakazawa G, Yazdani SK, Finn AV, Vorpahl M, Kolodgie FD, Virmani R. Pathological findings at bifurcation lesions: the impact of flow distribution on atherosclerosis and arterial healing after stent implantation. J Am Coll Cardiol. 2010;55(16):1679-87.
4. Medina A, Suarez de Lezo J, Pan M. A new classification of coronary bifurcation lesions. Rev Esp Cardiol. 2006;59(2):183.
5. Nomura T, Kikai M, Hori Y, Yoshioka K, Kubota H, Miyawaki D, et al. Tips of the dual-lumen microcatheter-facilitated reverse wire technique in percutaneous coronary interventions for markedly angulated bifurcated lesions. Cardiovasc Interv Ther. 2018;33:146-53.
6. Chen SL, Sheiban I, Xu B, Jepson N, Paiboon C, Zhang JJ, et al. Impact of the complexity of bifurcation lesions treated with drug-eluting stents: the DEFINITION study (Definitions and impact of complEx biFurcation lesIons on clinical outcomes after percutaNeous coronary IntervenTIOn using drug-eluting steNts). JACC Cardiovasc Interv. 2014;7(11):1266-76.
7. Erglis A. Coronary guidewires. EuroIntervention. 2010;6:168-9.
8. Aliabadi D, Tilli FV, Bowers TR, Benzuly KH, Safian RD, Goldstein JA, et al. Incidence and angiographic predictors of side branch occlusion following high-pressure intracoronary stenting. Am J Cardiol. 1997;80:994-7.
9. Gil RJ, Vassilev D, Formuszewicz R, Rusicka-Piekarz T, Doganov A. The carina angle-new geometrical parameter associated with periprocedural side branch compromise and the long-term results in coronary bifurcation lesions with main vessel stenting only. J Interv Cardiol. 2009;22:E1-E10.
10. Kawasaki T, Koga H, Serikawa T. New bifurcation guidewire technique: a reversed guidewire technique for extremely angulated bifurcation—a case report. Catheter Cardiovasc Interv. 2008;71:73-6.

11. Hildick-Smith D, de Belder AJ, Cooter N, Curzen NP, Clayton TC, Oldroyd KG, et al. Randomized trial of simple versus complex drug eluting stenting for bifurcation lesions: the British Bifurcation Coronary Study: old, new, and evolving strategies. Circulation. 2010;121:1235-43.
12. Burzotta F, De Vita M, Sgueglia G, Todaro D, Trani C. How to solve difficult side branch access? EuroIntervention. 2010;6 (Suppl J):J72-80.
13. McClure SJ, Wahr DW, Webb JG. Venture wire control catheter. Catheter Cardiovasc Interv. 2005;66:346-50.
14. Routledge H, Lefèvre T, Ohanessian A, Louvard Y, Dumas P, Morice MC. Use of a deflectable tip catheter to facilitate complex interventions beyond insertion of coronary bypass grafts: three case reports. Catheter Cardiovasc Interv. 2007;70:862-6.
15. Thomas M, Hildick-Smith D, Louvard Y, Albiero R, Darremont O, Stankovic G, et al. Percutaneous coronary intervention for bifurcation disease. A consensus view from the first meeting of the European Bifurcation Club. EuroIntervention. 2006;2:149-53.
16. Hasegawa K, Yamamoto W, Nakabayashi S, Otsuji S. Streamlined reverse wire technique for the treatment of complex bifurcated lesions. Catheter Cardiovasc Interv. 2020;96:E287-E291.
17. Watanabe S, Saito N, Bao B, Tokushige A, Watanabe H, Yamamoto E, et al. Microcatheter-facilitated reverse wire technique for side branch wiring in bifurcated vessels: an in vitro evaluation. EuroIntervention. 2013;9:870-7.
18. Nomura T, Higuchi Y, Kubota H, Miyawaki D, Urata R, Sugimoto T, et al. Practical usefulness of dual lumen catheter-facilitated reverse wire technique for markedly angulated bifurcated lesions. J Interv Cardiol. 2015;28:544-50.
19. Alegría-Barrero E, Foin N, Chan PH, Syrseloudis D, Lindsay AC, Dimopolous K, et al. Optical coherence tomography for guidance of distal cell recrossing in bifurcation stenting: choosing the right cell matters. EuroIntervention. 2012;8(2):205-13.
20. Atkinson TM, Davies CH, Truong HT, Latif F. (2022). Bifurcation Tips and Tricks: Tools for Managing Recross, Failed Provisional Stenting, and Optimizing One-vs. Two-Stent Strategies. [online] Available from https://scai.org/bifurcation-tips-and-tricks-tools-managing-recross-failed-provisional-stenting-and-optimizing-one. [Last accessed October, 2024]
21. Hoye A. The Proximal Optimisation Technique for Intervention of Coronary Bifurcations. Interv Cardiol. 2017;12(2):110-5.
22. Li L, Liu J, Jin Q, Chen S. Case report of a novel manoeuvre to facilitate wire access to the side branch in bifurcation intervention-balloon block and support technique. Medicine (Baltimore). 2018;97(3):e9673.
23. Aranzulla TC, Sangiorgi GM, Bartorelli A, Cosgrave J, Corbett S, Fabbiocchi F, et al. Use of the Venture wire control catheter to access complex coronary lesions: how to turn procedural failure into success. EuroIntervention. 2008;4:277-84.
24. Burzotta F, Sgueglia GA, Trani C, Talarico GP, Coroleu SF, Giubilato S, et al. Provisional TAP-stenting strategy to treat bifurcated lesions with drug-eluting stents: one-year clinical results of a prospective registry. J Invasive Cardiol. 2009;21:532-7.
25. Aminian A, Dolatabadi D, Lalmand J. Small balloon inflation over a jailed wire as a bailout technique in a case of abrupt side branch occlusion during provisional stenting. J Invasive Cardiol. 2010;22:449-52.

CHAPTER 19

Side Branch Preservation

Dilip Kumar

INTRODUCTION

Coronary bifurcation lesions (CBL) represent a challenge to the interventional cardiologist and account for up to 20% of all lesions encountered in clinical practice, and side branch (SB) compromise is a major complication of stenting these bifurcation lesions.[1] Medina classifications 1,0,1; 1,1,1; 0,1,1 are considered as true bifurcation lesion. Stenting techniques using complex two-stents or provisional one-stent technique have been developed.[2-4] The stepwise layered provisional stenting (PS) strategy is recommended for the vast majority of patients with non-true non-left main (non-LM) CBLs or true non-LM CBL with a SB lesion length.[5-9] Until now, a two-stent strategy has been shown to be superior in complex left main lesions only.[10] In addition to these techniques, several novel stenting systems for bifurcation lesions have been developed.[11] However, still even now, SB occlusion after MB stenting occurs in 7.4–8.4% of bifurcation lesions.[12,13] Importantly, any of these bifurcation techniques can work only after a guidewire is successfully recrossed to SB after MB stenting in case of a SB compromise. However, if SB is once occluded after MB stenting, it is very difficult to rewire through stent strut to SB.

SIDE BRANCH RELEVANCE

Consistent with the Bifurcation Academic Research Consortium (Bif-ARC) consensus,[14] an SB should be defined as "relevant" if the reference vessel diameter is ≥2.0 mm and represents a significant territory (>10%) of the myocardium, impacting prognosis. However, in common practice, many operators consider a relevant SB a vessel ≥2.0 mm that they are unwilling to lose in the context of a specific patient anatomy.

PREDICTORS OF SIDE BRANCH OCCLUSION

- Overdilatation of the distal part of the main vessel (MV) stent during the initial implantation
- A carina with a spiky morphology (an "eyebrow" sign) by intravascular ultrasound (IVUS)[15]

- High lipid content of the MV lesion and a contralateral location of lipid in the bifurcation area by optical coherence tomography (OCT)[16]
- A narrower carina tip angle, a shorter length between the proximal branching point to the carina tip and calcified plaque in the MV by OCT[17,18]
- The diameter stenosis in both branches, lesion length, bifurcation angle or a thrombus-containing lesion are also predictors.[19]

MEASURES TO PRESERVE SIDE BRANCH

- *Jailed wire technique:*[20-23] This technique consists of leaving a wire in the SB while implanting a stent in the MV. It has the following potential advantages:
  - The technique helps to keep the SB open, and, in case of occlusion, the guidewire is the only marker of the SB ostium.
  - It facilitates access to the SB by favorably changing the angle of the bifurcation.
  - The jailed wire can provide anchoring of the guide catheter which facilitates balloon crossing through the stent struts to the SB.
  - In case of SB occlusion, the jailed wire can be used to pass a low-profile balloon (or penetrative microcatheter) between the stent and the vessel wall to restore SB flow. The intervention can then be completed with the inverted crush or any other technique.[24,25]
- "Conventional" jailed balloon technique **(Figs. 1 and 2)**
- "Simplified" jailed balloon technique **(Fig. 3)**

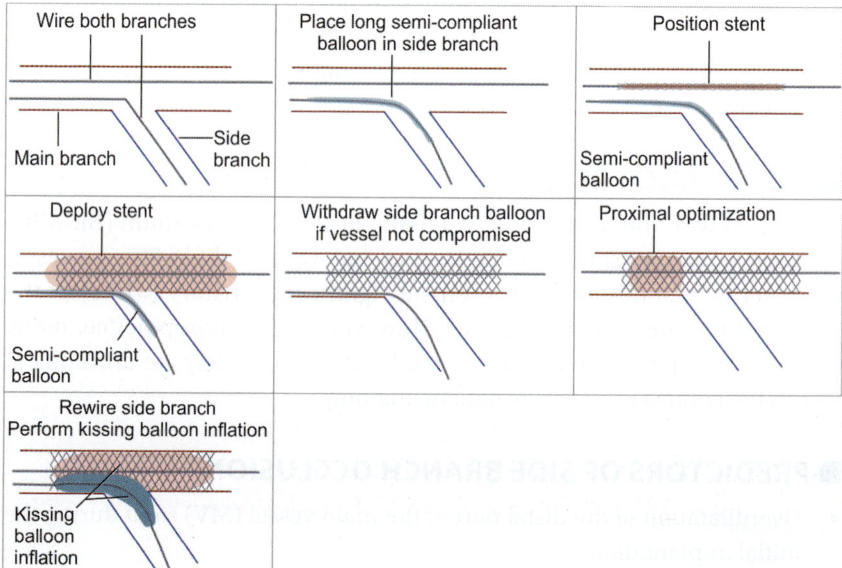

Fig. 1: Stepwise "conventional" jailed balloon technique without side branch is not compromised.

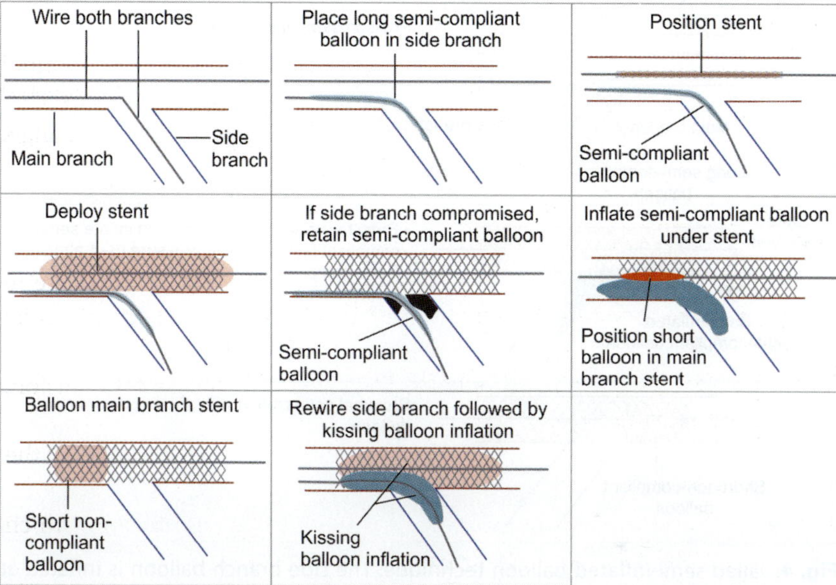

Fig. 2: Stepwise "conventional" jailed balloon technique with side branch compromise.

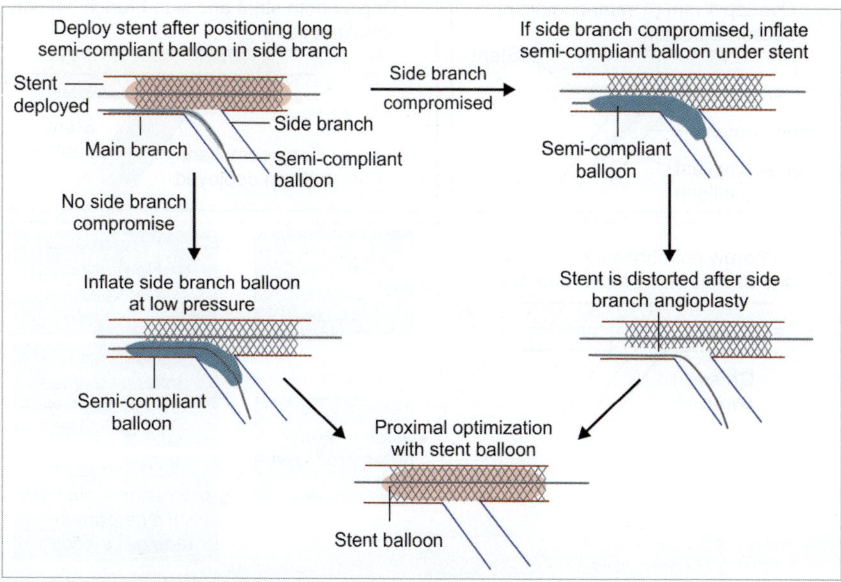

Fig. 3: "Simplified" jailed balloon technique with and without side branch compromise. Final proximal optimization is performed with stent balloon.

- Jailed semi-inflated balloon technique **(Fig. 4)**
- "Modified" jailed balloon technique and balloon stent kissing technique **(Fig. 5)**

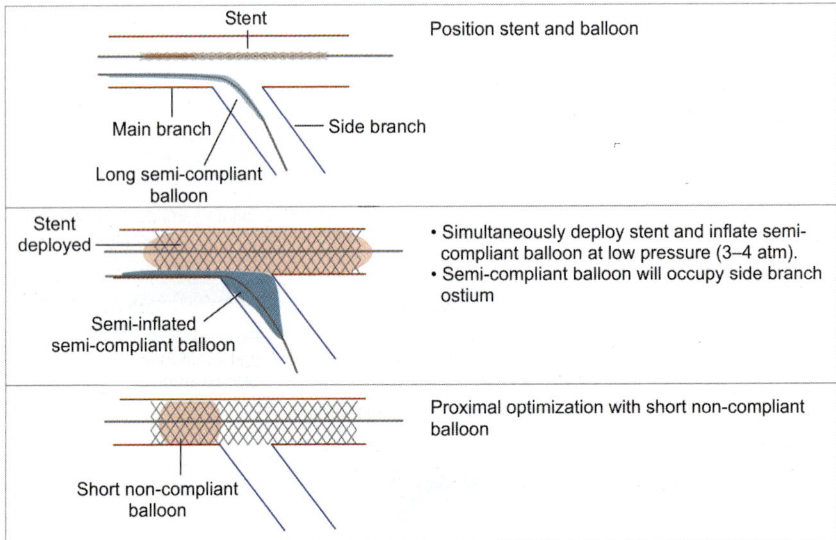

Fig. 4: Jailed semi-inflated balloon technique. The side branch balloon is inflated at low pressure during stent deployment. Final proximal optimization is performed with a short balloon.

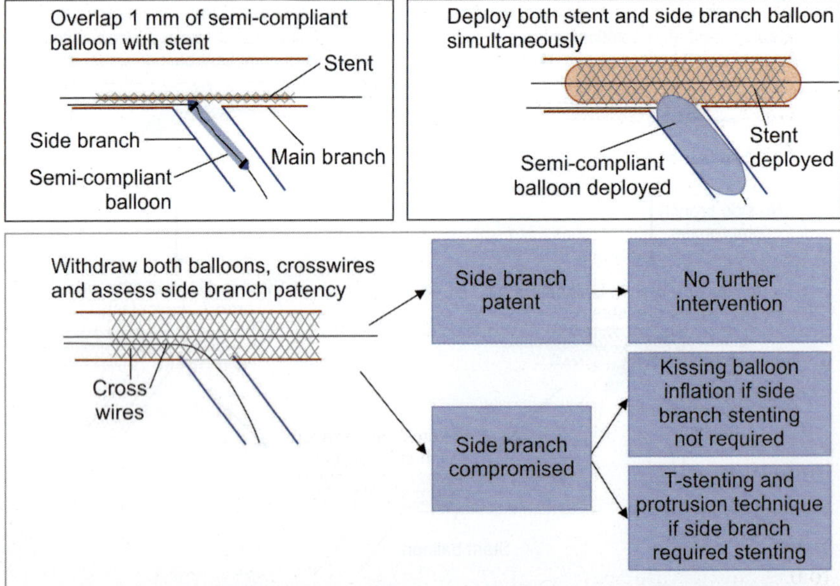

Fig. 5: Modified jailed balloon technique. Side branch balloon is positioned so that it protrudes about 1 mm into main branch. If the side branch is compromised, a kissing balloon inflation or T-stenting and protrusion is performed.

- Jailed stent balloon technique **(Fig. 6)**
- *Jailed balloon and Corsair trifurcation technique:* Limited to case reports, this technique integrates the jailed semi-inflated balloon technique with

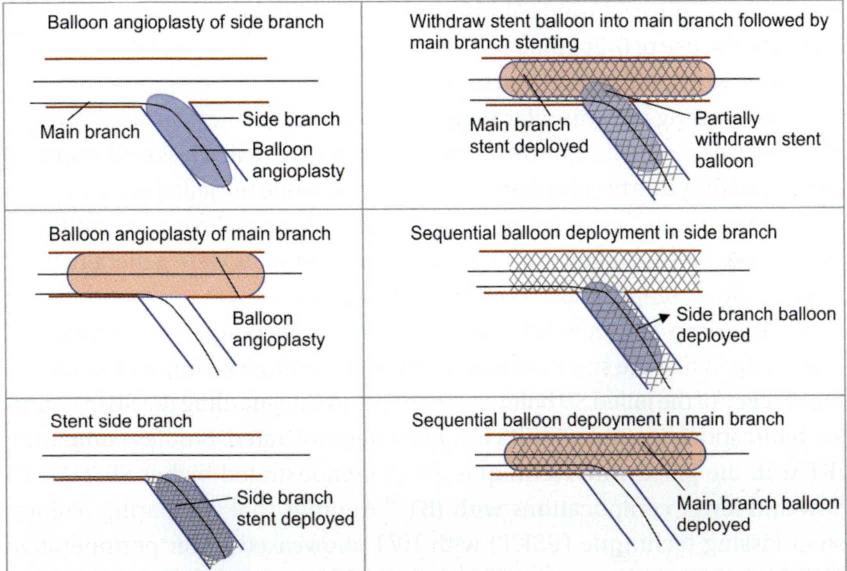

Fig. 6: Stepwise jailed stent balloon technique.

the "jailed Corsair technique" that was published in a 2017 case report by Numusawa et al.[26] The Corsair microcatheter's tip needs to move into the SB sufficiently downstream to prevent its tip from being cut during the removal process.

- *Complications of jailed balloon technique:*
  - The most dreaded complication of this technique is entrapment of the jailed balloon.
  - Repeated balloon inflation and deflation to rescue the trapped balloon itself will cause loss of balloon profile, and this loss of balloon profile may further hinder balloon withdrawal.
- *Complication of Corsair technique:*
  - Risk of guide wire entrapment.

The jailed balloon technique (JBT) was assessed for its efficacy in maintaining lumen patency in SBs after stenting, as highlighted in Omori et al.'s recent publication.[27] While initial measurements post-stenting showed suboptimal results (Pd/Pa of 0.34), the removal of the balloon improved this to 0.60, indicating the JBT's ability to secure SB lumen patency.

A summary of major trials revealed that most patients in these studies were hypertensive, nondiabetic males in their 1960s and 1970s without prior coronary intervention. However, differences existed among trials regarding patient characteristics and diagnoses, with some trials focusing on stable angina while others enrolled acute coronary syndrome patients. Lesions treated primarily involved left anterior descending (LAD)/diagonal bifurcations, with exclusion of LM lesions in certain trials. Procedure specifics included the use of 6-Fr guide catheters, transradial access, and various stent platforms with comparable outcomes.[28-32]

Studies using intravascular imaging showed differences in stent apposition based on the technique used. Simplified JBT[29] revealed less well-apposed stents, possibly due to compliant stent balloons, while the jailed semi-inflated balloon technique[30] reported more well-apposed stents through postdilation with a noncompliant balloon. Procedural success rates were generally high, with minimal complications reported across studies.

Comparison between different jailed balloon techniques was limited by scant data. While the standard jailed SB wire technique is simpler to execute, the efficacy of the jailed SB balloon technique in safeguarding the SB in complex bifurcations treated with PS has been demonstrated. Studies comparing JBT with the jailed wire technique (JWT) demonstrated higher SB TIMI III flow and fewer complications with JBT.[33] Another trial comparing balloon stent kissing technique (BSKT) with JWT showcased lower perioperative major adverse cardiac events (MACE) incidence with BSKT, emphasizing potential benefits.[34] Nonetheless, these findings were limited to specific centers and require larger, controlled studies with long-term follow-up for validation. Another randomized trial, the CIT-RESOLVE Trial,[35] involved lesions at high risk of SB occlusion. Patients were randomly assigned to either the conventional strategy utilizing the jailed SB wire technique or the SB protection strategy using the jailed SB balloon. The study revealed that the active SB protection strategy proved superior to the conventional approach, significantly reducing the incidence of SB occlusion and the loss of SB flow immediately after the full apposition of the main vessel (MV) stent.

CONCLUSION

The stepwise PS technique is applicable to the majority of complex bifurcation lesions. Nonetheless, occlusion of the SB subsequent to main vessel stenting may arise, posing challenges for resolution. Employing angiographic and intracoronary imaging criteria to anticipate the likelihood of SB closure could promote the implementation of SB protection strategies. These protective methodologies offer tactics aimed at preventing SB closure or addressing compromise subsequent to main vessel stenting. By minimizing procedural injury, these strategies ensure a lasting and robust outcome for patients with coronary lesions in bifurcation areas.

REFERENCES

1. Collins N, Seidelin PH, Daly P, Ivanov J, Barolet A, Mackie K, et al. Long-term outcomes after percutaneous coronary intervention of bifurcation narrowings. Am J Cardiol. 2008;102:404-10.

2. Lefèvre T, Louvard Y, Morice MC, Dumas P, Loubeyre C, Benslimane A, et al. Stenting of bifurcation lesions: Classification, treatments, and results. Catheter Cardiovasc Interv. 2000;49:274-83.
3. Latib A, Colombo A. Bifurcation disease: What do we know, what should we do?. JACC Cardiovasc Interv. 2008;1:218-26.
4. Melikian N, Di Mario C. Treatment of bifurcation coronary lesions: A review of current techniques and outcome. J Interven Cardiol. 2003;16:507-13.
5. Burzotta F, Lassen JF, Louvard Y, Lefèvre T, Banning AP, Darremont O, et al. European Bifurcation Club white paper on stenting techniques for patients with bifurcated coronary artery lesions. Catheter Cardiovasc Interv. 2020;96:1067-79.
6. Burzotta F, Lassen JF, Lefèvre T, Banning AP, Chatzizisis YS, Johnson TW, et al. Percutaneous coronary intervention for bifurcation coronary lesions: the 15th consensus document from the European Bifurcation Club. EuroIntervention. 2021;16:1307-17.
7. Banning AP, Lassen JF, Burzotta F, Lefèvre T, Darremont O, Hildick-Smith D, et al. Percutaneous coronary intervention for obstructive bifurcation lesions: the 14th consensus document from the European Bifurcation Club. EuroIntervention. 2019;15:90-8.
8. Lassen JF, Burzotta F, Banning A, Lefèvre T, Darremont O, Hildick-Smith D, et al. Percutaneous coronary intervention for the left main stem and other bifurcation lesions: 12th consensus document from the European Bifurcation Club. EuroIntervention. 2018;13:1540-53.
9. Di Gioia G, Sonck J, Ferenc M, Chen SL, Colaiori I, Gallinoro E, et al. Clinical Outcomes Following Coronary Bifurcation PCI Techniques: A Systematic Review and Network Meta-Analysis Comprising 5,711 Patients. JACC Cardiovasc Interv. 2020;13:1432-44.
10. Chen SL, Zhang JJ, Han Y, Kan J, Chen L, Qiu C, et al. Double Kissing Crush Versus Provisional Stenting for Left Main Distal Bifurcation Lesions: DKCRUSH-V Randomized Trial. J Am Coll Cardiol. 2017;70:2605-17.
11. Latib A, Colombo A, Sangiorgi GM. Bifurcation stenting: Current strategies and new devices. Heart. 2009;95:495-504.
12. Dou K, Zhang D, Xu B, Yang Y, Yin D, Qiao S, et al. An angiographic tool for risk prediction of side branch occlusion in coronary bifurcation intervention: The RESOLVE score system (Risk prEdiction of Side branch OccLusion in coronary bifurcation interVEntion). JACC Cardiovasc Interv. 2015;8:39-46.
13. Hahn JY, Chun WJ, Kim JH, Song YB, Oh JH, Koo BK, et al. Predictors and outcomes of side branch occlusion after main vessel stenting in coronary bifurcation lesions: Results from the COBIS II Registry (COronary BIfurcation Stenting). J Am Coll Cardiol. 2013;62:1654-9.
14. Lunardi M, Louvard Y, Lefèvre T, Stankovic G, Burzotta F, Kassab GS, et al. Definitions and Standardized Endpoints for Treatment of Coronary Bifurcations. EuroIntervention. 2023;19(10):e807-31.
15. Suárez de Lezo J, Medina A, Martín P, Novoa J, Suárez de Lezo J, Pan M, et al. Predictors of ostial side branch damage during provisional stenting of coronary bifurcation lesions not involving the side branch origin: an ultrasonographic study. EuroIntervention. 2012;7:1147-54.
16. Kini AS, Vengrenyuk Y, Pena J, Yoshimura T, Panwar SR, Motoyama S, et al. Plaque morphology predictors of side branch occlusion after provisional

stenting in coronary bifurcation lesion: Results of optical coherence tomography bifurcation study (ORBID). Catheter Cardiovasc Interv. 2017;89:259.

17. Watanabe M, Uemura S, Sugawara Y, Ueda T, Soeda T, Takeda Y, et al. Side branch complication after a single-stent crossover technique: prediction with frequency domain optical coherence tomography. Coron Artery Dis. 2014;25:321-9.
18. Fujino Y, Attizzani GF, Tahara S, Takagi K, Naganuma T, Wang W, et al. Impact of main-branch calcified plaque on side-branch stenosis in bifurcation stenting: an optical coherence tomography study. Int J Cardiol. 2014;176:1056-60.
19. Choi YJ, Lee SJ, Kim BK, Hong SJ, Ahn CM, Kim JS, et al. Effect of Wire Jailing at Side Branch in 1-Stent Strategy for Coronary Bifurcation Lesions. JACC Cardiovasc Interv. 2022;15:443-55.
20. Thomas M, Hildick-Smith D, Louvard Y, Albiero R, Darremont O, Stankovic G, et al. Percutaneous coronary intervention for bifurcation disease. A consensus view from the first meeting of the European Bifurcation Club. EuroIntervention. 2006;2:149-53.
21. Legrand V, Thomas M, Zelízko M, De Bruyne B, Reifart N, Steigen T, et al. Percutaneous coronary intervention of bifurcation lesions: state-of-the-art. Insights from the second meeting of the European Bifurcation Club. EuroIntervention. 2007;3:44-9.
22. Lassen JF, Holm NR, Stankovic G, Lefèvre T, Chieffo A, Hildick-Smith D, et al. Percutaneous coronary intervention for coronary bifurcation disease: consensus from the first 10 years of the European Bifurcation Club meetings. EuroIntervention. 2014;10:545-60.
23. Albiero R, Burzotta F, Lassen JF, Lefèvre T, Banning AP, Chatzizisis YS, et al. Treatment of coronary bifurcation lesions, part I: implanting the first stent in the provisional pathway. The 16th expert consensus document of the European Bifurcation Club. EuroIntervention. 2022;18:e362-76.
24. Pan M, Romero M, Ojeda S, Segura J, Mazuelos F, Suárez de Lezo J, et al. Inverted crush technique for uncrossable side branch occlusion during provisional side branch stenting: a new role for the jailed wire. Rev Esp Cardiol. 2011;64:718-22.
25. Lassen JF, Albiero R, Johnson TW, Burzotta F, Lefèvre T, Iles TL, et al. Treatment of coronary bifurcation lesions, part II: implanting two stents. The 16th expert consensus document of the European Bifurcation Club. EuroIntervention. 2022;18:457-70.
26. Numasawa Y, Sakakura K, Yamamoto K, Yamamoto S, Taniguchi Y, Fujita H, et al. A novel side branch protection technique in coronary stent implantation: Jailed Corsair technique. Cardiovasc Revasc Med. 2017;18:295-8.
27. Omori H, Kawase Y, Tanigaki T, Matsuo H. Pressure wire assessment of jailed balloon technique efficacy in a patient with complex bifurcated lesion. EuroIntervention. 2018;14:e316-7.
28. Burzotta F, Trani C, Sianos G. Jailed balloon protection: a new technique to avoid acute side-branch occlusion during provisional stenting of bifurcated lesions. Bench test report and first clinical experience. EuroIntervention. 2010;5:809-13.
29. Singh J, Patel Y, Depta JP, Mathews SJ, Cyrus T, Zajarias A, et al. A modified provisional stenting approach to coronary bifurcation lesions: clinical application of the "jailed-balloon technique". J Interv Cardiol. 2012;25:289-96.
30. Çaylı M, Şeker T, Gür M, Elbasan Z, Şahin DY, Elbey MA, et al. A Novel-Modified Provisional Bifurcation Stenting Technique: Jailed Semi-Inflated Balloon Technique. J Interv Cardiol. 2015;28:420-9.

31. Saito S, Shishido K, Moriyama N, Ochiai T, Mizuno S, Yamanaka F, et al. Modified jailed balloon technique for bifurcation lesions. Catheter Cardiovasc Interv. 2018;92:E218-26.
32. Qu W, Li X, Liu B. GW29-e1527 "Balloon-stent kissing" technique avoid side-branch compromise for simple true bifurcation lesions. J Am Coll Cardiol. 2018;72(16 Supplement):C130.
33. He P, Luo J, Gu M, Liu Y, Huang W, Tan N, et al. (2013). Effect of jailed balloon technique on side branch protection in percutaneous coronary intervention for bifurcation lesions. [online] Available from https://caod.oriprobe.com/articles/40422171/Effect_of_jailed_balloon_technique_on_side_branch_.htm. [Last accessed October, 2024].
34. Jin Z, Song L, Zheng Z, Zhang S, Wang M. Balloon-stent kissing technique versus jailed wire technique for interventional treatment of coronary bifurcation lesions: Comparison of short-and long-term clinical outcomes. Medicine (Baltimore). 2019;98:e15633.
35. Dou K, Zhang D, Pan H, Guo N, Li L, Li Y, et al. CIT-RESOLVE Investigators. Active SB-P Versus Conventional Approach to the Protection of High-Risk Side Branches: The CIT-RESOLVE Trial. JACC Cardiovasc Interv. 2020;13:1112-22.

CHAPTER 20

Double Kiss Culotte Stent Technique for Coronary Angioplasty

C Raghu

INTRODUCTION

Bifurcation lesions comprise 20% of coronary stenosis and represent one of the most challenging situations for interventional cardiologists.[1] The complexity is contributed by differing diameters of coronary vessels—main branch (MB) and side branch (SB) proximal and distal to the bifurcation, angulation between MB and SB, location of bifurcation stenosis—left main versus nonleft main and most importantly large vessel bifurcation lesion. Bifurcation variables involved illustrate the complexity of performing a bifurcation stenting.[2] These variables include lesion characteristics, patient-specific features, equipment availability, procedural technique planned, outcome determinants, and above all the operator expertise. Large vessel bifurcation lesions are defined as those lesions where the SB size is >2.5 mm.[3] Despite the recent algorithmic approach by the European Bifurcation Club (EBC), each case of bifurcation stenosis poses a unique challenge leading to intense discussions and planning before the angioplasty procedure.[4] In this article, we discuss a 2-stent strategy for complex, large vessel bifurcation—double kiss culotte (DK Culotte) stent technique, rationale for this technique, detailed description and need for each step of the procedure, bench testing studies' comparison with the established double kiss crush (DK Crush) technique and ongoing studies investigating the efficacy of DK Culotte technique.

Provisional T-stent strategy is considered the gold standard for bifurcation lesions because it is simple to perform with excellent short- and long-term outcomes. It has limitations in the presence of complex, large vessel bifurcation stenosis.[5]

Managing complex large vessel bifurcations has improved with various iterations involving multiple modifications. Initial approaches for complex large vessel bifurcations were the Crush technique and Culotte techniques. Crush technique has progressively been modified with mini to nano leading to the DK crush technique. Standard Culotte technique started with MB stent followed by the SB stent to evolve to the reverse Culotte where the SB gets the initial stent followed by the MB stent. The latest iterations, DK crush and DK Culotte, involve an initial optimization of the SB stent result with a kissing balloon followed by the MB stent and final kissing balloon inflation. These steps involving kissing balloon dilatation twice led to the term double kiss Culotte and Crush technique.

Determinants of a successful bifurcation coronary lesion stent with lower restenosis rates:

- Ensure adequate coverage of all vascular branches in the bifurcation lesion.
- Minimize the metal burden at the bifurcation lesion.[6]

The DK Culotte has borne out to fulfill the above objectives as a superior alternative to DK crush technique.

EVOLUTION OF THE CULOTTE TECHNIQUE

The Culotte technique was proposed by Chevalier in 1998, to protect against SB occlusion, by implantation of 2 similar stents in 2 steps in the main branch and in the side branch with overlapping of the 2 stents in the main branch before bifurcation. This process of MB stent followed by the SB stent is termed classic Culotte.[7] Subsequent iteration involved SB stent first followed by the MB stent which is termed as the reversed or inverted Culotte strategy. The inverted Culotte strategy is the most followed strategy in clinical practice. Inverted Culotte strategy which involves double kissing balloon inflation (DKI) at various steps is termed as DK Culotte strategy and is the commonly practiced version.[8]

Double kiss Culotte is useful in two clinical scenarios:

1. To protect a large side branch as a bail out during a provisional single stent strategy.
2. Complex large vessel bifurcation where the distal calibers of the MB and SB are identical.[5]

The limitations of the DK culotte technique are:

- Culotte may not be the optimal technique for bifurcation lesions with very different branch sizes.
- Involves multiple steps making the coronary angioplasty procedure complex.
- Double layer of metal in the proximal MB before the bifurcation lesion.
- If there is a large disparity between the SB distal vessel caliber and proximal MB caliber, DK Culotte is not a suitable strategy and DK crush is preferred.[5]

Advantages of DK Culotte over DK crush technique:

- Coverage of the SB ostium with a single layer of metal making access to SB and MB easier.
- When the distal SB caliber is like that of MB distal vessel, DK Culotte is a preferred strategy.

- Single metal layer at the bifurcation in DK Culotte compared to the three metal layers in the lateral wall of proximal MB in DK crush. This reduced metal burden at bifurcation theoretically should result in reduced restenosis rates.[8]

RATIONALE FOR THE DOUBLE KISSING BALLOON INFLATION

The kissing balloon inflation (KBI) involves double balloon inflation at 2 different steps—first KBI after the SB stent and the final KBI after the MB stent. The initial KBI of the SB stent prior to the MB stent optimizes the SB stent result. This protects against the SB stent deformation after the MB stent. In addition, access to the SB is straightforward and predictable after the MB stent as the SB stent struts are fully opened for the final kissing balloon inflation. In the two-stent technique, double KBI also plays a pivotal role in acquiring adequate expansion and apposition of the stents. Double KBI in the DK crush technique after SB and MB stentings provided a lower cumulative major adverse cardiovascular event (MACE) rate (11.4% vs. 24.4%, $p = 0.02$) than standard crush stenting with lower performance of final KBI only (100% vs. 78%, $p < 0.001$).[9]

STEPS IN DOUBLE KISSING CULOTTE TECHNIQUE (FIG. 1)

The European Bifurcation Club, in its white paper on stenting techniques for patients with bifurcated coronary artery lesions, provided a stepwise detail on how to perform a DK Culotte stent procedure.[5]

The recommended steps for inverted DK culotte are:

- After appropriate predilation of both branches, the first stent is implanted in the SB protruding inside the proximal MV. The stent is sized according to the diameter of the distal SB and long enough to allow POT in the proximal MV **(Figs. 1A and B)**.
- Postdilation of the stent at the level of proximal MV up to the carina level is performed with a balloon sized 1:1 according to the proximal MV [proximal optimization technique (POT)] **(Fig. 1C)**.
- Rewiring of the MV close to the carina is performed using the pullback technique from SB **(Figs. 1D to F)**.
- Distal MV balloon dilation (or kissing balloon inflation) is performed to open the struts into distal MV direction **(Figs. 1D to F)**.
- Second stent implantation in the distal MV covering up to the proximal MV is performed. DES diameter is selected 1:1 according to the distal MV size, DES length selected to ensure proximal MV lesion coverage **(Fig. 1G)**.
- Systematic postdilation of the stent at the level of proximal MV up to the carina level with a balloon diameter sized 1:1 according to the proximal MV (repeat POT) is recommended **(Fig. 1H)**.

- Distal rewiring of the SB by the pullback technique is performed **(Figs. 1I to K)**.
- Kissing balloon inflation (using short noncompliant balloons) is systematically needed. Usually, after having placed the two balloons in the proper position, sequential inflation at high pressure followed by simultaneous kissing balloon inflation is suggested **(Figs. 1L and M)**.
- Postdilation of the stent at the level of proximal MV up to the carina level with a balloon diameter sized 1:1 according to the proximal MV (final POT) is performed **(Figs. 1L to N)**.

The EBC strongly recommends systematic POT immediately after each stent deployment to avoid the presence of malapposed struts in the proximal MV that may cause abluminal rewiring.

My argument for DK Culotte strategy as a preferred strategy emerges from the vascular geometry achieved result in physiological vascular flows.

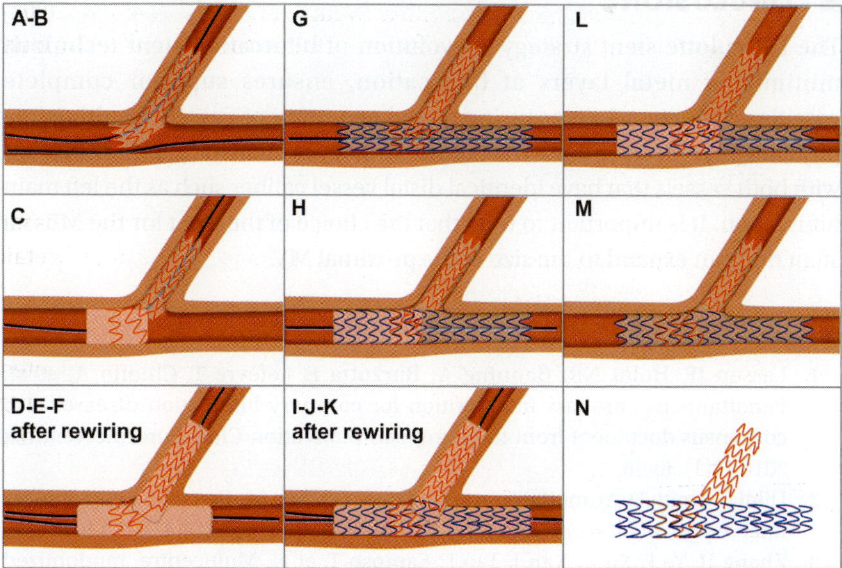

Figs. 1A to N: (A) Placement of 2 coronary guidewires in main and side branch vessels; (B) Deployment of first stent in the side branch; (C) POT in the side branch stent struts that are present in the main branch—first POT; (D) Exchange of coronary guidewires: rewiring of the main branch from the side branch by pullback technique; (E) Exchange of coronary guidewires: wiring of the side branch; (F) Kissing balloon inflation of main and side branch—first kissing balloon; (G) Main branch stent placement; (H) POT of the main branch stent—second POT; (I) Exchange of coronary guidewires: Rewiring of the side branch from the main branch by pull back technique; (J) Exchange of coronary guidewires: wiring of the main branch; (K) Kissing balloon inflation of main and side branch—second kissing balloon; (L) POT of the main branch stent—third POT; (M) Final control angiogram; (N) Image showing how both the stents are overlapped without any gap. (POT: proximal optimization technique)

From a structural point of view, the culotte technique might be considered as more "physiologic" compared to the other approaches for bifurcation stenosis.[8]

- Ensures full coverage in all three segments (as compared to T-stenting)
- Minimal or no neo carina (as compared to T-and-protrusion)
- No triple layer (as compared to DK-crush)
- Tubular architecture of the stents is maintained with fractal deformation only (as compared to DK-crush)
- Final vascular anatomy is ovoid, devoid of any floating stent struts without any massive stent deformation.

Recent case reports published attempt to further minimize the metal burden at the bifurcation location with single-cell coverage of the SB ostium, double kissing string culotte technique and double kissing nano culotte technique.[10-12]

CONCLUSION

The DK culotte stent strategy is evolution of bifurcation stent technique minimizing metal layers at bifurcation, ensures superior complete vascular coverage while ensuring fractal geometry of vessels resulting in a physiological vascular flow. DK Culotte strategy is ideal for those bifurcation with both vessels that have identical distal vessel caliber such as the left main bifurcation. It is important to note that the choice of the stent for the MB is a stent that can expand to the size of the proximal MV.

REFERENCES

1. Lassen JF, Holm NR, Banning A, Burzotta F, Lefèvre T, Chieffo A, et al. Percutaneous coronary intervention for coronary bifurcation disease: 11th consensus document from the European Bifurcation Club. EuroIntervention. 2016;12(1):38-46.
2. Hildick-Smith D, Arunothayaraj S, Stankovic G, Chen SL. Percutaneous coronary intervention of bifurcation lesions. EuroIntervention. 2022;18(4):e273-91.
3. Zhang JJ, Ye F, Xu K, Kan J, Tao L, Santoso T, et al. Multicentre, randomized comparison of two-stent and provisional stenting techniques in patients with complex coronary bifurcation lesions: the DEFINITION II trial. Eur Heart J. 2020;41(27):2523-36.
4. Lassen JF, Albiero R, Johnson TW, Burzotta F, Lefèvre T, Iles TL, et al. Treatment of coronary bifurcation lesions, part II: implanting two stents. The 16th expert consensus document of the European Bifurcation Club. EuroIntervention. 2022;18(6):457-70.
5. Burzotta F, Lassen JF, Louvard Y, Lefèvre T, Banning AP, Daremont O, et al. European Bifurcation Club white paper on stenting techniques for patients with bifurcated coronary artery lesions. Catheter Cardiovasc Interv. 2020;96(5):1067-79.

6. Raphael CE, O'Kane PD, Johnson TW, Prasad A, Gulati R, Sandoval Y, et al. Evolution of the Crush Technique for Bifurcation Stenting. JACC Cardiovasc Interv. 2021;14(21):2315-26.
7. Chevalier B, Glatt B, Royer T, Guyon P. Placement of coronary stents in bifurcation lesions by the "culotte" technique. Am J Cardiol. 1998; 82:943-9.
8. Toth GG, Sasi V, Franco D, Prassl AJ, Di Serafino L, Ng JCK, et al. Double-kissing culotte technique for coronary bifurcation stenting. EuroIntervention. 2020;16(9):e724-33.
9. Murasato Y, Finet G, Foin N. Final kissing balloon inflation: the whole story. EuroIntervention. 2015;11 Suppl V:V81-5.
10. Sandesara PB, Shekiladze N, Nicholson WJ, Jaber WA. A Novel Single-Cell, Double-Kissing Culotte Technique for Left Main Bifurcation Stenting. JACC Cardiovasc Interv. 2022;15(8):898-900.
11. Chan YH, Hospital PO, Kong H. "Double Kissing String Culotte Technique" for bifurcation PCI: Could we make it real with modern generation of stent? Available from https://www.apsic.net/%E2%80%9Cdouble-kissing-string-culotte-technique-bifurcation-pci-could-we-make-it-real-modern-generation%E2%80%9D-it-really-deal. [Last accessed October, 2024]
12. Kahraman S, Güner A, Çizgici AY, Ertürk M. Reply to Letter to the Editor: Provisional (Reverse) Double-Kissing Nano-Culotte Stenting. Anatol J Cardiol. 2023;27(5):292-4.

CHAPTER 21

Double Kiss Crush Technique: Step-by-Step Approach with Troubleshooting

K Sivaprasad

INTRODUCTION

The preferred approach in a coronary bifurcation lesion is provisional layered stenting strategy. However, there are high risk situations in which there exists a significant risk of side branch (SB) loss/reduced perfusion in certain complex coronary bifurcations, which can result in serious hemodynamic complications and higher adverse outcomes. DEFINITION II criteria provide a handy tool to categorize patients with bifurcation phenotype for upfront two stent strategy and the preferred approach therein is double kissing crush (DKC).[1]

The following is the step-by-step approach to double kissing crush with frequently ask questions and troubleshooting at each stage. Most important initial step is the study of coronary bifurcation.[2-4]

ANALYSIS OF THE ANGIOGRAM

A detailed analysis of the target lesion involving the main vessel and the side branch, often with the use of imaging with intravascular ultrasound (IVUS) or optical coherence tomography (OCT) to access the proximal to distal extent of the disease, minimal lumen diameter, lumen to lumen size at the landing zones or external elastic lamina to external elastic lamina sizing of the vessels, appropriate landing zones, degree and extent of SB disease, presence of thrombus, presence and extent of calcification, bifurcation angle, etc. are to be assessed.

ACCESS

Though radial access with 6F guide catheter (GC) can be used to perform double kiss crush stenting for simple bifurcation lesions, in lesions involving complex bifurcations such as severe calcification and tortuosity, using a large GC—7 or 8F through femoral artery access provide improved support and procedural ease. In DKC technique, GC should impart strong support and preferred choices for right coronary artery (RCA) is AL 1/AL 0.75 and for left coronary artery (LCA) is EBU/XB.

HARDWARE PLANNING

As stated earlier, 6F and/or 7F or 8F GC is selected according to the type of bifurcation and hardware planned.

- 2 regular work horse wires and also hydrophilic wires should be available in case of need.
- 2 × 10/12 mm, 2.5 × 10/12 mm, 3 × 10/12 and 3.5 × 10/12 mm semicompliant (SC) or noncompliant (NC) balloons, balloons as per requirement
- Be prepared with appropriate sized stents preferably with open cell design with less connectors across.
- Imaging catheters IVUS/OCT and rotablation are certain select cases.

While choosing the main vessel (MV) stent, the stent expansion characteristics have to be analyzed and is to be applied to the case.

STEP I

Wire both MV and SB using regular work horse wires.

Frequently Asked Questions

Which should be wired first?

The more critical, more tortuous/calcified vessel is to be wired first, where more wire manipulation is anticipated. This is because if planned as a second wiring, then torqueing of the wire to traverse the vessel where more manipulation is needed can result in wire wrap. Thus, there should not be too much twiddling or twisting torqueing of the wire (not beyond 180° in order to avoid wire wrapping during second wire manipulation).

Importantly, reducing the frame rate to 7.5 fps than the usual 15 fps during fluoroscopy will go a long way in reducing the radiation risk in time and fluoroscopy intensive procedures such as DKC.

In complex bifurcations and in left main coronary artery (LMCA) bifurcation, it is preferred to use imaging if available and the bifurcation MV lesion length, size, MLD and calcification bifurcation angle, etc. should be identified and information gathered can be utilized for better preparation of for DKC.

Troubleshooting

- *Wiring the difficult SB:* Can arise in situations such as the SB with unfavorable angulation and plaque at the ostium and severe side branch ostial disease.

  The difficult SB wiring can be done with the help of microcatheter (MC) or angled MC or dual lumen MC or deflectable tip MC with modifies wire tip bends suiting the anatomy of origin of the side branch.

- *Wire wrap: When to suspect and what to do?*

  When the advancing balloon halts at the any point in transit especially at the MV entry/side branch origin when the wires are truly luminal, suspect wire wrap. When wire wrap is suspected, advance the balloon to as much distal location as possible and with draw one of the wrapped wire entirely into the balloon proximal to the balloon tip (this will unwrap if any) and reenter the vessel, preferably with a loop, which often helps to advance the balloon.

STEP II: PREPARATION OF THE MV LESION AND THE SB LESION

Prepare the SB ostium and the main vessel lesion using appropriately sized NC balloons (for SB 1:1 or 1.1:1 NC balloon and for the main vessel, an NC balloon which matches the distal main vessel can be used and dilated up to 12–14 ATM).

Frequently Asked Questions

Balloon could not be passed to SB/MV. What next?

Use a small highly deliverable balloon such as—Sapphire II PRO 1 mm or 1.5 mm (OrbusNeich, Innvolution Healthcare Pvt. Ltd., Kaushambi Ghaziabad—UP, India), TAKERU balloon (TERUMO), THREADER (Boston Scientific) and after crossing and dilatation, incrementally larger balloons can be used for proper SB dilatation.

If the smallest balloon fails to cross, another method is to try MC such as FineCross MG to cross to SB and may modify the ostium and allow the advancement of balloon.

If the above methods fail, another support wire such as WIGGLE wire (Abbott vascular) can be used to aid balloon crossing.

Another important step is to increase the guide support, by using a guide extension catheter or balloon anchoring technique with balloon placed ideally in MV segment where later stenting is planned in order to avoid injury to the vessel.

If all the above methods are unsuccessful, consider the benefit versus risk of atherectomy of the SB if the branch is large and has a favorable angle with strong contention to defer from atherectomy in tortuous, angulated SB and which are small in caliber.

Another important reason for nonpassage of the balloon may be wire wrap. It is suspected when the balloon while advancing smoothly comes to a halt in the wire further push may pull back the wire/s.

Once recognized wire wrap "unwrap" as above.

STEP III: SIDE BRANCH STENTING

Side branch stenting is done with the placement of an NC balloon in the main vessel at the bifurcation point. The stent is sized 1:1 to the SB and MV balloon 1:1 to distal MV diameter (preferably judged by intravascular imaging) and deploy the SB stent with 2–3 mm into the MV confirmed by an appropriate orthogonal angiographic view/s to properly visualize the SB ostium. The SB stent is deployed at optimal pressure of deployment and after which the balloon is slightly withdrawn to MV and redilate to higher pressure for optimal ostial expansion of the SB stent. If inadequate ostial expansion is anticipated, 1:1 sized NC balloon should be used at 12–16 or more ATM to optimize the SB ostial stent apposition and this will aid in subsequent luminal crossing of the SB wire.

STEP IV: SIDE BRANCH STENT CRUSHING (THE "FIRST CRUSH")

Once the SB stent is well deployed, the MV portion of the SB stent in MV can be crushed using the prepositioned MV balloon at 12–14/16 ATM. If the proximal MV (pMV) segment is larger, another NC balloon which matches the pMV diameter (as evaluated by the IV imaging study) matched 1:1 sized short NC balloon sized to pMV diameter can be used optimize the proximal segment of the SB stent crush, but it is important to place the distal balloon marker in front of the SB carina to avoid distal MV injury and/or undesirable crushing of the SB stent to the ostium of the SB.

But it is important to avoid premature SB stent crushing. Before crushing the SB stent, an angiogram (if possible intravascular imaging to be done) to look for any distal stent edge complications, downstream geographical miss, and distal disease if any and is to be corrected before crushing.

STEP V: REWIRING THE SB STENT

Rewiring of the SB is to be done, not through the distal strut as is done in other bifurcation strategies, in DKC technique, it needs to be done preferably through the nondistal or proximal strut except in very narrow angle bifurcations where more metal may be shifted to distal carina by proximal wiring and in such situations careful distal wiring can be accepted.

Frequently Asked Questions

SB: Why fear distal wiring?

Attempt to pass the wire through the distal SB strut may take the wire through the abluminal surface of the SB stent and after a variable distance the wire renters the lumen and parked distally. Subsequent kissing balloon dilatations crush the portion of the stent where the wire was abluminal and the proximal segment of SB become devoid of stent. This can be overcome by intentional nondistal and proximal wiring.

Troubleshooting the difficulty in rewiring the SB after stenting the SB and crushing:

- Create or modify the wire tip shape of regular workhorse with sharpening of the primary curve adding smaller or larger secondary curves. Once the guidewire (GW) catches the ostium of the side branch, it is important to keep the tip free and by careful initial torqueing to secure the position of the wire tip within the stent struts, more rapid to and fro torqueing or twiddling the wire and pushing it carefully may help to advance the wire distally in the SB. Special care needs to be taken while advancing through heavily diseased segments to avoid dissection.
- If wiring with workhorse guidewires fails, different wire types, such as hydrophilic-coated, polymer-jacketed which allow easy cross ability or occasionally dedicated chronic total occlusion wires, can be used.
- If there is a highly angulated SB which does not permit direct wiring, large bend is made in the GW and advanced to the distal main vessel beyond the ostium of the side branch and then slowly and carefully withdraw it. As the bend in the wire uncoils often the tip gets engaged to the SB ostium and further careful uncoiling and torqueing of the wire helps to wire the SB. An extreme from this is hairpin technique.
- SB wiring can also be made possible using MC which helps to deliver the highly angulated GW to the SB ostium without having to navigate the highly bend wire through the pMV and thus losing the integrity of intended bend. Fixed angle tip MC such as Supercross can also be of aid in certain situations and for severely angled take off the SB, angulated steerable microcatheters [such as Venture® (Teleflex) or SwiftNINJA® (Merit Medica)] may also be used in selected situations.

STEP VI: THE "FIRST KISS"

Simultaneous kissing is given using noncompliant SB balloon 1:1 to the SB diameter and MV balloon 1:1 to distal MV diameter to 12–14 ATM. Initially each balloon is inflated individually at high pressures (16–20 ATM). This will optimize the SB and MV stents. Then both balloons are simultaneously inflated to 12–14 ATM and then the pressure is released simultaneously.

A modified kissing balloon inflation approach is also used where the SB is first inflated to 12 ATM, then partly deflated back to 4 ATM with simultaneous inflation of the MV balloon to 12 ATM which may reduce proximal stent deformation.

STEP VII: STENTING THE MV

There exists a debate regarding whether the SB wire be removed before MV stent for fear of entrapment. It is preferable to remove the SB wire. The MV stent length and the proximal and distal extension beyond the SB is partly determined by the MV disease, but it is preferable to leave at least 6–8 mm of the stent proximal to the SB for proximal optimization of the stent. The MV stent size is determined by the diameter of the distal MV.

Frequently Asked Questions

What can be done if the MV stent does not track across the crushed SB stent?
Increase the guide support by coaxial alignment, balloon anchoring, or guide extension catheters can be used to improve the deliverability of the stent. Additionally stents which are more malleable and trackable can be used such as Tetrilimus (Sahajanand Medical Technology Pvt. Ltd., Surat, India), Synergy (Boston scientific), Xience Sierra (Abbotts), Ultimaster Nagomi (Terumo), and Resolute Onyx (Medtronics) to name a few.

STEP VIII: PROXIMAL OPTIMIZATION TECHNIQUE

As the MV stent is matched to the size of the distal main vessel (dMV) proximal part of the stent should be postdilated to expand to the size of the pMV using 1:1 balloon which is matching the pMV diameter and at 12–14 ATM. It is important to use either a regular NC balloon of 6–8 mm length or dedicated POT NC balloons. The distal marker of the balloon should be at the carina or just in front. It is important to postdilate the full length of the pMV stent segment with POT balloon if the pMV segment stent is longer than 8 mm by pulling back the balloon till the ostium of the stent included.

STEP IX: REWIRING THE SB THROUGH THE CENTRAL/PROXIMAL STRUT IN MV STENT

Attempt rewiring of the side branch after second POT through the middle/proximal strut (can confirm by imaging and if not proper reattempt wiring through middle/proximal strut).

Frequently Asked Questions

What should be done in cases where rewiring the SB is difficult?

Troubleshooting: Difficulty is experienced due to multiple layers of stent at SB ostium and deformation of the cells.

Solutions:

- Reshape the wire tip and add secondary bends—larger/smaller bends
- Change to polymer jacketed hydrophilic or some of the CTO wires with increased torqueability, with a customized shape at the tip preferably with primary and secondary curves.
- MC may help to cross the struts at the ostium, increase the wire support and allows easier reshaping and wire exchanges.
- For very angulated take offs, preshaped angulated MC, steerable MC or dual lumen MC may help.

Difficulty in passing the balloon to even traverse the proximal segment of the MV stent: Suspect abluminal wiring of the MV by the wire used to cross to the side branch.

It often is the result of improperly done pMV POT which is not correctly done up to the proximal end of the MV stent with the POT balloon. This can be confirmed only by imaging the proximal stent segment or some times by stent enhancing techniques in fluoroscopy. In order to avoid this, pMV POT to be done meticulously as described earlier. Rewiring after repeat POT up to the proximal end of the pMV stent is the way to correct this event.

Difficulty in passing the desired balloon to SB:

- Wire wrap if identified correct it as described earlier.
- Use the smallest profile new balloon 1 mm or 1.5 mm in diameter to advance to the side branch stent and then serially optimize the SB stent.
- Use of MC to dilate/modify the SB stent deformity such that further advancements with balloon is possible.
- Increase the coaxial support by proper engagement of GC or careful deep engagement of the GC or using a guide extension catheter
- If all measures fail, consider rewiring through another strut of the MV.

The OCT/IVUS may done to confirm the wire positions and the distal stent deployment dissections apposition and expansions and the MLA achieved so that further action can be taken. Similarly wire crossing also can be verified.

STEP X: FINAL KISSING BALLOON

The SB and MV is dilated further with two NC balloons—SB balloon matching the side branch and MV balloon matching the distal MV diameter, individual high pressures >16 ATM initially and subsequently simultaneously both balloons to 12–14 ATM with balloons protruding about 2 mm into the pMV.

Problem: The SB stent may be inadvertently crushed after after kissing balloon inflation and this may cause neo carina formation.

This can happen due to two causes:

1. Nonsimultaneous deflation of the SB and DMV balloon during SKB dilatation.
2. Too much protrusion of the final POT balloon distally beyond the carina.

Avoidance of these two happenings and careful technique will avoid these mishaps.

STEP XI: POT OF THE MV STENT

Proximal POT of the MV stent using short appropriately sized PMV balloon. Unlike the first POT, it may be best to keep the distal balloon marker for the re-POT just proximal to the carina to avoid disruption of the bifurcation stent architecture.

Final imaging run to MV and SB to confirm stent apposition, expansion and the bifurcation area, polygon of confluence (POC) and the ostia of the branches distal or proximal dissections and after imaging final angiogram is to be done.

Activated clotting time (ACT) should be maintained above 280 ms during the procedure.

STEPS OF DK CRUSH TECHNIQUE

The essential steps in DKC:

1. *Wire both vessels* ***(Fig. 1)***
2. *Prepare both vessels* ***(Fig. 2)***
3. *Stent the SB with 2 mm protrusion to the MV with MV NC balloon (dMV diameter) in bifurcation across the SB origin* ***(Fig. 3)***
4. *First crush* ***(Fig. 4)***
5. *Rewiring through nondistal strut—proximal* ***(Fig. 5)***
6. *First kiss* ***(Fig. 6)***
7. *MV stenting (may remove the SB wire) (the second crush)* ***(Fig. 7)***
8. *First POT* ***(Fig. 8)***
9. *Rewiring the SB through the proximal strut* ***(Fig. 9)***
10. *Second kiss* ***(Fig. 10)***
11. *Final POT* ***(Fig. 11)***
12. *Final picture* ***(Fig. 12)***

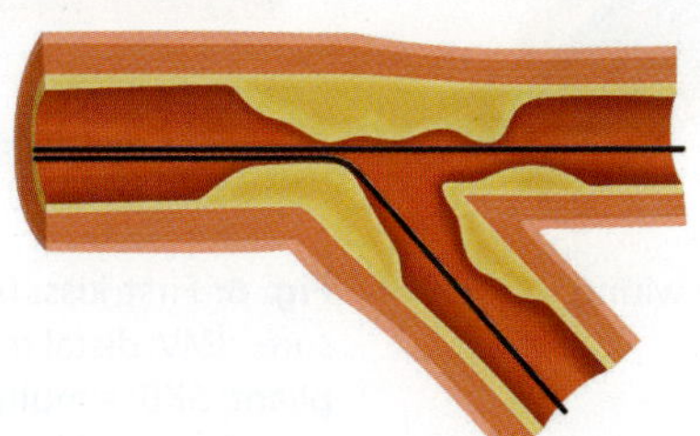

Fig. 1: *Step I:* Wire both vessels—work horse wires.

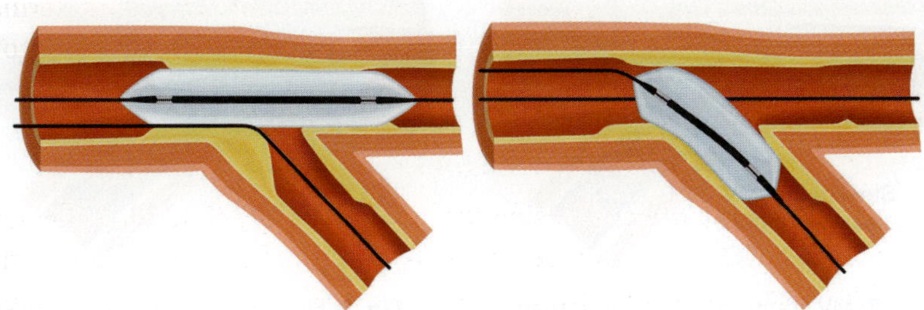

Fig. 2: Prepare both vessels.

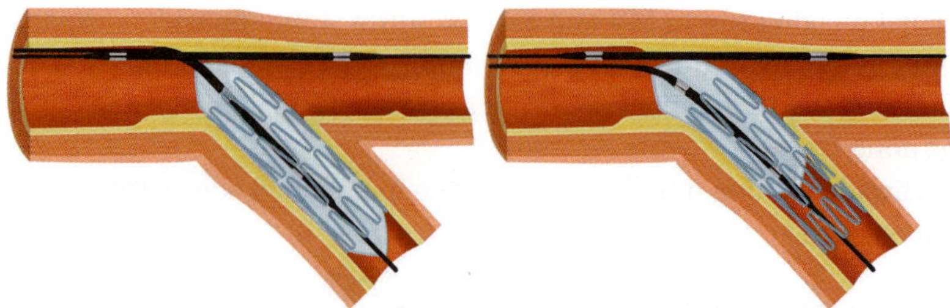

Fig. 3: Stenting the SB.

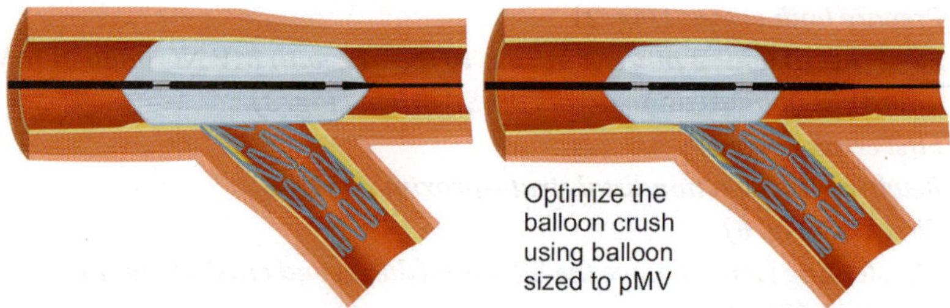

Fig. 4: First crush. (pMV: proximal main vessel)

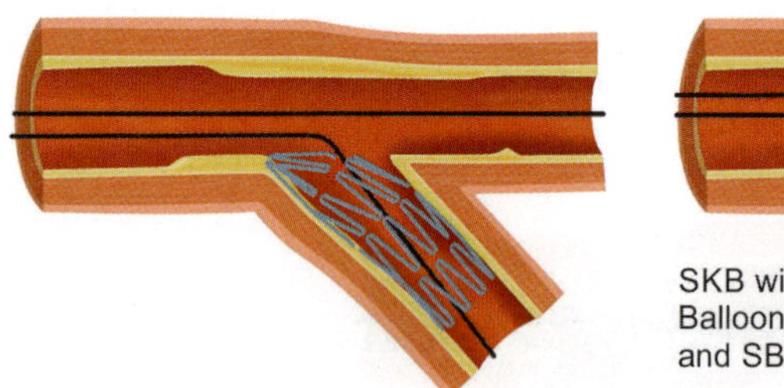

Fig. 5: First rewiring.

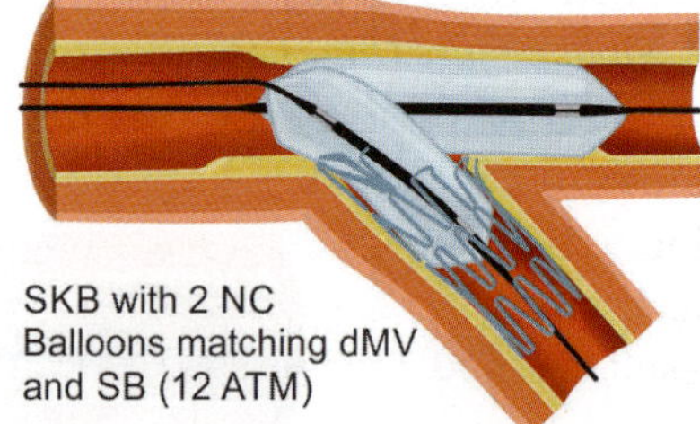

Fig. 6: First kiss. (ATM: atmosphere pressure; dMV: distal main vessel; NC: noncompliant; SKB: simultaneous kissing balloon; SB: side branch)

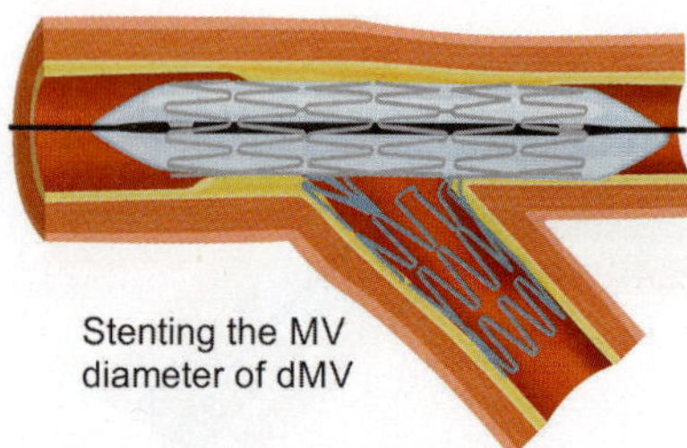

Fig. 7: MV stenting. (dMV: distal main vessel)

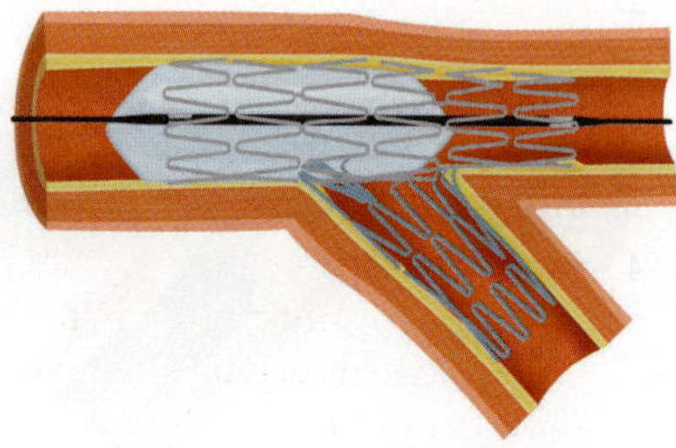

Fig. 8: First proximal optimization technique (POT).

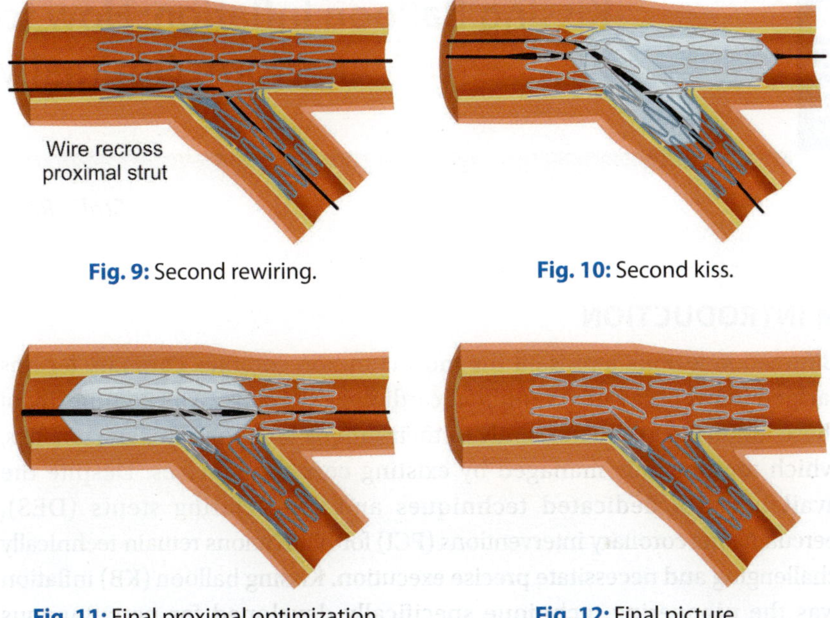

Fig. 9: Second rewiring.

Fig. 10: Second kiss.

Fig. 11: Final proximal optimization technique (POT).

Fig. 12: Final picture.

CONCLUSION

DK crush is the most extensively used two stent strategy in the modern interventional practice. It is consider superior to other two stent strategies due to the easier performance of final kissing balloon inflation. Though performance of DK crush is time consuming because of multiple steps, it results in good long term outcomes.

REFERENCES

1. Zhang JJ, Ye F, Xu K, Kan J, Tao L, Santoso T, et al. Multicentre, randomized comparison of two-stent and provisional stenting techniques in patients with complex coronary bifurcation lesions: the DEFINITION II trial. Eur Heart J. 2020;41(27):2523-36.
2. Hall AB, Chavez I, Garcia S, Gossi M, Poulose A, Sorajja P, et al. Double kissing crush bifurcation stenting: step-by-step troubleshooting. EuroIntervention. 2021;17:e317-25.
3. Zhang JJ, Chen SL. A step-by step description of DK crush technique. Cardiac Interv Today. 2020;14(5):38-41.
4. Lassen JF, Albeiro R, Johnson TW, Burzotta F, Lefevre J, Iles TL, et al. Treatment of coronary bifurcation lesions Part II: Implanting two stents. The 16th expert consensus document of European bifurcation club. EuroIntervention. 2022;18:457-70.

CHAPTER 22

Kissing Balloon Inflation: How to Perform Optimally

Stalin Roy J

INTRODUCTION

Bifurcation lesions represent the most common complex coronary lesions tackled in everyday interventional cardiology practice.[1] The complexity of these lesions lies predominantly in their unique anatomical characteristics, which are not fully managed by existing coronary devices. Despite the availability of dedicated techniques and drug-eluting stents (DES), percutaneous coronary interventions (PCI) for bifurcations remain technically challenging and necessitate precise execution. Kissing balloon (KB) inflation was the pioneering technique specifically developed for percutaneous bifurcation interventions and continues to be integral in these procedures. The KB technique aims to optimize stent apposition, improve side branch (SB) access, and rectify stent deformation or distortion. Extensive research over the years, ranging from bench testing and computer simulations to in vivo intravascular imaging and clinical studies, has generated substantial data regarding the benefits and limitations of the KB technique. This chapter provides a comprehensive overview of these aspects.

ANATOMY OF BIFURCATION LESIONS

A coronary bifurcation consists of a main vessel (MV) and a SB. The proximal segment of the MV precedes the SB origin, while the distal segment follows it. The flow divider, or carina, is the tissue membrane at the bifurcation point. The anatomical complexity of bifurcation lesions includes varying atherosclerosis distribution, spatial relation defined by angles A, B, and C, the tapered nature of the SB ostium, and the asymmetrical geometric reduction at the bifurcation site **(Fig. 1)**.

Bifurcation stenosis is defined as a narrowing near or involving the SB origin, with the SB being considered significant based on patient-specific factors like symptoms and left ventricular function.[2] Plaque distribution classifications have led to multiple schemes, with "true" bifurcations involving significant SB stenosis. Atherosclerotic plaques are primarily located in low shear stress areas, such as the lateral walls of the MV and SB, while the carina, subjected to high shear stress, is less affected.[3]

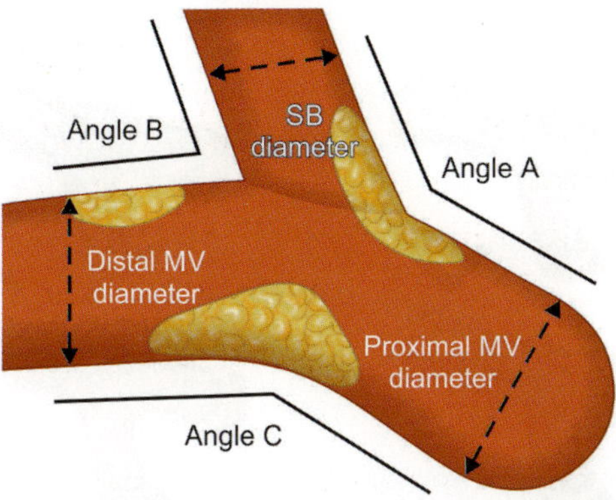

Fig. 1: The anatomy of bifurcations. (MV: main vessel; SB: side branch)

NEED FOR KISSING BALLOON TECHNIQUE

Bifurcation lesions pose a risk of SB damage, leading to worsened stenosis or occlusion. Mechanisms include plaque or carina shift, refractory spasm, or ostial dissection. SB occlusion can result in myocardial necrosis and elevated cardiac enzyme levels, impacting both short- and long-term outcomes. Even though most acutely occluded SBs eventually reperfuse, temporary occlusion causes myocardial enzyme elevation.[4] SB stenosis can lead to myocardial ischemia, persistent symptoms, or mechanical dysfunction. In cases of significant SB stenosis post-DES implantation, patients exhibit higher rates of late inducible ischemia and minor adverse coronary events.[5]

HISTORY OF KISSING BALLOON TECHNIQUE

The KB technique was first described by Gruentzig for iliac bifurcation stenosis treatment and later applied to coronary revascularization.[6] Early implementations required two guiding catheters and sequential balloon inflation to minimize vessel dissection risk. Technological advancements have simplified the technique, allowing KB through a single guiding catheter using various balloon configurations. The KB technique's adoption has increased with the introduction of coronary stents and subsequent technological improvements.

GAINING INSIGHT INTO KISSING BALLOON TECHNIQUE

Bench Testing

Bench testing has significantly enhanced our understanding of bifurcation stenting. Ormiston et al., demonstrated that SB balloon dilation through the MV stent side opens a cell toward the SB, causing marked stent distortion.[7] KB can prevent or correct this distortion, emphasizing the need for properly

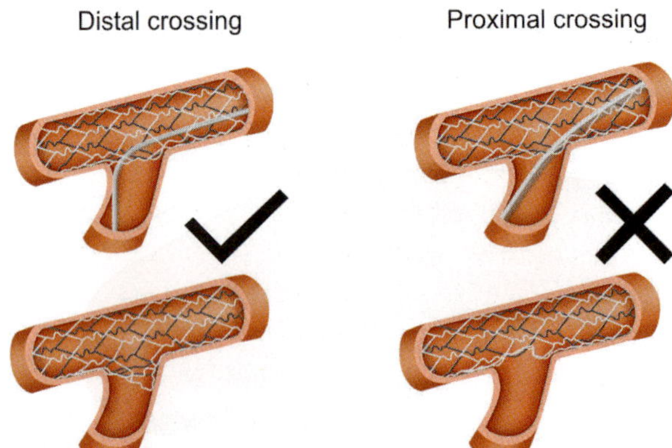

Fig. 2: Distal crossing in provisional technique gives optimal side branch ostial scaffolding after KB inflation. (KB: kissing balloon)

sized balloons and simultaneous balloon deflation. Additionally, proper SB rewiring through the cell closest to the carina ensures optimal scaffolding, as shown by bench testing **(Fig. 2)**.

Finite Element Analysis

Computer simulations using finite element analysis have provided valuable insights into bifurcation interventions. These simulations highlight the importance of the MV stent's relative position for optimal SB access and emphasize mandatory KB for open-cell stents. Simulations also reveal that KB induces elliptical deformation of the proximal MV stent, potentially causing vessel wall stress and injury at the SB entry.[3]

Computational Flow Dynamics

Numerical methods and algorithms applied to fluid interactions with stented bifurcations demonstrate the advantages of final KB in terms of better flow patterns and reduced hemodynamic disturbance. These studies show that KB improves flow by removing stent struts from the blood flow path, enhancing access to the SB and reducing disturbances.

SUCCESS AND SAFETY OF KISSING BALLOON TECHNIQUE

The BBC ONE study highlighted the higher success rates of KB in simple stenting procedures compared to complex procedures.[8] Only one complication, an intramural hematoma, was reported in published studies. Overall, KB has proven to be a safe and effective technique in bifurcation lesion interventions.

IMAGING ASSESSMENT OF KISSING BALLOON TECHNIQUE

One-stent Strategy

Intravascular ultrasound (IVUS) studies have shown that SB dilation introduces geometric distortion of the distal MV stent, with KB partially restoring stent geometry. The CORPAL Kiss trial suggested that KB results in a larger proximal stent cross-sectional area, indicating overexpansion of the proximal MV stent.[9] Recent OCT studies have reinforced the importance of KB after MV stenting, highlighting high rates of uncovered struts across the SB ostium without final KB.

Two-stent Strategy

Intravascular ultrasound analysis of the crushing technique revealed frequent incomplete stent apposition and SB ostial stenosis, with double-kissing (DK) crush techniques showing better outcomes. Proper execution of KB, particularly in terms of rewiring proximal to the carina, significantly impacts clinical outcomes following crush stenting.

FUNCTIONAL ASSESSMENT OF KISSING BALLOON TECHNIQUE

Fractional flow reserve (FFR) studies indicate that KB can significantly improve functional outcomes in SBs with severe stenosis.[10] Lack of KB inflation was associated with post-procedural inducible ischemia, highlighting the functional benefits of KB in bifurcation lesion treatment.

CLINICAL ASSESSMENT OF KISSING BALLOON TECHNIQUE

One-stent Strategy

The bare-metal stent era showed improved outcomes with KB in provisional stenting. THUEBIS and Nordic-Baltic Bifurcation Study III trials found no significant differences in major adverse cardiac events between KB and non-KB groups, although KB reduced angiographic SB restenosis in true bifurcation lesions. Real-world registry data suggested that the lack of final KB was associated with worse outcomes in patients treated with main mTOR inhibitor-eluting stents.[11] A recent meta-analysis suggests that while KBI might raise the risk of main vessel restenosis and lower the risk of SB restenosis, avoiding KBI in bifurcation lesions treated with a one-stent approach yields similar short- and long-term results, making routine KBI unnecessary.[12]

Two-stent Strategy

Ge et al., found that not performing a final KB in 181 patients treated with the crush technique predicted target lesion revascularization (TLR) at

9 months.[13] Dzavik et al., reported higher event-free survival at 386 days in patients who underwent final KB.[14] The DKCRUSH-1 study showed that the double-kissing crush technique had a higher final KB success rate and fewer adverse events at 8 months compared to classical crush.[15] In another study of 132 patients treated with the culotte technique, final KB tended to reduce binary restenosis at 6–8 months.

PRACTICAL TIPS FOR KISSING BALLOON INFLATION

Rewiring the SB:

- In the provisional technique, both in vitro and in vivo studies show that rewiring through the cell closest to the carina provides better scaffolding than proximal crossing.
- Balloon trackability into the SB is easier when recrossing through the distal cell.
- SB predilation is discouraged to avoid SB ostium dissection and to take advantage of the carina shift from MV stenting.
- Pullback rewiring is advised to increase the chance of crossing through the distal strut. The wire should be manually shaped, and careful steering allows crossing into the SB.
- Hydrophilic-coated wires reduce friction but increase the risk of SB dissection.

Balloon diameters:

- Bench tests emphasize the importance of appropriate KB diameters—balloons should be sized based on distal main and SB diameters.[7]
- Mitsudo's law, validated by IVUS, is a formula for selecting balloon diameters for simultaneous kissing inflation (Diameter of MV^2 = Diameter MB^2 + Diameter SB^2).[16] Murray's and Finet's laws show that the main vessel area is smaller than the combined areas of the two daughter branches, hence, using optimally sized balloons for each branch during KBI is likely to be oversized for the main vessel **(Fig. 3)**.

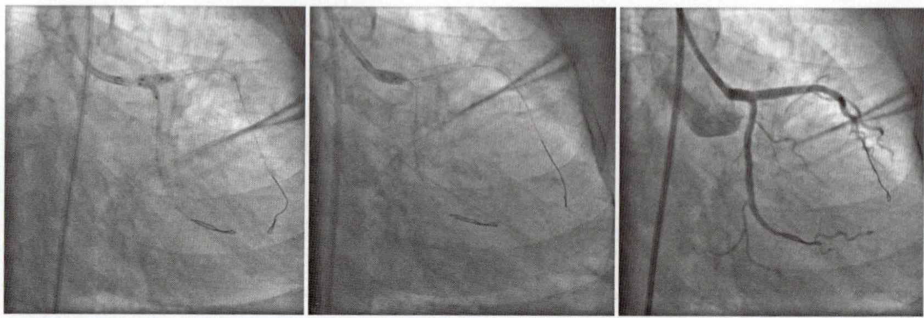

Fig. 3: Case example of KB inflation and POT techniques. (KB: kissing balloon; POT: proximal optimization technique)

- Protrusion of KBs into the main branch must be kept minimal to reduce oval deformation of proximal main vessel stent.

Tracking sequence:

- Due to the more complex pathway to the SB, the balloon directed to this branch should be tracked first.
- Easy navigability of the balloon to the SB often indicates optimal rewiring.
- Sequential removal starting from the last balloon tracked is advised.

Inflation duration:

- A Japanese study suggests that prolonged inflation times up to 60 seconds result in optimal stent expansion.[17]
- A recommended 2-step strategy involves 30-second sequential balloon inflation followed by another 30-second KB inflation. However, in bifurcations involving the left main coronary artery shorter inflation times are preferred.

Deflation sequence:

- Bench tests suggest deflating the SB balloon simultaneously with the MV balloon to avoid MV stent deformation.[7]
- Using a 3-way stopcock to connect both balloons to a single inflation device ensures simultaneous deflation which can be controlled by a single operator.

CONCLUSION

The KB technique remains a critical tool in the interventional cardiologist's arsenal for managing bifurcation lesions. While the technique is associated with certain challenges and requires precise execution, its benefits in optimizing stent apposition, improving SB access, and correcting stent deformation are well documented. Future research and technological advancements will continue to refine the KB technique, further improving clinical outcomes for patients with complex coronary bifurcation lesions.

REFERENCES

1. Sgueglia GA, Chevalier B. Kissing balloon inflation in percutaneous coronary interventions. JACC Cardiovasc Interv. 2012;5(8):803-11.
2. Lassen JF, Burzotta F, Banning AP, Lefèvre T, Darremont O, Hildick-Smith D, et al. Percutaneous coronary intervention for the left main stem and other bifurcation lesions: 12th consensus document from the European Bifurcation Club. EuroIntervention. 2018;13(13):1540-53.
3. Genuardi L, Chatzizisis YS, Chiastra C, Sgueglia G, Samady H, Kassab GS, et al. Local fluid dynamics in patients with bifurcated coronary lesions undergoing percutaneous coronary interventions. Cardiol J. 2021;28(2):321-9.
4. Poerner TC, Kralev S, Voelker W, Sueselbeck T, Latsch A, Pfleger S, et al. Natural history of small and medium-sized side branches after coronary stent implantation. Am Heart J. 2002;143:627-35.

5. Burzotta F, Trani C, Todaro D, Lanza GA, Mariani L, Tommasino A, et al. Prospective evaluation of myocardial ischemia related to post-procedural side-branch stenosis in bifurcated lesions treated by provisional approach with drug-eluting stents. Catheter Cardiovasc Interv. 2012;79:351-9.
6. Myler RK, McConahay DR, Stertzer SH, Johnson W, Cumberland DC, Boucher RA, et al. Coronary bifurcation stenoses: the kissing balloon probe technique via a single guiding catheter. Cathet Cardiovasc Diagn. 1989;16(4):267-78.
7. Ormiston JA, Webster MW, El Jack S, Ruygrok PN, Stewart JT, Scott D, et al. Drug-eluting stents for coronary bifurcations: bench testing of provisional side-branch strategies. Catheter Cardiovasc Interv. 2006;67:49-55.
8. Behan MW, Holm NR, de Belder AJ, Cockburn J, Erglis A, Curzen NP, et al. Coronary bifurcation lesions treated with simple or complex stenting: 5-year survival from patient-level pooled analysis of the Nordic Bifurcation Study and the British Bifurcation Coronary Study. Eur Heart J. 2016;37(24):1923-8.
9. Pan M, Medina A, Suárez de Lezo J, Romero M, Segura J, Martín P, et al. Coronary bifurcation lesions treated with simple approach (from the Cordoba & Las Palmas [CORPAL] Kiss Trial). Am J Cardiol. 2011;107(10):1460-5.
10. Koo BK, Park KW, Kang HJ, Cho YS, Chung WY, Youn TJ, et al. Physiological evaluation of the provisional side-branch intervention strategy for bifurcation lesions using fractional flow reserve. Eur Heart J. 2008;29(6):726-32.
11. Sgueglia GA, Burzotta F, Trani C, Todaro D, Talarico GP, Niccoli G, et al. Comparative assessment of mammalian target of rapamycin inhibitor-eluting stents in the treatment of coronary artery bifurcation lesions: the CASTOR-Bifurcation registry. Catheter Cardiovasc Interv. 2011;77:503-9.
12. Zhong M, Tang B, Zhao Q, Cheng J, Jin Q, Fu S. Should kissing balloon inflation after main vessel stenting be routine in the one-stent approach? A systematic review and meta-analysis of randomized trials. PLoS One. 2018;13(6):e0197580.
13. Ge L, Airoldi F, Iakovou I, Cosgrave J, Michev I, Sangiorgi GM, et al. Clinical and angiographic outcome after implantation of drug-eluting stents in bifurcation lesions with the crush stent technique: importance of final kissing balloon post-dilation. J Am Coll Cardiol. 2005;46:613-20.
14. Dzavik V, Kharbanda R, Ivanov J, Ing DJ, Bui S, Mackie K, et al. Predictors of long-term outcome after crush stenting of coronary bifurcation lesions: importance of the bifurcation angle. Am Heart J. 2006;152:762-9.
15. Chen SL, Zhang JJ, Ye F, Chen YD, Patel T, Kawajiri K, et al. Study comparing the double kissing (DK) crush with classical crush for the treatment of coronary bifurcation lesions: the DKCRUSH-1 Bifurcation Study with drug-eluting stents. Eur J Clin Invest. 2008;38:361-71.
16. Morino Y, Yamamoto H, Mitsudo K, Nagaoka M, Takeuchi H, Okamoto N, et al. Functional formula to determine adequate balloon diameter of simultaneous kissing balloon technique for treatment of bifurcated coronary lesions: clinical validation by volumetric intravascular ultrasound analysis. Circ J. 2008;72: 886-92.
17. Kawasaki T, Koga H, Serikawa T, Orita Y, Ikeda S, Mito T, et al. Impact of a prolonged delivery inflation time for optimal drug-eluting stent expansion. Catheter Cardiovasc Inter. 2009;73:205-11.

CHAPTER 23

Proximal Optimization Technique

Keshava Ramaiah

INTRODUCTION

Coronary bifurcations constitute approximately 15–20% of percutaneous coronary interventions (PCIs) and are primary sites of atherosclerosis, they are classified as complex PCI group, involving single stent strategy or double stent strategy. Proximal optimization technique (POT) was designed to preserve the ellipticity of the proximal part of the main vessel stent and to restore ideal bifurcation anatomy. It was proposed by Dr Olivier Darremont and is fully supported by the European Bifurcation Club and is a key part of the consensus statement produced by this group of experts.[1]

Postdilatation of stent just before the carina in the main vessel with reference to proximal diameter of the main vessel in bifurcation lesions is called proximal optimization technique (POT) **(Fig. 1)**. It is also called as the sequential POT-SIDE-POT technique.

THE PROBLEM

In provisional stenting strategy, to avoid carina shift toward the SB ostium and to avoid distal main vessel dissection, stent size is selected with reference to distal main vessel. As a drawback, stent will probably be "undersized", leading to stent malapposition in the proximal main vessel.[2]

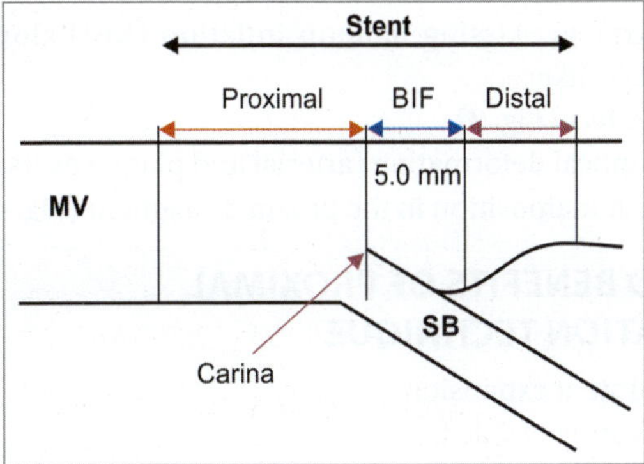

Fig. 1: Bifurcation (BIF) anatomy of a vessel showing proximal main vessel (MV), distal main vessel, and side branch (SB). POT is done in the proximal main vessel. (POT: proximal optimization technique)

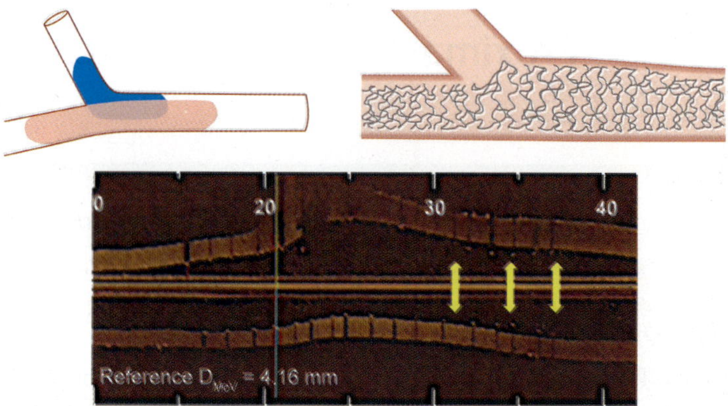

Fig. 2: Bottle neck effect in the proximal most part of the stent as shown in yellow arrows.

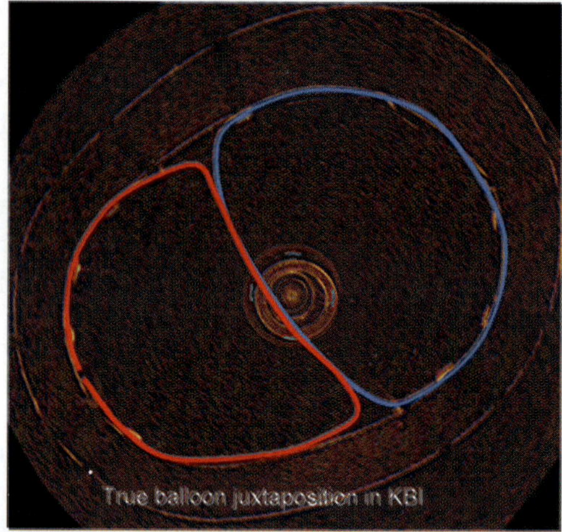

Fig. 3: Elliptical deformation is seen in the proximal main vessel segment where both balloons overlap. (KBI: kissing balloon inflation)

In two-stent strategy, kissing balloon inflation (KBI) alone can lead to detrimental effects like:

- Bottle neck effect **(Fig. 2)**
- Proximal elliptical deformation (arterial and plaque overstretch) **(Fig. 3)**
- Opposite strut malposition in the proximal segment **(Fig. 4)**

INTENDED BENEFITS OF PROXIMAL OPTIMIZATION TECHNIQUE

- Symmetrical stent expansion
- Facilitate rewiring of side branch
- Opening of side branch struts
- To prevent detrimental side effects of KBI

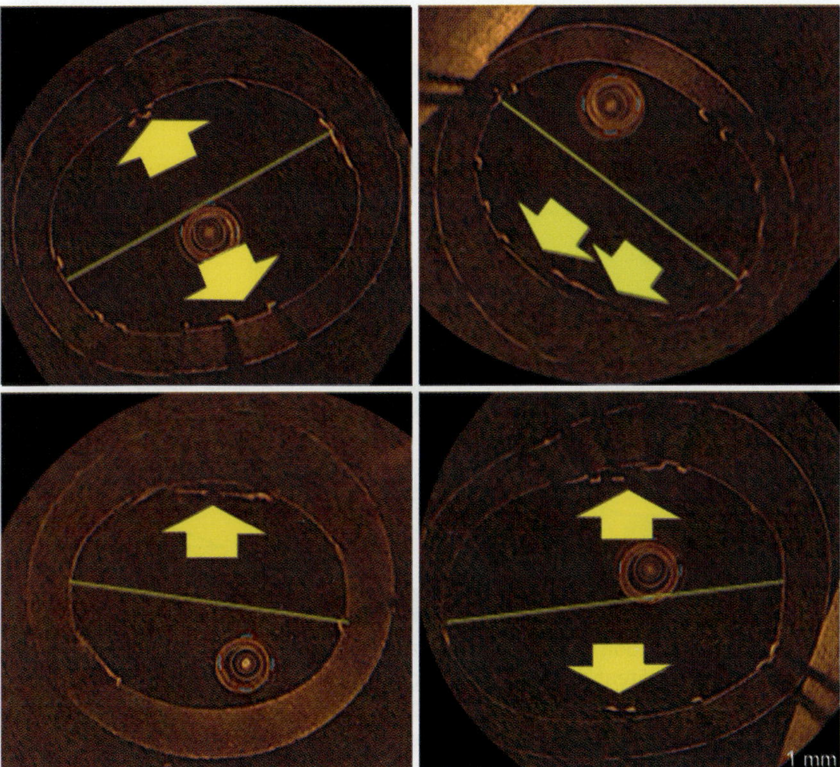

Fig. 4: Yellow arrows indicate strut malposition.

METHOD OF PROXIMAL OPTIMIZATION TECHNIQUE

- A short noncompliant or a short semicompliant balloon can be used.
- Balloon diameter is of utmost importance and should be sized in reference with proximal main vessel **(Figs. 5A to D)**.
- A practical test to ascertain optimal POT balloon diameter is the PUFF test, administer a small amount of contrast during POT balloon dilatation, if contrast medium does not percolate beyond the balloon, good stent apposition is likely to be achieved.
- A POT immediately after main vessel stenting and final re-POT give more optimal results.
- The distal balloon should be placed just before carina.
- Position can be confirmed on orthogonal views.
- If positioned too distal, it can cause carinal shift, if it is too proximal then this will not appropriately expand the stent overlying the side branch ostium.

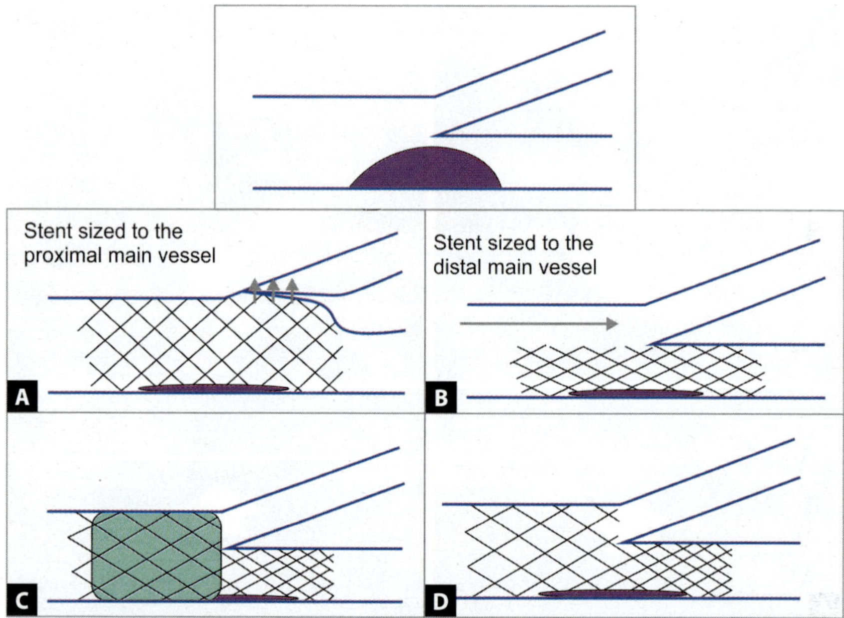

Figs. 5A to D: Bifurcation lesion. (A) The stent is sized to the proximal reference diameter of the main vessel. Stent deployment will displace the carina thereby compromising flow into the side branch; (B) The stent is sized to the distal reference diameter of the main vessel. Following stent deployment, the proximal part of the stent is malapposed; (C) Illustration of the proximal optimization technique. A short balloon sized to the proximal main vessel diameter is positioned just up to the carina and inflated; (D) Following POT, there is good apposition of the stent throughout its length and without shifting of the carina. (POT: proximal optimization technique)

EVIDENCE TO FAVOR PROXIMAL OPTIMIZATION TECHNIQUE

Bench models demonstrated the benefits of proximal optimization technique. Further, Foin et al.[3] evaluated the concept of proximal optimization technique in a bench model of commercially available stents. They showed that a final POT was improved the anatomical result following single stent implantation for a bifurcation, by reducing malapposition of the stent in the proximal main vessel **(Figs. 6A to C)**. They also showed the detrimental effects of final kissing balloon inflation which has traditionally been recommended in clinical practice. Foin and colleagues further proposed a step-wise postdilation strategy in preference to KBD. They performed POT followed by side branch balloon-inflation immediately after stent implantation. The final step was either KBI or a final POT.

Murasato et al.[4] used a bench model to suggest that a compliant balloon may be preferable to the use of a noncompliant balloon to optimize strut

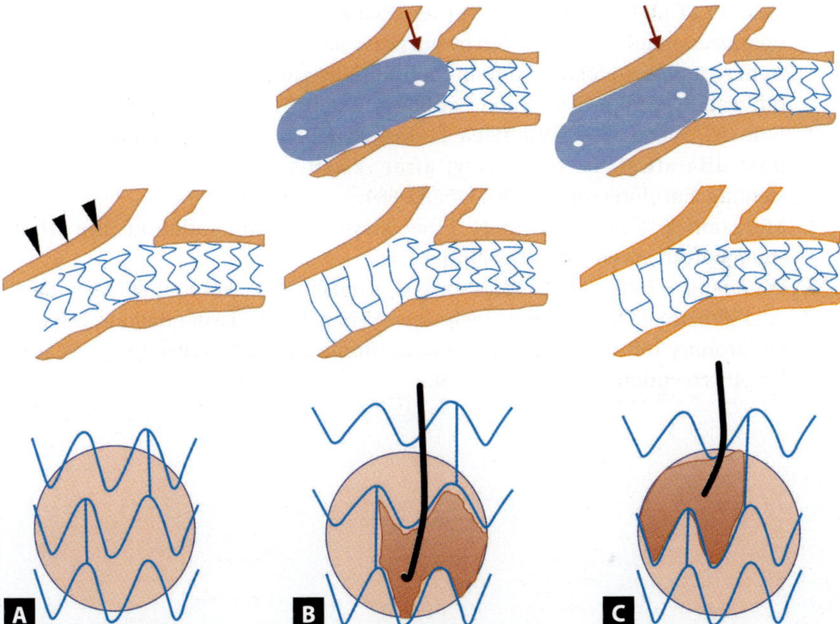

Figs. 6A to C: Final POT improves the malapposition of the stent in the proximal main vessel segment in provisional strategy. (POT: proximal optimization technique)

apposition during POT. It is not mandatory to do a high-pressure dilatation as the balloon merely needs to dilate the unopposed stent; however, a larger balloon diameter is obligatory.

Recently, the PROPOT trial[5] investigated whether POT is superior in terms of stent apposition compared with the conventional kissing balloon technique (KBT) in real-life bifurcation lesions using optical coherence tomography (OCT). POT followed by side branch dilation did not show any advantages over conventional KBT in terms of stent apposition; however, excellent midterm clinical outcomes were observed in both strategies.

CONCLUSION

Proximal optimization technique is easy and safe technique employed in bifurcation lesions, involving either a single stent or two stent strategy. The right technique is of utmost importance, balloon sizing and positioning just before the carina provides optimal results.

REFERENCES

1. Hoye A. The proximal optimisation technique for intervention of coronary bifurcations. Interv Cardiol Rev. 2017;12(2):110-5.

2. Hakim D, Chatterjee A, Alli O, Turner J, Sattar A, Foin N, et al. Role of proximal optimization technique guided by intravascular ultrasound on stent expansion, stent symmetry index, and side-branch hemodynamics in patients with coronary bifurcation lesions. Circulation Cardiovasc Interv. 2017;10(10):e005535.
3. Foin N, Secco GG, Ghilencea L, Krams R, Di Mario C. Final proximal post-dilatation is necessary after kissing balloon in bifurcation stenting. EuroIntervention. 2011;7:597-604.
4. Murasato Y, Finet G, Foin N. Final kissing balloon inflation: the whole story. EuroIntervention. 2015;11:81-5.
5. Watanabe Y, Murasato Y, Yamawaki M, Kinoshita Y, Okubom YK, Masuda N, et al. Proximal Optimisation Technique Versus Final Kissing Balloon Inflation in coronary bifurcation lesions: the randomised, multicentre PROPOT trial. EuroIntervention. 2021;17(9):747-56.

CHAPTER 24

Contemporary Management of Isolated Ostial Side Branch Disease (Medina 0,0,1)

Arun Mohanty

INTRODUCTION

In intervention cardiology, coronary bifurcation lesions (CBLs) are one of the most challenging and frequently encountered lesion subsets and account for 20% of all percutaneous coronary intervention (PCI) procedures.[1] A bifurcation lesion is defined by the European Bifurcation Club as a "coronary artery narrowing occurring adjacent to, and/or involving, the origin of a significant side branch". CBLs are classified using Medina classification, endorsed by European Bifurcation Club.[2] In this classification, binary value (0 or 1) is assigned to the proximal, distal main branches (MBs) and the side branch (SB), in that respective order, based on the presence (1) or absence (0) of significant plaque burden (≥50% stenosis) in that vascular segment **(Fig. 1)**. Isolated side branch ostial lesions (Medina type 0,0,1) represent <5% of CBLs.[3] In a large-sized multicenter registry-based study evaluating

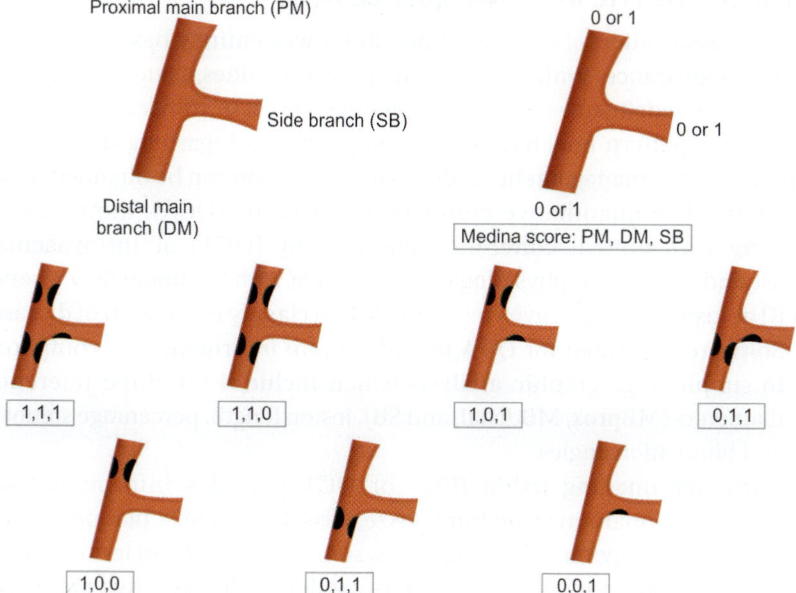

Fig. 1: Medina classification of coronary bifurcations.[4] (PMB: proximal main branch; DM: distal main branch; SB: side branch)

the clinical outcomes of PCI for bifurcation lesions according to the Medina classification showed the worst clinical outcome for Medina 0,0,1 subtype at 1 year compared with other bifurcation types.[4] Due to the uniqueness and rarity of such lesions, there is limited evidence regarding the optimal treatment strategy for Medina 0,0,1 bifurcation lesions. Hence, treatment of these lesions poses a great challenge, especially for those with involvement of the unprotected left main coronary artery. This paper aims to discuss the importance of technical aspects for the management of Medina 0,0,1 lesions along with the latest published data supporting the various proposed interventional treatment strategies.

LAWS OF BIFURCATION ANATOMY

Coronary artery tree exhibits "fractal geometry" as it branches into smaller vessels. Murray's law states that: "When a parent blood vessel branches into daughter vessels, the cube of the radius of the parent vessel is equal to the sum of the cubes of the radii of daughter blood vessels".[5] So, a branch of radius r dividing into two branches with radii r1 and r2, then $r^3 = r_1^3 + r_2^3$. Estimation of coronary size in bifurcation lesions is done using this law. Another formula has been proposed by Finet et al., for estimation of the diameter of the mother vessel (Dm) and daughter vessels (D_{d1}, D_{d2}) based on a simple fractal ratio, and this rule has also been used to estimate vessel sizes: $D_m = 0.678 \times (D_{d1} + D_{d2})$.[6]

DEFINING THE MEDINA 0,0,1 LESION

Earlier classification of coronary bifurcation was entirely based on angiographic appearance. With advent of imaging modalities, pattern of bifurcation may be redefined especially for Medina 0,0,1 lesions because defining the disease pattern may have clinical implications regarding the optimal approach for its management. Additional information can be obtained using modalities like quantitative coronary angiography (QCA), intravascular imaging with optical coherence tomography (OCT) or intravascular ultrasound (IVUS) and physiological assessment with fractional flow reserve (FFR) or instantaneous wave-free ratio (iFR) to classify the pattern of disease.

- Software dedicated for QCA provides more information as compared to simple angiographic analysis which includes the three reference diameters (MBprox, MBdistal, and SB), lesion length, percentage stenosis and bifurcation angles.
- Coronary imaging using IVUS or OCT provides information on bifurcation anatomy: true lumen size, vessel diameters, plaque burden and morphology, stent landing zones, stenosis severity and lesion length. But, both OCT and IVUS parameters can have a low positive predictive value for determining the functional significance of SB ostial lesions in Medina 0,0,1.[7]

- FFR or iFR provides additional "functional information" regarding a lesion by physiological assessment of bifurcation anatomy, further guiding the management.

MANAGEMENT OF CORONARY BIFURCATION (MEDINA 0,0,1)

Before any invasive intervention, the physician must consider the morphology of the lesion (with angiographic/intravascular imaging guidance), the presence of ischemia in the associated territory (noninvasive/invasive documentation), and the clinical scenario (acute coronary syndrome, chronic coronary syndrome, etc.). The interventionist should also anticipate the complex interplay between angiographic appearances, symptom burden, and documented myocardial ischemia.

Considering the risk of compromising the MB in Medina 0,0,1 bifurcation lesions, it is imperative to have PCI approach reserved for patients in whom it is truly indicated, and treatment decisions must be made on individual basis and clinical presentation.

- In a study by Koo et al., 65 patients with left anterior descending (LAD) artery bifurcation lesions, lower rates of anginal chest pain (40% vs. 100%; $p = 0.001$), ST segment change (37% vs. 92%; $p = 0.001$), and arrhythmia were seen with diagonal branch occlusion in comparison to LAD occlusion.[8]
- In a study by Hachamovitch et al., revascularization showed greater survival benefit (absolute and relative) in patients with moderate to large amounts of inducible ischemia (>10% ischemia) in comparison to optimal medical therapy.[9]

Thus, optimal medical therapy remains the preferred first-line treatment, particularly for single-vessel coronary artery disease and in presence of stable angina, while PCI should be reserved for patients with refractory anginal symptoms.

TECHNICAL CONSIDERATIONS IN TREATING MEDINA 0,0,1 LESIONS

Compared with the other bifurcation lesion subtypes, an isolated SB lesion has some unique features that complicate treatment with PCI.[10]

- Risk of injuring main vessel (MV) while treating the SB.
- These lesions often have fibrocalcific characteristics with significant risk of recoil, resulting in a lower acute gain after PCI.
- A relatively small SB vessel size induces a small stent size, which is a well-known risk factor for restenosis and stent thrombosis.
- Concepts of "ostial miss" and "MB protrusion": "Ostial miss" refers to too distal placement of the stent thus, missing the ostium of the SB whereas "MB protrusion" refers to too proximal placement of the stent such that

it protrudes into the MB. Restenosis risk increases in the MV and SB in presence of ostial miss and MV protrusion, hence, must be avoided.

TECHNIQUES

Interventional strategies for the management of Medina 0,0,1 lesions can be categorized into techniques that include stenting and those that do not. Lesion preparation is important prior to stenting, especially in the presence of a fibrotic or calcified lesion. In a nonstenting approach, one must be careful not to dissect the vessel and be ready for a bail-out stenting strategy **(Flowchart 1)**.

NONSTENTING TECHNIQUES

- *Plain old balloon angioplasty:*
  - Plain old balloon angioplasty (POBA) has been used for the management of CBLs as an earlier treatment strategy. However, POBA procedures were associated with a low rate of procedural success and frequent complications, such as recoil, dissection and restenosis secondary to intimal disruption.[11] There has been no dedicated randomized control study on POBA in Medina 0,0,1 lesions.

Flowchart 1: Proposed treatment algorithm for Medina 0,0,1 lesions.[10]

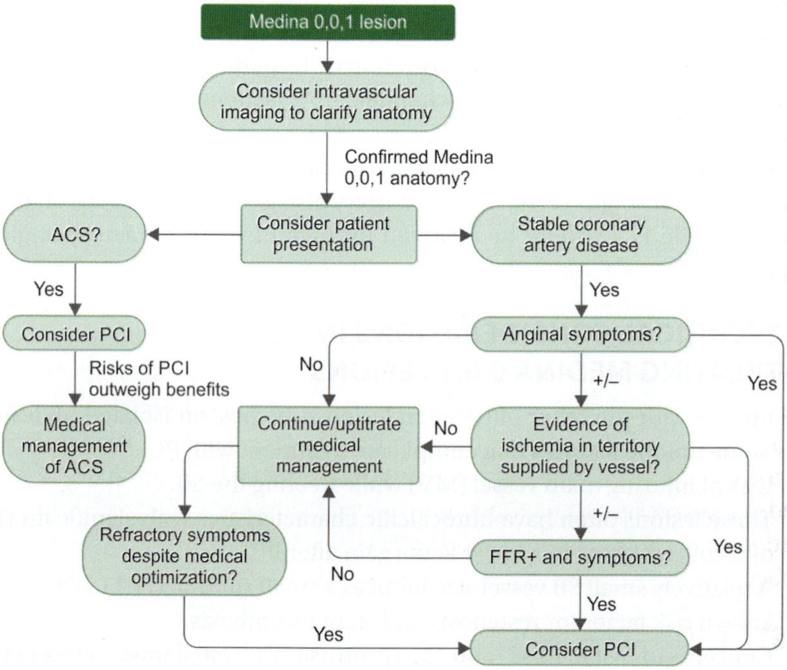

(ACS: acute coronary syndrome; FFR: fractional flow reserve; PCI: percutaneous coronary intervention)

- *Drug-eluting balloon treatment:* Drug-eluting balloons (DEBs) are semicompliant angioplasty balloons coated with an antiproliferative drug (usually paclitaxel) that is rapidly released upon contact with the vessel wall. Stenotic lesions are pretreated with standard balloon angioplasty, a noncompliant balloon and/or scoring or cutting balloons prior to the use of a DEB. Once an adequate initial balloon angioplasty result is obtained, the DEB can be inflated for up to 60–90 s to permit sufficient drug transfer. DEBs have emerged as a potential alternative to drug-eluting stents.

Advantage: Use of a DEB in the management of bifurcation lesions includes homogeneous administration of the drug to the coronary wall, which may negate some of the restenosis seen in comparison with POBA. Others are—less disruption of the carinal anatomy compared with stenting and short duration of dual antiplatelet therapy is required.

Challenges/disadvantage: These include issues with antiproliferative drug release, elastic recoil of lesions and coronary dissection.

A 3-year multicenter observational registry by Vaquerizo et al., with a study population of 49 patients anf Medina 0,0,1 lesions, evaluated DEB without stenting. After preparing lesion, a paclitaxel DEB (5 mm longer than the predilating balloon) was inflated for >45 seconds. Bail-out stent implantation was only required in 14% of patients. At 1 year, the rate of target lesion revascularization was 14%. Thus, study concluded that DEBs are a safe and technically feasible therapeutic option for the treatment of Medina 0,0,1 lesions.[12]

Another similar multicenter prospective study by Erdoğan et al., which included 30 patients, assessed the safety and efficacy of DEBs in patients with acute coronary syndrome (ACS) and de novo Medina type 0,1,0 or 0,0,1 left main stem bifurcation lesions. 22 patients were treated only with DEBs and provisional drug-eluting stent implantation and 8 had drug-eluting stent implantation followed by DEBs therapy of the ostium of the left main stem major branch. 22 patients were treated only with DEBs and provisional drug-eluting stent implantation and 8 had drug-eluting stent implantation followed by DEBs therapy of the ostium of the left main stem major branch. The procedural success rate was 100%, with no MACE during the index hospitalization. None of the patients experienced an adverse event during clinical follow-up (mean duration—7.7 ± 6.0 months).[13] Currently, DEBs represent a potential option for the management of Medina 0,0,1 lesions, especially when SB stenting is not desired. However, randomized studies are required to make definitive recommendations in its favor.

STENTING STRATEGIES

- *Flush ostial technique:* Also known as "nailing the ostium", involves placing the stent exactly at the ostium of the SB. There will inevitably be some degree of ostial miss or MB stent protrusion with this technique unless the angle of the bifurcation lesion is at 90°, which may increase restenosis risk of the MB and SB.

- *Szabo technique:* A bifurcation technique for the treatment of isolated ostial bifurcation lesions by using the target wire and the anchor wire. In this technique, the anchor wire which passes through the most proximal stent strut helps to prevent excessive progression of the stent beyond the ostium and facilitates the precise stenting of the ostium. Recently, Gutiérrez-Chico et al., reported that the Szabo technique is more accurate than the conventional technique in avoiding malpositioning of the stent. However, the Szabo technique is not the ideal technique due to technical difficulties. The anchor wire can be prolapsed into the target branch and the stent can advance excessively into the target branch, leading to incomplete coverage of the target branch ostium in the Szabo technique.[14]
- *"Inverted" provisional T stenting technique:*

Procedure: The main steps followed during procedure are—insertion of two 0.014" wires: one in the DMB (recommended) and one in the SB, the diseased vessel is predilated followed stent implantation from the proximal MV to the side branch, over the side branch 0.014" wire. The second wire is left in the distal MV and jailed. Then, the SB wire is advanced distally through the mesh of the stent from the proximal MV to the DMB. A kissing balloon inflation is systematically performed to open the strut at the diameter of the MV and without deformation of the stent at the SB ostium **(Fig. 2)**. If a satisfactory result is achieved, the procedure is stopped.

A retrospective study of 40 patients by Brunel et al., showed 100% procedural success with no MACE (death, myocardial infarction, stent

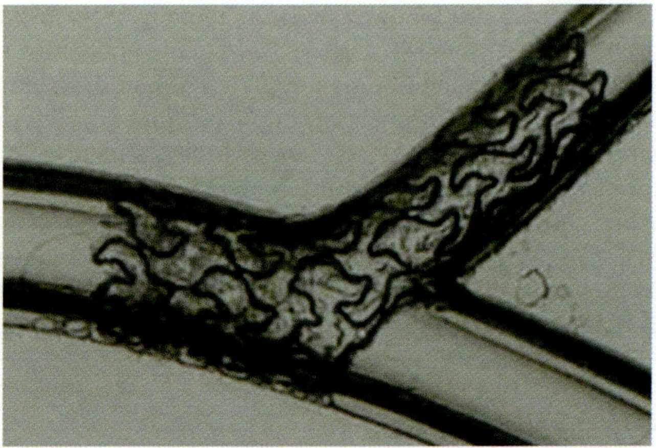

Fig. 2: Provisional T stenting and kissing balloon for the treatment of a Medina 0,0,1 type lesion. Final position, note that this allows a total ostial coverage.[3]

thrombosis, or repeat revascularization) within first 30 days of follow-up. About 92.5% of the cases underwent implantation of a single stent and was associated with a very low target lesion revascularization (TLR) rate of 2.5% and an acceptable reintervention rate of 5%. This procedure must be done only if optimal medical therapy is effective. These encouraging results need to be verified by larger trials over longer periods of observation.[3]

Advantage: Complete coverage of the ostium.

Challenges/disadvantage: (1) Complete apposition of the stent despite different diameters of PMB and SB, and (2) an optimal opening of the strut in front of the DMB. The systematic kissing balloon maneuver helps overcome these hurdles.

- *Modified flower petal technique:*

Procedure: A large (7 or 8 Fr) and strong back-up support guiding catheter must be selected for this technique. First, wiring of both the branches, i.e., MB and SB (the first wire into the target branch and second wire into the other branch as an anchor wire). A stent-balloon system is prepared outside of the guiding catheter as shown in **Figures 3A to D**. The stent-balloon system becomes more flexible and allows easy advancement of the stent or balloon into high take-off vessels. The prepared stent-balloon system is advanced through the guiding catheter to the target lesion until the anchor balloon stops the advancement of the stent **(Fig. 4A)**. Thereby, the anchor balloon can prevent excessive stent advancement into the target branch and provide complete coverage of the lesion by the stent struts. First, the stent balloon is inflated and deflated **(Fig. 4B)**. Second, the anchor balloon is inflated and deflated **(Fig. 4C)**. Then, the stent balloon is inflated again **(Fig. 4D)**.

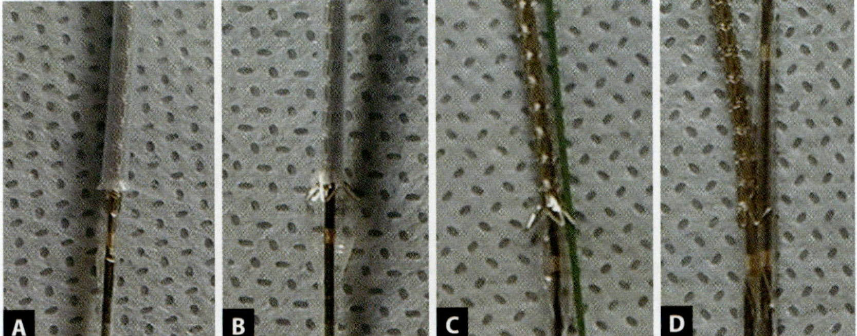

Figs. 3A to D: Preparation of the stent-balloon system. (A) The plastic stent cover is pulled back slightly to expose the final proximal stent strut; (B) The stent delivery system balloon is inflated to 5–6 atmospheres and deflated; (C) The proximal end of the second wire is passed through the final proximal stent strut; (D) Another balloon is loaded onto the second wire as an anchor balloon. The proximal markers of the stent and balloon are aligned. Then, the final proximal strut of the stent is re-crimped by hand.[15]

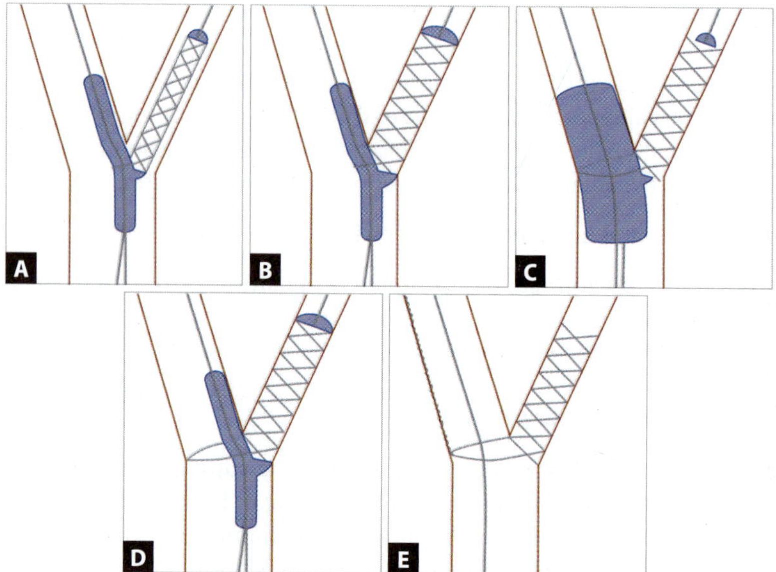

Figs. 4A to E: Schematic model presentation of the new technique.[15]

Thus, the protruding final proximal strut is in contact with the opposite side of the adjacent vessel wall **(Fig. 4E)**.

In a study of 64 patients with Medina type 0,0,1 or 0,1,0 lesions who underwent PCI using modified flower petal technique were followed up for 9 months after the intervention. QCA analyses were done at baseline, post-PCI procedure, and at 9-month follow-up for both the main and the side branch. 20 patients (31.2%) had ostial left anterior descending artery lesions, 9 patients (14.1%) had ostial circumflex artery lesions, and the other patients had isolated ostial nonleft main bifurcation lesions. The procedural success rate was 100%.[15]

Advantage: Complete coverage of the ostial bifurcation by stent struts without protruding into the adjacent vessel, and a lower metallic burden at the carina region. It does not require routine final kissing balloon inflation (FKBI).

Challenges/disadvantage: Decreased flexibility of the stent during advancement of the stent-balloon system.

- *Bifurcation and ostial optical coherence tomography mapping (BOOM):* This is a novel technique using OCT-guided angiographic coregistration termed "bifurcation and ostial OCT mapping" (BOOM). This technique uses coregistration for exact identification and mapping of ostium of the side branch to minimize protrusion of stent struts into the MB thus, ensuring complete ostial coverage in the side branch.[16]

CONCLUSION

Medina 0,0,1 bifurcated lesions are the least prevalent in real-world practice, and the prognosis after PCI was the worst of the bifurcation subtypes. The interpretation and comparison of published studies are further complicated by heterogeneity of various characteristics such as lesion size and location, degree of calcification, and angulation between arterial branches. Additionally, the variable expertise among interventional cardiology centers adds to the complexity. When risk-benefit ratio is considered, one must remember that Medina 0,0,1 lesions will tend to be of lesser prognostic importance than the MB and will supply a relatively small myocardial territory. Nevertheless, the optimal treatment strategy for Medina 0,0,1 lesion remains a subject of debate.[16,17]

REFERENCES

1. Burzotta F, Lassen JF, Lefèvre T, Banning AP, Chatzizisis YS, Johnson TW, et al., Percutaneous coronary intervention for bifurcation coronary lesions: the 15th consensus document from the European bifurcation Club. EuroIntervention. 2021;16:1307-17.
2. Sawaya FJ, Lefèvre T, Chevalier B, Garot P, Hovasse T, Morice MC, et al., Contemporary approach to coronary bifurcation lesion treatment. JACC Cardiovasc Interv. 2016;9:1861-78.
3. Brunel P, Martin G, Bressollette E, Leurent B, Banus Y. "Inverted" provisional T stenting, a new technique for Medina 0,0,1 coronary bifurcation lesions: feasibility and follow-up. EuroIntervention. 2010;5:814-20.
4. Mohamed MO, Lamellas P, Roguin A, Oemrawsingh RM, Ijsselmuiden AJJ, Routledge H, et al., Clinical outcomes of percutaneous coronary intervention for bifurcation lesions according to medina classification. J Am Heart Assoc. 2022;11:e025459.
5. Murray CD. The physiological principle of minimum work: I. The vascular system and the cost of blood volume. Proc Natl Acad Sci USA. 1926;12:207-14.
6. Finet G, Gilard M, Perrenot B, Rioufol G, Motreff P, Gavit L, et al., Fractal geometry of arterial coronary bifurcations: a quantitative coronary angiography and intravascular ultrasound analysis. EuroIntervention. 2008;3:490-8.
7. Koh JS, Koo BK, Kim JH, Yang HM, Park KW, Kang HJ, et al., Relationship between fractional flow reserve and angiographic and intravascular ultrasound parameters in ostial lesions: major epicardial vessel versus side branch ostial lesions. JACC Cardiovasc Interv. 2012;5:409-15.
8. Koo BK, Lee SP, Lee JH, Park KW, Suh JW, Cho YS, et al., Assessment of clinical, electrocardiographic, and physiological relevance of diagonal branch in left anterior descending coronary artery bifurcation lesions. JACC Cardiovasc Interv. 2012;5:1126-32.
9. Hachamovitch R, Hayes SW, Friedman JD, Cohen I, Berman DS. Comparison of the short-term survival benefit associated with revascularization compared with medical therapy in patients with no prior coronary artery disease undergoing stress myocardial perfusion single photon emission computed tomography. Circulation. 2003;107:2900-7.

10. Suleiman S, Coughlan JJ, Touma G, Szirt R. Contemporary management of isolated ostial side branch disease: an evidence-based approach to medina 001 bifurcations. Interv Cardiol. 2021;16:e06.
11. Zack PM, Ischinger T. Experience with a technique for coronary angioplasty of bifurcational lesions. Cathet Cardiovasc Diagn. 1984;10:433-43.
12. Vaquerizo B, Fernández-Nofreiras E, Oategui I, Suarez de Lezo J, Rumoroso JR, Martín P, et al., Second-generation drug-eluting balloon for ostial side branch lesions (001-bifurcations): mid-term clinical and angiographic results. J Interv Cardiol. 2016;29:285-92.
13. Erdoğan E, Li Z, Zhu YX, Tufaro V, Feng SL, Li Q, et al., DCB combined with provisional DES implantation in the treatment of De Novo Medina 0, 1, 0 or 0, 0, 1 left main coronary bifurcation lesions: A proof-of-concept study. Anatol J Cardiol. 2022;26:218-25.
14. Kern MJ, Ouellette D, Frianeza T. A new technique to anchor stents for exact placement in ostial stenoses: the stent tail wire or Szabo technique. Catheter Cardiovasc Interv. 2006;68:901-6.
15. Çayli M, Elbasan Z, Gür M, Seker T, Uçar H, Kuloglu O, et al., Modified flower petal technique in the treatment of Medina type 0, 0, 1 or 0, 1, 0 lesions. EuroIntervention. 2015;11:772-9.
16. Hlofmitz E, Sosa F, Goldberg A, Maehara A, Ali ZA, Mintz GS, et al., Bifurcation and ostial optical coherence tomography mapping (BOOM) - Case description of a novel bifurcation stent technique. Cardiovasc Revasc Med. 2018;19(8S):47-9.
17. Stankovic G, Darremont O, Ferenc M, Hildick-Smith D, Louvard Y, Albiero R, et al. Percutaneous coronary intervention for bifurcation lesions: 2008 consensus document from the fourth meeting of the European Bifurcation Club. EuroIntervention. 2009;5:39-49.

CHAPTER 25

Left Main Coronary Intervention

Prasant Kr Sahoo, Pankaj Manoria

INTRODUCTION

The highest risk subset of the coronary artery disease (CAD) is the left main coronary artery (LMCA) disease. This heightened risk is attributed to:

- *High ischemic and hemodynamic instability:* A substantial proportion, approximately 70%, of myocardium is at risk, leading to significantly increased cardiovascular morbidity and mortality compared to other forms of obstructive CAD.[1,2]
- *Complex anatomy:* The incidence of significant LMCA disease, marked by angiographic narrowing exceeding 50%, is notable, affecting approximately 4–6% of individuals undergoing coronary angiography.[3] This prevalence underscores the clinical importance of recognizing and addressing LMCA pathology. Furthermore, patients diagnosed with medically untreated unprotected LMCA (ULMCA) disease face a concerning 3-year mortality rate of approximately 50%, emphasizing the severity and potential life-threatening consequences associated with this condition.[4]

ANATOMY

Left aortic coronary sinus is typically the source of left main (LM):

- Bifurcating into left circumflex (LCX) artery and left anterior descending (LAD) (85% of cases)
- Trifurcating into LAD, LCX, and ramus (15% of cases)

Length

It typically falls between 1 and 15 mm. In about 0.02–0.07% of instances with distinct ostium of LCX and LAD from the coronary sinus, LM is absent.

Structures supplied by LM: Anterior two-fifths of interventricular septum (IVS), left ventricle, left atrium, and sinoatrial (SA) node in approximately 40% of people.

Diseases of the LM: 80% of LM percutaneous coronary intervention (PCI) involves bifurcation. Other diseases of the LM include ostial disease, body disease, and diffusely diseased **(Fig. 1)**.

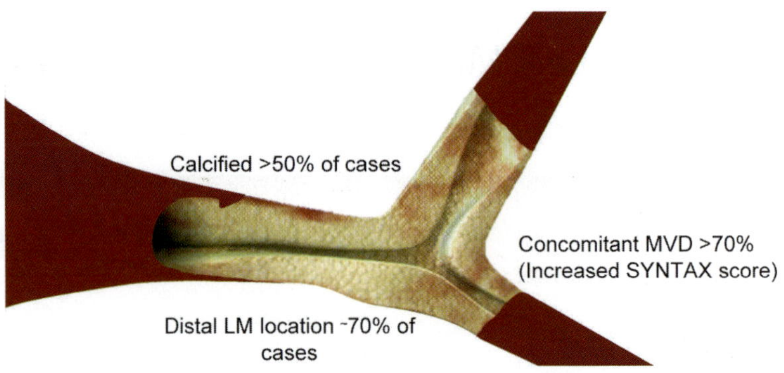

Fig. 1: Characteristics of LMCA disease. (LM: left main; MVD: multivessel disease)

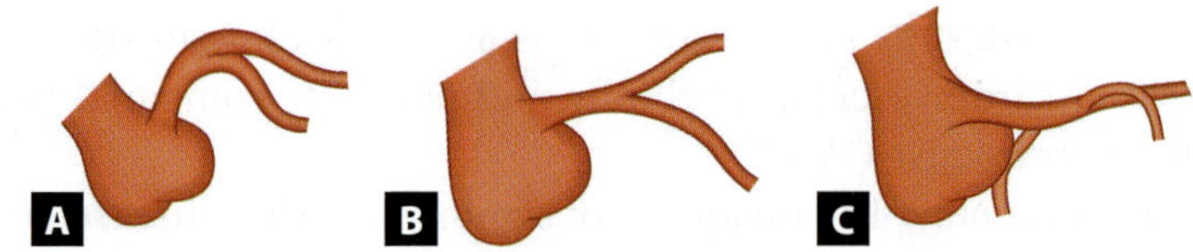

Figs. 2A to C: Angle of take off. (A) Acute take off; (B) Right angle left main coronary artery (LMCA) take off; (C) Obtuse take off.

Diameter

Men's nondiseased LMCA diameters are reported to be 4.5 ± 0.5 mm, whereas women's diameters are 3.9 ± 0.4 mm.[5] Postmortem examinations, however, have found that nondiseased hearts can have sizes of up to 10 mm.[6] A study of 106 hearts at autopsy revealed that the length of the LMCA varies significantly, from 2 to 40 mm.[7] A bicuspid aortic valve has been linked to short LMCA,[8] yet the majority of research show little association between LMCA length and patient height or heart size.

Parts

The ostium, the mid portion (body), and the distal portion or bifurcation are the important parts of LMCA.[5] The ostium, located just above the left sinus of Valsalva, is characterized by a greater proportion of smooth muscle and elastic tissue compared to the rest of the coronary vessels **(Fig. 2)**.[6] The course of the LMCA forms an angle of about 90° from ostium and is typically leftward, posterior, and superior. It traverses about 2–4 mm through the wall of the aorta and emerges posterior to the pulmonary trunk **(Figs. 3 and 4)**. Subsequently, it travels in the left atrioventricular groove, dividing before reaching the base of the left atrial appendage.[5]

Lesions associated to the LMCA create a number of clinical challenges since it supplies a significant portion of the heart. Blood flow constraints

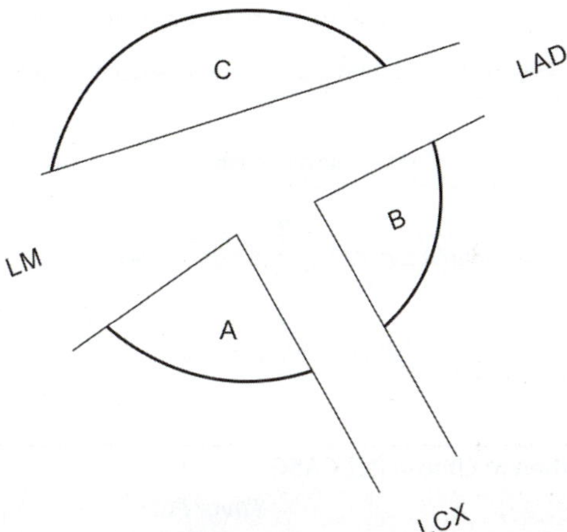

Fig. 3: LM bifurcation (bifurcation angles). (LAD: left anterior descending; LCX: left circumflex; LM: left main)

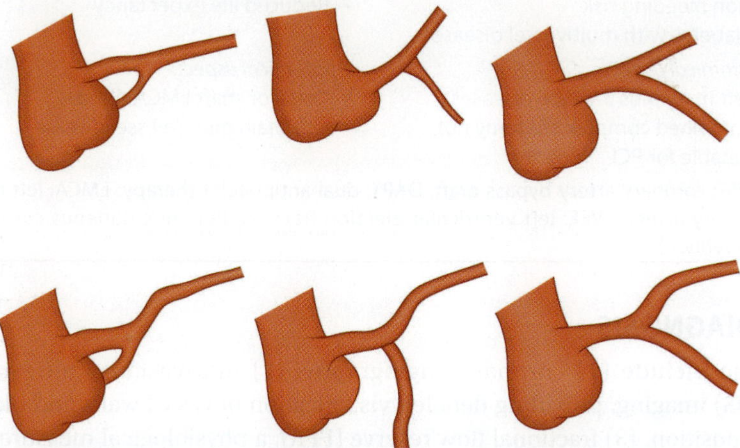

Fig. 4: Types of left main coronary artery (LMCA) bifurcation.

resulting from ostial lesions close to the origin of the LMCA, body lesions in the midportion, and bifurcation lesions during division into the LAD and LCX arteries may affect myocardial perfusion. Treatments may be more challenging as the blood flow to multiple coronary arteries may be affected by diffuse lesions. These lesions are more prevalent close to places where trifurcations occur. Calcification in the LMCA exacerbates atherosclerosis and complicates stent placement and angioplasty. Prompt medical intervention is important because life-threatening acute thrombosis in the LMCA can cause significant obstructions and myocardial infarction.[9] Management of the LMCA disease is decided by the 'Heart team' **(Flowchart 1)** and the advantages and disadvantages of PCI and CABG are given below **(Table 1)**.

Flowchart 1: Heart team approach to left main coronary artery (LMCA) lesions.[10]

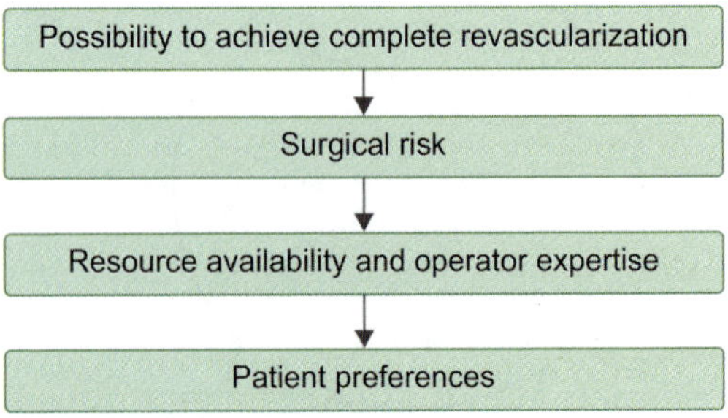

Possibility to achieve complete revascularization
↓
Surgical risk
↓
Resource availability and operator expertise
↓
Patient preferences

TABLE 1: LMCA: When to choose PCI/CABG?

Favor CABG	*Favor PCI*
Clinical characteristics: • Low LVEF • Concomitant cardiac surgery • Doubtful DAPT adherence including high bleeding risk • Diabetes with multivessel diseases	*Clinical characteristics:* • Urgent revascularization • Serious comorbidity, high surgical, and frailty • Reduced life expectancy
Anatomical aspect: • Left main plus 3-vessel diseases • Combined complex anatomy not suitable for PCI	*Anatomical aspect:* • Ostial or shaft LMCA disease • Left main plus 1-vessel disease

(CABG: coronary artery bypass graft; DAPT: dual antiplatelet therapy; LMCA: left main coronary artery; LVEF: left ventricular ejection fraction; PCI: percutaneous coronary intervention)

DIAGNOSIS

These include (1) coronary angiography, (2) intravascular ultrasound (IVUS) imaging, providing detailed visualization of vessel walls and plaque composition, (3) fractional flow reserve (FFR), a physiological measure that assesses the functional severity of coronary stenosis, (4) optical coherence tomography (OCT) evaluation, which offers a high resolution image for detailed assessment of plaque morphology; and (5) identification of borderline lesions, where the combination of these technologies aids in comprehensive lesion evaluation.

Angiographic Evaluation

Significant interpersonal variation exists for 30–70% of left major lesions, which can be attributed to the disease's widespread nature and short length of the reference segment.

The best angiographic view for evaluating the primary LM lesion:

- *LM ostial lesions:* Anteroposterior (AP) cranial and left anterior oblique (LAO) cranial

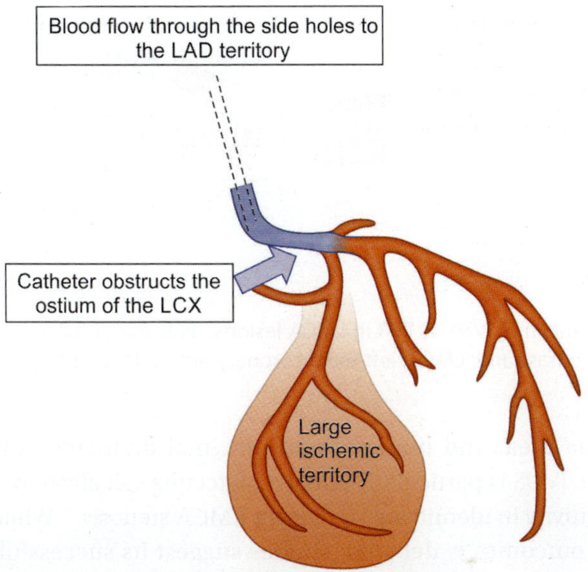

Fig. 5: Guide catheter engagement of LM. (LCX: left circumflex; LAD: left anterior descending)

- *LM distal lesion:* AP caudal, right anterior oblique (RAO) caudal, and LAO caudal (spider view)

The gold standard for diagnosing clinically significant LMCA is coronary angiography despite its potential limitations. While angiography is sensitive, it is not without interobserver variabilities, leading to occasional false-positive and false-negative results. Operators aim to evade precipitating myocardial ischemia in severe cases of LMCA and often limit angiographic shots and dye injections, potentially impacting diagnostic accuracy, especially for less experienced operators. Ostial LMCA stenosis, challenging to visualize angiographically, relies on detecting pressure damping upon catheter engagement with the ostia alongside an absence of the dye reflux into the coronary sinus during the injection **(Fig. 5)**. Assessing LMCA stenosis and bifurcation depends on a normal segment for comparison, potentially leading to underestimation of concentric stenoses. Additionally, angiography struggles to accurately assess lesion calcification, a crucial factor influencing visual assessment accuracy and a significant risk factor for dissection following PCI.[11]

Intravascular Ultrasound Imaging

Intravascular ultrasound imaging plays a crucial role in the assessment and intervention of LMCA disease. Offering a comprehensive 360° sagittal scan, IVUS provides detailed visualization from the lumen to the vessel wall through the media. It surpasses angiography by measuring cross sectional

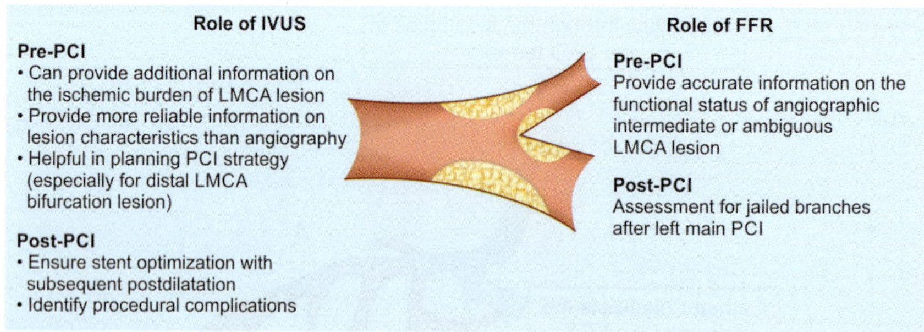

Fig. 6: Comparison of IVUS vs FFR in LMCA lesions. (FFR: fractional flow reserve; IVUS: intravascular ultrasound; LMCA: left main coronary artery; PCI: percutaneous coronary intervention)

area, plaque area, and minimal and maximal diameters, offering vital information. IVUS is particularly adept at detecting calcification and exhibits higher sensitivity in identifying significant LMCA stenosis.[12] While its routine use in PCI outcomes is debated, studies suggest its successful utilization as an adjunct to stent implantation. IVUS is recommended throughout LMCA PCI, before, during, and after the intervention, enhancing accuracy at each step **(Fig. 6)**. Notably, IVUS-guided LMCA PCI has demonstrated a mortality advantage compared to procedures guided solely by angiography, underlining its significance in improving patient outcomes. IVUS emerges as an indispensable tool in the management of LMCA disease, providing precise imaging and valuable quantitative assessments for informed decision-making and enhanced intervention strategies.[13]

Fractional Flow Reserve

Fractional flow reserve is a well-validated and a lesion specific index and offers a precise reflection of the functional impact of the coronary stenosis on the blood flow. It provides an accurate estimation of the blood supply to specific myocardial territories, which is independent of hemodynamic parameters including blood pressure, heart rate, or changes in myocardial contractility **(Table 2)**. Large randomized studies conducted in recent years consistently demonstrate that employment of an FFR-guided revascularization strategy with a cut-off value of 0.80 reduces costs and results in excellent clinical outcomes. These advantages extend to the functional assessment of LMCA disease, providing a valuable tool for informed decision-making in the management of LMCA lesions.[14]

Optical Coherence Tomography

Optical coherence tomography, an advanced imaging technique plays a crucial role in evaluating LMCA disease. By utilizing light waves, OCT produces cross sectional images of high resolution, allowing for detailed

TABLE 2: Role of IVUS and FFR in pre- and post- LMCA assessment.

	Pre-PCI	*Post-PCI*
Role of IVUS	• Additional information on the ischemic burden of LMCA lesion • Reliable lesion characteristics information compared to angiography • Devise PCI strategy, especially for distal LMCA bifurcation lesion	• Ensure stent optimization with subsequent postdilatation • Identify procedural complications
Role of FFR	Accurate information on the functional status of angiographic intermediate or ambiguous LMCA lesion	Assessment for jailed branches after left main PCI

(FFR: fractional flow reserve; IVUS: intravascular ultrasound; LMCA: left main coronary artery; PCI: percutaneous coronary intervention)

TABLE 3: Comparison of intravascular imaging: IVUS vs OCT in LMCA.

Lesion type	*Intravascular ultrasound (IVUS)*	*Optical coherence tomography (OCT)*
Ostial left main	++	–
Neointimal hyperplasia	+	++
Calcified	++	+
Thrombus	+	++
Stent apposition	+	++
Dissection	+	++
Thin-capped atheroma	–	++
Vessel diameter >5 mm	++	+

(++: excellent lesion assessment; +: good lesion assessment; –: difficult lesion assessment)

visualization of the coronary artery lumen **(Table 3)**. It excels in providing precise measurements of luminal dimensions, offering valuable insights into plaque morphology and composition. OCT's strengths lie in its superior imaging resolution, enabling clear visualization of the LMCA and surrounding structures. It further facilitates quantitative measurements, including minimal and maximal luminal diameters and plaque thickness, contributing to a comprehensive assessment of LMCA lesions. In interventions like PCI, OCT guides the procedure in real-time, aiding in decision-making for lesion preparation, stent selection, and optimal stent deployment. While OCT is a powerful diagnostic tool for LMCA, its routine use is influenced by factors such as availability, expertise, and specific clinical indications, prompting a tailored and judicious approach in clinical decision-making.[15]

Flowchart 2: Algorithm for intermediate LMCA lesions.

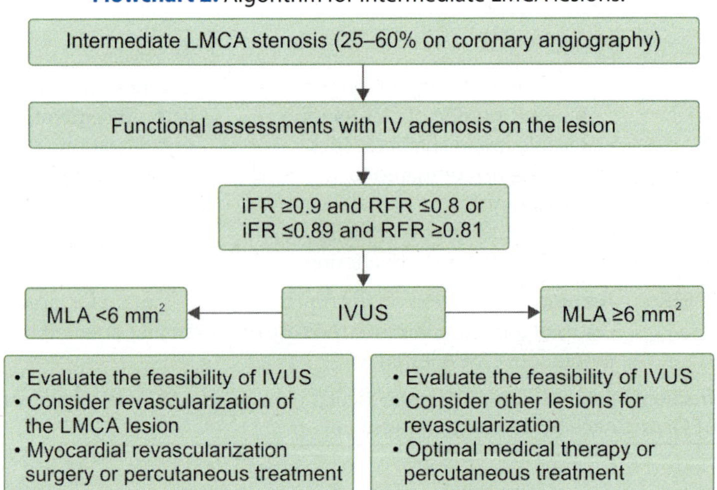

(iFR: instantaneous wave-free ratio; IV: intravenous; IVUS: intravascular ultrasound; LMCA: left main coronary artery; MLA: minimum lumen area; RFR: resting full cycle ratio)

Borderline Lesion Diagnosis

The diagnosis of borderline lesions, especially in the context of LMCA, is a critical aspect of cardiovascular care. Borderline lesions refer to those with mild or moderate stenosis that may not be immediately classified as requiring intervention but still merit careful consideration. In LMCA diagnosis, identifying borderline lesions involves assessing the degree of stenosis and considering various factors, such as plaque characteristics and patient symptoms. Diagnostic modalities such as FFR, IVUS, and angiography may be employed to evaluate borderline lesions in the LMCA **(Flowchart 2)**. The goal of employing these techniques is to determine the functional significance of the lesion and guide appropriate management, whether it is medical therapy, closer monitoring, or intervention. Decisions regarding borderline lesions in the LMCA necessitate a comprehensive evaluation, balancing the potential risks and benefits to ensure optimal patient outcomes.[16]

RADIAL APPROACH

In the last few decades, the radial approach has gained prominence as the preferred vascular access for coronary angiography, with a continuous increase in procedural adoption since its introduction in 1989.[17] This method offers distinct advantages, including effective hemostasis, reduced vascular complications, and immediate postexamination ambulation, contributing to shorter hospital stays and decreased costs.[18] Notably, studies have even suggested an enhanced quality of life for patients undergoing radial procedures.[19] Despite these benefits, challenges such as a longer learning curve, a higher crossover rate, and limitations in feasibility, especially with repeated procedures, underscore the need for careful consideration and operator expertise. The success rates reported in studies, such as those by Abdelaal et al.,[20] demonstrate the efficacy of radial access, with success rates of 93% for a second attempt, 81% for a third attempt, and a decline to 60% for eight or more procedures.

FEMORAL APPROACH

Conversely, the femoral approach continues to be relevant, offering advantages for operators, including reduced radiation exposure and the ability to use larger catheters in complex PCI, ensuring better catheter control.[20] However, the approach may result in higher rates of bleeding and vascular complications. While the radial approach has shown benefits in reducing bleeding complications,[21] especially in PCI, the femoral route remains a viable option. Numerous trials and meta-analyses have validated the radial approach's efficacy, demonstrating its superiority in certain clinical scenarios, particularly in acute coronary syndrome (ACS) and ST-segment elevation myocardial infarction (STEMI) cases, as observed in studies such as the RIFLE-STEACS trial.[22] Despite the short-term advantages reported, the long-term impact of these approaches on patient outcomes remains an area that necessitates further investigation beyond the often limited 30-day follow-up periods in existing studies.[23]

HEMODYNAMIC SUPPORT

Hemodynamic support devices are typically infrequently necessary when the left ventricular ejection fraction (LVEF) exceeds 50%. Our recommendation aligns using an intra-aortic balloon pump (IABP) in cases where the ejection fraction (EF) ranges between 35 and 50%, while an Impella device is advised for EF below 30%. Notably, in exceptional situations involving complex distal LM lesions coupled with an occluded right coronary artery (RCA) or a nondominant RCA, our guidance suggests considering the deployment of an IABP or Impella. This proactive approach is aimed at preventing hemodynamic deterioration, even in instances where the left ventricular (LV) function is ostensibly within the normal range. Emerging devices like the Impella LP 2.5 and LP 5.0 offer a potential solution, representing minimally invasive and easily deployable mechanical assist devices that may provide superior hemodynamic support when compared to the extensively used IABP.[24]

CHOICE OF HARDWARE

Guide Catheter Strategies

Selecting an appropriate guide catheter is crucial for successful PCI. Optimal outcomes are often achieved with smaller (6 Fr) catheters, minimizing pressure dampening risks upon engagement. Choosing less aggressive catheters, like Judkins, proves effective in controlled stent manipulation and reduces the likelihood of inadvertent movements **(Figs. 7A to C)**. Caution is warranted with side-hole catheters, especially in unprotected LM or RCA scenarios, where they may obscure pressure signals and hinder lesion visualization, necessitating a larger contrast volume. The Ostial Pro device enhances procedural control by keeping the guide catheter outside the ostium. Advanced techniques, including the "floating wire" method and small guide catheter extensions, contribute to successful coronary artery engagement and facilitate catheter disengagement. The "independent-hand" technique emerges as a valuable approach for enhanced precision in aorto-ostial lesion stenting.[25]

Guidewire Choices (Table 4)[26]

For LMCA percutaneous therapy, a soft-tipped spring wire (BMW or comparable) is typically utilized. Due to the vessel's great diameter and proximity to the aorta, this guidewire—whose primary characteristic is that it offers exceptional flexibility and mild support—makes lesion crossing easy. A guidewire which is hydrophobic (ideally medium tipped) is highly suggested and recommended when a major vessel calcification is present, in lesion eccentricity, when there are extremely acute angles between the

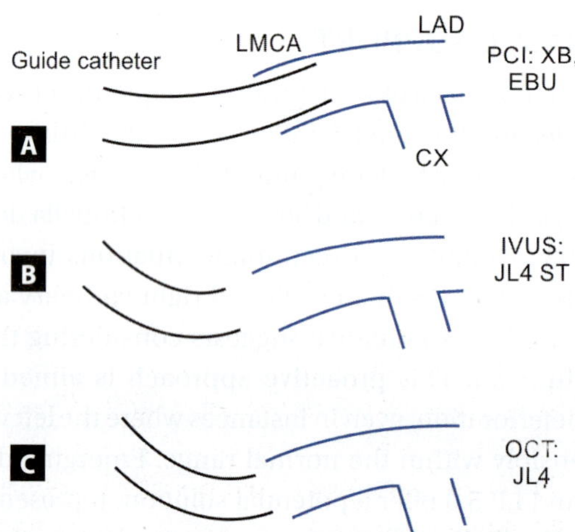

Figs. 7A to C: Guide catheter choice for PCI and imaging of LMCA. (IVUS: intravascular ultrasound; LAD: left anterior descending; LMCA: left main coronary artery; OCT: optical coherence tomography; PCI: percutaneous coronary intervention).

TABLE 4: Guidewire choices.

Manufacturer	*Wire*	*Diameter tip (inches) and stiffness (g)*	*Stiffness (g)*	*Coating characteristics*
Abbott vascular	BMW, BMW universal	0.014	1	Nonhydrophilic
Asahi Intec	Prowater flex	0.014	1	Nonhydrophilic
Terumo	Runthrough NS floppy	0.014	1	Hydrophilic
	Runthrough NS floppy	0.014	1	Hyperhydrophilic

LMCA and LAD or LCX, during excessive endings, or in the presence of an ulcerated plaque which is at risk of destabilization **(Table 4)**. This is because the hydrophilic guidewire reaches the periphery more easily and offers greater support during the procedure.[27]

Debulking Strategies

Percutaneous transluminal rotational atherectomy (PTRA) was introduced in 1988 by David Auth, primarily to achieve mechanical debulking of atherosclerotic plaque.[28] Debulking strategies in LMCA interventions involve techniques to address significant atherosclerotic burden and optimize vessel preparation. Atherectomy devices, such as rotational atherectomy or orbital atherectomy, may be employed to reduce plaque burden and enhance stent delivery. These debulking techniques aim to create a more favorable vascular environment, allowing for improved stent expansion and apposition. The choice of debulking strategy in LMCA interventions is influenced by the specific characteristics of the lesion, including calcification and plaque morphology, and is often determined through careful consideration by the interventional cardiologist based on the individual patient's anatomy and clinical presentation.[29]

STENT AND ITS EXPANSIBILITY

A stent is a mesh-like tube used in medical procedures to support narrowed blood vessels. Stent expansibility is crucial for effective deployment, ensuring it opens sufficiently and maintain optimal patency of the vessel and blood flow. Factors such as stent material, design, and deployment technique influence expansibility **(Table 5)**. Modern stents are designed to be flexible and possess radial strength to reduce restenosis risk. During a PCI, the stent is expanded using a balloon catheter. The choice of stent and its successful expansibility are critical for positive outcomes in coronary interventions, improving revascularization and long-term vessel patency. Advances in stent technology aim to enhance expansibility and overall performance.[30]

ROLE OF PROXIMAL OPTIMIZATION TECHNIQUE

The proximal optimization technique (POT) was introduced by Dr Olivier Darremont, addresses diameter differences in bifurcation lesions during stenting. This technique, endorsed by the European Bifurcation Club and outlined in their consensus statement, involves expanding a short balloon in the proximal main vessel (MV) up to the carina.[32] This approach ensures full stent expansion and complete apposition in the proximal MV. Additionally, POT facilitates recrossing into the side branch (SB), allowing for further optimization of the final result if necessary. Embraced by experts in the field, POT stands as a key strategy for achieving optimal outcomes in bifurcation lesion interventions.[33]

Ostial Left Main Coronary Artery Intervention

When there is adequate pressure, nitroglycerin intracoronary (IC) injection is required to differentiate between an actual ostial lesion and an ostial spasm caused by a catheter **(Fig. 8)**.

TABLE 5: Choice of stent for LMCA stenting.[31]

Stent size	*Xience Sierra*	*Xience Alpine*	*Skypoint*	*Synergy™*	*Megatron™*	*Onyx™*	*Orsiro*	*Orsiro Mission*
2.0								
2.25		3.25				3.25		
2.5				3.5				
2.75	3.75		3.75			3.75	3.5	3.59
3.0		3.75						
3.25				4.25				
3.5	5.5	4.5				4.75	4.5	4.42
4.0			5.75	5.75	6.0			
4.5						5.75		
5.0								

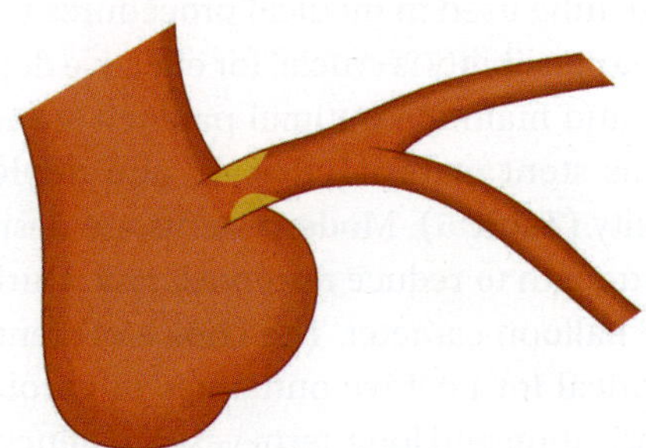

Fig. 8: Ostial left main anatomy.

Since pressure damping frequently occurs, pressure needs to be closely watched, and contrast should never be injected when there is dampening.

Sporadic catheter guidance: To expedite the process, disengagement is recommended with the guiding wire preloaded (*hit and run approach*) **(Figs. 9 and 10)**.

Lead the way, cath: In order to demarcate and isolate an area and avoid pressure dampening, extension or floating wire may be required **(Fig. 11)**.

To guarantee ostial coverage, it should be aorto ostial with a 2–3 mm protrusion into the aorta.

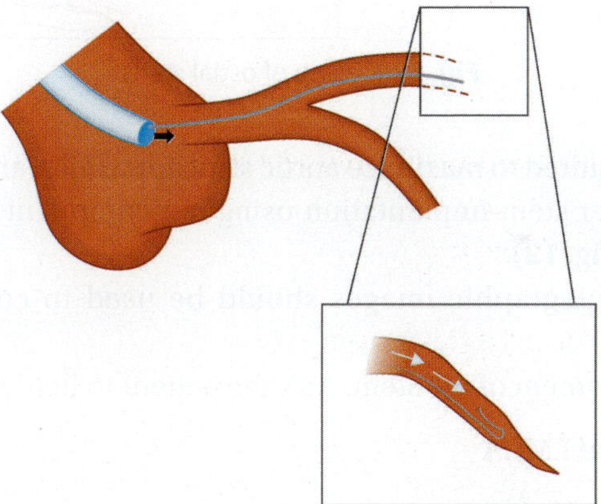

Fig. 9: Passing the wire with catheter floating.

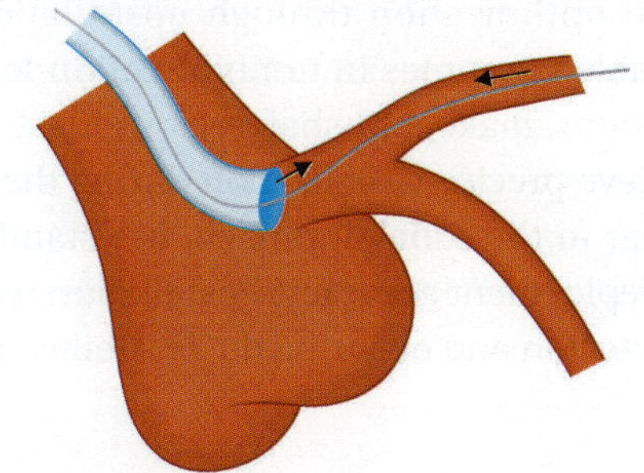

Fig. 10: Making catheter coaxial to osteum.

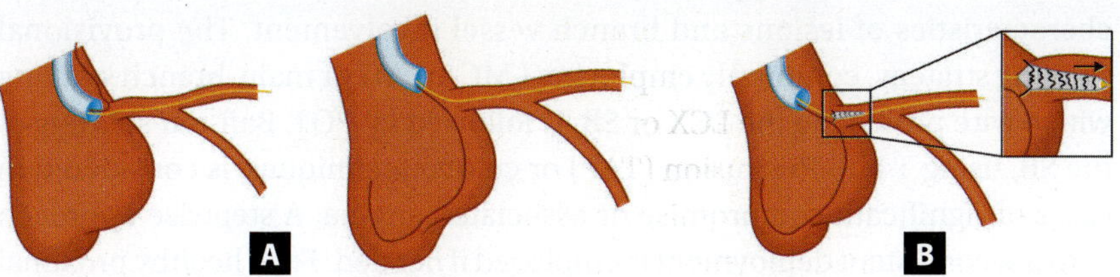

Figs. 11A and B: (A) Sepal wire technique; (B) Szabo technique.

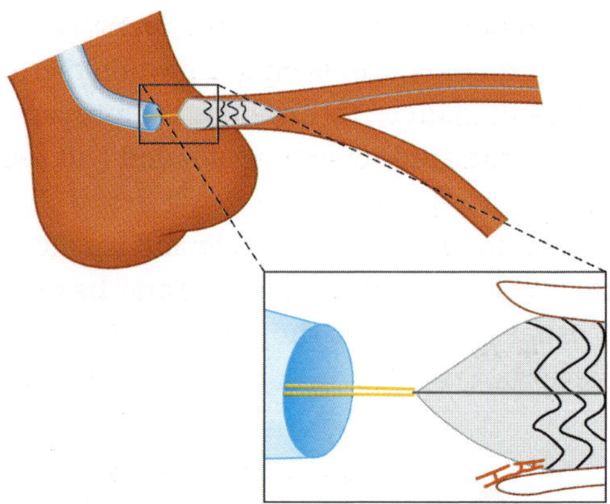

Fig. 12: Flaring of ostial stent.

Flaring is required to maximize aortic strut apposition and enable further engagement after stent implantation using noncompliant (NC) balloon or Flash balloon **(Fig. 12)**.

Multiple angiographic images should be used to confirm the stent location.[34]

Before deployment of the stent, ASK the patient to hold their breath.

Stenting of Ostial LMCA

SHAFT LEFT MAIN CORONARY ARTERY STENTING

For mid-shaft LMCA lesions, a single appropriately sized stent suffices for PCI, with additional optimization through postdilation guided by IVUS or OCT.[35] The favorable outcomes in nonbifurcation lesions, attributed to larger lumen dimensions, make mid-shaft regions ideal for PCI. Employ the cranial views to achieve precise visualization during the intervention (LAO, AP, and RAO). Similar to the ostial approach, use standard guides without side holes for stent deployment accuracy. Postdilation remains a key step for optimizing stent expansion and ensuring the feasibility of future procedures **(Figs. 13A to E)**.[36]

DISTAL LEFT MAIN CORONARY ARTERY

The distal LMCA PCI approach involves consideration of vessel anatomy, characteristics of lesions and branch vessel involvement. The provisional stenting strategy, commonly employing LMCA-LAD or main-branch stenting with a wire protecting the LCX or SB, is followed by POT. Bail-out stenting of the SB, using T and Protrusion (TAP) or culotte techniques, is considered in cases of significant compromise or associated angina. A stepwise approach with a second stent deployment is employed if needed. For a healthy proximal LMCA, studies suggest no benefits in extending the stent into the ostium.

Dedicated short POT balloons are available for healthy ostioproximal LMCA. The two-stent strategy may be considered for LCX-dominant vessels or LCX ostial disease. Techniques such as T-stenting, TAP, culotte, or double kissing (DK) crush is preferred. Imaging-guided procedures, mandatory final kissing balloon inflation (FKBI), and additional final POT enhance clinical outcomes. The DEFINITION criteria are commonly used for strategy selection, helping stratify lesions based on complexity.[36]

SIMULTANEOUSLY KISSING STENT/V STENT

The SKS/V stent, also known as the "simultaneous kissing stents with a V-stent" technique, is a bifurcation stenting strategy used in the PCI of complex LMCA bifurcation lesions **(Fig. 14)**. This approach involves the simultaneous deployment of two stents—one in the MV and the other in the SB—followed by the creation of a V-shaped configuration to cover the bifurcation area **(Fig. 15)**. The SKS/V stent technique aims to provide optimal coverage and support for both the main and SBs, reducing the risk of restenosis and improving procedural success. This strategy is one of several

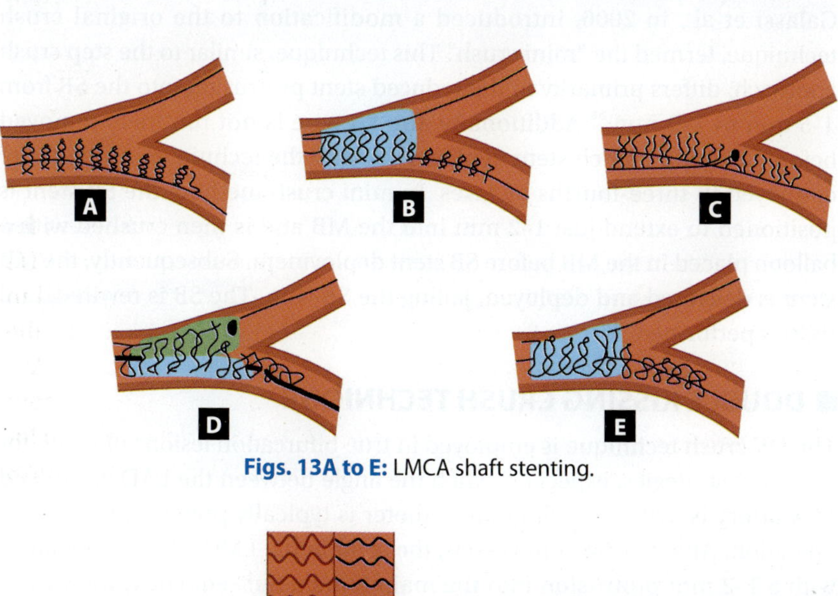

Figs. 13A to E: LMCA shaft stenting.

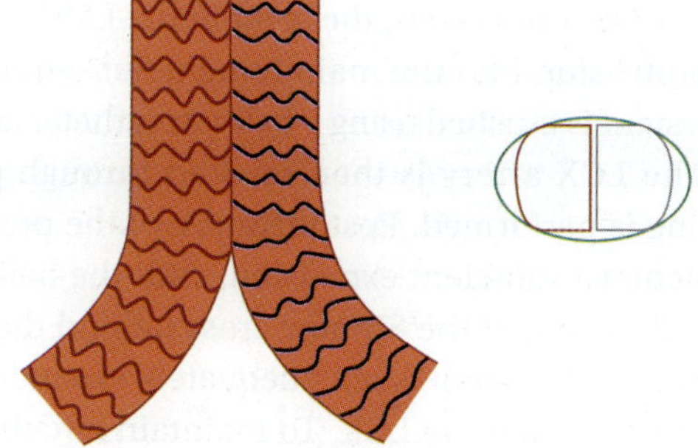

Fig. 14: Simultaneously kissing stent (SKS) technique.

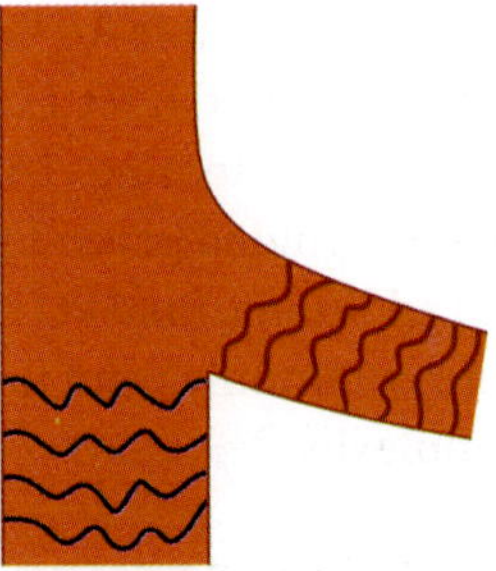

Fig. 15: V stenting.

options available for managing complex LMCA bifurcation lesions and is chosen based on the specific anatomical and clinical characteristics of the lesion. The selection of bifurcation stenting techniques, including SKS/V stent, requires careful consideration and may vary depending on individual patient factors and lesion complexity.[37]

MINI CRUSH

Galassi et al., in 2006, introduced a modification to the original crush technique, termed the "mini crush". This technique, similar to the step crush approach, differs primarily in the reduced stent protrusion into the SB from 4–5 mm to 1–2 mm.[38] Additionally, the SB wire is not routinely removed before the main branch stent deployment, with the technique of jailed wire employed in three-fourths of cases. In mini crush method, the SB stent is positioned to extend just 1–2 mm into the MB and is then crushed with a balloon placed in the MB before SB stent deployment. Subsequently, the MB stent is delivered and deployed, jailing the SB wire. The SB is rewired, and FKBI is performed.[39]

DOUBLE KISSING CRUSH TECHNIQUE

The DK crush technique is employed in true bifurcation lesions planned for two-stent strategies, especially when the angle between the LAD artery and LCX artery is <70°.[40] A 7 Fr guide catheter is typically preferred for ease of operation. After wiring both vessels, the stent in the LMCA-LCX is deployed with a 1–2 mm protrusion into the main lumen. Subsequently, the wire is removed, and the stent is crushed using a balloon catheter across the LMCA-LAD **(Fig. 16)**. The LCX artery is then rewired through proximal struts, and the first kissing is performed. Postdilatation of the proximal stent may be necessary to achieve sufficient expansion, with the balloon sized 1:1 to the proximal MV. Rewiring of the SB may cross behind the MV stent if the proximal portion of the MV stent is not adequately expanded. FKBI/second kissing follows after rewiring the LCX. To maintain circular geometry and reduce SB ostium strut obstruction, POT is repeated at the end of the DK crush technique. Retaining the distal balloon marker for re-POT just proximal to the carina is advisable to preserve the bifurcation stent design.[36,41]

CULOTTE TECHNIQUE

The culotte technique is suitable for bifurcation lesions with a shallow angle (<70°) between the LAD artery and LCX artery, where the vessels typically have similar diameters.[42] After predilatation, a stent is deployed from the LAD to the left main stem (LMS) across the LCX ostium, positioning the proximal portion in the LMCA. POT with a larger balloon at the LMS portion follows. Subsequently, the LCX is rewired, and the balloon is inflated at the ostium of the LCX to open the stent struts, facilitating stent advancement into the LCX **(Fig. 17)**. The second stent is then advanced into the LCX, with the proximal portion positioned in the LMCA, overlapping the first stent. Deployment occurs after removing the LAD wire. The wire is readvanced through the stent struts into the LAD to perform FKBI and reshape the carina. The sequence of stenting the LAD can be reversed if the LCX is large and there is severe angulation.[36]

T AND SMALL PROTRUSION (TAP) TECHNIQUE

The TAP technique is utilized for LMCA bifurcation lesions with an angle >70° between the LAD artery and LCX artery.[43] After wiring both vessels, a stent is placed in the LCX, protruding into the LMCA, covering its ostium.

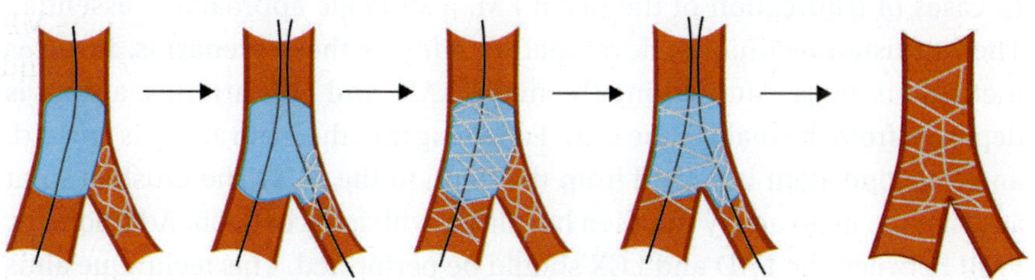

Fig. 16: Double kissing (DK) crush.

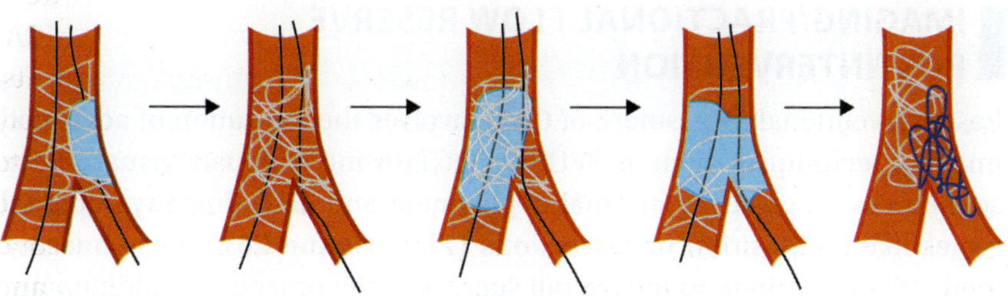

Fig. 17: Culotte technique.

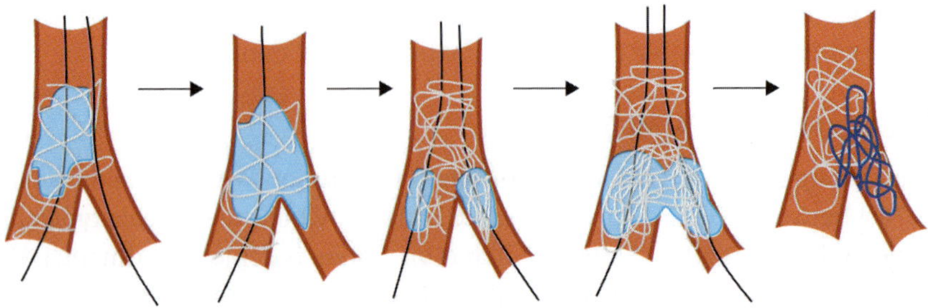

Fig. 18: T and protrusion (TAP).

The stent is then crushed with a prepositioned balloon in the LAD-LMCA, and another stent is deployed in the LM-LAD across the LCX. FKBI completes the procedure.

In provisional TAP, after LMCA predilatation, an LMCA-LAD stent is deployed. If the LCX ostium is compromised, a wire is advanced through the distal stent strut into the LCX, and balloon dilatation widens the stent strut at the LCX origin. Subsequently, a stent is placed in the LCX, with the proximal margin protruding into the LM, covering the ostial LCX. FKBI is performed by inflating a pre-positioned balloon in the LMCA-LAD to conclude the procedure **(Fig. 18)**.[36]

TRIFURCATION OF DISTAL LEFT MAIN AND KURDISTAN TECHNIQUE

In cases of trifurcation of the distal LM, a strategic approach is essential. The Kurdistan technique, developed to address these scenarios, involves meticulous steps. After wiring the main, LAD, and LCX arteries, a stent is deployed from the main to the LAD. Following this, the main artery is rewired, and a second stent is placed from the main to the LCX. The crushed stent struts in the main artery can then be dilated with a NC balloon. Additionally, FKBI between the LAD and LCX should be performed. This technique aims to optimize stent placement and enhance procedural success in challenging distal LM trifurcation cases.[44]

IMAGING/FRACTIONAL FLOW RESERVE POSTINTERVENTION

Postinterventional assessment of CAD involves the utilization of advanced imaging techniques such as IVUS or OCT to meticulously visualize the stented vessel, ensuring optimal deployment and detecting any potential issues like malposition or dissections **(Figs. 19 and 20)**. These imaging modalities contribute to the overall success of the procedure. Additionally, FFR is employed for functional evaluation, measuring pressure gradients

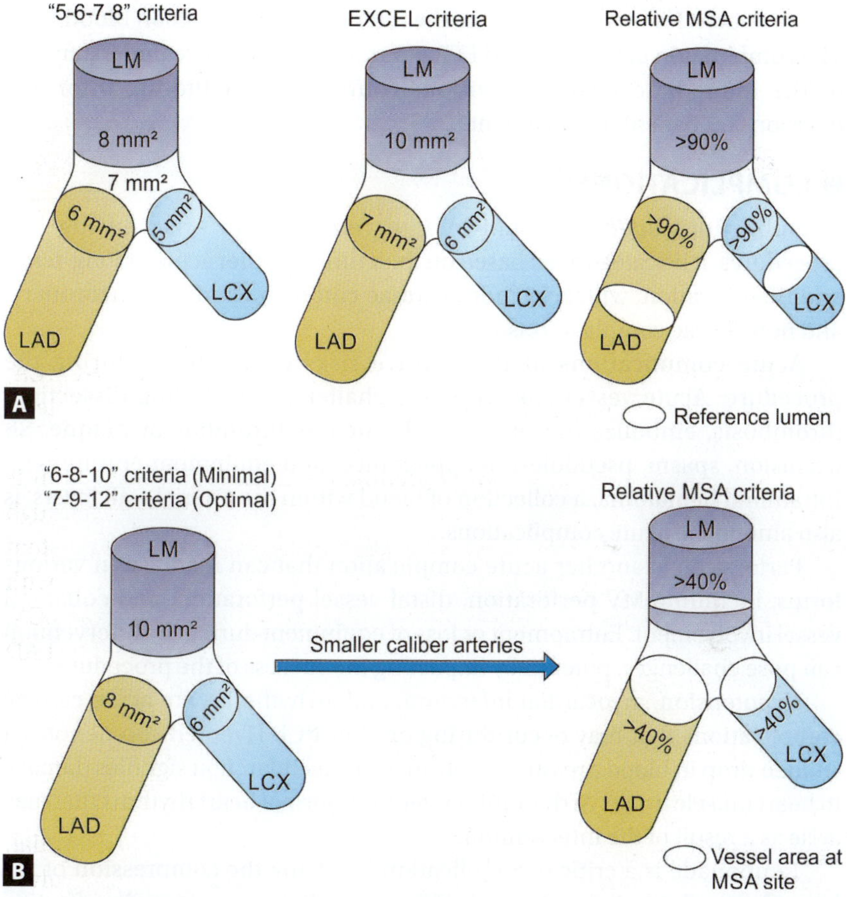

Figs. 19A and B: Expansion criteria. (A) Existing stent expansion criteria for distal left main (LM) bifurcation stenting; (B) Proposed stent expansion criteria for LM stenting. (LAD: left anterior descending; LCX: left circumflex; MSA: minimal stent area)

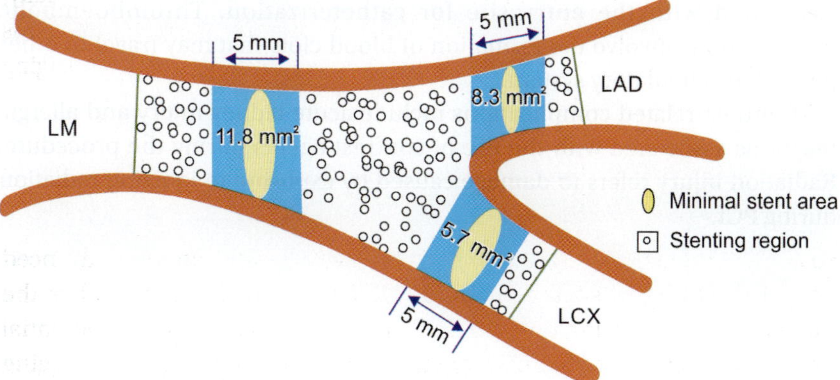

Fig. 20: The optimal minimal stent area within each left main segment. (LAD: left anterior descending; LCX: left circumflex; LM: left main)

across treated lesions to determine the intervention's impact on blood flow. The combination of imaging and FFR offers a comprehensive understanding of the immediate postinterventional outcomes, facilitating informed decisions on patient management.[13-15]

COMPLICATIONS[25]

Complications specific to LMCA interventions can arise during PCI procedures. It be categorized based on their timing, either acute or long-term, and their location, which includes cardiac coronary, cardiac noncoronary, and noncardiac complications.

Acute complications of PCI involve risks encountered during the procedure. Acute vessel closure poses challenges, including dissection, thrombosis, embolization of materials such as thrombus or plaque, SB occlusion, spasm, pseudolesion appearance, and equipment entrapment. Intramural hematoma, a collection of blood within the arterial wall layers, is also among the acute complications.

Perforation is another acute complication that can manifest in various forms, including MV perforation, distal vessel perforation, and collateral vessel involvement. Entrapment or loss of equipment during the intervention can pose challenges, potentially impacting the success of the procedure.

Hypotension, myocardial infarction, and arrhythmias are acute cardiac complications that may occur during or after PCI. Hypotension denotes a sudden drop in blood pressure, while myocardial infarction signifies damage to heart muscle tissue. Arrhythmias refer to abnormal heart rhythms that may arise as a result of the intervention.

Tamponade is a critical complication involving the compression of the heart due to fluid accumulation in the pericardial sac, potentially affecting cardiac function.

Noncoronary complications encompass issues not directly related to the coronary arteries. Vascular access complications pertain to problems associated with the entry site for catheterization. Thromboembolic complications involve the formation of blood clots that may travel to other parts of the circulatory system.

Contrast-related complications include acute kidney injury and allergic reactions associated with the use of contrast agents during the procedure. Radiation injury refers to damage caused by exposure to ionizing radiation during PCI.

CASE STUDIES

Case 1: LMCA Shaft Stenting (Pre- and Poststenting with Single Stent Strategy)

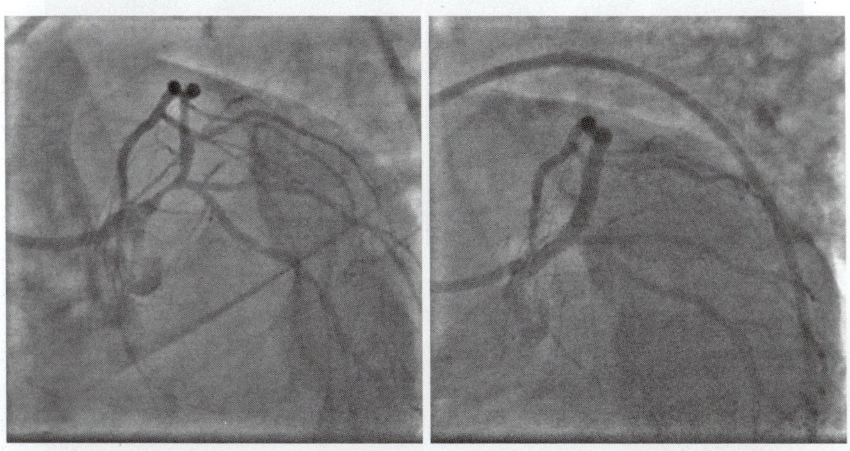

Case 2: LMCA Osteal Stentig (Pre- and Poststenting with IVUS Evaluation)

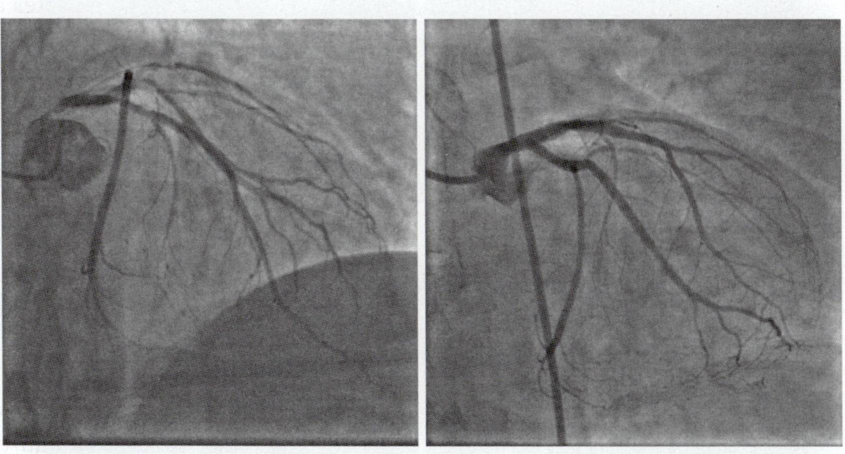

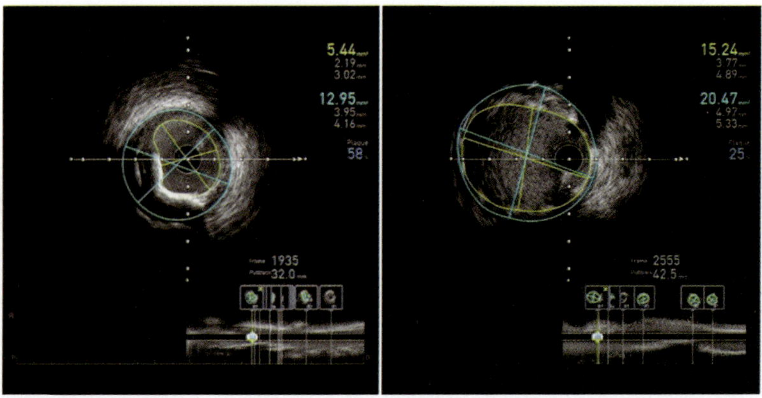

Case 3: LMCA Distal Bifurcation (DKC—Pre- and Poststenting)

Prestenting

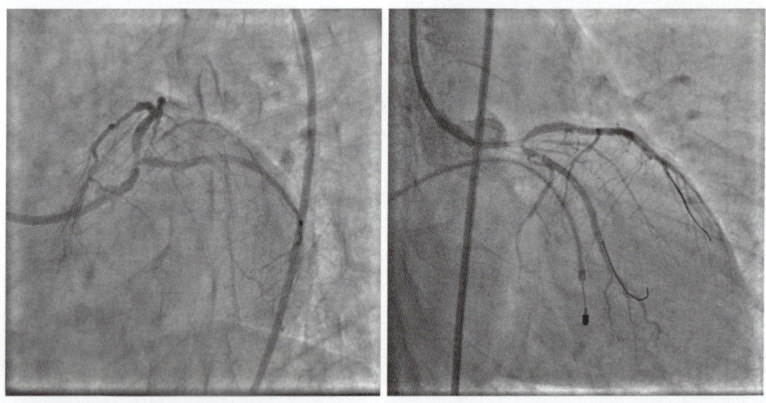

Poststenting (with Intravascular Ultrasound Images)

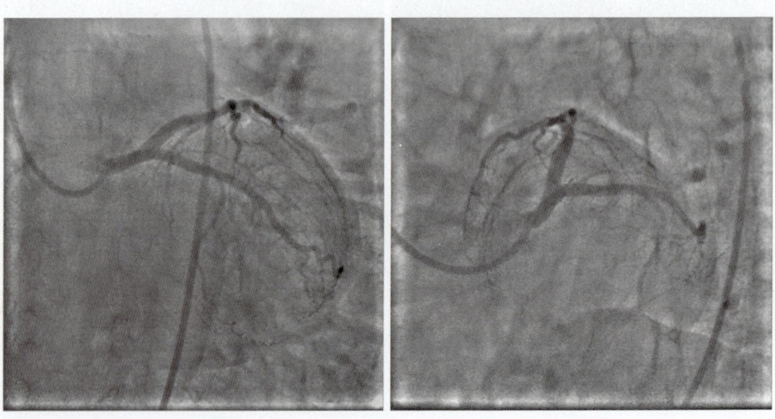

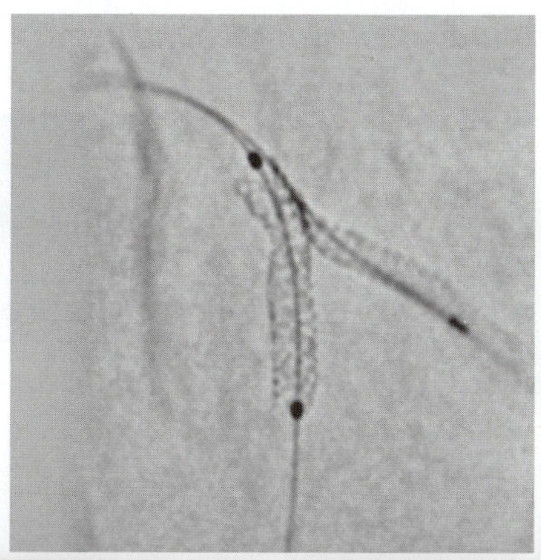

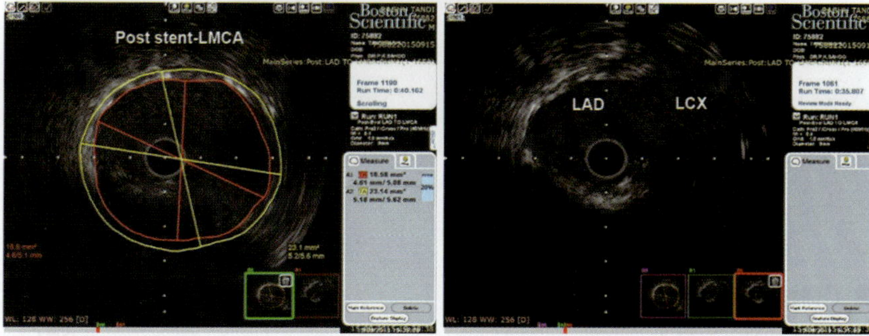

Case 4: LMCA Trifurcation Senting—Kurdistan Technique

Prestenting with Intravascular Ultrasound (IVUS)

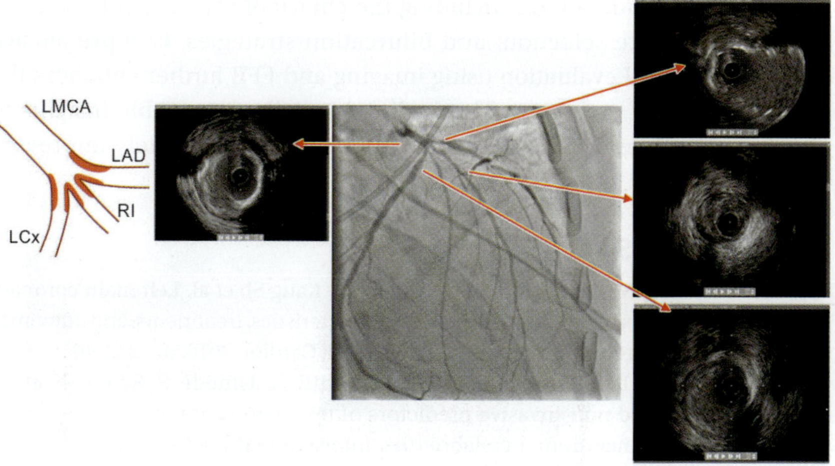

Poststenting with Intravascular Ultrasound Results

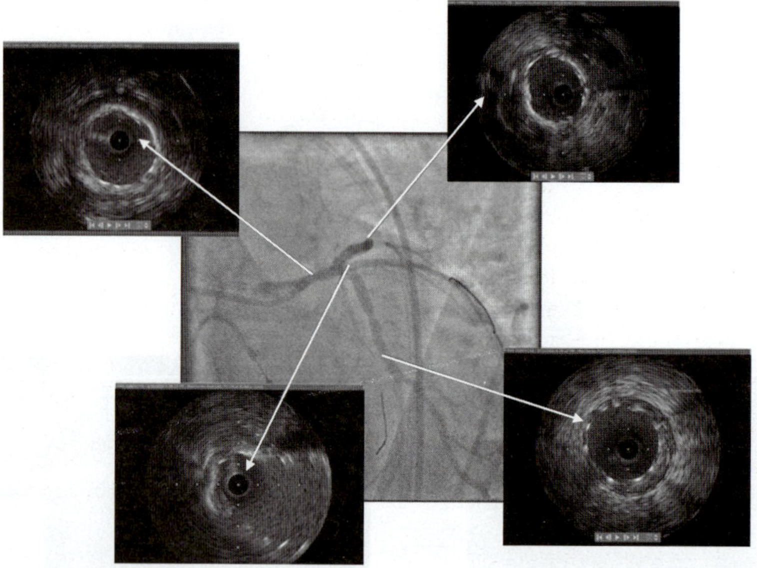

CONCLUSION

In conclusion, this review underscores the safety and efficacy of PCI in LMCA disease, particularly with drug-eluting stents, as demonstrated in a retrospective analysis of Indian patients. The study emphasizes the importance of assessing patient characteristics, utilizing advanced diagnostic modalities, and employing precise procedural techniques. The review outlines key considerations, including the choice of access, hemodynamic support, hardware selection, and bifurcation strategies. Comprehensive postinterventional evaluation using imaging and FFR further enhances the understanding of outcomes. The findings contribute valuable insights to guide clinicians in optimizing LMCA interventions, ultimately improving patient care.

REFERENCES

1. Lee PH, Ahn JM, Chang M, Baek S, Yoon SH, Kang SJ, et al. Left main coronary artery disease: secular trends in patient characteristics, treatments, and outcomes of left main coronary artery disease. J Am Coll Cardiol. 2016;68:1233-46.
2. D'Ascenzo F, Presutti DG, Picardi E, Moretti C, Omedè P, Sciuto F, et al. Prevalence and non-invasive predictors of left main or three-vessel coronary disease: evidence from a collaborative international meta-analysis of 22,740 patients. Heart. 2012;98:914-9.
3. Ragosta M, Dee S, Sarembock IJ, Lipson LC, Gimple LW, Powers ER, et al. Prevalence of unfavorable angiographic characteristics for percutaneous

intervention in patients with unprotected left main coronary artery disease. Catheter Cardiovasc Interv. 2006;68:357-62.
4. Taylor HA, Deumite NJ, Chaitman BR, Davis KB, Killip T, Rogers WJ, et al. Asymptomatic left main coronary artery disease in the Coronary Artery Surgery Study (CASS) registry. Circulation. 1989;79:1171-9.
5. Dodge JT Jr, Brown BG, Bolson EL, Dodge HT. Lumen diameter of normal human coronary arteries. Influence of age, sex, anatomic variation, and left ventricular hypertrophy or dilation. Circulation. 1992;86:232-46.
6. James TN. Anatomy of Coronary Arteries. New York: Paul B. Hoeber; 1961. pp. 12-8.
7. Johnson AD, Detwiler JH, Higgins CB. Left coronary artery anatomy in patients with bicuspid aortic valves. Br Heart J. 1978;40:489-93.
8. Bergelson BA, Tommaso CL. Left main coronary artery disease: assessment, diagnosis, and therapy. Am Heart J. 1995;129:350-9.
9. Libby P. Braunwald's Heart Disease: A Textbook of Cardiovascular Medicine, 12th edition. Netherlands: Elsevier Health Sciences; 2021.
10. Gannon S. (2018). Intravascular Imaging: Understanding the Role of IVUS and OCT. [online] Available from https://www.acc.org/latest-in-cardiology/articles/2018/08/28/14/42/cover-story-intravascular-imaging-understanding-the-role-of-ivus-and-oct. [Last accessed October, 2024].
11. Mintz GS, Popma JJ, Pichard AD, Kent KM, Satler LF, Chuang YC, et al. Patterns of calcification in coronary artery disease. A statistical analysis of intravascular ultrasound and coronary angiography in 1155 lesions. Circulation. 1995;91:1959-65.
12. Tanyeli O. Left Main Coronary Artery Disease: Current Treatment Options. London: IntechOpen; 2017.
13. Case BC, Yerasi C, Forrestal BJ, Shlofmitz E, Garcia-Garcia HM, Mintz GS, et al. Intravascular ultrasound guidance in the evaluation and treatment of left main coronary artery disease. Int J Cardiol. 2021;325:168-75.
14. Hamilos M. (2014). The Use of Fractional Flow Reserve in Left Main Coronary Artery Lesion Assessment. Available from https://doi.org/10.15420/rc.2014.wp01. [Last accessed October, 2024].
15. Miura K, Tada T, Shimada T, Ohya M, Murai R, Kubo S, et al. Three-dimensional optical coherence tomography versus intravascular ultrasound in percutaneous coronary intervention for the left main coronary artery. Heart Vessels. 2021;36(5):630-7.
16. Ruzsa Z, Pálinkás A, Forster T, Ungi I, Varga A. Angiographically borderline left main coronary artery lesions: correlation of transthoracic Doppler echocardiography and intravascular ultrasound: a pilot study. Cardiovasc Ultrasound. 2011;9:19.
17. Campeau L. Percutaneous radial artery approach for coronary angiography. Cathet Cardiovasc Diagn. 1989;16:3-7.
18. Amin AP, House JA, Safley DM, Chhatriwalla AK, Giersiefen H, Bremer A, et al. Costs of transradial percutaneous coronary intervention. JACC Cardiovasc Interv. 2013;6:827-34.
19. Cooper CJ, El-Shiekh RA, Cohen DJ, Blaesing L, Burket MW, Basu A, et al. Effect of transradial access on quality of life and cost of cardiac catheterization: a randomized comparison. Am Heart J. 1999;138:430-6.

20. Abdelaal E, Molin P, Plourde G, Machaalany J, Bataille Y, Brousseau-Provencher C, et al. Successive transradial access for coronary procedures: experience of Quebec Heart-Lung Institute. Am Heart J. 2013;165:325-31.
21. Andò G, Capodanno D. Radial access reduces mortality in patients with acute coronary syndromes: results from an updated trial sequential analysis of randomized trials. JACC Cardiovasc Interv. 2016;9:660-70.
22. Romagnoli E, Biondi-Zoccai G, Sciahbasi A, Politi L, Rigattieri S, Pendenza G, et al. Radial versus femoral randomized investigation in ST-segment elevation acute coronary syndrome: the RIFLE-STEACS (radial versus femoral randomized investigation in ST-elevation acute coronary syndrome) study. J Am Coll Cardiol. 2012;60:2481-9.
23. Le May MR, Singh K, Wells GA. Efficacy of radial versus femoral access in the acute coronary syndrome: is it the operator or the operation that matters? JACC Cardiovasc Interv. 2015;8:1405-9.
24. Mehta R, Sharma SK. Left main coronary interventions. In: Kini A, Sharma SK (Eds). Practical Manual of Interventional Cardiology. New York: Springer, Cham; 2021.
25. Brilakis E. Manual of Percutaneous Coronary Interventions: A Step-by-Step Approach. Netherlands: Elsevier Science; 2020.
26. Baba Y. (2023). Guidewires. [online] Available from https://doi.org/10.53347/rID-163388. [Last accessed October, 2024].
27. Brilakis ES, Mashayekhi K, Tsuchikane E, Abi Rafeh N, Alaswad K, Araya M, et al. Guiding principles for chronic total occlusion percutaneous coronary intervention: a global expert consensus document. Circulation. 2019;140(5):420-33.
28. Auth D. Percutaneous Transluminal Rotational Atherectomy. Circulation. 1988;78(2):442-4.
29. Barbato E, Shlofmitz E, Milkas A, Shlofmitz R, Azzalini L, Colombo A, et al. State of the art: evolving concepts in the treatment of heavily calcified and undilatable coronary stenoses—from debulking to plaque modification, a 40-year-long journey. EuroIntervention. 2017;13(6):696-705.
30. Chieffo A, Colombo A. Treatment of unprotected left main coronary artery disease with drug-eluting stents: is it time for a randomized trial? Nat Rev Cardiol. 2005;2:396-400.
31. Dash D, Mody R, Ahmed N, Mylarappa YP, Kejariwal M, Mody B. Left main bifurcation stenting: a 2023 appraisal. J Transcat Intervent. 2023;31:eA202302.
32. Lassen JF, Holm NR, Banning A, Burzotta F, Lefèvre T, Chieffo A, et al. Percutaneous coronary intervention for coronary bifurcation disease: 11th consensus document from the European Bifurcation Club. EuroIntervention. 2016;12:38-46.
33. Hoye A. The Proximal Optimization Technique for Intervention of Coronary Bifurcations. Interv Cardiol. 2017;12(2):110-5.
34. Di Mario C, Sutaria N. Coronary angiography in the angioplasty era: projections with a meaning. Am Heart J. 2005;91:968-76.
35. Showkathali R, Yalamanchi RP. Contemporary Left Main Percutaneous Coronary Intervention: A State-of-the-art Review. Interv Cardiol. 2023;18:e20.
36. Khalil I. Coronary artery intervention techniques. London: IntechOpen; 2020.

37. Ghosh P, Shah A, Sporn D, Kaluski E. Two-Step V-Stenting and Simultaneous Kissing Stent via 6F Guides: Simple Just Got Simpler. Cardiovasc Revasc Med. 2022;45:63-6.
38. Galassi AR, Colombo A, Buchbinder M, Grasso C, Tomasello SD, Ussia GP, et al. Long-term outcomes of bifurcation lesions after implantation of drug-eluting stents with the "mini-crush technique". Catheter Cardiovasc Interv. 2007;69:976-83.
39. Moroni F, Shue-Min Yeh J, Attallah A, Santiago R, Martins Filho E, Hall J, et al. Crush techniques for percutaneous coronary intervention of bifurcation lesions. EuroIntervention. 2022;18(1):71-82.
40. Zhang JJ, Ye F, Xu K, Kan J, Tao L, Santoso T, et al. Multicenter, randomized comparison of two-stent and provisional stenting techniques in patients with complex coronary bifurcation lesions: the DEFINITION II trial. Am Heart J. 2020;41:2523-36.
41. Rab T, Sheiban I, Louvard Y, Sawaya FJ, Zhang JJ, Chen SL. Current interventions for the left main bifurcation. JACC Cardiovasc Interv. 2017;10(9):849-65.
42. Chevalier B, Glatt B, Royer T, Guyon P. Placement of coronary stents in bifurcation lesions by the "culotte" technique. Am Heart J. 1998;82:943-9.
43. Dahdouh Z, Fadel BM, Roule V, Sarkis A, Grollier G. Snuggle T and protrusion (S-TAP) technique for coronary bifurcation stenting: a step-by-step angiographic and illustration demonstration. Am Heart J. 2017;18:14-6.
44. Mirza AJ. "Kurdistan" Technique for the Treatment of Unprotected Trifurcation Left Main Stem Coronary Artery Lesion: Case Report. World J Cardiovasc Dis. 2014;4(9):58-66.

CHAPTER 26

Chronic Total Occlusion Percutaneous Coronary Intervention Toolbox

Roopali Khanna

INTRODUCTION

Chronic total occlusion (CTO) percutaneous coronary intervention (PCI) has grown and evolved over the past few decades in terms of myriad techniques and overall procedural success rate.[1] Much of this owes to recent advances in technology involving hardware used in CTO procedures, with major developments coming in the form of newer, safer, and stiffer hydrophilic guidewires and more negotiable varied-length small caliber microcatheters.

Herein, we enumerate various CTO-specific hardware essentials for the successful intervention of CTO PCI.

ESSENTIAL CTO PCI TOOLBOX

- Guide catheters (GCs)
- CTO guidewires
- Microcatheters
- Low profile and special balloons
- Miscellaneous

Guide Catheters

The first key to success for CTO PCI is the selection of a GC. For effective guidewire manipulation, the coaxial orientation of the GC and stability and backup force are crucial. Usually, multiple hardware are needed to facilitate CTO crossing, which requires the presence of a large GC, 7 Fr GCs are preferred; in selected cases, 8 Fr GCs may be needed. For right coronary artery (RCA) CTO intervention, Amplatzer 1 or 2 or short Amplatzer GCs are preferred guides. For the left anterior descending (LAD) artery, CTO's extra backup (EBU or XBU) guides are usually preferred, and Amplatzer guides are useful in LCx interventions.[2]

Chronic Total Occlusion Guidewires

In recent years, significant advances have been made in CTO wire technology, resulting in wires with better torque transmission, penetration force, and wire control.[3] This has led to an increase in the success rate of antegrade wiring and thus decreased the need for a retrograde approach. Puncturing the proximal cap is the most crucial step in CTO PCI. The CTO wires have

Flowchart 1: Chronic total occlusion (CTO) guidewires classification according to their characteristics

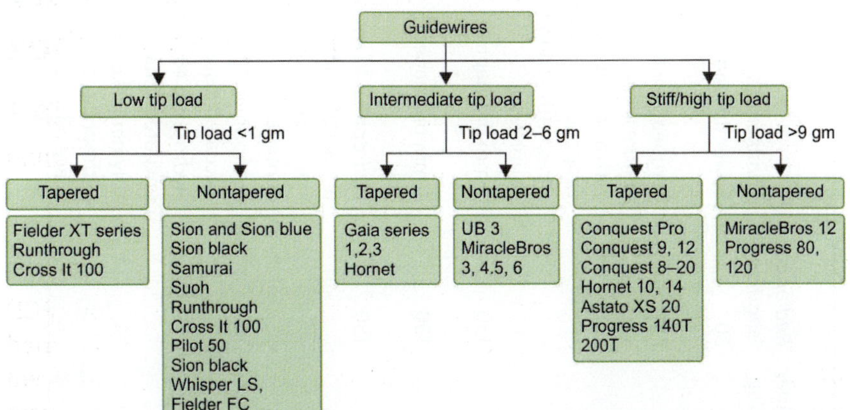

been divided into low, intermediate, and high penetration wires based on their tip load **(Flowchart 1)**. The operator should be aware of at least one wire from each category.

The choice of initial wire depends upon the proximal cap morphology and course of the CTO segment. Different CTO crossing techniques have been described, and three commonly used methods are the loose tracking/sliding technique, the drilling/redirecting method, and the penetration method for crossing the wire intimally. In subintimal tracking, the knuckle wiring technique can be used in cases of long, angulated, and calcified lesions. Usually, a hydrophilic or polymer jacketed intermediate nontapered is preferred for knuckling. **Table 1** summarizes the different CTO wires and their indications. We should have a low threshold to switch to the appropriate wire with the appropriate shape for each proximal cap puncture, CTO body crossing, and distal true lumen exit.

Microcatheters

Backup support is the secret to good wire control and penetration force. It is always better to improve backup support before increasing wire penetration force. A high penetration force (HPF) wire without good backup support becomes uncontrollable and is, therefore, dangerous. Microcatheters increase backup support and are useful in CTO procedures for wire exchange without losing vessel access.

They can be categorized into single-lumen, double-lumen, and special catheters designed for specific purposes.[4]

- *Single-lumen microcatheters (SLMs):* SLMs are standard microcatheters intended to provide good support, improve guidewire penetration power, and exchange or reshape guidewires without sacrificing access.
    - The FineCross microcatheter (Terumo, Japan) is a low-profile tapered-end microcatheter with a short distal tapered end and an outer

TABLE 1: Properties of guidewires.

Wire	*Core*	*Tip*	*Tip coat*	*Tip diameter (inches)*	*Tip load (g)*	*Polymer coating*	*Radiopaque length (mm)*	*Comments*
Sion black	High tensile steel	Dual-core coil 200 mm	Hydrophilic	0.014	0.5	Yes	30	Lower tip load
Gaia first	Stainless steel	Composite core, Micro-cone tip	Hydrophilic	0.010	1.7	No	150	Torqueable wire, main feature is composite coil with a central core wire wrapped by six acetone wires, with spring coil in periphery
Gaia second	Stainless steel	Composite core, micro-cone tip	Hydrophilic	0.011	3.5	No	150	1-mm preshaped
Gaia third	Stainless steel	Composite core, micro-cone tip	Hydrophilic	0.012	4.5	No	150	1-mm preshaped
Gaia Next First	Stainless steel	Xtrand coil, micro-cone tip	Hydrophilic	0.011	2.0	No	150	Hydrophilic 40 cm with uncoated distal tip, lower risk of wire damage
Gaia next second	Stainless steel	Xtrand coil, micro-cone tip	Hydrophilic	0.012	4.0	No	150	Hydrophilic 40 cm with uncoated distal tip
Gaia next third	Stainless steel	Xtrand coil, micro-cone tip	Hydrophilic	0.012	6.0	No	150	Hydrophilic 40 cm with uncoated distal tip
Gladius mongo	Stainless steel		Hydrophilic	0.014	3	Yes	30	Polymer jacket and hydrophilic, subintimal space advancement

Contd...

Contd…

Wire	*Core*	*Tip*	*Tip coat*	*Tip diameter (inches)*	*Tip load (g)*	*Polymer coating*	*Radiopaque length (mm)*	*Comments*
Ultimate Bros 3	Stainless steel	Core to tip design	Hydrophilic	0.014	3		110	Hydrophilic with uncoated distal tip
Choice PT	Unibody stainless steel	No coil	Hydrophilic	0.014	2.1	Yes	350	
Pilot 150	High tensile steel (Durasteel)	45 mm coil	Hydrophilic	0.014	2.5	Yes, 290 mm	30	Hydrophilic wire
Pilot 200	High tensile steel (Durasteel)	45 mm coil	Hydrophilic	0.014	3.9	Yes, 290 mm	30	
Fielder FC	Stainless steel	110 mm spring coil	Hydrophilic	0.014	0.8	Yes, 220 mm	30	Polymer jacket, useful in highly tortuous or stenosed lesions
Fielder XT	Stainless steel	110 mm spring coil	Hydrophilic	0.009	0.8	Yes, 220 mm	160	Good choice for narrow channel crossing
Fielder XT-R	Stainless steel	Composite coil, 160 mm	Hydrophilic	0.010	0.6	Yes, 170 mm	160	Fielder family but composite coil, microchannel crossing
Fielder XT-A	Stainless steel	Composite coil, 160 mm	Hydrophilic	0.010	1	Yes, 170 mm	160	Fielder family but composite coil, tapered proximal cap of CTO
Cross-IT 100XT	Stainless steel	300 mm coil	Hydrophilic	0.0105	1.7	No	30	
Cross-IT 200XT	Stainless steel	300 mm coil	Hydrophilic	0.0105	4.7	No	30	

Contd…

Contd…

Wire	*Core*	*Tip*	*Tip coat*	*Tip diameter (inches)*	*Tip load (g)*	*Polymer coating*	*Radiopaque length (mm)*	*Comments*
Cross-IT 300XT	Stainless steel	300 mm coil	Hydrophilic	0.0105	6.2	No	30	
Cross-IT 400XT	Stainless steel	300 mm coil	Hydrophilic	0.0105	8.7	No	30	
Miracle Brother-3	Stainless steel	110 mm spring coil	Hydrophobic	0.014	3.9	No	110	Hydrophobic (silicone), useful in lesions at a bend or some tortuosity
Miracle Brother-4.5	Stainless steel	110 mm spring coil	Hydrophobic	0.014	4.4	No	110	Hydrophobic (silicone)
Miracle Brother-6	Stainless steel	110 mm spring coil	Hydrophobic	0.014	8.8	No	110	Hydrophobic (silicone)
Miracle Brother-12	Stainless steel	110 mm spring coil	Hydrophobic	0.014	13	No	110	Hydrophobic (silicone)
Conquest 9	Stainless steel	200 mm coil	Hydrophobic	0.009	8.6	No	200	Hydrophilic with uncoated distal tip
Conquest 12	Stainless steel	200 mm coil	Hydrophobic	0.009	12	No	200	Hydrophilic with uncoated distal tip
Conquest Pro 9	Stainless steel	200 mm coil	Hydrophilic	0.009	9.3	No	200	Distal most 1 mm of tip is uncoated
Conquest Pro 12	Stainless steel	200 mm coil	Hydrophilic	0.009	12	No	200	Distal most 1 mm of tip is uncoated
Conquest Pro 8–20	Stainless steel	200 mm coil	Hydrophilic	0.008	20	No	200	Highest penetrating wire
RG3	Stainless steel	80 mm platinum coil	Hydrophilic	0.010	3	No	30	For externalization

diameter of 1.8 Fr. This makes navigating tortuous but short vessel segments easy due to the coating of polytetrafluoroethylene (PTFE). Further, it has a distal tip marker. The catheter is advanced simply by *threading* over the fixed guidewire.

- Corsair (Asahi, Japan) has a "SHINKA" shaft with 10 stainless steel (8 thin and 2 thick) braided wires that enable high push and rotational manipulation. This maneuvering is further enhanced by 60 cm of distal hydrophilic coating with a distal soft tungsten tip. The microcatheter is advanced by rotating motion, but overtorque may lead to kinking.
- The Caravel (Asahi, Japan) microcatheter is a low-profile, specially-designed microcatheter for negotiating collaterals, microchannels, and tortuous small-caliber vessels. It supports only push movement and is a nontorque microcatheter.
- The SuperCross microcatheter has an angulated distal end, facilitating difficult or angulated wiring more easily. It sometimes scores better than a double-lumen catheter, avoiding reverse wire shaping (resulting in wire torque loss).[5]
- The Turnpike microcatheter has a unique five-layered design with a dual-layer bidirectional central coil, enabling better torque transfer from hub to tip. It is useful for navigating tortuous and highly stenotic lesions.
- The Tornus microcatheter (by Asahi, Japan) has eight distinct spirally wound stainless steel wires in its middle layer with tapered distal parts. The catheter is negotiated with anticlockwise rotations for a maximum of 20 rotations, after which it must be released to prevent wire fractures. Due to its limited length, it is preferred for an antegrade CTO approach rather than retrograde and works well with resistant CTO lesions.

Other microcatheters, such as MAMBA Flex (Boston, USA), Teleport (Cardiovascular, USA), and MicroCross (Roxwood, USA), are less often used due to limited availability.

The comparative properties of these SLMs are summarized in **Table 2**.

- *Double-lumen microcatheters (DLMs):* DLMs are specially designed with two lumens, one for a rapid delivery system over which it threaded onto the guidewire in place, and the other lumen is over the wire (OTW) to introduce the second purposed guidewire, thus facilitating simultaneous and independent maneuvering of two different guidewires. There are two radiopaque markers denoting exit ports of two lumens **(Fig. 1)**.[6]

  These DLMs include Twin-Pass (by Teleflex, USA), SASUKE (Asahi, Japan), Crusade (Kaneka, Japan), FineDuo (Terumo, Japan), ReCross (IMDS, Netherlands) and NHancer (IMDS, Netherlands).[4]
- *Special catheters:*
  - The CrossBoss and Stingray catheter (Boston, USA) are used in subintimal reentry. CrossBoss is a microcatheter with a distal

TABLE 2: Single-lumen microcatheter characteristics and advancement technique.

Trade name/ properties	*Distal tip*	*Distinguishing properties*	*Available lengths*	*Advancement*
Finecross (Terumo, Japan)	1.8 Fr	Short distal tapered profile	130 cm, 150 cm	Nontorqueable
Corsair Pro (Asahi, Japan)	1.3 Fr with distal shaft profile of 2.6 Fr	"Shinka" shaft with distal long tapered end	135 cm, 150 cm	Torqueable
Corsair Pro XS (Asahi, Japan)	1.3 Fr with distal shaft profile of 2.1 Fr	"Shinka" shaft with lower profile and more flexible tip	135 cm, 150 cm	Torqueable
Caravel (Asahi, Japan)	1.4 with distal shaft profile of 1.9 Fr	Low profile	135 cm, 150 cm	Nontorqueable
Supercross (Teleflex, USA)	1.8 Fr	Distal angulated segment	130 cm, 150 cm	Nontorqueable
Turn pike (Teleflex, USA)	1.6 Fr with distal shaft of 2.6 Fr	Dual-layered central coil	135 cm, 150 cm	Torqueable
Turnpike LP (Teleflex, USA)	1.6 Fr tip with distal shaft of 2.2 Fr	Lower profile and more flexibility with ability to negotiate extreme tortuosities	135 cm, 150 cm	Torqueable

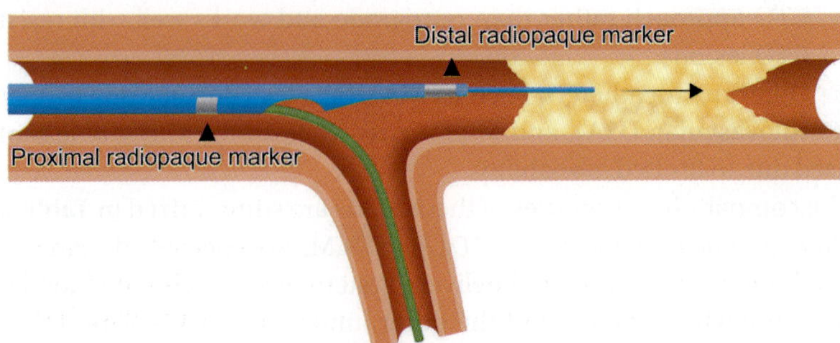

Fig. 1: Pictorial representation of double lumen catheter Crusade microcatheter with one monorail wire and other over the wire (OTW) exit port.

blunt end and a multiwire core that enables rapid rotation, causing controlled dissection at the distal end without causing hematoma, a technique employed in antegrade dissection and reentry. Stingray has a distally placed balloon with the central lumen connected with two communicating side port exits on either side of the distal balloon.

The side ports are identifiable with radiopaque markers and enable guidewire negotiation at an angle from the central lumen **(Figs. 2A and B)**. Stingray and CrossBoss catheters work as a system for the antegrade dissection and reentry technique. CrossBoss achieves blunt dissection and drilling in the subintimal plane, and a steering guidewire from the appropriate side port of the Stingray catheter manages further reentry into the true lumen.

- ReCross catheter (IMDS, Netherlands) is a dual-lumen OTW microcatheter with a low crossing profile. It has two distinct OTW lumens and three exit ports, enabling the operator to navigate through CTO from different angles (180° apart) **(Figs. 2A and B)**. This helps in the hematoma decompression, subintimal guidewire redirection, reentry of the wire from the subintimal space to the intimal lumen.

Selection of microcatheter: Selection of microcatheter for a particular case scenario factors variables such as tortuosity of the vessel, complexity of the

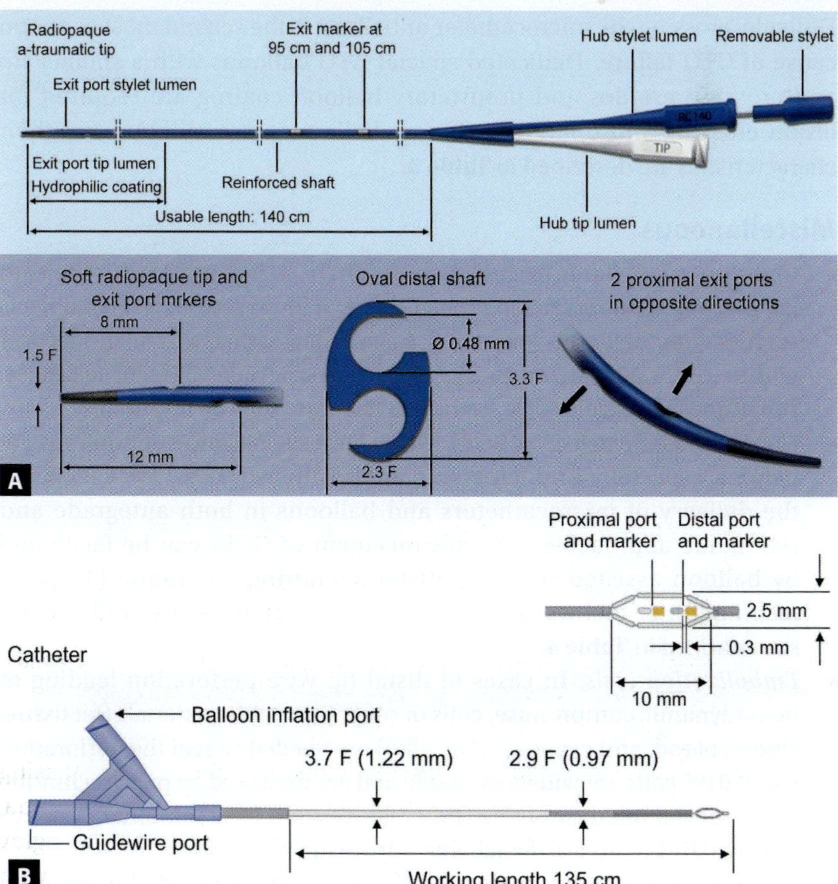

Figs. 2A and B: (A) ReCross microcatheter; (B) Stingray balloon showing the exit port.

CTO lesion, presence/absence of severe calcium, angulation involving the entry into CTO lesion, guidewire distal tip diameter, distal tip and shaft profile of the microcatheter, and technique employed (antegrade wire escalation/ antegrade dissection and reentry/retrograde).[4]

Employing long tapered tip profile microcatheters such as Caravel and Corsair for narrow, long channels/long tortuous vessels are recommended. On the other hand, CTO lesion in an ectatic vessel or maneuvering in a shorter segment requires the use of a short-tapered tip microcatheter like FineCross.

Angulated microcatheters like SuperCross can help negotiate lesions at angulation or in proximal tortuous vessels with an angulated distal tip profile.

In the antegrade parallel wiring approach, DLM-like Crusade can help with entry into the true lumen plane. Low-profile catheters such as Caravel and Corsair support wire crossing through collaterals for retrograde CTO procedures.

Low-profile Special Balloon

Difficulty crossing the microcatheter or balloon is the second most common cause of CTO failure. Dedicated special CTO balloons with a smaller tip and crossing profiles and proprietary balloon coating are required for lesion crossing and dilation. Different balloons are available, and their characteristics are described in **Table 3**.

Miscellaneous

- *Coronary snare:* Endovascular and coronary snares must be in the cath lab inventory. Retrieval and repositioning of intravascular foreign objects such as coils, balloons, lost stents, fragmented catheters, and guidewires within the cardiovascular system. In retrograde CTO procedures, sometimes retrograde wire snaring in the aorta may be required.
- *Guide catheter extension (GCE):* GCEs increase backup support and are helpful, especially in uncrossable and tortuous CTOs.[7] They facilitate the delivery of microcatheters and balloons in both antegrade and retrograde approaches. The advancement of GCEs can be facilitated by balloon-assisted tracking, distal anchoring technique (Torpedo technique), or inchworming method. The various GCEs available are summarized in **Table 4**.
- *Embolization coils:* In cases of distal tip wire perforation leading to hemodynamic compromise, coils or other injectable materials (fat tissue, clotted blood, and cyanoacrylate glue) are needed to seal the perforation site. 0.018″ coils are widely available and are delivered by push technique using special microcatheters (Progreat, Terumo Interventional Systems, Japan). 0.014″ coils are detachable but are more expensive.
- *Covered stents:* Coronary perforation is a most dreaded complication in CTO PCIs and can be seen in up to 5–6% of cases. It is usually due to

TABLE 3: Low-profile special balloon for CTO crossing.

	Tip profile	*Crossing profile*	*Diameter*	*Length*	*Maker*	*Special characteristics*
NIC Nano	0.016″	0.019″	0.85 mm	6 mm	SIS medical, Switzerland	Proximal single radiopaque—better crossability, high rated burst pressure (RBP)
ACROSS CTO RX	0.016″ with 4 mm distal tip	0.87 mm	0.83 mm	10 mm	Acrostak, CH, Switzerland	Short tip (ST) model, good performance in tortuous and calcified lesions
ACROSS CTO OTW	0.016″ with 4 mm distal tip	1.16 mm	0.87 mm	10 mm, 15 mm, 20 mm	Acrostak, CH, Switzerland	Improved force transmission and high pushability
SAPPHIRE-II PRO	1.75 mm with distal tip length 1.5–2.5 mm	2 mm	1.75 mm	10 mm	OrbusNeich, Netherlands	Hydrophilic distal shaft for better crossability
Ikazuchi zero	0.78 mm	0.78 mm	1 mm	6 mm	Kaneka Medicals, Japan	Good option of the microcatheter uncrossable lesion
RYUREI	1 mm	0.41 mm	1 mm	5 mm	Terumo, Japan	Excellent trackability and crossability
ALVEO HP 0.75	0.0156″	0.0184″	0.75 mm	5 mm, 8 mm, 10 mm, 12 mm	Brosmed Medical, China	Ultra-low tip profile with high RBP of 20 atm, good in calcified lesions

(CTO: chronic total occlusion)

TABLE 4: Properties of various guide extension catheters.

S. No.	*Feature*	*GuideLiner V3*	*GuideZilla II*	*Telescope*	*GuidePlus II ST*	*GuidePlus II EL*	*TrapLiner*
1	Tip OD (inch) and compatible guide catheter	0.053″ (5 F), 0.063″ (5.5 F), 0.067″ (6 F), 0.075″ (7 F), 0.085″ (8 F)	0.06″ (6 F), 0.073″ (7 F), 0.083″ (8 F)	0.067″ (6 F), 075″ (7 F)	0.06″ (6 F)	0.07″ (6 F)	0.067″ (6 F), 0.075″ (7 F), 0.085″ (8 F)
2	Catheter ID (inch) and compatible guide catheter	0.046″ (5 F), 0.051″ (5.5 F), 0.056″ (6 F), 0.062″ (7 F), 0.071″ (8 F)	0.057″ (6 F), 0.063 (7 F), 0.072 (8 F)	0.056″ (6 F), 0.062″ (7 F)	0.052″ (6 F)	0.056″ (6 F)	6 Fr. (0.070″), 7 Fr. (0.078″), 8 Fr (0.088″)
3	Catheter type	Straight	Straight	Straight	Tapered—5.3 F to 4.7 F	Tapered—5.5 F to 5 F	Straight
4	Coating	Silicone wipe	Z glide hydrophilic coating	Hydrophilic coating	Hydrophilic coating	Hydrophilic coating	Hydrophilic coating
5	Available size (F)	5, 5.5, 6, 7, 8	6, 6 F Long, 7, 8	6, 7	6	6	6, 7, 8
6	Rapid exchange length (cm)	25	25 (standard), 40 (6 F long)	25	25	25	13
7	Working length (cm)	150	150	150	145	145	150
8	Marker	Metallic	Metallic	Metallic	Nonmetallic resin	Nonmetallic resin	Nonmetallic resin

oversizing a balloon or subintimal balloon dilation at high pressures. In cases of hemodynamic collapse with type 3 coronary perforation, a covered stent needs to be deployed.

- *Imaging:* Intravascular imaging [intravascular ultrasound (IVUS) and Optical coherence tomography (OCT)] guides us in the pre-assessment of lesion morphology and optimal stent deployment. In cases of CTO PCIs, IVUS helps in the side branch method to identify the proximal cap in ambiguous cap morphology lesions. IVUS identification and differentiation of true vessel lumen from false lumen, thereby assisting reentry into the true lumen with a guidewire. IVUS-guided subintimal reentry can be tried as a last resort to get a subintimal wire into the distal true lumen.

Thus, to summarize, the development and evolution of contemporary guidewires and microcatheters have been parallel and often played a crucial role in the success of these procedures. Technical and procedural success rates have risen tremendously over the past few years due to operator experience, improved equipment, refinements of the retrograde approach, and the introduction of "putting it all together". Ensuring the inventory availability discussed earlier can achieve a good CTO PCI success rate and a decreased risk of complications.

REFERENCES

1. Wu EB, Brilakis E, Mashayekhi K, Tsuchikane E, Alaswad K, et al. Global Chronic Total Occlusion Crossing Algorithm: JACC State-of-the-Art Review. J Am Coll Cardiol. 2021;78(8):840-53.
2. Dash D. Interventional Management of "Balloon-Uncrossable" Coronary Chronic Total Occlusion: Is There Any Way Out? Korean Circ J. 2018;48(4):e53.
3. Wu EB, Tsuchikane E, Sidney Lo, Lim ST, Ge L, Chen JY, et al. Chronic Total Occlusion Wiring: A State-of-the-Art Guide From The Asia Pacific Chronic Total Occlusion Club. Heart Lung and Circ. 2019;28:1490-500.
4. Vemmou E, Nikolakopoulos I, Xenogiannis I, Megaly M, Hall A, Wang Y, et al. Recent advances in microcatheter technology for the treatment of chronic total occlusions. Expert Rev Med Devices. 2019;16(4):267-73.
5. Chan YH, Cheng VYH, Wong CW, Lam CS. A simplified reverse wire technique using an angulated supercross microcatheter. Catheter Cardiovasc Interv. 2020;96(1):E93-7.
6. Oreglia JA, Garbo R, Gagnor A, Gasparini GL. Dual lumen microcatheters for complex percutaneous coronary interventions. Cardiovasc Revasc Med. 2018;19(3 Pt A):298-305.
7. Garbo R, Iannaccone M, Werner GS, Mashayekhi K, Boudou N, Bufe A, et al. Utility of Guiding Catheter Extensions for Recanalization of Chronic Total Occlusions: A EuroCTO Club Expert Panel Report. JACC Cardiovasc Interv. 2023;16(15):1833-44.

CHAPTER 27

Chronic Total Occlusion Wiring: A State-of-the-Art Guide

Surya Prakash

INTRODUCTION

Due to advances in wire technology, in terms of better torque transmission, penetration force and wire control, the success rate of antegrade approach has increased significantly. Wiring technique remains a core part of chronic total occlusion (CTO) intervention. The aim of this chapter is to review this CTO wiring techniques systematically.

CHRONIC TOTAL OCCLUSION WIRES

Simple method of classifying CTO wires as high penetration force (HPF), intermediate penetration force (IPF), and low penetration force (LPF) depends upon tip load and further divided as blunt or tapered tip **(Table 1)**[1] and **Table 2**[2] gives additional information above polymer jacket.

BASICS OF A WIRING

Chronic total occlusion wires usually have primary curve of 40–60° within 1 mm of tip, and a variable secondary curve made 4–6 mm proximal to primary curve. Primary curve preshaped in Gaia series, whereas secondary curves angles made depending on angle between proximal vessel and CTO

TABLE 1: Classification of wires into high, intermediate, and low penetration force and blunt versus tapered tip.

	Blunt tip	*Tapered tip*
High penetration force	Miracle 12 g	Gaia Third, Gaia Next Third, Conquest or Confianza Pro 9 g, 12 g, 8/20, and Hornet 14
Intermediate penetration force	Ultimate Bros 3 g and Pilot 200	Gaia Second and Gaia Next Second
Low penetration force	Pilot 50 and Fielder FC	XTA, XTR, XT, and Fighter

Note: Miracle 12 g, Gaia Third, Next Third, Conquest or Confianza Pro 9 g, 12 g, 8/20, Ultimate Bros 3 g, Gaia Second, Gaia Next Second, Fielder FC, XTA, XTR, XT—Asahi Intecc. Pilot 200, Pilot 50—Abbott Vascular, St Paul, MN, USA. Hornet 14, Fighter—Boston Scientific.

TABLE 2: Wire category.

Wire category	*Wire name*	*Polymer jacket*	*Tapered tip (inch)*	*Tip load (gf)*	*Manufacturer*
Low penetration force	Fielder XT*	✓	0.009	0.8	Asahi Intecc
	Fielder XT-R*	✓	0.010	0.6	Asahi Intecc
	Fielder XT-A*	✓	0.010	1.0	Asahi Intecc
	Pilot 50	✓	×	1.5	Abbott Vascular
	Fighter	✓	0.009	1.5	Boston Scientific
	Hornet	×	0.008	1.0	Boston Scientific
	Gaia 1st	×	0.010	1.7	Asahi Intecc
	Cross-it 100XT	×	0.010	2.0	Abbott Vascular
Intermediate penetration force	Pilot 150	✓	×	2.7	Abbott Vascular
	Pilot 200*	✓	×	4.1	Abbott Vascular
	Gladius	✓	×	3.0	Asahi Intecc
	Miracle 3	×	×	3.0	Asahi Intecc
	Ultimate 3*	×	×	3.0	Asahi Intecc
	Gaia 2nd*	×	0.010	3.5	Asahi Intecc
	Cross-it 200	×	0.011	3.0	Abbott Vascular
High penetration force	Conquest Pro*	✓	0.009	9.0	Asahi Intecc
	Conquest Pro 12*	✓	0.009	12.0	Asahi Intecc
	Gaia 3rd*	×	0.012	4.5	Asahi Intecc
	Hornet 10	×	0.008	10.0	Boston Scientific
	Hornet 14	×	0.008	14.0	Boston Scientific
	PROGRESS 200T	×	0.009	13.0	Abbott Vascular
	Miracle 12	×	×	12.0	Asahi Intecc

*Most commonly used guidewires

body so called angle of attack (AOA). If AOA is steep, then acute secondary curve is given. Before escalating wire to HPF always ensure solid backup support of guide catheter (e.g., Amplatzer), adequate microcatheter support, a side branch balloon anchor support if feasible or even guide extension catheters also. Going on escalating wire to HPF without addressing the earlier mentioned issue is as bad as firing in the dark.

ANTEGRADE WIRING

Proximal Cap

As shown in **Flowchart 1**, the morphology of proximal cap decides the wire selection. Tapered proximal cap with residual channels wire of choice is XT-R (Asahi Intecc). In tapered proximal cap without residual channel, the wire of choice is XT-A (Asahi Intecc). In blunt cap, a HPF wire is usually helpful. Order of escalation of wire for puncturing proximal cap is IPF blunt, HPF blunt, and HPF tapered.

Flowchart 1: Algorithm for CTO crossing.[2]

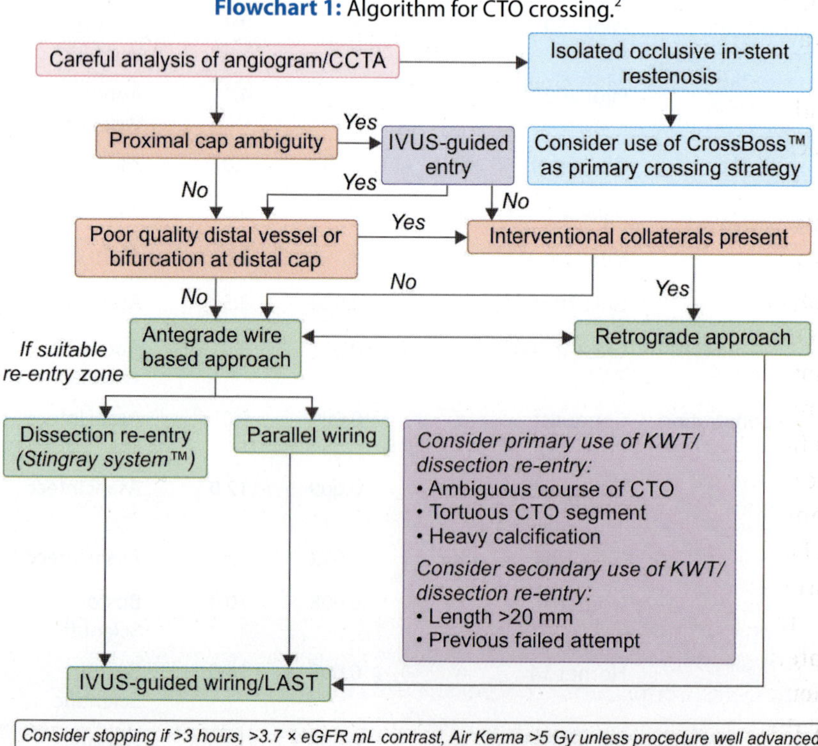

(CCTA: coronary computed tomography angiography; CTO: chronic total occlusion; eGFR: estimated glomerular filtration rate; IVUS: intravascular ultrasound; KWT: knuckle wire technique; LAST: limited antegrade subintimal tracking)

When you encounter blunt proximal cap, and if there is a side branch nearby, use it for intravascular ultrasound (IVUS) or a dual lumen catheter. The latter for better support as well as directing the penetration force of HPF wire. Use penetrating force for tips to enter cap, till the secondary curve, after this further use of penetrating force may direct primary curve into subintimal space.

CHRONIC TOTAL OCCLUSION BODY WIRING

Aims of CTO body crossing includes (1) get to the distal cap, (2) no wire perforation outside the vessel architecture, (3) avoid a wire going into the subintimal space, (4) avoid enlarging the subintimal space and forming a hematoma, and (5) avoid enlarging the peri-wire space, which reduces antegrade wire control.

Avoiding wire perforations and getting into distal cap are predictors of CTO success, however last three aims (3, 4, and 5) can be ignored when dealing CTOs which have ambiguous course, calcific, and are tortuous, here intentional subintimal wiring is advised to get into distal true lumen in order to avoid perforation. One such example is knuckle wire technique.

Three methods of CTO crossing explained by Sumitsuji et al.,[3] are loose body tracking, intentional intraplaque tracking, and intentional subintimal tracking.

Loose Body Tracking

As the name suggests wire will track the loose tissue within the CTO body, polymer jacketed wires of LPF namely XT-A series, are the wire of choice. SION Black can also be used for this purpose. Very important to use rotational movement and allow torque to transmit to tip, this itself generates minimal force enough to track down the loose tissue, in other way allow the "wire to finds its way". Never use push force with XT-A wire, because of soft tip it loops and forms peri-wire space, which eventually results in losing the wire control. Other popular wire for this purpose is Pilot wire (Abbott Vascular, St Paul, Minnesota, USA). It has stiffer tip than XT-A which results in less-loop forming tendency.

In case if you are suspicious of wire position in subintimal space or entering side branch then simply redirect. If you encounter resistance, then ensure better support either by adjusting guide catheter position or by threading down the microcatheter till the tip of wire. In spite of these measures, if you are not progressing that means you are hitting the hard plaque, and that is the time to escalate wire to IPF or HPF, so called intentional intimal plaque tracking.

Intentional Intimal Plaque Tracking

Loose tissue tracking fails when you come across continuous hard plaque path and tortuosity. Unlike in loose tissue tracking, knowing anatomical course of CTO is very important for intimal plaque tracking success. There are three ways to know about this: (1) Pre-procedural computed tomography angiography (CTA), gives idea about course; (2) IVUS guided, directing of wire; and (3) knowing calcium course on fluoroscopy. Going forward the best way is to have CTA and fluoroscopy interface images to exactly guide the path (possible in near future). We use IVSU guide, when first wire inadvertently enters the subintimal space, here 1.5 mm balloon tracked before advancing the IVUS catheter over subintimal wire, then second wire is used for intimal tracking under IVUS guidance. Note in this technique there is always risk of subintimal space expansion, because of hematoma after IVUS catheter placement. For most well-trained eyes the calcium on fluoroscopy gives best guess of CTO path; however, knowledge of CTA beforehand will be much helpful. HPF wires are commonly used, because of calcium and tortuosity, HPF wire usually finds subintimal path, which forms spiral cage around the vessel, keeping this wire in situ (acts as roadmap), take another wire to find intimal path.

Why it is Important to Step-up or Step-down in Intimal Plaque Tracking?

Whenever resistance is felt, the wire is abutting the hard plaque, then advance microcatheter till tip of wire, exchange wire to HPF, once progress is made, step down to IPF/LPF to continue tissue tracking. Idea is to enter distal true lumen.

■ INTRAVASCULAR ULTRASOUND GUIDED

A 1.5 mm balloon inflated on the subintimal wire, then IVUS catheter parked, under its guidance a second wire—preferably Conquest and Confianza (Asahi Intecc). Because of soft core, the Gaia wires have tendency to prolapse into subintimal space therefore not the preferred second wire in IVUS-guided intimal plaque tracking.

Why Intimal Plaque Tracking Less Successful?

- Imprecise knowledge of CTO course (unless there is CT and fluoroscopy superimposition), ambiguity, and tortuosity.
- HPF most often prolapses into subintimal space, causing expansion and hematoma formation without the knowledge of operator.
- It is time consuming. Keep a check on radiation dose and duration.

For reasons earlier mentioned, experienced operators skip intimal tracking when loose tissue wiring fails and proceed to subintimal tracking (stingray re-entry or knuckle wire).

ANTEGRADE SUBINTIMAL TRACKING

"Long plus" CTO constitutes long length of CTO, presence of calcium, tortuosity, and ambiguity of course of CTO. In this particular subset, antegrade subintimal tracking works better with low risk of complication. Wire of choice is IPF hydrophilic coated or polymer jacketed. Wire is manipulated to direct into subintimal space, not to use strong pushing force in order to avoid perforation. Another way is to form wire knuckle, which is discussed in detail in later part of this chapter.

CROSSING THE DISTAL CAP

One needs to identify the hard distal cap by following characteristics:

- Rounded distal cap
- Presence of large side branch as distal cap
- Rapid filling of distal cap by well-formed collaterals (good collateral reconstituted pressure hardens the distal cap)
- Presence of calcium

Track microcatheter all the way till distal cap, then use HPF wires preferably Conquest or Confianza Pro 9 g, 12 g, or Hornet 14 or Conquest Pro. Wire of good torque and force transmission is the key. Gaia 3 next also fulfills these criteria; however, because of slippery tip it finds way into subintima.

What to do when Antegrade Wire Fails to Puncture into Distal True Lumen? (Flowchart 2)

- Redirection
- Parallel wire
- Stingray

Flowchart 2: Various dissection re-entry techniques.

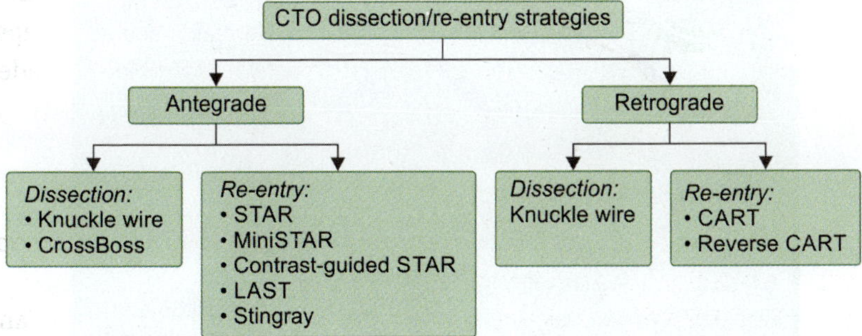

(CART: controlled antegrade and retrograde tracking; CTO: chronic total occlusion; LAST: limited antegrade subintimal tracking)

Redirection

In this technique, redirect the wire from subintimal space into true lumen. Mainly works when wire is near to the distal true lumen which is of good size and not much wiring done beforehand (short length CTO) without much tortuosity. Always keep low threshold to shift to parallel wire or stingray. If redirection fails, it often results in expansion of subintimal space.

Parallel Wire

First wire which is in subintimal space now acts as roadmap to use second wire. Using this roadmap primary, secondary wire directed into the body of CTO.

Feature favoring use of parallel wiring are:

- Identified wire deflection point into sub-intimal space
- Heavy calcification and/or diffusely diseased distal bed
- Important side branch near distal cap

Stingray System (Fig. 1)

Salient features of Stingray system are:

- Flat balloon
- One exit each side
- 3.2Fr shaft
- Stingray guidewire's angled tip and distal probe
- Two radiopaque marker bands for exact placement

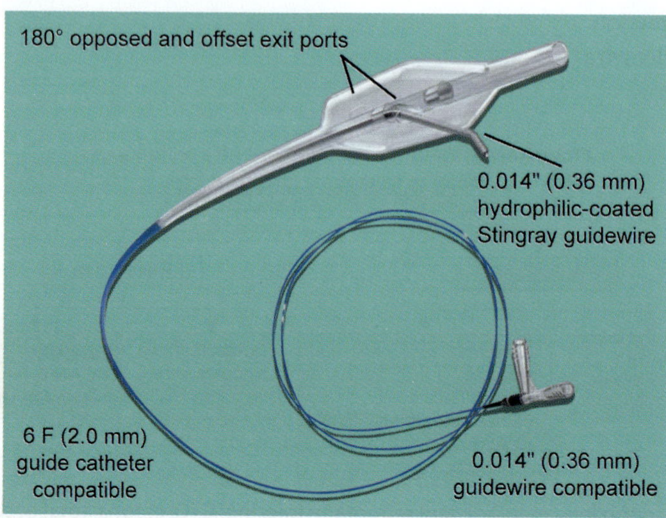

Fig. 1: Stingray CTO re-entry system.

- 014” guidewire compatible
- 6 Fr guide catheter compatible

Features favoring the use of Stingray are:

- Ambiguous vessel course
- Long, calcified, and tortuous CTO lesion
- If wire is in subintimal space at the proximal cap
- Good landing zone without a major side branch and calcification
- Tip of wire is <500 μm from distal true lumen

KNUCKLE WIRE TECHNIQUE (FIGS. 2A TO C)

Polymer jacket or hydrophilic wires with LPF like XT-A, SION black (Asahi Intecc), and the Pilot series (Abbott Vascular, Santa Clara, CA, USA) are best suited for knuckle wiring. To create a knuckle, the wire must loop on itself such that the leading edge is usually the junction between the stiff shaft and the floppy distal segment **(Fig. 2B)**. The knuckle loop can be initiated by preshaping the wire tip as an “umbrella handle” and by applying forward pressure on the wire once it is within the CTO **(Fig. 2A)**. Never rotate wire at this stage to avoid knot formation.

Always advance the knuckle wire over the microcatheter for following reasons:

- As shown in **Figure 3**, to control the knuckle width and length
- If wire gets stuck or broken within the calcific segment
- To exchange for HPF wire for re-entry into distal true lumen once knuckle wire crosses the CTO segment.

Further advancement of knuckle should be done keeping the microcatheter near the junction of stiff and floppy junction (knuckle point),

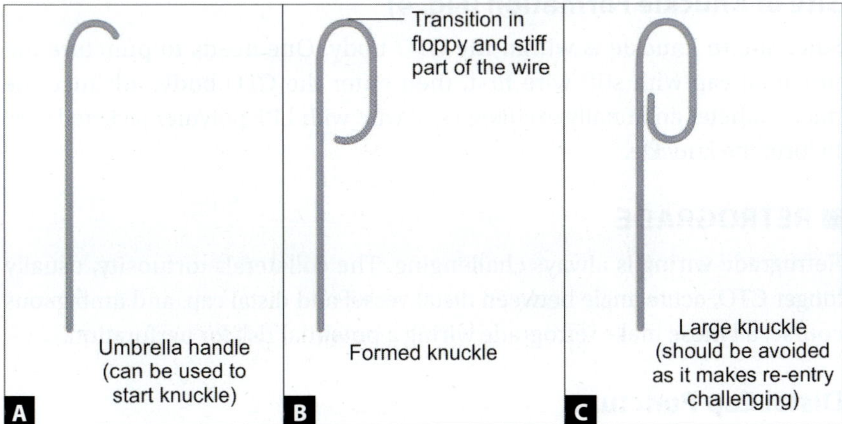

Figs. 2A to C: Wire and tip shaping. (A) Umbrella handle; (B) Formed knuckle; (C) Large knuckle.[4]

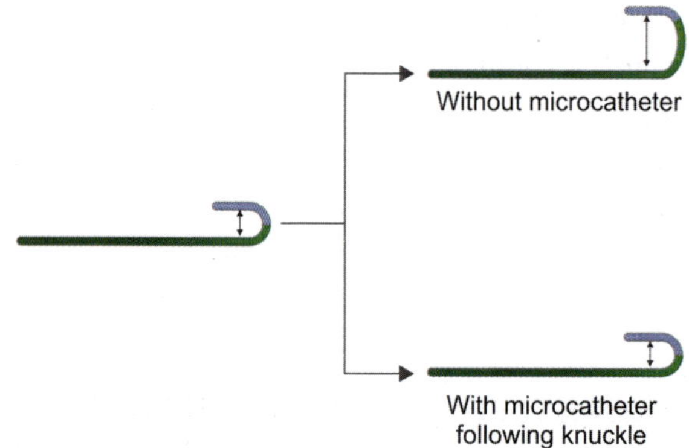

Fig. 3: Controlling the knuckle.[4]

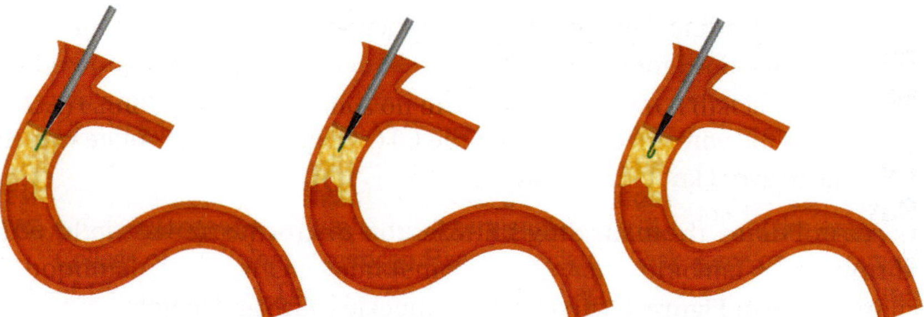

Fig. 4: Puncture of proximal cap with stiffer wire over microcatheter allows exchange of it to low penetration force (LPF) for knuckle formation.[4]

if this is not followed the knuckle shifts proximal to stiffer part, which in turn widens the knuckle and split open the vessel **(Fig. 3)**.

Site of Knuckle Formation (Fig. 4)

Safer site to knuckle is within the CTO body. One needs to puncture the proximal cap with stiff wire first, then enter the CTO body, advance the microcatheter and finally exchange stiff wire with LPF polymer jacketed wire to form the knuckle.

RETROGRADE

Retrograde wiring is always challenging. The collaterals tortuosity, usually longer CTO, acute angle between distal vessel and distal cap, and ambiguous course, all these make retrograde wiring a potential risk for perforation.

Distal Cap Puncture

Usually distal cap is softer, LPF with tapered tip usually (XT-A) is first wire of choice.

Rarely, the distal cap is tough which requires HPF wire with microcatheter support. Even the presence of significant side branch at distal cap often results in prolapse of LPF wire into it. One can use IPF wire stiffer pre-tip shaft like pilot 200 (Abbott Vascular) or even UB-3 (Asahi Intecc) is also suitable for this purpose. Other way is to use low profile dual lumen catheter like Sasuke (Asahi Intecc), in which one can step up the wire to HPF (rarely required) wires like Confianza 12 or Conquest Pro.

Retrograde Chronic Total Occlusion Body Wiring

Loose tissue tracking, first method used to wire the body. Being retrograde advantages are softer distal end and retroflex angle of side branches (rarely the wire prolapses to these branches). Most of the times wiring is successful by this method.

In long plus CTO's (length >20 mm, ambiguous course, tortuosity, and calcification) best method is subintimal tracking (less time/radiation and also less perforation risk).

Reverse Controlled Antegrade and Retrograde Tracking Wiring

For successful reverse CART, wire of choice is often HPF with excellent direction control (like Gaia 2 and 3). Antegrade wire being intraplaque and retrograde wire in subintimal space, the retrograde wire is simply directed toward the end of inflated balloon on antegrade wire, so called "end balloon wiring". If this technique fails, then "side balloon entry" technique used, in which antegrade wire balloon inflated and retrograde wire is directed facing the side of inflated balloon, the moment balloon is deflated a void is created and retrograde wire is simply pushed into this void to complete so called "directed reverse CART" **(Figs. 5A to F)**.

Rendezvous and Tip-in Technique

One important step of CTO retrograde wiring is externalization of retrograde wire. At times it is difficult, in such cases we can adopt tip-in technique or Rendezvous technique.

Tip-in Method

The retrograde wire is advanced into antegrade microcatheter within the antegrade guide catheter.

Rendezvous Technique

An antegrade wire is advanced into the retrograde microcatheter.

In both these techniques, retrograde system now converted into antegrade to finally complete the procedure.

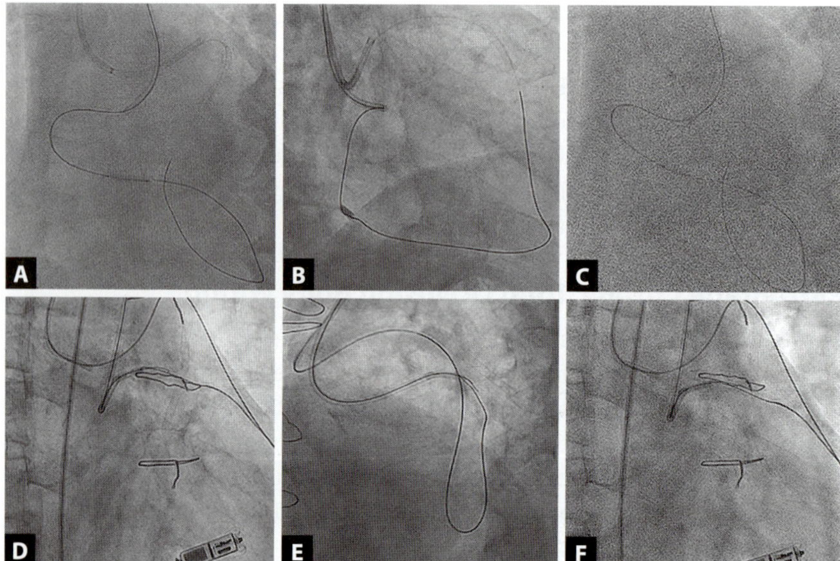

Figs. 5A to F: Directed reverse controlled antegrade and retrograde tracking (CART) methods. (A) End balloon wiring left anterior oblique view; (B) End balloon wiring right anterior oblique view; (C) Successful end balloon wiring; (D) Side balloon entry technique; (E) Side balloon entry in orthogonal view; (F) Successful side balloon entry.

Tip Detection Method

The tip detection process entails maneuvering the transducer between the distal tip and the transition point of the guidewire's tip and shaft. This allows for the visual construction of a 3D image within the vessel, revealing the direction (clockwise or counterclockwise) and the extent of the second guidewire's rotation toward the target.[5]

CONCLUSION

Wiring of CTO involves three parts, i.e., proximal cap puncture, CTO body wiring, and distal true lumen wiring. Each step needs different set of wires for successful recanalization. Any attempt to use single wire to address all three steps often fails and lands up in complicating the procedure. Knowing the merits and demerits of these different sets of wires is essential for its optimal use.

REFERENCES

1. Wu EB, Tsuchikane E, Lo S, Lim ST, Ge L, Chen JY, et al. Chronic total occlusion wiring: a state-of-the-art guide from the Asia Pacific Chronic Total Occlusion Club. Heart Lung Circ. 2019;28(10):1490-500.

2. Harding SA, Wu EB, Lo S, Lim ST, Ge L, Chen JY, et al. A new algorithm for crossing chronic total occlusions from the Asia Pacific Chronic Total Occlusion Club. JACC Cardiovasc Interv. 2017;10(21):2135-43.
3. Sumitsuji S, Inoue K, Ochiai M, Tsuchikane E, Keno F. Fundamental wire technique and current standard strategy of percutaneous intervention for chronic total occlusion with histopathological insights. JACC Cardiovasc Interv. 2011;4:941-51.
4. Reddy SA, Pillai AA, Reddy B, Rao V, Deshpande A. Knuckle wire technique in percutaneous coronary intervention of chronic total occlusion: Knuckle wire technique. AsiaIntervention. 2020;6(2):91-101.
5. Okamura A, Iwakura K, Iwamoto M, Nagai H, Sumiyoshi A, Tanaka K, et al. Tip detection method using the new IVUS facilitates the 3-dimensional wiring technique for CTO intervention. JACC Cardiovasc Interv. 2020;13:74-82.

CHAPTER 28

Antegrade Chronic Total Occlusion Crossing Techniques

Blessvin Jino

INTRODUCTION

The hybrid algorithm has increased the success rate of chronic total occlusion (CTO) percutaneous coronary intervention (PCI), as shown in multiple registries.[1-3] Antegrade approach, particularly antegrade wire escalation (AWE), remains the most common initial wire crossing strategy, despite the increasing trend of retrograde approach.[4] The initial wire crossing strategy requires meticulous analysis of the coronary angiogram, and it depends on the proximal cap morphology, lesion length, distal vessel quality, and the presence of interventional collaterals.[5] Histopathological examination of the CTO segment frequently shows microchannels with dense fibrous tissue in the earlier stages and more calcification with fewer microchannels in the later stages. Antegrade wire tracking may be intimal or subintimal. However, the success rate of entering the distal true lumen is higher with intimal or intraplaque wire tracking than subintimal wire tracking. The resistance for the guidewire tip in the subintimal layer is less than the resistance for it to enter the true lumen. The principle of "loose tissue tracking" helps in successful intraplaque wiring even with intermediate stiffness wires. Additionally, even during intraplaque wire tracking, dense calcium can resist the advancement of the wire and result in technical failure.[6]

SELECTING THE APPROPRIATE STRATEGY: FACTORS INVOLVED

Proximal cap morphology is an important factor involved in strategy selection in the antegrade approach. The global CTO crossing algorithm advocates "move the cap" technique, retrograde approach, or intravascular ultrasound (IVUS)-guided proximal cap puncture in ambiguous proximal caps.[5] Ambiguous or blunt proximal caps are important predictors of failure to cross, as shown in various studies,[7] and a tapered proximal cap favors antegrade wire crossing. Similarly, lesion length >20 mm and calcific CTO are important reasons for technical failure. Lesion length can be assessed by dual angiography or a CT coronary angiogram (CTCA). CTCA can also assess the course of the vessel, including the tortuosity, extent of calcium, proximal cap morphology, and possible reentry area.[8,9]

commercially available devices for ADR: The Stingray LP and the ReCross catheter. Both are OTW devices and can be used in 6F guide catheters. The BridgePoint system consists of three parts: A CrossBoss catheter, a Stingray balloon, and a dedicated reentry wire. The CrossBoss, a dedicated coronary catheter with a blunt atraumatic 1 mm tip, crosses the CTO segment true-to-true lumen in one-third of cases.[21] If the catheter enters the subintimal space, it is advanced to the reentry site, and a wire is inserted and exchanged for a Stingray LP balloon for reentry. The CrossBoss catheter limits the size of the dissection and hematoma compared to the wire based subintimal entry. However, CrossBoss may track along the smaller side branches over greater curvature, and may lead to perforation. Stingray LP, a flat, self-orienting balloon that automatically positions one exit port toward the true lumen, helps to accurately target the distal reentry.

The balloon can be taken into the required reentry position once an antegrade rotational microcatheter dilates the tract (Bougie technique). A stiff guidewire is then advanced through the side port of the stingray LP balloon to puncture the vessel wall, and then it is tracked down into the distal true lumen (stick and drive), or the stiff wire may be exchanged to a polymer-jacketed wire after puncturing for true lumen entry (stick and swap). Visualizing the distal true lumen in relation to the stingray balloon is important for successful reentry.[22,23] If there is difficulty in visualizing the distal true lumen due to hematoma, the "double-blind stick-and-swap technique" may be used. In this technique, a stiff wire is used to puncture through both side ports of the stingray LP balloon, followed by the advancement of a polymer jacketed wire through any of these ports until it enters the distal true lumen. When there is difficulty entering the distal true lumen, the stingray LP balloon may be moved to a different position (bobsledding). ReCross is a dual lumen microcatheter with three exit ports and the possibility to simultaneously exchange two guidewires due to the availability of two separate OTW lumens. The stingray balloon often requires predilatation to take it into the desired position. However, ReCross can be taken without predilatation. Once the wire enters subintimal space, ReCross may be taken inside, and a second CTO wire may be taken as a parallel wire through the other OTW lumen. Similarly, the ReCross catheter may be taken distal to the occlusion in the subintimal space, and a stiff wire may be taken through side ports for reentry. ReCross can be used in the STRAW technique for decreasing the subintimal hematoma.[24]

IMPENETRABLE PROXIMAL CAP

Heavily calcified and fibrotic proximal caps often cause difficulty in wire entry. Increasing the backup support and penetration force of the wires may help in successful wire entry. However, when these techniques fail, "move the cap" techniques or a retrograde approach help. By entering the subintimal space proximal to the cap and treating it as a virtual cap (move the cap), the original cap along with the CTO segment may be crossed. After entering the subintimal space proximally, reentry is done as with other ADR techniques. The various techniques described are:

- Scratch and go
- Balloon-assisted subintimal entry (BASE)
- Carlino technique

In the "scratch and go" technique, a HPF wire like Conquest Pro-12 is used to puncture 1–2 mm into the subintimal space. Then, using a tapered microcatheter such as corsair and soft polymer jacketed wire, further steps of ADR are done. This technique is done on a diseased proximal vessel. However, in a nondiseased proximal vessel, the BASE technique is used. An oversized balloon is used to create a limited dissection, and then subintimal entry is done using a polymer jacketed wire. In the Carlino technique, after entering the subintimal space, contrast is injected through a microcatheter, which in turn creates a dissection plane.

INTRAVASCULAR ULTRASOUND-GUIDED ANTEGRADE APPROACH

Intravascular ultrasound helps to localize the ambiguous proximal cap, facilitates reentry into the true lumen after subintimal wire crossing, and confirms the distal wire position in the true lumen.[25] IVUS may be parked in a side branch just proximal to the ambiguous proximal cap and then pulled manually until the cap is located **(Fig. 3)**. The location of the proximal cap is marked by dry cine, and it is kept as a roadmap. However, in larger guide catheters, a live puncture can be done. When FineCross is used along with

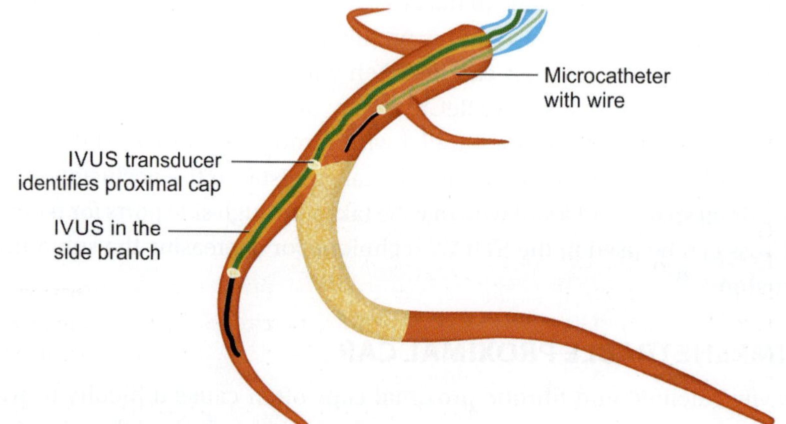

Fig. 3: Intravascular ultrasound (IVUS)-guided puncture of ambiguous proximal cap.

IVUS, a 7F guide catheter is required, and for other microcatheters, an 8F guide catheter is needed. The bulky IVUS catheter often deflects the wire away and may preclude simultaneous contrast injection when a live IVUS-guided puncture is done. These problems are avoided with intermittent IVUS guidance. Comparing the conventional microcatheters, a dual lumen microcatheter offers better support force and better visualization of guidewire by IVUS. Entering the true lumen from subintimal space, under IVUS guidance, is one of the most difficult techniques to learn. A HPF wire like the Conquest Pro-12 is used for reentry, and a short tip volcano eagle eye is better for IVUS guidance. IVUS-guided reentry is used when all the techniques of antegrade and retrograde approaches fail. IVUS-guided reentry may expand the subintimal space and may lead to vessel perforation in tortuous vessels.

CONCLUSION

Advances in technique and equipment have led to significant improvements in the success rate of the antegrade approach. The technical success rate of the antegrade approach has reached >95% in an Asia-Pacific CTO registry.[26] The strategy of switching from one approach to another often helps to minimize the radiation dose, contrast volume, and it increases the success rate. Operator experience is vital to achieve a high success rate.

REFERENCES

1. Christopoulos G, Karmpaliotis D, Alaswad K, Yeh RW, Jaffer FA, Wyman RM, et al. Application and outcomes of a hybrid approach to chronic total occlusion percutaneous coronary intervention in a contemporary multicenter US registry. Int J Cardiol. 2015;198:222-8.
2. Wilson WM, Walsh SJ, Yan AT, Hanratty CG, Bagnall AJ, Egred M, et al. Hybrid approach improves success of chronic total occlusion angioplasty. Heart. 2016;102:1486-93.
3. Maeremans J, Walsh S, Knaapen P, Spratt JC, Avran A, Hanratty CG, et al. The Hybrid algorithm for treating chronic total occlusions in Europe: The RECHARGE Registry. J Am Coll Cardiol. 2016;68:1958-70.
4. Konstantinidis NV, Werner GS, Deftereos S, Di Mario C, Galassi AR, Buettner JH, et al. Euro CTO Club. Temporal trends in chronic total occlusion interventions in Europe. Circ Cardiovasc Interv. 2018;11(10):e006229.
5. Wu EB, Brilakis ES, Mashayekhi K, Tsuchikane E, Alaswad K, Araya M, et al. Global Chronic Total Occlusion Crossing Algorithm: JACC State-of-the-Art Review. J Am Coll Cardiol. 2021;78(8):840-53.
6. Sumitsuji S, Inoue K, Ochiai M, Tsuchikane E, Ikeno F. Fundamental wire technique and current standard strategy of percutaneous intervention for chronic total occlusion with histopathological insights. JACC Cardiovasc Interv. 2011;4(9):941-51.
7. Lembo NJ, Hatem R, Karmpaliotis D. Predictive Scores of Success in CTO PCI: There Is No Substitute for Operator Experience and Skill. JACC Cardiovasc Interv. 2017;10(11):1099-101.

8. Werner GS. Use of coronary computed tomographic angiography to facilitate percutaneous coronary intervention of chronic total occlusions. Circ Cardiovasc Interv. 2019;12(10):e007387.
9. Yassin F, Khan J, Mozid A, Connolly D, Sharma V. The utility of CT coronary angiography in chronic total occlusion percutaneous coronary intervention. Eur Cardiol. 2023;18:e48.
10. Zhong X, Gao W, Hu T, Chen J, Tang X, Huang S, et al. Impact of subintimal plaque modification on reattempted chronic total occlusions percutaneous coronary intervention. JAAC Cardiovasc Interv. 2022;15:1427-37.
11. Megaly M, Xenogiannis I, Abi Rafeh N, Karmpaliotis D, Rinfret S, Yamane M, et al. Retrograde approach to chronic total occlusion percutaneous coronary intervention. Circ Cardiovasc Interv. 2020;13:e008900.
12. Mohandes M, Guarinos J, Sans J, Bardaji A. Intravascular ultrasound in percutaneous coronary intervention for chronic total occlusion. Int Cardiovasc Res J. 2010;4(3):101-6.
13. Fujii K, Ochiai M, Mintz GS, Kan Y, Awano K, Masutani M, et al. Procedural implications of intravascular ultrasound morphologic features of chronic total coronary occlusions. Am J Cardiol. 2006;97(10):1455-62.
14. Wu EB, Tsuchikane E, Lo S, Lim ST, Ge L, Chen JY, et al. Chronic total occlusion wiring: a state-of-the-art guide from the Asia Pacific Chronic Total Occlusion Club. Heart Lung Circ. 2019;28:1490-500.
15. Harding SA, Wu EB, Lo S, Lim ST, Ge L, Chen JY, et al. A New Algorithm for Crossing Chronic Total Occlusions from the Asia Pacific Chronic Total Occlusion Club. JACC Cardiovasc Interv. 2017;10:2135-43.
16. Reddy SA, Pillai AA, Reddy B, Rao V, Deshpande A. Knuckle wire technique in percutaneous coronary intervention of chronic total occlusion: Knuckle wire technique. AsiaIntervention. 2020;6(2):91-101.
17. Colombo A, Mikhail GW, Michev I, Iakovou I, Airoldi F, Chieffo A, et al. Treating chronic total occlusions using subintimal tracking and reentry: the STAR technique. Catheter Cardiovasc Interv. 2005;64:407-11.
18. Carlino M, Godino C, Latib A, Moses JW, Colombo A. Subintimal tracking and re-entry technique with contrast guidance: a safer approach. Catheter Cardiovasc Interv. 2008;72:790-6.
19. Michael TT, Papayannis AC, Banerjee S, Brilakis ES. Subintimal dissection/reentry strategies in coronary chronic total occlusion interventions. Circ Cardiovasc Interv. 2012;5(5):729-38.
20. Smith EJ, Di Mario C, Spratt JC, Hanratty CG, de Silva R, Lindsay AC, et al. Subintimal TRAnscatheter Withdrawal (STRAW) of hematomas compressing the distal true lumen: a novel technique to facilitate distal reentry during recanalization of chronic total occlusion (CTO). J Invasive Cardiol. 2015;27(1):E1-4.
21. Whitlow PL, Burke MN, Lombardi WL, Wyman RM, Moses JW, Brilakis ES, et al; FAST-CTOs Trial Investigators. Use of a novel crossing and re-entry system in coronary chronic total occlusions that have failed standard crossing techniques: results of the FAST-CTOs (Facilitated Antegrade Steering Technique in Chronic Total Occlusions) trial. JACC Cardiovasc Interv. 2012;5(4):393-401.
22. Christopoulos G, Kotsia AP, Brilakis ES. The Double-Blind Stick-and-Swap Technique for True Lumen Reentry After Subintimal Crossing of Coronary Chronic Total Occlusions. J Invasive Cardiol. 2015;27(9):E199-202.

23. Wu EB, Brilakis ES, Lo S, Kalyanasundaram A, Mashayekhi K, Kao HL, et al. Advances in CrossBoss/Stingray use in antegrade dissection reentry from the Asia Pacific Chronic Total Occlusion Club. Catheter Cardiovasc Interv. 2020;96(7):1423-33.
24. Garbo R, Iannaccone M, Sánchez JS, Oreglia JA, Gagnor A, Gasparini GL, et al. The ReCross dual-lumen microcatheter versatility during percutaneous coronary intervention of chronic total coronary occlusions. REC Interv Cardiol. 2022;4(1):63-71.
25. Galassi AR, Sumitsuji S, Boukhris M, Brilakis ES, Di Mario C, Garbo R, et al. Utility of intravascular ultrasound in percutaneous revascularization of chronic total occlusions: an overview. JACC Cardiovasc Interv. 2016;9:1979-91.
26. Wu EB, Tsuchikane E, Ge L, Harding SA, Lo S, Lim ST, et al. Retrograde Versus Antegrade Approach for Coronary Chronic Total Occlusion in an Algorithm-Driven Contemporary Asia-Pacific Multicentre Registry: Comparison of Outcomes. Heart Lung Circ. 2020;29(6):894-903.

CHAPTER 29

Retrograde Chronic Total Occlusion Crossing: Techniques

Byju Cheriya Kacheri

INTRODUCTION

This chapter describes the techniques for successfully crossing the chronic total occlusion (CTO) once the retrograde guidewire is successfully delivered to the distal cap of the CTO through a suitable interventional collateral channel.

BASIC METHODS OF RETROGRADE WIRE CROSSING

There are four basic methods of retrograde wire crossing:[1]

1. Kissing wire technique
2. Retrograde true lumen penetration [retrograde wire escalation (RWE)]
3. Reverse controlled antegrade and retrograde tracking (CART)
4. CART (controlled antegrade and retrograde wire tracking)

Rest of the crossing methods are modifications and variations of these basic techniques.

PLANES OF CROSSING AND CONNECTION IN EACH BASIC METHOD OF CROSSING

There are two "planes" (this should in reality be mentioned as "space" in a three-dimensional sense which really is the case in the CTO lesion) through which wires cross through the CTO lesion.

Intraplaque or True Lumen Crossing

In kissing wire technique and retrograde true lumen tracking, antegrade and retrograde wires remain inside the plaque and does not exit into the extraplaque (otherwise known as subintimal) space.

Extraplaque (Subintimal)

In reverse CART and CART, antegrade and retrograde wires exit and traverse through the extraplaque (subintimal) space in some part of their journey through the CTO lesion.

SPATIAL RELATIONSHIP BETWEEN ANTEGRADE AND RETROGRADE WIRE IN THE CTO LESION

There can be four types of relationships between antegrade and retrograde guidewire inside the CTO lesion:

1. Both antegrade and retrograde guidewires in intraplaque space (true lumen). Connection between the spaces and crossing can be done by either kissing wire technique or retrograde true lumen tracking. In kissing wire technique, retrograde guidewire can be used as a marker wire to guide the antegrade guidewire so that it remains in the intraplaque space and exits the distal cap successfully, leading to an antegrade true lumen crossing. This works successfully in cases with short, straight CTO segments, and soft lesions which are less calcific and fibrotic. Success rate of kissing wire technique is better with a distal CTO segment which is favorable for antegrade wire crossing (softer distal CTO segment, less angulation at the exit segment of the CTO, and good distal exit vessel which is not diffusely diseased). Kissing wire technique is primarily chosen in situations where retrograde microcatheter cannot be delivered to the distal CTO cap as presence of a micro catheter is a necessity in most cases to successfully achieve a retrograde wire placement into the antegrade guide catheter.[2] Retrograde true lumen crossing (RWE) can be done when a microcatheter also can be delivered to the distal CTO cap along with the retrograde guidewire. Like kissing wire technique, this also works successfully when the CTO lesion is soft, straight and short, with a proximal exit vessel which is not diseased diffusely without much angulation. In right coronary artery (RCA) or left main coronary artery (LMCA) ostial CTO, retrograde true lumen crossing is achieved in many cases when the CTO is short, as a favorable exit into the proximal larger vessel (aorta) occurs while the retrograde guidewire comes through the intraplaque space.
2. Antegrade guidewire and retrograde guidewire in extraplaque (subintimal) space. Making a connection between the antegrade and retrograde spaces is relatively easy in this situation. Controlling the size, extent, and position of the extraplaque space available for the guidewires to pass through is of paramount importance in achieving a successful connection between the spaces. Facilitation of entry of retrograde guidewire from extraplaque (subintimal) space into the antegrade extraplaque (subintimal space) can be facilitated by a balloon dilatation of the antegrade extraplaque space. This technique is known as reverse CART.[3] In conventional reverse CART, balloon used is larger in diameter as the technique depends on creating an adequately large extraplaque space antegradely into which the retrograde extraplaque guidewire can be directed for entry. Accurate sizing of the balloon can be determined by use of intravascular ultrasound (IVUS).

This technique is known as IVUS-guided reverse CART. When IVUS is not used, a balloon approximately about the same diameter of the proximal vessel is used to dilate the extraplaque (subintimal) space around the antegrade guidewire. In "directed reverse CART", a smaller diameter balloon is used to dilate the extraplaque space. Thereafter, retrograde guidewire in extraplaque space is directed to this antegrade extraplaque space achieving successful connection. Proper timing of deflation of the smaller antegrade balloon helps in achieving this connection. Antegrade balloon is deflated just when the retrograde guidewire aims at the balloon. This helps the retrograde guidewire to enter the smaller antegrade extraplaque space before it gets closed off. In stent-assisted reverse CART, a stent deployed in the extraplaque space is sometimes used to keep the antegrade extraplaque space patent for facilitating retrograde guidewire entry. In mother and child (MAC) catheter-assisted reverse CART, a MAC catheter like GuideLiner or Guidezilla can be used to keep the antegrade extraplaque space patent for facilitating retrograde guidewire entry. In cases where retrograde microcatheter could not be negotiated into the extraplaque space along with the retrograde guidewire, CART is a useful technique. In this, a balloon introduced retrogradely is used to dilate and expand the retrograde extraplaque space into which the antegrade guidewire can be negotiated to achieve the connection and complete the angioplasty.

3. Antegrade guidewire in intraplaque space (true lumen) and retrograde guidewire in extraplaque (subintimal) space. Connection is difficult in this scenario unless antegrade guidewire is directed intentionally into extraplaque space and subsequently antegrade extraplaque space is expanded by balloon. Methods described to enter the antegrade extraplaque space include knuckle wire technique, "scratch-and-go" technique, balloon-assisted subintimal entry (BASE), contrast-assisted creation of subintimal dissection plane, etc. In knuckle wire technique, a polymer jacket-coated guidewire like Fielder XT, Pilot 50, or Pilot 150 is introduced into the subintimal space by forceful pushing of the guidewire without rotations. In scratch-and-go technique, a hard penetrating guidewire like Conquest Pro with a small bend at the tip is used to make an entry point into the subintimal space from the true lumen. Into this entry point, a polymer jacket guidewire can be directed to enter the subintimal space. In BASE, a balloon with a diameter similar to the vessel, is used to dilate the proximal segment to create dissection planes. A hydrophilic guidewire can be directed into this dissection plane to enter the subintimal space. Once the subintimal space is entered antegradely, any of the variations of reverse CART can be used to successfully make the connection of retrograde and antegrade extraplaque spaces.

4. Antegrade guidewire in extraplaque (subintimal) space and retrograde guidewire in intraplaque space (true lumen). This is the situation which gives maximum challenge to achieve connection of antegrade and retrograde spaces. Direction of retrograde guidewire into the extraplaque space is often challenging. Excellent support from a retrograde microcatheter like Corsair Pro is essential in forcely directing the retrograde guidewire into the subintimal space. A balloon introduced through the retrograde route may be inflated in distal cap or nearby region to create dissection plane to achieve the entry of retrograde guidewire into extraplaque space in very challenging scenarios. Once retrograde wire is directed into the extraplaque space, connection can be achieved easily. Once a connection is made between the antegrade and retrograde spaces, externalization of the guidewire is done in most cases to complete the angioplasty. In some cases, antegrade guidewire is introduced to distal vessel and angioplasty is completed over the antegrade guidewire.

CONCLUSION

Retrograde approach increases the success rate of a CTO PCI. However, optimal case selection and operator experience are essential for the technical success. Newer devices and wires help to achieve a higher success rates even in complex CTO lesions.

REFERENCES

1. Michael Megaly, IosifXenogiannis, Nidal Abi Rafeh, et al. Retrograde Approach to Chronic Total Occlusion Percutaneous Coronary Intervention. Circ Cardiovasc Interv. 2020;13:e008900.
2. Wu EB, Tsuchikane E, Lo S, Lim ST, Ge L, Chen JY, et al. Retrograde algorithm for chronic total occlusion from the Asia Pacific Chronic Total Occlusion club. AsiaIntervention. 2018;4(2):98-107.
3. Matsuno S, Tsuchikane E, Harding SA, Wu EB, Kao HL, Brilakis ES, et al. Overview and proposed terminology for the reverse controlled antegrade and retrograde tracking (reverse CART) techniques. EuroIntervention. 2018;14(1):94-101.

CHAPTER 30

Wire Externalization Techniques in Retrograde CTO PCI

Manu Rajendran

INTRODUCTION

Wire externalization is a final crucial step after crossing the chronic total occlusion (CTO) lesion retrogradely during percutaneous coronary intervention (PCI). Wire externalization means advancing the retrograde guidewire into and through the antegrade guiding catheter to serve as an antegrade route for balloon and stents followed by safe removal of externalized equipment.

OPTIONS

Two options are available for wire externalization:

1. *Wiring the antegrade guide:* Simple and preferable method. Facilitated by coaxial guide position, using large guide catheters and advancing a guide catheter extension through the antegrade guide catheter.
2. *Snaring:* If antegrade guide wiring fails as in aorto-ostial CTO and in noncoaxial guide engagement.

Wiring the Antegrade Guide

Directly wiring the antegrade guide catheter with the retrograde wire is the simplest technique and should be the first choice to externalize a guidewire whenever possible.[1,2]

Steps involved are:

1. Once the retrograde wire (that crossed the CTO lesion) advances into the antegrade guide, a trapping balloon is inflated within the antegrade guide adjacent to the wire to facilitate advancement of the retrograde microcatheter into the antegrade guide catheter **(Figs. 1A to C)**.[3]
2. The retrograde guidewire is then removed after deflating the trapping balloon keeping the retrograde microcatheter within the antegrade guide catheter **(Fig. 2A)**.
3. The dedicated externalization wire (RG3 or R350) is then inserted and advanced through the retrograde microcatheter **(Fig. 2B)**.
4. The antegrade Y-connector is disconnected from the antegrade guide catheter and a finger is placed over the antegrade guide catheter hub,

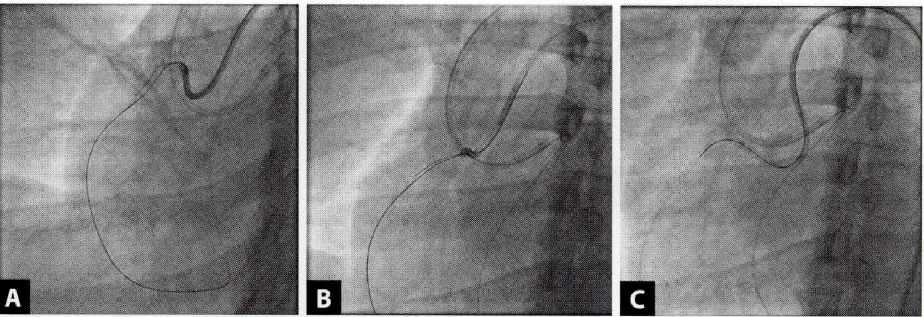

Figs. 1A to C: (A) Directly wiring the antegrade guide catheter with retrograde wire; (B) Balloon trapping the retrograde wire; (C) Advancing the retrograde microcatheter through the trapped retrograde wire into antegrade guide catheter.

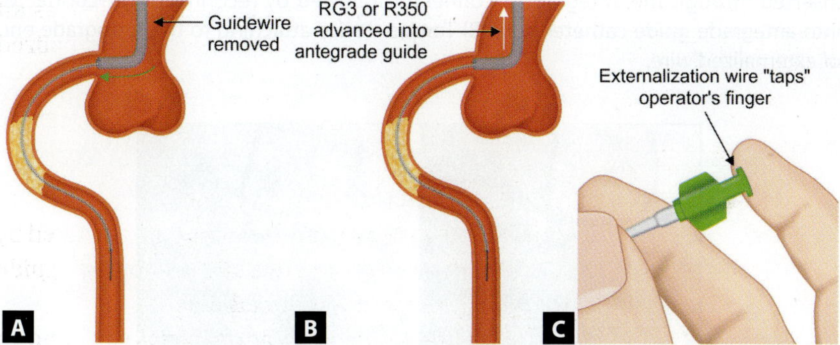

Figs. 2A to C: (A) Removing the retrograde wire; (B) Advancing the dedicated externalization wire through the retrograde microcatheter; (C) Pushing the externalized wire until it is felt tapping on the finger placed over antegrade guide catheter hub.

until the retrograde externalization guidewire is felt tapping on the finger **(Fig. 2C)**.

5. A wire introducer is then inserted through the antegrade Y-connector and the retrograde guidewire tip is threaded through the introducer. To minimize bleeding the same balloon used for trapping the retrograde wire can also be used for trapping the retrograde microcatheter proximally to the side holes of guiding catheter, to stop the bloody filling of the antegrade guide catheter **(Fig. 3A)**.[4]
6. The antegrade Y-connector is then reconnected to the guide catheter hub **(Fig. 3A)**.
7. Push the retrograde guidewire until 20–30 cm has come out through the Y-connector **(Fig. 3A)**.
8. A torque device should be attached to the retrograde guide end of the externalized wire to prevent losing the retrograde ending of the externalization wire by inadvertently pulling through the retrograde

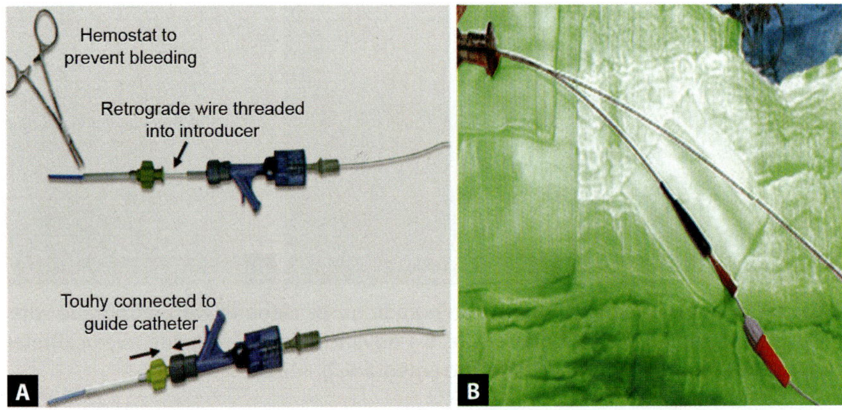

Figs. 3A and B: (A) Exiting retrograde wire is advanced into the introducer needle inserted through the antegrade Y-connector followed by reconnecting Y-connector into antegrade guide catheter hub; (B) Torque device attaching to the retrograde end of externalized wire.

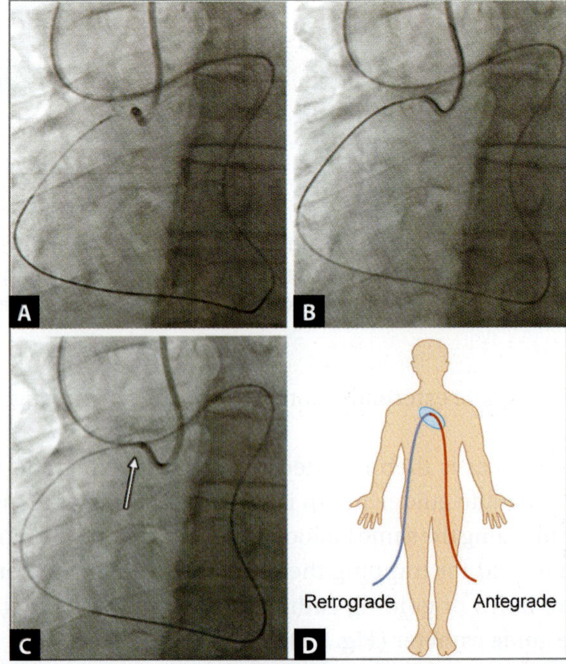

Figs. 4A to D: Conventional wire externalization creating a loop between antegrade and retrograde catheter.

microcatheter during PCI **(Fig. 3B)**. **Figures. 4A to D** showed the final retrograde loop created by wire externalization in retrograde CTO PCI.

Standard single trapping balloon and double trapping balloon for trapping the retrograde wire for providing support to advance the retrograde

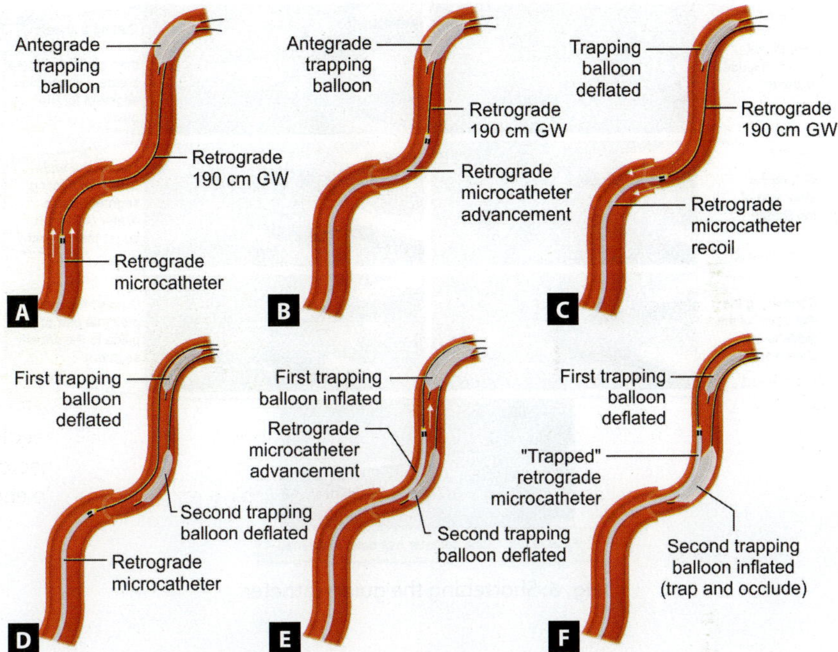

Figs. 5A to F: Single and double balloon trapping technique. (A to C) Standard trapping balloon; (D to F) Double trapping balloon

microcatheter into antegrade guide. Double trapping balloon method is used to trap the retrograde microcatheter with a distal balloon once it enters the antegrade catheter to counteract microcatheter recoil during trapping balloon deflation **(Figs. 5A to F)**. Balloon diameter of 2.5 mm for 6–7 Fr guiding catheters and 2.75–3 mm for 8 Fr guiding catheters inflated at 8 atm are used for trapping.

Shortening the Guide Catheter (Fig. 6)

With the advent of short guiding catheters (90 cm), guide extension catheters, long retrograde microcatheters (>150 cm) and dedicated externaliaztion wires of 300 cm routine shortening of the guide catheter is not required now. But if the distance between the antegrade and retrograde guiding catheter exceed the length of the microcatheter it may be impossible to exchange the wires safely as in retrograde cases via bypass grafts or apical epicardial collaterals. Utilizing a shorter guide catheter extends the reach of balloons, wires, and microcatheters advanced retrogradely. If manufactured short guide catheters (90 cm) are not available, a 100 cm long guide can be shortened by cutting a segment of sheath 1 Fr smaller than the guide and inserting the cut sheath into proximal and distal ends of the cut guide catheter after flaring the ends of the connected sheath segment with a dilator 1 Fr larger than the sheath size.[5]

Another option is to use a guide catheter extension deeply intubated into the CTO target vessel **(Figs. 7A to C)**, which is especially useful for retrograde

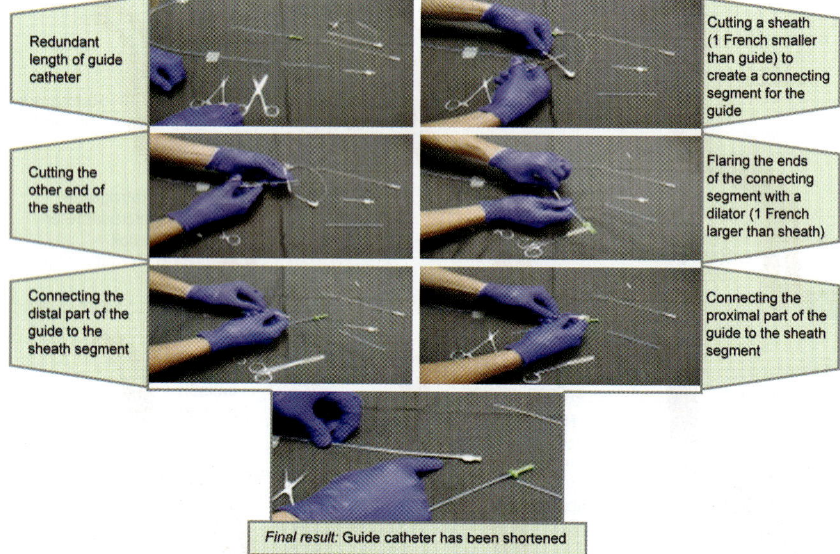

Fig. 6: Shortening the guide catheter.

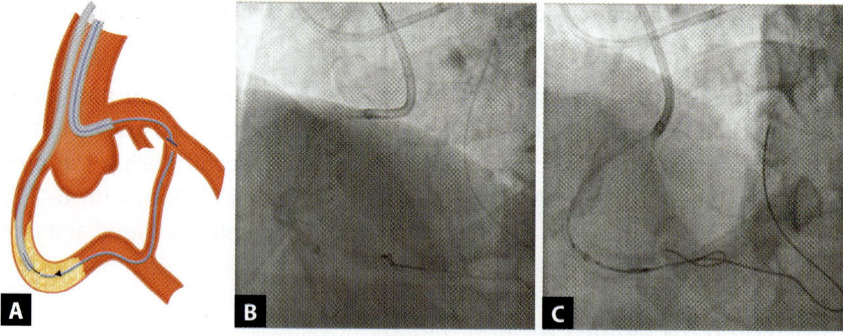

Figs. 7A to C: Shortening the retrograde externalization route. Insertion of an antegrade child catheter toward the proximal cap of the chronic total occlusion (CTO).

crossing through epicardial collaterals or (left or right) internal mammary artery grafts.[6]

Types of externalization guidewires are given in **Flowchart 1**.

Snaring the Retrograde Guidewire

Direct retrograde guidewire engagement to antegrade guiding catheter cannot be performed in:

- Aorto-ostial CTO
- CTO in vessels with anomalous origin
- Poor retrograde wire control

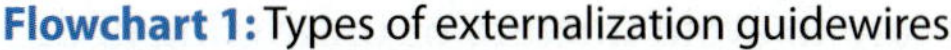

Flowchart 1: Types of externalization guidewires.

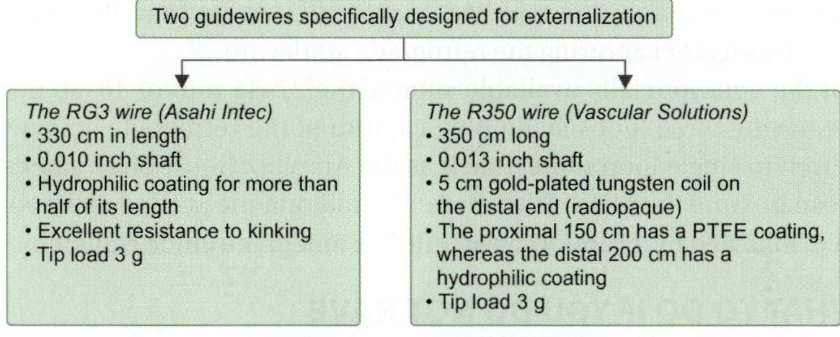

(PTFE: polytetrafluoroethylene)

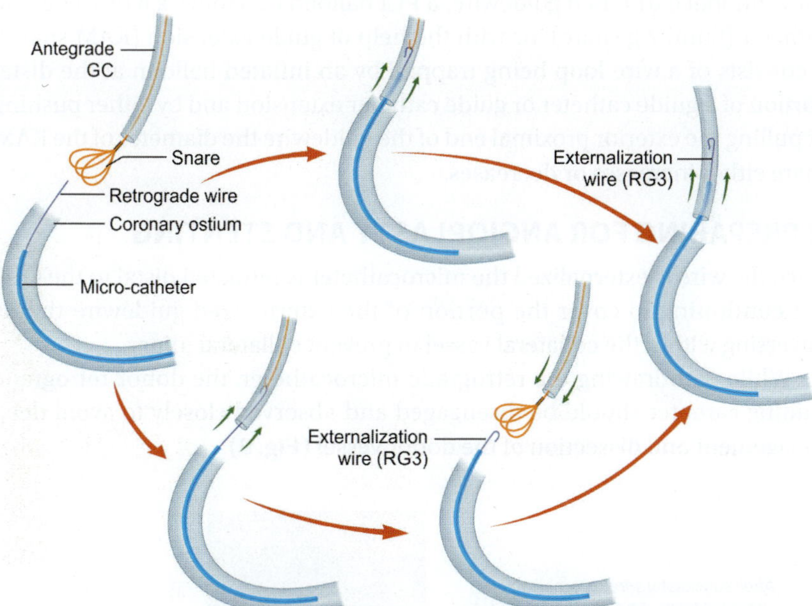

Fig. 8: Snaring the retrograde wire. (GC: guiding catheter)

- Noncoaxial guide engagement
- If the vessel caliber is much larger than the antegrade guide

Externalization requires guidewire engagement within the aortic root or ascending aorta by means of an antegrade coronary snare device **(Fig. 8)**. After snaring the wire into the antegrade guide catheter the retrograde microcatheter is then advanced into the antegrade guide either directly using the snaring as support or with trapped balloon support after releasing the snare followed by exchanging with a dedicated externalization wire. If it is not possible to advance the microcatheter through the CTO and into the aorta, then a standard 300 cm long wire or externalization wire may need to be snared taking care to avoid fracture or unraveling of the distal part of the guidewire. The snare is then pulled back, until it exists from the antegrade guide Y-connector capturing the retrograde guidewire.

Of the commercially available snares, the 27–45 mm or 18–30 mm EN Snare having three loops facilitating capture of the retrograde guidewire is preferred to single loop snares, such as the Amplatz Goose Neck snares and microsnares and the Micro Elite snare. The radiopaque portion of the wires is snared, followed by a careful sweep into the antegrade guide catheter.

WHAT TO DO IF YOU DO NOT HAVE A COMMERCIAL SNARE?

If a commercial snare is not available, a homemade snare can be created by a conventional 0.014 inch guidewire, a PCI balloon (2.5 mm), a 6 or 7 Fr guide catheter (Sumi 2 g snare)[7] or with the help of guide extension (KAM snare). It consists of a wire loop being trapped by an inflated balloon at the distal portion of a guide catheter or guide catheter extension and by either pushing or pulling the exterior proximal end of the guidewire the diameter of the KAM snare either increases or decreases.

PREPARING FOR ANGIOPLASTY AND STENTING

Once the wire is externalized the microcatheter is retracted distal to the CTO but continuing to cover the portion of the externalized guidewire that is traversing within the collateral vessel to prevent collateral injury.

While withdrawing the retrograde microcatheter, the donor retrograde guiding catheter should be disengaged and observed closely to avoid deep engagement and dissection of the donor vessel **(Fig. 9)**.

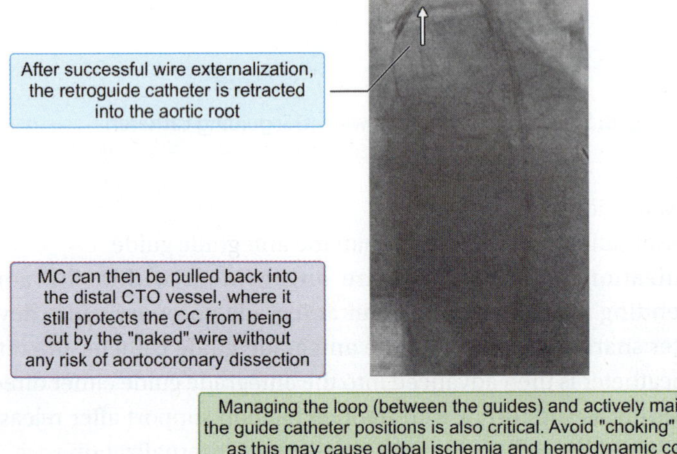

Fig. 9: Precautions to be taken while stenting. (CC: collateral channel; CTO: chronic total occlusion; MC: microcatheter)

A torquer or hemostat is attached at the proximal end of the externalized guidewire to avoid the risk for inadvertent withdrawal of the wire into the retrograde microcatheter.

Chronic total occlusion lesion is then predilated and stented antegradely through the externalization wire which offers excellent support for antegrade delivery of balloons and stents.

"PING-PONG" GUIDE CATHETER TECHNIQUE FOR RETROGRADE INTERVENTION OF A CHRONIC TOTAL OCCLUSION THROUGH AN IPSILATERAL COLLATERAL

- The retrograde approach via ipsilateral collateral channels (CCs) is very challenging, mainly because collaterals are mostly very fragile epimyocardial CCs.
- 7 Fr guides are often too narrow to host the antegrade and retrograde devices.
- Retrograde CTO PCI through an ipsilateral collateral can be accomplished by using a second ipsilateral guiding catheter (ping-pong catheter) for retrograde wire externalization **(Fig. 10).**[8]
- Engagement of the target coronary artery alternated between the antegrade and retrograde guide catheter in a "ping-pong" fashion enabling lesion crossing and equipment delivery.
- Excessive shear stress due to alternating ostial intubation at the coronary ostium as well as simultaneous ostial intubation of both guiding catheters should be avoided.

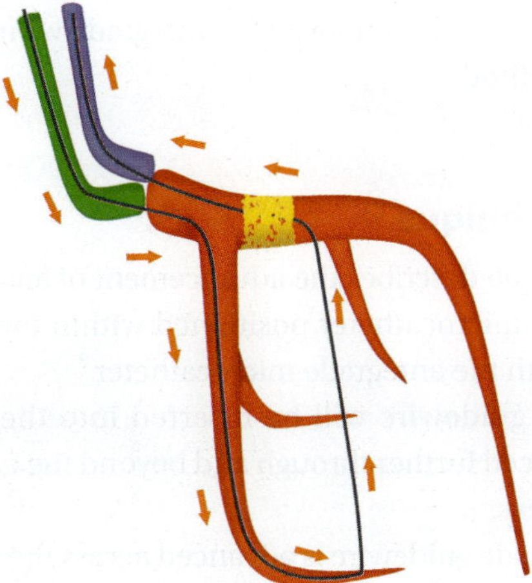

Fig. 10: Retrograde chronic total occlusion (CTO) percutaneous coronary intervention (PCI) through an ipsilateral collateral can be accomplished by using a second ipsilateral guiding catheter (ping-pong catheter) for retrograde wire externalization.

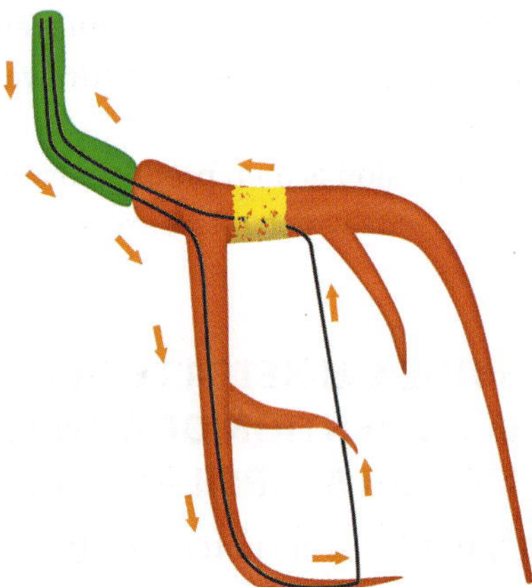

Fig. 11: "Single-guiding technique" using only one single 8Fr guiding catheter might offer sufficient space for both the antegrade and retrograde guidewires and devices.

- "Single-guiding technique" using only one single 8 Fr guiding catheter might offer sufficient space for both the antegrade and retrograde guidewires and devices **(Fig. 11)**.

ALTERNATIVES TO WIRE EXTERNALIZATION

In some cases, wire externalization may be impossible or should be avoided such as when:

- Wire or microcatheter may not easily advance into the antegrade guide, usually due to tortuosity or calcified retrograde course.
- Retrograde equipment resulting in ischemia and needs to be removed.

Two techniques commonly employed for antegrade wiring are:

1. Rendezvous method
2. Tip-in technique

Rendezvous Technique

Rendezvous technique describes the advancement of an antegrade guidewire into the retrograde microcatheter positioned within the antegrade guiding catheter alinged with the antegrade microcatheter.[9]

The antegrade guidewire will be inserted into the retrograde microcatheter and advanced further through and beyond the CTO to the distal end of the coronary artery.

Once the antegrade guidewire is advanced across the CTO, the retrograde microcatheter is pulled, followed by advancement of the antegrade microcatheter. Finally, the antegrade guidewire may be exchanged for a soft-tipped conventional guidewire to finalize the procedure.

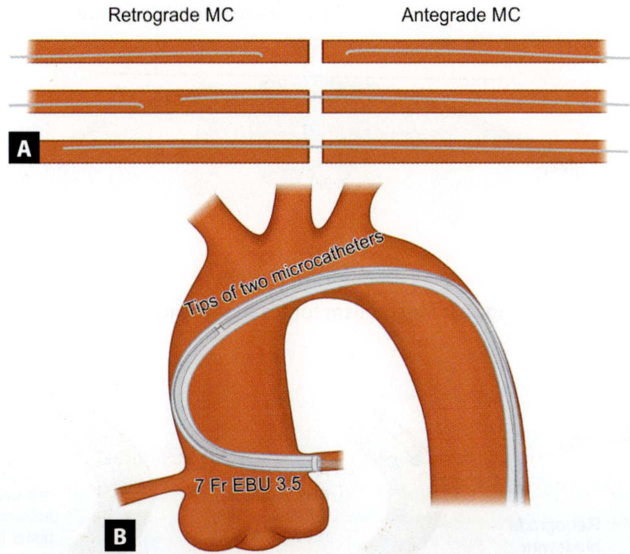

Figs. 12A and B: Illustration of bridge or rendezvous method. (A) Two microcatheters (MCs) were aligned within the guiding catheter at the level of the ascending aorta; (B) Illustration of bridging process. Antegrade guidewire is inserted through the bridge of two aligned MCs within the guiding catheter, which can be progressed further down beyond the totally occluded site through the retrograde MC.

The rendezvous method is more easily performed using two microcatheters at the curvature of the aortic arch or secondary curvature of the guiding catheter **(Figs. 12A and B)**.

If the wire-crossing of the rendezvous becomes difficult due to misalignment of the microcatheters, a 2.5-mm balloon can be placed under their tips and inflated at 6–10 atm, to enable optimal alignment.

The "rendezvous" technique was described originally to be performed within the antegrade guiding catheter, this maneuver can also be modified and performed at any site of the coronary artery, always provided that optimal alignment of the retrograde and antegrade microcatheters can be achieved.

In the case of Corsair usage, the inner lumen diameter of the tapered tip is 0.38 mm, which is slightly smaller than the FineCross microcatheter (0.45 mm at distal portion), and therefore it can require a slightly longer crossing time.

Tip-in Technique

Once the retrograde wire crosses the CTO lesion and entered the antegrade guiding catheter, and if there is inability to advance the retrograde microcatheter into the antegrade guide catheter due to difficult anatomy, such as proximal calcification and severe tortuosity may result in procedural failure during CTO PCI. In such situations, tip-in method can be adopted and

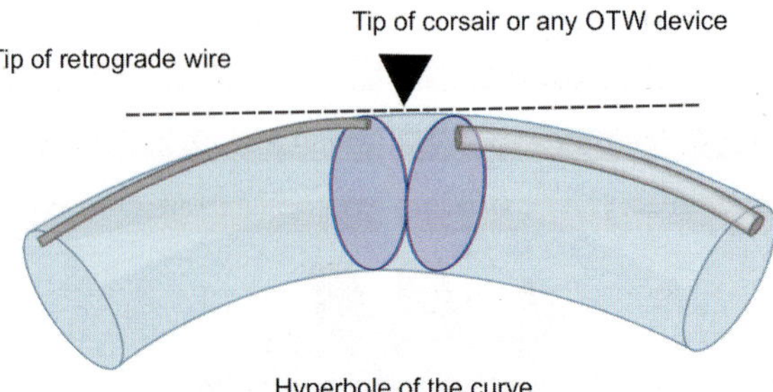

Fig. 13: Mechanism for tip-in technique.

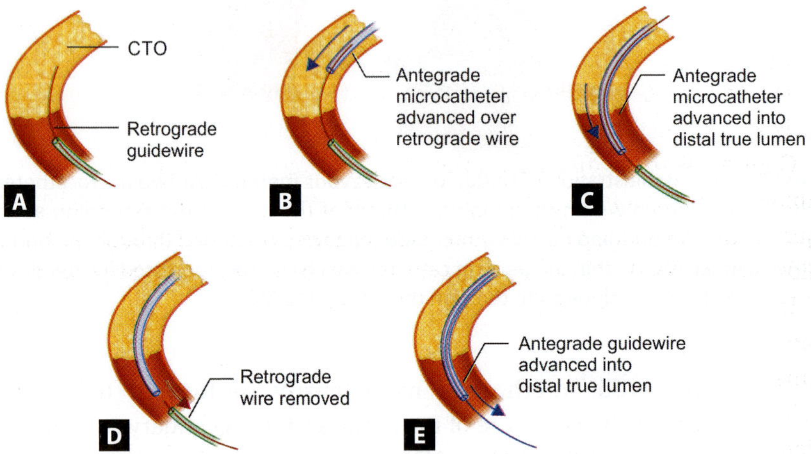

Figs. 14A to E: Tip-in technique. (CTO: chronic total occlusion)

overcomes shortcomings of the contemporary retrograde recanalisation in need of "bail-out" situation.

In tip-in method **(Fig. 13)**, place an antegrade microcatheter at the outer curvature of guiding catheter in aortic arch and deliver the retrograde wire into it and then advancing antegrade microcatheter through the retrograde wire beyond the CTO lesion followed by removal of retrograde wire and then insertion of an antegrade guidewire and antegrade delivery of balloons and stents **(Figs. 14A to E)**.[10]

Advantages of antegrade wiring methods are simplicity and safety. This method saves time, contrast, cost, and there is less chance of intracoronary loop shear stress and hence collateral damage and guide catheter-induced ostial dissection during wire externalization can be avoided.

The limitation of antegrade wiring method is that this method cannot provide the strong support in delivering a balloon or a stent as externalization method can, due to inherent nature of the antegrade system.

EXTERNALIZED GUIDEWIRE REMOVAL

Once the stenting of the CTO is over, the retrograde wire should be removed safely because lot of complications can occur during this stage.

- First the retrograde microcatheter is advanced back into the antegrade guide (across the recently deployed stents) unless resistance is met.
- Both guide catheters are then disengaged to minimize the risk for deep guide catheter advancement into the coronary ostia, likely causing dissection. The retrograde guide is disengaged by holding the microcatheter and using it as rail for guide retraction. The antegrade guide is disengaged by pushing the externalized guidewire.
- The retrograde guidewire is then withdrawn paying careful attention to the position of the tip of the donor guide catheter (to prevent deep engagement and coronary artery dissection).

The retrograde microcatheter is then withdrawn into the donor vessel leaving the retrograde guidewire across the collateral.

Contrast is then injected via the retrograde guide to make sure that no damage (perforation or rupture) of the collateral vessel has occurred. If injury is detected, the microcatheter can be readvanced over the retrograde guidewire to seal the CC perforation and possibly deliver coils or gelfoam.

If no collateral vessel injury is detected, the guidewire is removed after readvancing the microcatheter over the guidewire to lessen the risk for CC damage, mainly in tortuous epicardial collaterals.

The antegrade balloons or stents should not meet the retrograde microcatheter or balloon in order to minimize the risk of catheter interlocking and entrapment.

CONCLUSION

This chapter summarizes the essential steps of default wire externalization during retrograde PCI of CTOs which is the crucial final step and the bail out techniques of alternatives to wire externalization. Important tips and tricks are also outlined in order to avoid potential complications and improve the chance of successful retrograde CTO PCI intervention.

REFERENCES

1. Sianos G, Barlis P, Di Mario C, Papafaklis MI, Büttner J, Galassi AR, et al; EuroCTO Club. European experience with the retrograde approach for the recanalisation of coronary artery chronic total occlusions. A report on behalf of the EuroCTO club. EuroIntervention. 2008;4:84-92.
2. Ozawa N. A new understanding of chronic total occlusion from a novel PCI technique that involves a retrograde approach to the right coronary artery via a septal branch and passing of the guidewire to a guiding catheter on the other side of the lesion. Catheter Cardiovasc Interv. 2006;68:907-13.

3. Ge JB, Zhang F, Ge L, Qian JY, Wang H. Wire trapping technique combined with retrograde approach for recanalization of chronic total occlusion. Chin Med J (Engl). 2008;121:1753-6.
4. Gasparini GL, Oreglia JA, Garbo R. The trap and occlude technique for retrograde wire externalization during chronic total occlusion revascularization. Catheter Cardiovasc Interv. 2018;91:57-63.
5. Kim TH, Jang Y. A new technique for shortening a guiding catheter during retrograde recanalization of a chronic total occlusion. Catheter Cardiovasc Interv. 2011;77:358-62.
6. Mozid AM, Davies JR, Spratt JC. The utility of a guideliner catheter in retrograde percutaneous coronary intervention of a chronic total occlusion with reverse cart-the "capture" technique. Catheter Cardiovasc Interv. 2014;83:929-32.
7. Yokoi K, Sumitsuji S, Kaneda H, Siegrist PT, Okayama K, Ide S, et al. A novel homemade snare, safe, economical and size-adjustable. EuroIntervention. 2015;10:1307-10.
8. Brilakis ES, Grantham JA, Banerjee S. "Ping-pong" guide catheter technique for retrograde intervention of a chronic total occlusion through an ipsilateral collateral. Catheter Cardiovasc Interv. 2011;78:395-9.
9. Muramatsu T, Tsukahara R, Ito Y. "Rendezvous in coronary" technique with the retrograde approach for chronic total occlusion. J Invasive Cardiol. 2010;22:E179-82.
10. Vo MN, Ravandi A, Brilakis ES. "Tip-in" technique for retrograde chronic total occlusion revascularization. J Invasive Cardiol. 2015;27:E62-4.

CHAPTER 31

Management of In-Stent Restenosis

A Sreenivas Kumar

INTRODUCTION

The incidence of in-stent restenosis (ISR) has significantly declined in the past two decades with predominant use of drug-eluting stents (DESs), advancements in coronary stent designs with biodegradable polymer coating, implantation techniques, and pharmacotherapies and use of imaging modalities. ISR of bare-metal stents (BMSs) tends to occur within the first year after implantation; but with current-generation, DESs are associated with an ongoing risk of stent failure of around 1–2% per year.[1] In US CathPCI registry from 2009 to 2017, 5,100,394 patients underwent percutaneous coronary intervention (PCI), and 10.6% of patients underwent PCI for ISR lesions. Patients with BMS ISR declined from 2.6% in 2009 to 0.9% in 2017, and DES ISR rose from 5.4% in 2009 to 6.3% in 2017.[2] The clinical presentation of ISR can vary from chronic stable angina to acute coronary syndrome with ST elevation myocardial infarction (STEMI). In US CathPCI registry patients who underwent ISR-PCI, around 25% presented with an acute myocardial infarction.[2] The rates of recurrent stent failures remain a challenging aspect in clinical practice. From previous registries, the reported rates of recurrence of ISR after a first, second, and third reintervention were 8.3%, 17.1%, and 22.8%, respectively.[3] Multiple metallic stent layers are associated with a progressively higher risk of recurrent ISR, after treatment with DES or drug-coated balloons (DCBs), particularly in the presence of 3-layer ISR.[4,5] Various anatomic, patient and procedure-related factors that contribute to ISR were described in **Figure 1**.

Metallic stent implantation within a coronary artery induces a local trauma with endothelial injury and activation of an inflammatory foreign body reaction. Persistence of local inflammation after 90 days is associated with a subsequent high risk of delayed endothelialization, ISR, and late or very late stent thrombosis (ST).[6] Hypersensitivity and inflammatory reactions promote the formation of neointimal hyperplasia (NIH), thereby leading to ISR. Previous studies with BMS showed a strong association between the extent of medial damage, inflammation with leukocyte infiltration, and restenosis. Autopsy studies with first-generation DES reported delay

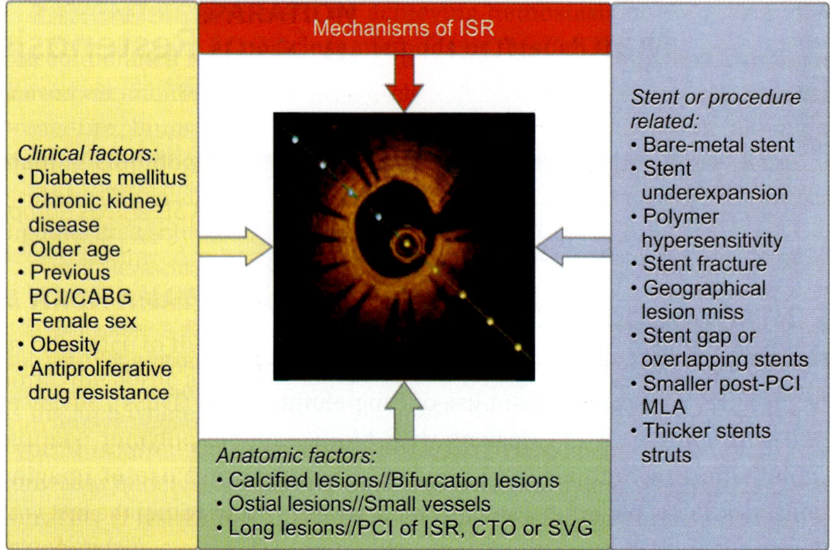

Fig. 1: Mechanisms of ISR due to various patient, procedure and stent related factors. (CABG: coronary artery bypass grafting; CTO: chronic total occlusion; ISR: in-stent restenosis; MLA: minimal luminal area; PCI: percutaneous coronary intervention; SVG: saphenous vein graft)

in arterial healing characterized by persistent inflammatory reaction with fibrin deposition and delayed re-endothelialization compared with BMS, explaining the increased risk of late and very late ST with first-generation DES.[7] Second-generation DESs have been shown to be associated with less vascular inflammation, less fibrin deposition and faster and more uniform stent strut endothelialization compared with first-generation DES.[8] Neoatherosclerosis is an increasingly recognized mechanism of stent restenosis seen with current generation DES. It is characterized by accumulation of lipid-laden foamy macrophages sometimes with necrotic core formation within stented segments with or without calcification.

CLASSIFICATIONS OF IN-STENT RESTENOSIS

In-stent restenosis is angiographically defined as recurrent diameter stenosis at the stent segment >50% of the vessel diameter or the vessel segments 5 mm proximal and distal to the stent (the "stent edges"), as assessed by coronary angiography. Using intravascular imaging (IVI), which acquires data in three dimensions, ISR has been defined as a renarrowing of ≥75% of the reference vessel area in cross-section.[9] There were various proposed classifications for ISR **(Boxes 1, 2 and Table 1)**.

BOX 1: Mehran classification of in-stent restenosis (ISR) based on angiogram. May not hold good for drug-eluting stent (DES) ISR.

Mehran classification based on angiograms[10]
This system classified patients with bare-metal stents (BMS)-ISR into groups based on three characteristics: (1) ISR length (≤10 mm: focal, >10 mm: diffuse), (2) ISR location (within or beyond stent borders), and (3) occlusion (yes or no).
- Type I: Focal
- Type II: Diffuse, within stent
- Type III: Diffuse, within and beyond stent
- Type IV: Occlusive

BOX 2: Waksman classification based on intracoronary imaging.

In-stent restenosis (ISR)-Waksman classification: Five groups (based on intracoronary imaging):[11]
1. Mechanical (type I; underexpansion IA, stent fracture IB)
2. Biologic (type II; intimal hyperplasia IIA, neoatherosclerosis noncalcified IIB, neoatherosclerosis calcified IIC)
3. Mixed pattern (type III)
4. Chronic total occlusions (type IV)
5. Lesions previously treated with >2 stents (type V)

TABLE 1: SCAI proposed classification[12] for ISR based on time course and cause.

Classification	*Time interval*	*Morphological substrate*
Early	<30 days	• Undersizing • Underexpansion • Stent fracture
Late	30 days to 1 year	• Delayed healing (including drug induced) • Uncovered stent struts • Intimal hyperplasia (especially in BMS ISR)
Very late	>1 year	• Neoatherosclerosis • Intimal hyperplasia • Stent fracture

(BMS: bare-metal stent; ISR: in-stent restenosis; SCAI: Society for Cardiovascular Angiography and Interventions)

ROLE OF IMAGING IN IN-STENT RESTENOSIS MANAGEMENT

Identifying the cause of ISR is very important in management of these complex patient subgroups. With IVI, we can determine the cause of ISR, to inform therapeutic strategy, and to confirm effective treatment after PCI.

Stent Enhancement

Stent boost or clear stent fluoroscopic stent enhancement technique is useful for identification of stent underexpansion, and stent fracture can be easily and quickly performed during index PCI procedure.[13]

Intravascular Ultrasound and Optical Coherence Tomography

Some limitations of coronary angiography can be overcome by IVI, which enables us accurately assess the underlying pathophysiologic mechanism for ISR and degree of ISR.[9] IVI allows for more precise assessment of extent and nature of ISR, and thereby guiding us for more targeted treatment options with consequent better outcomes. With the available evidence, the use of IVI has been a class IIa recommendation[14] of ISR assessment. Most commonly used imaging modalities in current clinical practice are IVUS and OCT.

Intravascular ultrasound imaging **(Figs. 2A to F)** helps in assessing the deeper tissue characteristics including external elastic lamina (EEL), in comparison to OCT, but detailed tissue characterization is not possible with IVUS. However, IVUS can still demonstrate several findings relevant to ISR, including, mature neoatherosclerosis, neointimal hyperplasia, stentundersizing, underexpansion, and vessel calcification. With IVUS, the EEL is usually well delineated, both at the reference segment and beyond the stent struts, allowing accurate vessel sizing. Virtual histology IVUS has also been used to demonstrate neoatherosclerosis in both BMS-ISR and DES-ISR.[15]

Optical coherence tomography imaging **(Figs. 3A to F)** provides 10 times the spatial resolution of IVUS and thereby allows detailed assessment of neointimal tissue characterization including neoatherosclerosis, calcification, and thrombus. But OCT imaging needs blood-free field with higher contrast requirement and difficult to image in tight or ostial ISR lesions, particularly challenging in patients with multiple metal stent layers with limited tissue penetration. Advantages of OCT assessment are expected to outweigh the risk of complications, especially in patients with ISR.

With OCT imaging, homogeneous tissue pattern is often considered typical of early-onset BMS-ISR. The other three patterns (heterogeneous, attenuated, and layered) may represent part of the neoatherosclerotic disease spectrum, which is more commonly seen in DES-ISR. Hisopathologically, a homogenous tissue appearance on OCT has been shown to correspond to neointima and fibrous connective tissue as a result of smooth muscle cell proliferation.[16] Conversely, heterogeneous tissue patterns are associated with increased fibrin depositions and loose connective tissue and large lipid pools characteristic of neoatherosclerosis.[9]

MANAGEMENT OF IN-STENT RESTENOSIS

The use of DES and DCB **(Figs. 2 and 3)** are the two therapeutic strategies recommended by current revascularization guidelines. The conventional coronary angiography measures to assess and compare the outcomes of stent- and balloon-based treatment modalities in treating coronary stenosis

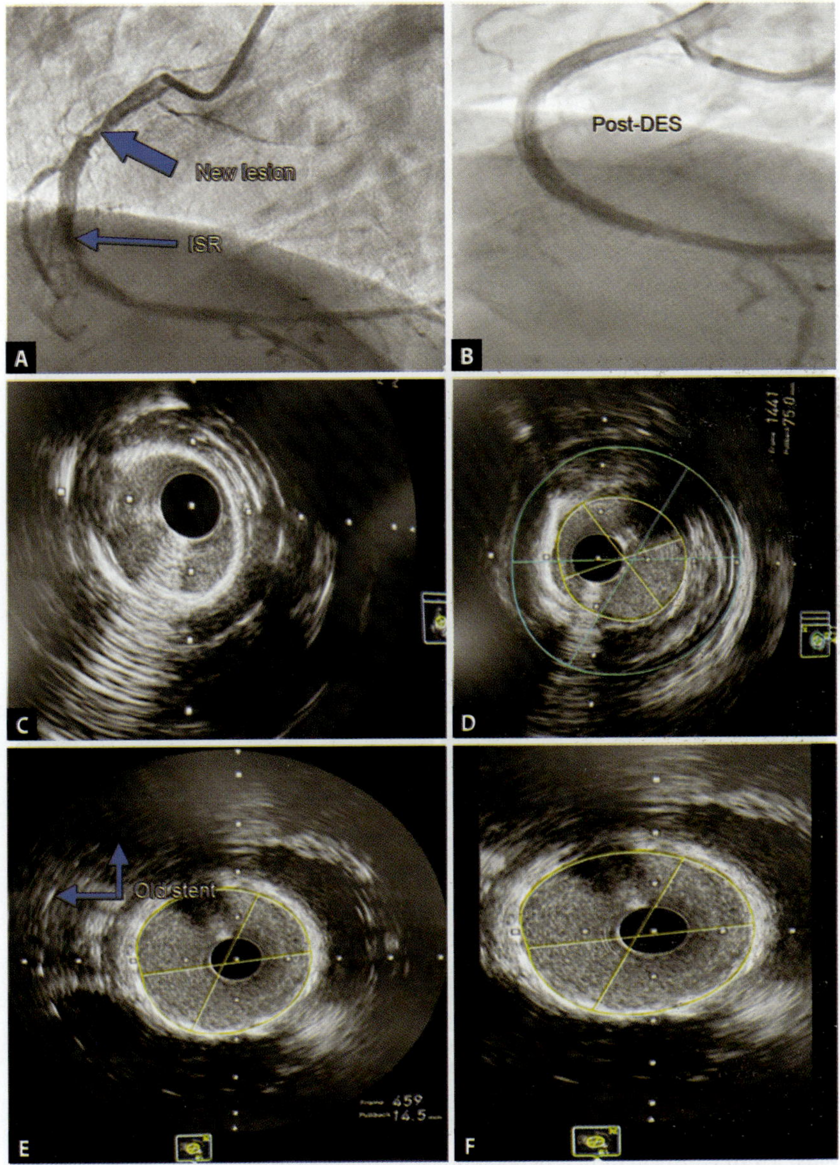

Figs. 2A to F: (A) Mid RCA stent ISR with new lesion at proximal RCA; (B) Post-balloon angioplasty and DES; (C) IVUS imaging of proximal RCA; (D) IVUS imaging at ISR segment; (E and F) Poststenting at ISR with DES. (DES: drug-eluting stent; ISR: in-stent restenosis; IVUS: intravascular ultrasound; RCA: right coronary artery)

include minimum lumen diameter (MLD), percentage diameter stenosis (%DS), acute gain, and late lumen loss (LLL). Acute gain is defined as the difference between the MLD preprocedure and the MLD immediately post-procedure. LLL is defined as the difference between the MLD immediately

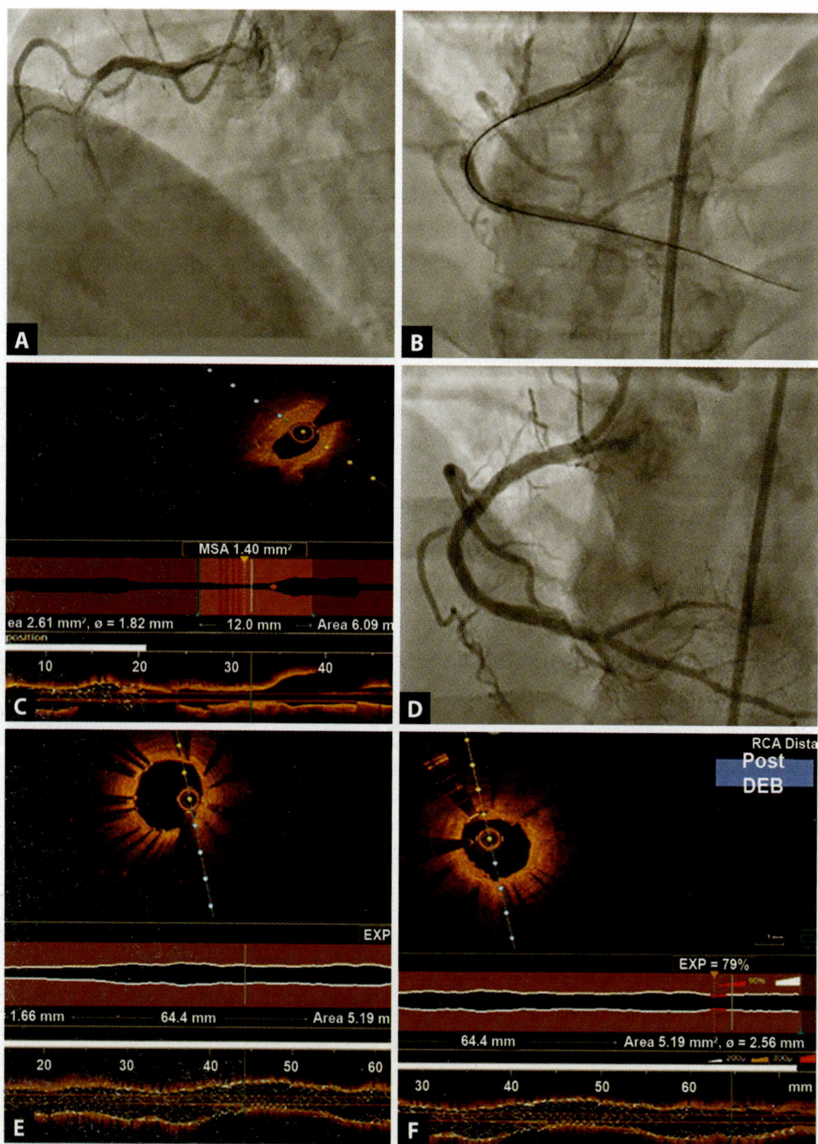

Figs. 3A to F: (A) ISR of first-generation DES; (B) Wire crossing with fielder wire and balloon angioplasty; (C) OCT imaging suggestive of (S/O) heterogeneous pattern ISR; (D) Final angiographic result after DEB and DES implantation; (E) final OCT imaging suggestive of good apposition with acute luminal gain with DES; (F) OCT imaging S/O good luminal gain with DEB in distal portion of stent. (DCB: drug-coated balloon; DES: drug-eluting stent; ISR: in-stent restenosis; OCT: optical coherence tomography; RCA: right coronary artery)

postprocedure and the MLD at follow-up angiography. When treating ISR, the aim is to maximize acute gain and minimize LLL. DES-based treatment is associated with more acute gain with increased late lumen loss, whereas

DCB-based treatment is associated with reduced acute gain and reduced LLL. In the setting of treating ISR lesions, the LLL and acute gain are not only dependent on lesion characteristics but also on extrinsic mechanical factors such as vessel calcification and calcific neoatherosclerosis.[17,18] Suboptimal treatment of ISR can result in risk of recurrence and subsequent management becomes more and more challenging, especially when patients are treated with an second DES (the so-called "sandwich strategy"), leading to multiple stent layers or the "onion skin phenomenon".[19]

Role of Drug-eluting Stents in In-Stent Restenosis

Use of DES is very attractive for ISR management **(Figs. 2 and 3)** due to acute gain at target lesion and for their antiproliferative properties. Based on various meta-analyses, the use of DES for ISR is the most effective treatment strategy.[20,21] Other head on comparison trials have demonstrated the superiority of DES implantation to several other therapeutic modalities for ISR, such as paclitaxel DCBs,[22] balloon angioplasty,[23] and intravascular brachytherapy (IVBT).[24] In treating ISR of previous DES lesions, it is hypothesized that treating DES-ISR with an alternative antiproliferative agent (the "hetero-DES" strategy) might provide superior outcomes to using a DES with the same antiproliferative agent (the "homo-DES" strategy). The ISAR DESIRE-2, only randomized trail did not show a benefit to the hetero-DES strategy for the treatment of sirolimus-eluting stent ISR.[25] Other trail comparing this strategy, RIBS-III study had suggested a hetero-DES strategy may provide superior outcomes and based on meta-analysis, a hetero-DES may provide a superior outcome for ISR lesions.[26]

Table 2 shows the advantages and disadvantages of drug-eluting stent (DES) for in-stent restenosis (ISR).

Drug-coated Balloons

Drug-coated balloons (DCBs) provide antiproliferative therapy to lesion site without requirement for an additional metal stent layer **(Figs. 4A to C)**. DCBs may be particularly useful for clinical situations where the addition of another stent layer is undesirable (i.e., multiple previous stent layers and the presence of a major side branch). DCB is particularly useful in patients with higher bleeding risk with short duration of dual antiplatelet therapy (DAPT).

TABLE 2: Advantages and disadvantages of drug-eluting stent (DES) for in-stent restenosis (ISR).

Advantages with DES for ISR	*Disadvantages with DES for ISR*
• Better acute luminal gain • Strong antiproliferative properties	• Rapid late lumen loss • Second layer of metal leading higher ISR • Very difficult to treat subsequent ISR

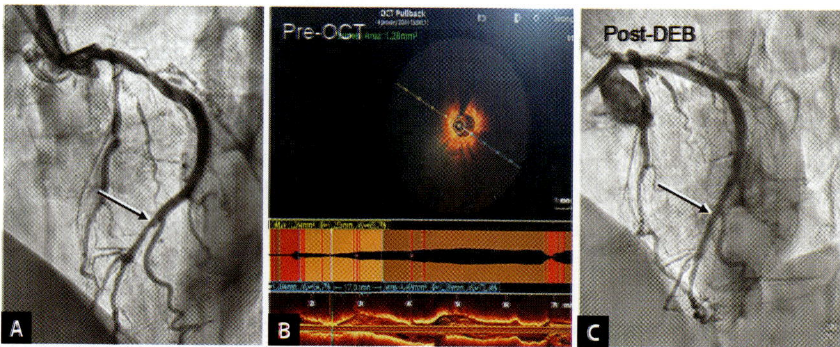

Figs. 4A to C: A 72-year-old male with post-PTCA to distal LCX 8 years back now exertional angina with TMT positive for ischemia. (A) ISR of distal LCX stent (arrow); (B) OCT image suggesting critical narrowing with luminal area of 1.28 mm^2; (C) post-DEB to distal LCX stent. (DEB: drug-eluting balloon; ISR: in-stent restenosis; LCX: left circumflex artery; OCT: optical coherence tomography; PTCA: percutaneous transluminal coronary angioplasty; TMT: treadmill test)

Adequate preparation of target lesion is very important for effective utilization of DCB with use of various options such as balloon angioplasty alone with use of cutting or scoring balloons or atherectomy devices. The efficacy of a DCB relies on rapid initial drug transfer of the antiproliferative drug and subsequent tissue retention in the restenotic area. Currently there are two types of DES available for clinical use such as paclitaxel DCB and sirolimus DCB. Limus-eluting stents have shown superior outcomes when compared to paclitaxel-eluting stents, and similar outcomes were expected from DCB with sirolimus. However, a small RCT comparing a novel sirolimus DCB to a paclitaxel DCB reported similar 6-month angiographic and 12-month clinical outcomes and further randomized studies are needed.[27] Drug-coated scoring balloons are being developed combining both treatment strategies of adequate lesion modification with drug release at lesion site.[28]

Studies comparing the DES with DCB for ISR lesions demonstrated that repeat DES implantation is moderately more effective in reducing the rate of target lesion revascularization (TLR) at 3 years.[9] The DAEDALUS study, a meta-analysis of patient-level data from 10 randomized clinical trials (RCTs) which included 1,976 patients, demonstrated that DESs reduced the need for subsequent TLR compared with paclitaxel DCBs at 3 years.[22]

Adjunctive therapies:
- Balloon angioplasty (BA)
- Cutting and scoring balloons
- IVBT
- Ablative strategies—rotational atherectomy (RA)/excimer laser coronary atherectomy (ELCA)

- Intravascular (IV) lithotripsy
- BMS
- Bioresorbable vascular scaffold (BVS)
- Coronary artery bypass grafting (CABG)
- Adjunctive medical therapy

Balloon angioplasty: This was the earlier treatment option for ISR but became inferior to DES or DCB.

Balloon angioplasty results in tissue extrusion (both longitudinal and axial) along with stent expansion, resulting ultimately in acute gain of lumen, but this could be short lived. Main disadvantage with BA is recurrent tissue proliferation. BA is used for focal ISR lesions where the risk of recurrence is expected to be low and where DCB is not available.[29] In an under deployed stent, noncompliant or ultra-high-pressure noncompliant balloons such as OPN NC at high pressures should be used to improve stent expansion. However, based on data till now, isolated BA is not commonly recommended for the treatment of ISR, and this is regarded as a method for lesion preparation before the use of other therapies or for final optimization of DES implantation.[9]

Cutting and scoring balloons: **Table 3** shows cutting and scoring balloons.

The main advantages to their use in lesion preparation are:

The incision of the blades into the stenotic plaque tissue may favor subsequent tissue preparation, and the interaction of the blades with the plaque serves to anchor the balloon in the plaque.[30] Use of scoring or

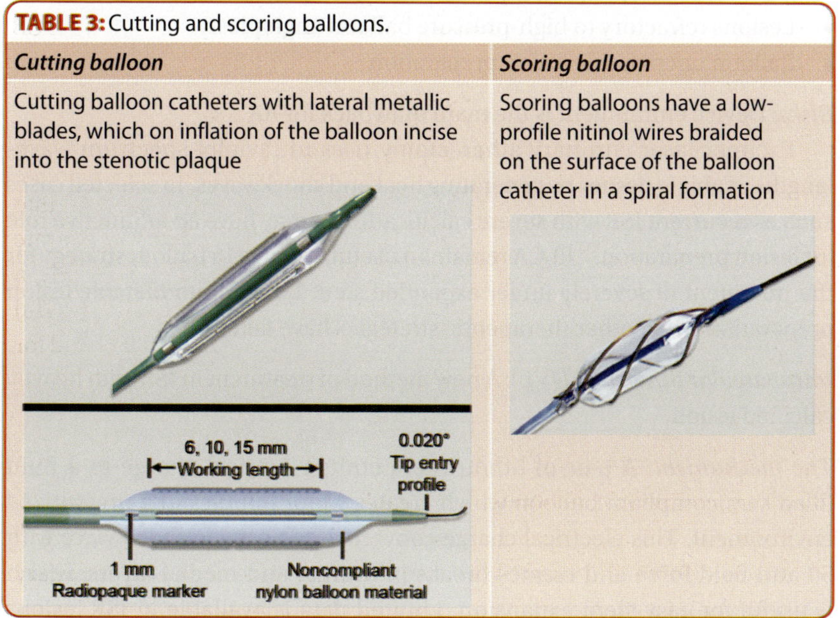

TABLE 3: Cutting and scoring balloons.

Cutting balloon	*Scoring balloon*
Cutting balloon catheters with lateral metallic blades, which on inflation of the balloon incise into the stenotic plaque	Scoring balloons have a low-profile nitinol wires braided on the surface of the balloon catheter in a spiral formation

cutting balloon prevents water melon seeding phenomenon during lesion preparation of diffuse ISR. Both the balloon types play a significant role in lesion preparation prior to DESs or DCBs in the treatment of ISR based on imaging finding of ISR mechanism.

Disadvantage: Higher lesion crossing profile and inability to inhibit neointimal proliferation similar to balloon angioplasty.

In the ISAR-DESIRE 4 trial, the use of a scoring balloon prior to a DCB has been shown to improve the antirestenotic efficacy of the DCB.[31] Drug-coated scoring balloons are under development by combining both the properties of adequate lesion preparation with release of antiproliferative agent at lesion site.[28]

Intravascular brachytherapy: Vascular brachytherapy delivers radioactive strontium-90 β-radiation which decreases proliferation by inhibiting neointimal formation in desired area. It was used in bare metal ISR, but no long-term benefits were demonstrated;[32] it is less effective if more than three stent layers are there. There are no randomized trail data available for use of IVBT in DES ISR.[9]

Ablative strategies: Rotational atherectomy and ELCA are two available ablative treatment methods for ISR; but in clinical trail, data for both methods have not demonstrated any significant benefits over long-term follow-up. Main indications are:

- When IVI confirms the presence of severe calcification within neo-atherosclerotic plaques, especially for lesion preparation
- Lesions refractory to high-pressure balloon angioplasty
- Balloon uncrossable lesion preparation

Risks: Device entrapment is the main drawback for RA.[17]

Excimer laser coronary atherectomy uses ultraviolet spectrum wavelengths to ablate tissues by generating heat and shockwaves. In selected cases such as recurrent ISR with severe calcification, it may have an adjunctive role for lesion preparation.[33] ELCA remains a useful option as a bailout strategy for the treatment of severely under expanded stent ISR with undilatable lesion preparation when other therapeutic strategies have failed.

Intravascular lithotripsy (IVL): A new method of treatment in ISR with heavily calcified lesion.

The mechanism: A pair of lithotripters emits electrical charge in a fluid filled semicompliant balloon which creates vapor bubbles in a pressurized environment. This electrical charge converts into acoustic shock wave with 50 atm field force and creates breaks in intimal and medial layers, which is useful for easy stent expansion. Limited data is available in ISR lesions than denovo lesions. IVL may be used for undilatable ISR resistant to conventional strategies, especially in the setting of stent underexpansion due to circumferential coronary artery calcification. When compared to ablative methods, it is user friendly and less dependent on operators.[34] IVL has also been combined with VBT, which needs further studies.

BMS: It has better results than plain BA, especially in large vessels (>3 mm) and edge ISR. No long-term benefits are observed in studies.[9]

Bioresorbable vascular scaffolds: BVS appears potentially useful for ISR lesion, but usage in ISR has high TLR rates when compared to DES.[35]

Coronary artery bypass grafting may be a reasonable treatment option in selected patients such as: recurrent ISR in a major vessel, ISR of the left main coronary artery or ostial LAD lesion, and ISR-associated multivessel disease in other coronary arteries. According to some observational analyses, CABG has superior outcomes compared to percutaneous therapies.[9]

Adjunctive medical therapy: Anti-inflammatory or antiproliferative therapy; according to OSIRIS study, oral sirolimus showed good improvement in 6-month follow-up in ISR lesions but failed to show long-term benefits with potential adverse effects of long-term antiproliferative therapy.[36]

Management of Recurrent In-Stent Restenosis

Patients with recurrent ISR are refractory to usual treatment modalities and in most instances associated with under expanded initial stent.

Drug-coated balloons may have benefits, but failure rates are also high with multiple metallic layers. The 1-year TLR incidence rate was reported as 14.5%, 14.9%, and 41.2% in 1-stent, 2-stent, and 3-stent layer groups, respectively.

Vascular brachytherapy is a choice in refractory ISR with multilayered stent. Recurrent ISR in the setting of calcification of neoatherosclerosis and stent underexpansion needs calcium modification with RA, ELCA, IVL, and high pressure balloon dilatation to modify calcium and facilitate stent expansion to get optimal results with maximum acute luminal gain.

Other options such as CABG or optimal medical therapy may be indicated in refractory ISR to avoid multiple procedures and its related complications.

Antiplatelet medication: DAPT also needed in ISR-PCI patients same as denovo lesions; but there is insufficient data for patients undergoing ISR-PCI for optimal DAPT and duration of DAPT. PRODIGY trial has suggested that a prolonged 2-year DAPT regimen may be beneficial for patients undergoing ISR-PCI compared to 6 months needs further trials to show benefits.[37] **Figure 5** summarizes the management of ISR lesions.

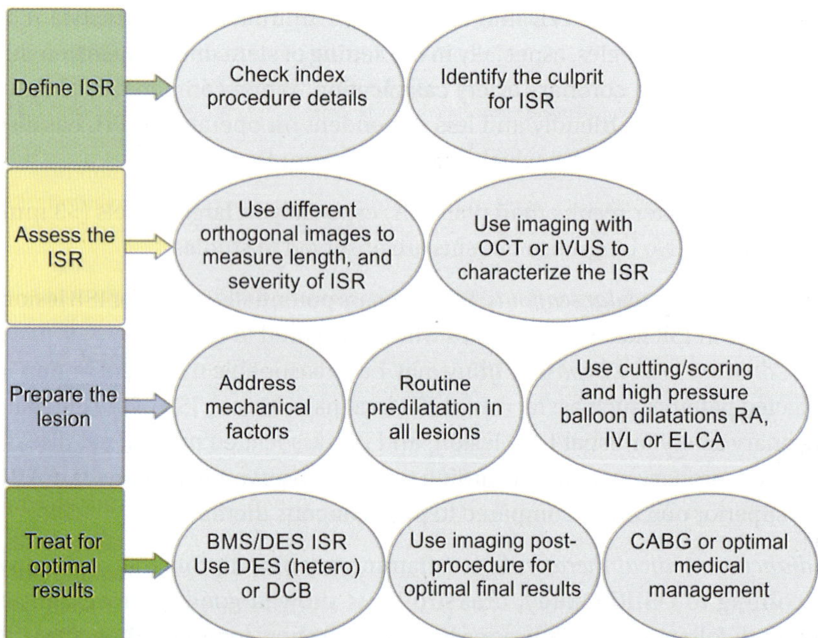

Fig. 5: Summary of management of ISR lesions. (BMS: bare-metal stent; CABG: coronary artery bypass grafting; DCB: drug-coated balloon; DES: drug-eluting stent; ELCA: excimer laser coronary atherectomy; ISR: in-stent restenosis; IVL: intravascular lithotripsy; IVUS: intravascular ultrasound; OCT: optical coherence tomography; RA: rotational atherectomy)

CONCLUSION

In-stent restenosis contributes to 5–10% of all interventional procedures of modern era despite use of advanced DES. DESs or DCBs are the optimal treatment modalities as per available evidence in majority of ISR PCI. Use of IVI is mandatory in all ISR cases for identifying the mechanism of ISR and for optimal treatment based on tissue characteristics. Other adjunctive therapies are useful for optimal preparation of the target lesions.

REFERENCES

1. Madhavan MV, Kirtane AJ, Redfors B, Généreux P, Ben-Yehuda O, Palmerini T, et al. Stent-related adverse events >1 year after percutaneous coronary intervention. J Am Coll Cardiol. 2020;75:590-604.
2. Moussa ID, Mohananey D, Saucedo J, Stone GW, Yeh RW, Kennedy KF, et al. Trends and outcomes of restenosis after coronary stent implantation in the United States. J Am Coll Cardiol. 2020;76:1521-31.
3. Kastrati A, Cassese S. In-stent restenosis in the United States: time to enrich its treatment armamentarium. J Am Coll Cardiol. 2020;76:1532-5.
4. Yabushita H, Kawamoto H, Fujino Y, Tahara S, Horikoshi T, Tada M, et al. Clinical outcomes of drug-eluting balloon for in-stent restenosis based on the number of metallic layers. Circ Cardiovasc Interv. 2018;11:e005935.

5. Kawamoto H, Ruparelia N, Latib A, Miyazaki T, Sato K, Mangieri A, et al. Drug-coated balloons versus second-generation drug-eluting stents for the management of recurrent multimetal-layered in-stent restenosis. JACC Cardiovasc Interv. 2015;8:1586-94.
6. Dangas GD, Claessen BE, Caixeta A, Sanidas EA, Mintz GS, Mehran R. In-stent restenosis in the drug-eluting stent era. J Am Coll Cardiol. 2010;56:1897-907.
7. Joner M, Finn AV, Farb A, Mont EK, Kolodgie FD, Ladich E, et al. Pathology of drug-eluting stents in humans: delayed healing and late thrombotic risk. J Am Coll Cardiol. 2006;48:193-202.
8. Otsuka F, Vorpahl M, Nakano M, Foerst J, Newell JB, Sakakura K, et al. Pathology of second-generation everolimus-eluting stents versus first-generation sirolimus- and paclitaxel-eluting stents in humans. Circulation. 2014;129:211-23.
9. Alfonso F, Coughlan JJ, Giacoppo D, Kastrati A, Byrne RA. Management of in-stent restenosis. EuroIntervention. 2022;18(2):e103-e123.
10. Mehran R, Dangas G, Abizaid AS, Mintz GS, Lansky AJ, Satler LF, et al. Angiographic patterns of in-stent restenosis: classification and implications for long-term outcome. Circulation. 1999;100:1872-8.
11. Shlofmitz E, Iantorno M, Waksman R. Restenosis of drug-eluting stents: a new classification system based on disease mechanism to guide treatment and stateof-the-art review. Circ Cardiovasc Interv. 2019;12(8):e007023.
12. Klein LW, Nathan S, Maehara A, Messenger J, Mintz GS, Ali ZA, et al. SCAI Expert Consensus Statement on Management of In-Stent Restenosis and Stent Thrombosis. J Soc Cardiovasc Angiogr Interv. 2023;2(4):100971.
13. Mishell JM, Vakharia KT, Ports TA, Yeghiazarians Y, Michaels AD. Determination of adequate coronary stent expansion using StentBoost, a novel fluoroscopic image processing technique. Catheter Cardiovasc Interv. 2007;69:84-93.
14. Neumann FJ, Sousa-Uva M, Ahlsson A, Alfonso F, Banning AP, Benedetto U, et al. 2018 ESC/EACTS Guidelines on myocardial revascularization. Eur Heart J. 2019;40(2):87-165.
15. Kang SJ, Mintz GS, Park DW, Lee SW, Kim YH, Lee CW, et al. Tissue characterization of in-stent neointima using intravascular ultrasound radiofrequency data analysis. Am J Cardiol. 2010;106:1561-5.
16. Kim JS, Afari ME, Ha J, Tellez A, Milewski K, Conditt G, et al. Neointimal patterns obtained by optical coherence tomography correlate with specific histological components and neointimal proliferation in a swine model of restenosis. Eur Heart J Cardiovasc Imaging. 2014;15:292-8.
17. Bastante T, Rivero F, Cuesta J, Alfonso F. Calcified Neoatherosclerosis Causing Undilatable In-Stent Restenosis: Insights of Optical Coherence Tomography and Role of Rotational Atherectomy. JACC Cardiovasc Interv. 2015;8:2039-40.
18. Garcia-Guimaraes M, Antuña P, Maruri-Sanchez R, Vera A, Cuesta J, Bastante T, et al. Calcified neoatherosclerosis causing in-stent restenosis: prevalence, predictors, and implications. Coron Artery Dis. 2019;30:1-8.
19. Alfonso F, Scheller B. Management of recurrent in-stent restenosis: onion skin full metal jacket? EuroIntervention. 2013;9:781-5.
20. Giacoppo D, Gargiulo G, Aruta P, Capranzano P, Tamburino C, Capodanno D. Treatment strategies for coronary in-stent restenosis: systematic review and hierarchical Bayesian network meta-analysis of 24 randomised trials and 4880 patients. BMJ. 2015;351:h5392.

21. Siontis GC, Stefanini GG, Mavridis D, Siontis KC, Alfonso F, Pérez-Vizcayno MJ, et al. Percutaneous coronary interventional strategies for treatment of in-stent restenosis: a network meta-analysis. Lancet. 2015;386:655-64.
22. Giacoppo D, Alfonso F, Xu B, Claessen B, Claessen BE, Adriaenssens T, et al. Paclitaxel-coated balloon angioplasty vs. drug-eluting stenting for the treatment of coronary in-stent restenosis: a comprehensive, collaborative, individual patient data meta-analysis of 10 randomized clinical trials (DAEDALUS study). Eur Heart J. 2020;41:3715-28.
23. Chevalier B, Moulichon R, Teiger E, Brunel P, Metzger JP, Pansieri M, et al. Cristal Investigators. One-year results of the CRISTAL Trial, a randomized comparison of cypher sirolimus-eluting coronary stents versus balloon angioplasty for restenosis of drug-eluting stents. J Interv Cardiol. 2012;25:586-95.
24. Park SW, Lee SW, Koo BK, Park DW, Lee SW, Kim YH, et al. Treatment of diffuse in-stent restenosis with drug-eluting stents vs. intracoronary beta-radiation therapy: INDEED Study. Int J Cardiol. 2008;131:70-7.
25. Mehilli J, Byrne RA, Tiroch K, Pinieck S, Schulz S, Kufner S, et al. ISAR-DESIRE 2 Investigators. Randomized trial of paclitaxel- versus sirolimus-eluting stents for treatment of coronary restenosis in sirolimus-eluting stents: the ISAR-DESIRE 2 (Intracoronary Stenting and Angiographic Results: Drug Eluting Stents for In-Stent Restenosis 2) study. J Am Coll Cardiol. 2010;55:2710-6.
26. Vyas A, Schweizer M, Malhotra A, Karrowni W. Meta-analysis of same versus different stent for drug-eluting stent restenosis. Am J Cardiol. 2014;113:601-6.
27. Ali RM, Abdul Kader M, Wan Ahmad WA, Ong TK, Liew HB, Omar AF. Treatment of Coronary Drug-Eluting Stent Restenosis by a Sirolimus- or Paclitaxel-Coated Balloon. JACC Cardiovasc Interv. 2019;12:558-66.
28. Scheller B, Fontaine T, Mangner N, Hoffmann S, Bonaventura K, Clever YP, et al. A novel drug-coated scoring balloon for the treatment of coronary in-stent restenosis: Results from the multi-center randomized controlled PATENT-C first in human trial. Catheter Cardiovasc Interv. 2016;88:51-9.
29. Mehran R, Mintz GS, Popma JJ, Pichard AD, Satler LF, Kent KM, et al. Mechanisms and results of balloon angioplasty for the treatment of in-stent restenosis. Am J Cardiol. 1996;78:618-22.
30. Takano M, Yamamoto M, Murakami D, Takano H, Asai K, Yasutake M, et al. Optical coherence tomography after new scoring balloon angioplasty for in-stent restenosis and de novo coronary lesions. Int J Cardiol. 2010;141:e51-3.
31. Kufner S, Joner M, Schneider S, Tölg R, Zrenner B, Repp J, et al.; ISAR-DESIRE 4 Investigators. Neointimal modification with scoring balloon and efficacy of drug-coated balloon therapy in patients with restenosis in drug-eluting coronary stents: a randomized controlled trial. JACC Cardiovasc Interv. 2017;10:1332-40.
32. Waksman R, Cheneau E, Ajani AE, White RL, Pinnow E, Torguson R, et al.; Washington Radiation for In-Stent Restenosis Trial for Long Lesions Studies. Intracoronary radiation therapy improves the clinical and angiographic outcomes of diffuse in-stent restenotic lesions: results of the Washington Radiation for In-Stent Restenosis Trial for Long Lesions (Long WRIST) Studies. Circulation. 2003;107:1744-9.
33. Sato T, Tsuchida K, Yuasa S, Taya Y, Koshikawa T, Tanaka K, et al. The effect of the debulking by excimer laser coronary angioplasty on long-term outcome compared with drug-coating balloon: insights from optical frequency domain imaging analysis. Lasers Med Sci. 2020;35:403-12.

34. Alfonso F, Bastante T, Antuña P, de la Cuerda F, Cuesta J, García-Guimaraes M, et al. Lithoplasty for the Treatment of Undilatable Calcified De Novo and In-Stent Restenosis Lesions. Cardiovasc Interv. 2019;12:497-9.
35. Alfonso F, Cuesta J, García Del Blanco B, Bosa F, de Prado AP, Masotti M, et al.; Restenosis Intrastent: Bioresorbable Vascular Scaffolds Treatment with Scoring Balloon Pre-dilatation (RIBS VI 'Scoring') Study Investigators (under the auspices of the Interventional Cardiology Working Group of the Spanish Society of Cardiology). Scoring balloon predilation before bioresorbable vascular scaffold implantation in patients with in-stent restenosis: the RIBS VI 'scoring' study. Coron Artery Dis. 2021;32:96-104.
36. Kufner S, Hausleiter J, Ndrepepa G, Schulz S, Bruskina O, Byrne RA, et al.; OSIRIS Trial Investigators. Long-term risk of adverse outcomes and new malignancies in patients treated with oral sirolimus for prevention of restenosis. JACC Cardiovasc Interv. 2009;2:1142-8.
37. Campo G, Tebaldi M, Vranckx P, Biscaglia S, Tumscitz C, Ferrari R, et al. Short-versus long-term duration of dual antiplatelet therapy in patients treated for in-stent restenosis: a PRODIGY trial substudy (Prolonging Dual Antiplatelet Treatment After Grading Stent-Induced Intimal Hyperplasia). J Am Coll Cardiol. 2014;63:506-12.

CHAPTER 32

Drug-coated Balloon in Clinical Practice

Rishi Sethi

INTRODUCTION

The field of interventional cardiology has evolved significantly since the first percutaneous coronary intervention (PCI) was performed 40 years ago.[1] This evolution began with the invention of a balloon catheter mounted on a fixed wire to open the stenosis in the coronary artery. It then progressed into bare-metal stents (BMSs), first-generation drug-eluting stents (DESs), and second- and third-generation biodegradable polymer-based DES and culminated with the advent of bioabsorbable stents (BRSs), which are currently underdevelopment.

Although each technological advancement led to improved outcomes, each also had its challenges. Despite the promising technological advances made in stent technology, managing the balance between reductions in target vessel revascularization (TVR), stent thrombosis (ST), and bleeding remains a highly complex issue. BRSs were designed with a view to avoid permanent metal in vessels, but they had a high incidence of ST due to thick stent struts, and they can be used only in simple lesions, so were removed from the market. Further advancement is needed in BRS technology to avoid its complications which are currently ongoing.[2] The latest advancement in the field of coronary intervention is the advent of drug-coated balloon (DCB), which can be used for treating a variety of coronary lesions while avoiding extra metal in coronaries. This review summarizes the evolution of DCB, their uses, and efficacy in coronary intervention.

PROBLEMS OF METAL IN CORONARY ARTERIES

Although the evidence-based use of new generation DESs has brought an era of excellent clinical outcomes, their rampant use has brought more and more metal to be placed in the coronaries. On the other hand, the mandatory use of long duration of dual antiplatelet therapy (DAPT) after DES may be prohibitory in certain cohorts of patients. More importantly, certain clinical settings may not be ideal for metallic stents.

DEVELOPMENT OF BIODEGRADABLE STENT

Bioabsorbable vascular scaffold (BVS) was designed to represent the fourth revolution in interventional cardiology. The concept behind their development is the idea that stent scaffolds are only transiently necessary to the vessel after their implantation to prevent acute recoil and maintain vessel integrity. Further, the degradation of stent scaffolds could allow restoration of the vasomotor and endothelial functions, thus reducing neoatherosclerosis and promoting positive remodeling. In addition, the absence of long-term metal reduces the risk of ST, allowing less duration of DAPT and room for coronary bypass grafting if the need arises.[3,4]

Although the concept of BVS was an attractive idea that raised global enthusiasm in the field of interventional cardiology, its use encountered several concerns that led to its withdrawal from the market after the disappointing results of the ABSORB III trial, which showed higher rates of target lesion failure (TLF) compared with the latest generation of DES. The TLFs were mainly due to increased risk of target-related myocardial infarction (MI) and higher ST rates.[5,6] The reasons behind its failure were improper lesion preparation, lesion selection with reference vessel size ≥2.50 mm, higher strut thickness, and stent base composition (poly-L-lactide was found to trigger thrombogenicity, inflammatory cell adhesion, and delayed endothelialization in porcine models). Despite these drawbacks, companies are still running BVS development programs for the improvement of the devices to overcome these drawbacks.

DRUG-COATED BALLOON FOR PERCUTANEOUS TRANSLUMINAL CORONARY ANGIOPLASTY

Drug-coated balloon is a novel device for percutaneous transluminal coronary angioplasty (PTCA). The rapid healing of the vessel wall due to the fast release of the drug is the basic concept for DCB. It is postulated that DCB could result in satisfactory results in certain lesions. Although dissection causing acute vessel closure was the major concern with the use of plain old balloon angioplasty (POBA), a study done by Takhiro Nishida et al., way back in 2002 has demonstrated that nonflow limiting dissection demonstrated on intravascular ultrasound performs better than BMS.[7] Thus, POBA is not bad, and strengthening it with the use of DCB in coronary interventions seems an intuitive step forward.

Why We need Stentless Percutaneous Transluminal Coronary Angioplasty: Challenges of Drug-eluting Stent

- *Need for pronged DAPT:* Use of DES although decreases the chances of in-stent restenosis (ISR), there is still a chance of late and very late ST, so patients need prolonged DAPT for up to 12 months till the stent is completely endothelialized. Although with the advancement in the stent platform and use of biocompatible or biodegradable polymer, a shorter duration of DAPT is possible in some cases and still it is preferable to give at least 6 months of DAPT. The use of DAPT is associated with an increased risk of hemorrhagic complications which lead to higher mortality, especially in the elderly, and those with a prior history of hemorrhage and bleeding diathesis. Patients on anticoagulation due to various reasons are also at heightened risk of major bleeding complications due to the combined use of DAPT and in patients requiring major surgery. On the other hand, withholding DAPT exposes them to the risk of ST and its sequelae.[8]

- *Adverse effects of permanent metal in coronaries:* Another potential limitation of DES is the permanent presence of both a metallic foreign body within the artery and often a durable polymer. Either of them may cause vascular inflammation, neoatherosclerosis, and restenosis or the risk of very late ST.[9] Metallic stents also impair the physiological vasomotor function of the vessel and impair the phenomenon of late luminal enlargement, and if placed in the distal coronary segment, the potential for grafting within this stented segment is also lost. The vessel size is a strong predictor of restenosis, thus placing a stent in them poses a risk of ISR and should be avoided.[9] Despite improvement in stent technology, coronary bifurcation lesions are still a challenge for PCI due to unsatisfactory clinical outcomes, mostly in the side branch (SB). Although in the DES era, ISR incidence in the main branch is reduced from up to 40–60% to 2.5%, restenosis at the ostium of the SB remains an obstinate problem and causes repeated revascularizations. ST is present in up to 4.4% of patients after PCI of bifurcation lesions compared with around 1.4% of patients with nonbifurcation lesions. The risk of subacute ST has been higher using two-stent techniques in the majority of trials.[10] Similarly, the presence of diffuse coronary lesions is again a challenge as a longer stent increases the odds of ST.

DRUG-COATED BALLOON: LEAVE NOTHING BEHIND

Drug-coated balloon is a novel treatment strategy for coronary artery disease (CAD) based on fast homogeneous transfer of antiproliferative drugs into the vessel wall by single inflation. The basic concept of DCB is rapid healing of the vessel wall due to the fast release of the drug. Furthermore, due to full exposure of drugs to smooth muscle cells in a short duration, there is a sustained effect in the first hours to days after angioplasty. DCB is a semicompliant angioplasty balloon which is coated with an antiproliferative agent and unlike the long-term drug release of DES, DCB transiently releases the drug in 30–60 seconds.[11]

Although DESs were introduced to reduce ISR by a controlled, sustained release of antiproliferative drugs. However, late occurrence of neoatherosclerosis and ST is a persistent concern even with second-generation DES. Therefore, the use of DCBs has been an attractive alternative as they fulfill the concept of "leaving nothing behind" without the elevated thrombotic risk seen even with temporary implants such as BVS.[12]

Technical Aspects

It has been demonstrated from initial experimental work that a rapid drug uptake by the tissue and drug persistence in the vessel wall to compensate for a short contact time is the main prerequisite for nonstent-based approaches for local drug delivery. Initially, a variety of different coatings on balloon catheters were tested, but taxane compounds were investigated finally. Further ahead, the combination of a highly lipophilic drug and a specific coating matrix was finally tested in a small first-in-human trial of coronary ISR, in which a significantly lower incidence of restenosis was demonstrated.[13] An important aspect of local paclitaxel therapy is the positive remodeling phenomenon, resulting in late luminal increase after DCB.

Recently, sirolimus and its derivatives were also investigated for the use in DCBs. However, the limitations of "limus" substances are the poorer transfer rate compared with paclitaxel and reversible binding to rapamycin receptor. Several approaches have been developed to solve the sirolimus drug delivery system.[12,14] One is the liquid formulation in a porous balloon. The SABRE (Sirolimus Angioplasty Balloon for Coronary In-Stent Restenosis) trial was the first clinical study with sirolimus in a liquid formulation delivered by a porous balloon for coronary ISR.[15] However, a crystalline sirolimus coating with butylated hydroxytoluene as an excipient led to persistent vessel concentrations of up to 50% of the initial concentration at 1 month, and a clinical randomized trial using this formulation in DES ISR showed comparable in-segment late lumen loss (LLL) after 6 months between the paclitaxel- and the sirolimus-coated balloon groups. Also, there was no difference in clinical events between the groups up to 12 months.[14,16]

Choice of Drug-coated Balloon: Paclitaxel or Sirolimus

Several different DCBs are commercially available for coronary use. Paclitaxel is still considered to be the drug of choice with a typical dose between 2 and 3.5 mg/mm^2 on the balloon surface. The reason is that the interaction among drug doses, formulations, release kinetics, and lesions is crucial for the vascular response after DCB therapy. However, since no evidence of a "class effect" is seen among different platforms, current guidelines recommend both.[17]

Lesion Preparation

To gain the proper benefits of DCB, the lesion should be adequately prepared. For uncomplicated lesion, predilatation using a semicompliant or a noncompliant balloon with a 1:1 balloon-to-artery ratio is adequate.

BOX 1: Practical tips for using drug-coated balloon.

- Proper guide catheter support or use of guide catheter extension to ensure drug-coated balloon (DCB) delivery in one attempt
- Optimal lesion preparation (noncompliant/cutting balloon)
- Quick and smooth delivery of DCB to the target site
- Prolong inflation of a fully inflated balloon of correct size
- <30% residual stenosis
- Thrombolysis in myocardial infarction (TIMI) flow >3
- Absence of flow-limiting dissections

For lesions with difficulty in balloon negotiation or underfilled or undersized vessels, serial dilatation starting from a smaller balloon size and re-assessing after administering vasodilatation should be done. In case the lesion does not open with a standard semicompliant or noncompliant balloon, high pressure noncompliant or scoring or cutting balloon should be used; this is especially helpful in dealing with ISR patients. In certain patients, adjunctive therapy such as rotablation, orbital atherectomy, laser, or lithotripsy can be employed in addition to balloon dilatation. An optimally prepared lesion is confirmed if: (1) Correct vessel size balloon inflates fully; (2) ≤30% residual stenosis; (3) thrombolysis in myocardial infarction (TIMI) flow grade 3; and (4) the absence of a flow-limiting dissection (type A and B dissections are acceptable) are present. For delivery of DCB, a properly engaged guide catheter with good support is paramount to ensure it reaches the target lesion in one attempt. It should be of the correct vessel size and inflated for a prolonged duration. Extreme caution should be exercised in handling DCB as some brands may shed drug after coming in contact with liquid. The tips for using DCB have been described in **Box 1.**[13]

CURRENT INDICATIONS OF DRUG-ELUTING BALLOON

- *Small coronary vessels:* The interventional treatment of coronary small-vessel disease, defined as lesions in vessels ≤2.5 mm in diameter, usually accounts for 30–50% of total coronary procedures. The clinical feasibility of DCB was first tested in several nonrandomized trials followed by randomized controlled trials (RCTs). The PEPCAD I study was the first RCT which assessed the performance of a DCB (SeQuent Please) in small vessels. It consisted of 114 patients with lesions in vessels <2.8 mm.[18] At 6 months, the in-segment LLL with a BMS was 0.62 ± 0.73 mm. In contrast, LLL was 0.16 ± 0.38 mm in DCB-only treated patients. The rate of major adverse cardiovascular events (MACEs) at 12 months was 6.1% versus 37.5%, which was mainly due to the need for target lesion revascularization (TLR). Excellent clinical outcome was demonstrated at 36 months follow-up in the DCB-only group.[19] BELLO trial was the first RCT of 182 patients with lesions in vessels <2.8 mm randomized to either an IN.PACT Falcon balloon and the TAXUS DES. After 6 months of follow-up, LLL was significantly lower in the DCB-arm than in DES-arm (0.08 ± 0.38 mm vs. 0.29 ± 0.44 mm; $p = 0.001$), ultimately translating into a reduction in MACEs at 3 years of follow-up.[20,21] In SeQuent SVD Registry of 479 patients with de novo lesions of small reference diameters (≥2.0 mm and ≤2.75 mm), TLR and MACE rates were lower with DCB at 9 months (4.7% and 3.6%, respectively), suggesting DCB to be an alternative treatment option to DES in small vessel disease.[22] In the BASKET -SMALL 2 trial, also DCB was noninferior for the treatment of native small coronary vessel disease with similar event rates at 12 months.[23]

- *Coronary in-stent-restenosis:* The pathophysiology of restenosis after stenting is different from POBA and is characterized by neointimal hyperplasia (BMS) and neoatherosclerosis plus hyperplasia (DES). DCB has shown superiority in both BMS and DES-ISR patients in various trials **(Table 1)**. Patients with DES ISR are a high-risk population because of the primary failure of local drug delivery by the stent.[24] Thus, the potential relative efficacy of DCBs versus DES according to the underlying tissue substrate (e.g., neointimal hyperplasia vs. neoatherosclerosis) may be different, which is also demonstrated in large meta-analysis of RCTS where DCBs were equivalent to DES in reducing revascularization for BMS ISR but were somewhat less efficacious in DES ISR. Patients with multiple previous stent layers particularly are the most suitable candidates for DEB use as it will protect relevant side branches emerging from the stent with ISR, and those who are candidates for shorter DAPT because of high bleeding risk.[25] Based on this, current guidelines on myocardial revascularization recommend the use of DCB for ISR treatment *(Class I, Level of Evidence: A)*.[17]
- *Bifurcation disease:* Treatment of coronary bifurcation lesions is still challenging due to unsatisfactory angiographic clinical outcomes, mostly in the SB. Even with the use of the latest generation DES restenosis risk remains, especially if more complex techniques are used. Due to this reason, provisional bifurcation approach with implanting a stent in the main branch (MB) only has become the preferred approach based on recent trial results. However, DCB treatment in the SB may be superior when compared with POBA.[26] The DEBUT study is RCT of 117 patients categorized into three arms: DEB pretreatment + BMS; BMS with an uncoated balloon; and paclitaxel DES with an uncoated balloon.[27] Although good results were achieved with DCB + BMS arm, it was not superior to BMS, mainly because of good results of the POBA-treated SB in both BMS and DES arms. In the multicentric BABILON RCT MACE and TLR rates were higher in the DCB group than the DES group (17.3% vs. 7.1%; $p = 0.105$ and 15.4 vs. 3.6%; $p = 0.045$) because DCB

bifurcation pretreatment with BMS implantation in MB showed greater and nonsignificant LLL compared with everolimus DES.[28] The DCB-only strategy has been studied by some investigators for bifurcation lesions. The PEPCAD BIF trial is a multicenter RCT, which compared the DCB-only strategy with POBA in 64 patients with coronary bifurcation lesions. The restenosis rate was significantly lower with the DCB strategy (6% in the DCB-only group vs. 26% in the POBA group, $p = 0.045$). The results demonstrated that the DCB-only strategy can be used for bifurcation lesions with acceptable angiographic results after careful lesion preparation.[29]

- *High bleeding risk:* Bleeding after PCI is an important cause of mortality as well as ischemic events such as nonfatal MI.[8] DCBs can be preferred over stent implantation in patients at high bleeding risk such as frail elderly patients, patients on anticoagulants or patients having chronic kidney disease or those with bleeding diathesis. Although with the latest generation DES, DAPT duration after PCI can be shortened, but antithrombotic can be stopped in case of severe life-threatening bleeding earlier after DCB than after DES. The recommended duration of DAPT after DCB-only strategy in de novo vessels is 4 weeks based on expert opinion, with good results in recent clinical trials for stable patients.[30] According to some RCTs and registry data of 1,500 patients, there was no incidence of acute or subacute thrombosis after a DCB-only treatment.[31] Some studies have reported an acute thrombosis risk of only 0.2% after DCB-only PCI.[32] Therefore, in a situation where a patient requires PCI and is at high bleeding risk (previous life-threatening bleeding or upcoming major surgery), only the DCB strategy can be employed because of the low thrombotic risk with them.
- *Diffuse coronary disease:* Stent length is an independent predictor of TLF in the form of ISR and ST.[33] In another study PCI of coronary lesions >25 mm in length, the outcomes of DCB (DES used as bailout) were comparable to DES-only approach. Thus, DCB alone using DES as a bailout to limit stent length in vessels with diffuse disease may be an alternative and useful approach.[34] The use of DCB in diffuse distal disease of left anterior descending (LAD) and right coronary artery (RCA) allows these vessels to remain targets of a surgical graft in future.

CONCLUSION

To summarize DCB is an appealing technology for coronary interventions, and its efficacy appears to be credible in patients with ISR, especially those with multiple layers of stents and other coronary de novo lesions. Although there are ample studies done on various applications of DCB, there is a lack of large RCTs and meta-analysis. Still because of a variety of clinical situations that prohibit the use of metallic stents or DAPT, the use of DCB is becoming an increasingly interesting preposition.

REFERENCES

1. Gruntzig A. Transluminal dilatation of coronary-artery stenosis. Lancet. 1978;311:1093.
2. Canfield J, Totary-Jain H. 40 Years of Percutaneous Coronary Intervention: History and Future Directions. J. Pers. Med. 2018;8:33.
3. Oberhauser JP, Hossainy S, Rapoza RJ. Design principles and performance of bioresorbable polymeric vascular scaffolds. EuroIntervention. 2009;5:F15-22.
4. Gogas BD. Bioresorbable scaffolds for percutaneous coronary interventions. Glob Cardiol Sci Pract. 2014;2014:55.
5. Wykrzykowska JJ, Kraak RP, Hofma SH, Van Der Schaaf RJ, Arkenbout EK, IJsselmuiden AJ, et al. Bioresorbable Scaffolds versus Metallic Stents in Routine PCI N Engl J Med. 2017;376:2319-28.
6. Kereiakes DJ, Ellis SG, Metzger C, Caputo RP, Rizik DG, Teirstein PS, et al. 3-Year Clinical Outcomes with Everolimus-Eluting Bioresorbable Coronary Scaffolds. J Am Coll Cardiol. 2017;70:2852-62.
7. Nishida T, Colombo A, Briguori C, Stankovic G, Albiero R, Corvaja N, et al. Outcomes of non-obstructive residual dissections detected by intravascular ultrasound following percutaneous coronary intervention. Am J Cardiol. 2022;89(11):1257-62.
8. Sorrentino S, Sartori S, Baber U, Claessen BE, Giustino G, Chandrasekhar J, et al. Bleeding Risk, Dual Antiplatelet Therapy Cessation, and Adverse Events After Percutaneous Coronary Intervention: The PARIS Registry. Circ Cardiovasc Interv. 2020;13(4):e008226.
9. Pelliccia F, Zimarino M, Niccoli G, Morrone D, De Luca G, Miraldi F, et al. In-stent restenosis after percutaneous coronary intervention: emerging knowledge on biological pathways. Eur Heart J Open. 2023;3(5):oead083.
10. Narbute I, Jegere S, Kumsars I, Juhnevica D, Knipse A, Erglis A. Real-life Bifurcation - Challenges and Potential Complications. Eur Cardiol. 2011;7(4):283-7.
11. Gao L, Chen YD. Application of drug-coated balloon in coronary artery intervention: challenges and opportunities. J Geriatr Cardiol. 2016;13(11):906-13.
12. Jeger RV, Eccleshall S, Wan Ahmad WA, Ge J, Poerner TC, Shin ES, et al. Drug-Coated Balloons for Coronary Artery Disease: Third Report of the International DCB Consensus Group. J Am Coll Cardiol Intv. 2020;13 (12):1391-402.
13. Scheller B, Hehrlein C, Bocksch W, Rutsch W, Haghi D, Dietz U, et al. Treatment of coronary in-stent restenosis with a paclitaxel-coated balloon catheter. N Engl J Med. 2006;355:2113-24.
14. Lemos PA, Farooq V, Takimura CK, Gutierrez PS, Virmani R, Kolodgie F, et al. Emerging technologies: polymer-free phospholipid encapsulated sirolimus nanocarriers for the controlled release of drug from a stent-plus-balloon or a stand-alone balloon catheter. EuroIntervention. 2013;9:148-56.
15. Verheye S, Vrolix M, Kumsars I, Erglis A, Sondore D, Agostoni P, et al. The SABRE trial (Sirolimus Angioplasty Balloon for Coronary In-Stent Restenosis): angiographic results and 1-year clinical outcomes. J Am Coll Cardiol Intv. 2017;10:2029-37.

16. Ali RM, Abdul Kader MASK, Wan Ahmad WA, Ong TK, Liew HB, Omar AF, et al. Treatment of coronary drug-eluting stent restenosis by a sirolimus- or paclitaxel-coated balloon. J Am Coll Cardiol Intv. 2019;12:558-66.
17. Neumann FJ, Sousa-Uva M, Ahlsson A, Alfonso F, Banning AP, Benedetto U, et al. 2018 ESC/EACTS guidelines on myocardial revascularization. Eur Heart J. 2019;40:87-165.
18. Unverdorben M, Kleber FX, Heuer H, Figulla HR, Vallbracht C, Leschke M, et al. Treatment of small coronary arteries with a paclitaxel-coated balloon catheter. Clin Res Cardiol. 2010;99:165-74.
19. Unverdorben M, Kleber FX, Heuer H, Figulla HR, Vallbracht C, Leschke M, et al. Treatment of small coronary arteries with a paclitaxel-coated balloon catheter in the PEPCAD I study: are lesions clinically stable from 12 to 36 months? EuroIntervention. 2013;9:620-8.
20. Latib A, Colombo A, Castriota F, Micari A, Cremonesi A, De Felice F, et al. A randomized multicenter study comparing a paclitaxel drug-eluting balloon with a paclitaxel-eluting stent in small coronary vessels: the BELLO (Balloon Elution and Late Loss Optimization) study. J Am Coll Cardiol. 2012;60:2473-80.
21. Latib A, Ruparelia N, Menozzi A, Castriota F, Micari A, Cremonesi A, et al. Three-year follow-up of the balloon elution and late loss optimization study (BELLO) JACC Cardiovasc Interv. 2015;8:1132-4.
22. Zeymer U, Waliszewski M, Spiecker M, Gastmann O, Faurie B, Ferrari M, et al. Prospective 'real world' registry for the use of the 'PCB only' strategy in small vessel de novo lesions. Heart. 2014;100:311-6.
23. Jeger RV, Farah A, Ohlow MA, Mangner N, Möbius-Winkler S, Leibundgut G, et al. Drug-coated balloons for small coronary artery disease (BASKET-SMALL 2): an open-label randomised non-inferiority trial. Lancet 2018;392:849-56.
24. Byrne RA, Cassese S, Windisch T, King LA, Joner M, Tada T, et al. Differential relative efficacy between drug-eluting stents in patients with bare metal and drug-eluting stent restenosis; evidence in support of drug resistance: insights from the ISAR-DESIRE and ISAR-DESIRE 2 trials. EuroIntervention. 2013;9:797-802.
25. Alfonso F, Byrne RA, Rivero F, Kastrati A. Current treatment of in-stent restenosis. J Am Coll Cardiol. 2014;63:2659-73.
26. Herrador JA, Fernandez JC, Guzman M, Aragon V. Drug-eluting vs. conventional balloon for side branch dilation in coronary bifurcations treated by provisional T stenting. J Interv Cardiol. 2013;26:454-62.
27. Belkacemi A, Stella PR, Chunlai S, Uiterwijk M, Ali D, Agostoni P. Angiographic fate of side branch dissections in bifurcation lesions treated with a provisional single stenting strategy: a post-hoc analysis of the international multicenter randomized DEBIUT study. Catheter Cardiovasc Interv. 2014;83:539-44.
28. López Mínguez JR, Nogales Asensio JM, Doncel Vecino LJ, Sandoval J, Romany S, Romero PM, et al. A prospective randomised study of the paclitaxel-coated balloon catheter in bifurcated coronary lesions (BABILON trial): 24-month clinical and angiographic results. EuroIntervention. 2014;10:50-7.
29. Kleber FX, Rittger H, Ludwig J, Schulz A, Mathey DG, Boxberger M, et al. Drug eluting balloons as stand alone procedure for coronary bifurcational lesions: results of the randomized multicenter PEPCAD-BIF trial. Clin Res Cardiol. 2016;105:613-21.

30. Kleber F, Scheller B, Ong P, Rissanen T, Zeymer U, Wöhrle J, et al. TCT-776 Duration of dual antiplatelet therapy after drug-coated balloon implantation. J Am Coll Cardiol. 2018;72 (13Suppl): B309-10.
31. Rissanen TT, Uskela S, Eränen J, Mäntylä P, Olli A, Romppanen H, et al. Drug-coated balloon for treatment of de-novo coronary artery lesions in patients with high bleeding risk (DEBUT): a single-blind, randomised, non-inferiority trial. Lancet. 2019;394:230-9.
32. Uskela S, Kärkkäinen JM, Eränen J, Siljander A, Mäntylä P, Mustonen J, et al. Percutaneous coronary intervention with drug-coated balloon-only strategy in stable coronary artery disease and in acute coronary syndromes: an all-comers registry study. Catheter Cardiovasc Interv. 2019;93:893-900.
33. D'Ascenzo F, Bollati M, Clementi F, Castagno D, Lagerqvist B, De La Torre Hernandez JM, et al. Incidence and predictors of coronary stent thrombosis: evidence from an international collaborative meta-analysis including 30 studies, 221,066 patients, and 4276 thromboses. Int J Cardiol. 2013;167:575-84.
34. Venetsanos D, Lawesson SS, Panayi G, Tödt T, Berglund U, Swahn E, et al. Long-term efficacy of drug coated balloons compared with new generation drug-eluting stents for the treatment of de novo coronary artery lesions. Catheter Cardiovasc Interv. 2018;92:E317-26.

CHAPTER 33

Complex High-risk Indicated Percutaneous Coronary Intervention Clinical Approach

Manoj Sivaraman

INTRODUCTION

Coronary artery disease is prevalent in vast and global scale, leading the mortality figures consistently. Coronary artery bypass grafting (CABG) and percutaneous coronary intervention (PCI) have addressed the need for coronary revascularization aiming to improve the symptom class, reduce the adverse event rates, and improve the quality of life.

Percutaneous coronary intervention has come a long way to offer effective mode of coronary revascularization since Dr Andreas Roland Gruntzig successfully carried out balloon dilatation of "widow maker" lesion in the left anterior descending (LAD) artery in 1974. Earlier days, many lesion types, and patient characteristics were considered unsuitable for PCI which was often offered for type A and B1 category of coronary artery lesions.[1] The significant leaps of advancements in the development of various tools applied in PCI namely guide catheters, guidewires, balloon and stent delivery systems, stent design, guide extension catheters, calcium modifying devices—atherectomy and lithotripsy, excimer laser coronary angioplasty (ELCA), etc. have allowed application of PCI in many difficult lesion types as type B2, type 3 categories[1] with acceptable procedural success, and long-term results minimizing the procedural complications as well. In the current practices, these subsets of patient would have not been offered PCI solution few decades ago. As the operator skill achievement could be acquired with familiarity in using the newer devices, technical success of PCI, in these erstwhile considered unsuitable lesions, improved remarkably after the advent of the current generation of drug-eluting stent (DES) platforms and antiplatelet usages. These practices led to the need for dedicated approaches for addressing the various higher risk profiles of lesions as well as clinical condition of patient with additional medical comorbidity conditions adding complexity to the whole profile of the treatment delivery. In the current era, left main PCI, PCI in acute coronary presentation, chronic total occlusion (CTO), bifurcation PCI, etc., with or without poor coronary reserve and hemodynamically unstable subset of subjects were increasingly undergoing PCI due to poor surgical subjects or rejects or from the understanding of comparable outcomes vis-à-vis CABG surgery option.

Complex high-risk indicated PCI (CHIP-PCI) concept was born, thereby addressing the systematic need for training and safe approaches in aiming for favorable procedural outcome. To specifically address the need for focused care and training in this high-risk subjects with complex lesions and poor hemodynamic conditions, Ajay Kirtane et al. brought out the white paper on this felt need in 2016[2] and led to more consensus initiation and guided directions in the approach to CHIP-PCI. CHIP-PCI is known to be an independent predictor of mortality.[3]

The definition of CHIP-PCI refers to offering PCI to complex lesion subsets in a multicomorbidity subject with or without adverse hemodynamic conditions. The various attributes in CHIP-PCI subject can be considered as shown in **Figure 1**.[2]

The individual complexity characteristics of each of the considered factors are detailed in **Figure 2**.

The patient-related factors adding to the complexity and high-risk characteristics can be further elaborated in **Table 1**.

Coronary anatomy lesion characteristics that add high-risk complexity features to PCI are described in **Table 2**.

When hemodynamics is unstable, life is at stake and in jeopardy. Hemodynamics is the key to sustain life. Identifying any adverse hemodynamic conditions at the baseline in the high-risk PCI subjects which need to be addressed upfront for support and protection to prevent further deterioration of the existing hemodynamic status are mentioned in **Table 3**.

Patients may have acute or chronic LV decompensation with *poor cardiac reserve* to sustain any further reduction in the coronary flow. Adverse hemodynamics will lead to incomplete revascularization with poor short/intermediate term outcomes–catheterization laboratory disasters. *Hemodynamic support has become an indispensable part of many CHIP-PCI* procedures. Proficiency with percutaneously implanted LV support devices is essential part of skillset of the team.

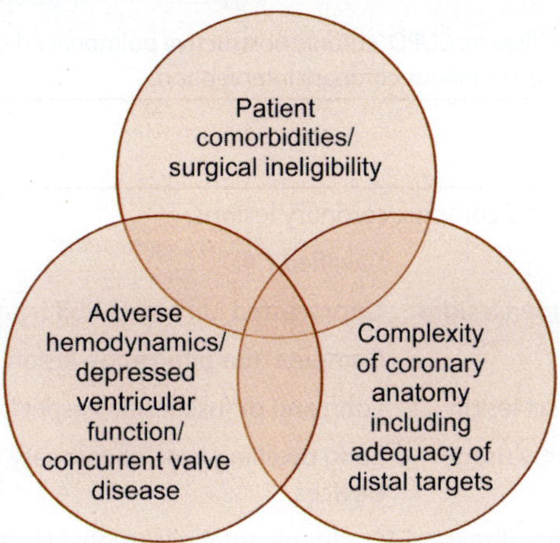

Fig. 1: Defining complex high-risk indicated percutaneous coronary intervention (CHIP-PCI) subject.[2]

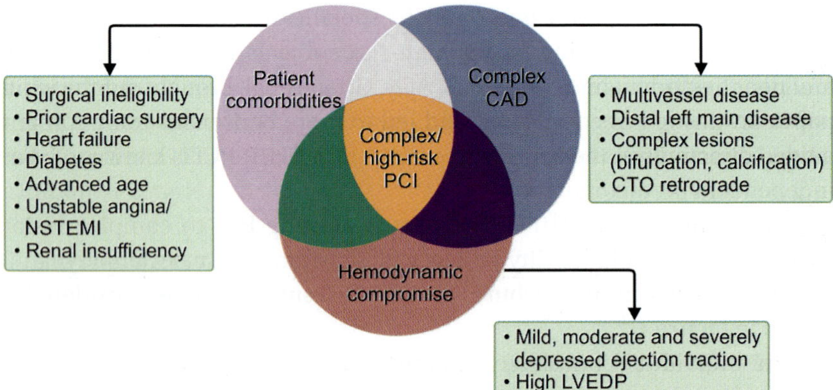

Fig. 2: Complex high-risk indicated percutaneous coronary intervention (CHIP-PCI) factors.
(CAD: coronary artery disease; CTO: chronic total occlusion; LVEDP: left ventricular end-diastolic pressure; NSTEMI: non-ST elevation myocardial infarction; PCI: percutaneous coronary intervention)
Source: Adapted from Simonton et al.[7]

TABLE 1: Patient related high risk features.

Advanced age	Frailty
Surgical reject	Acute coronary syndrome
Acute or chronic heart failure	Previous cardiac surgery
CKD	PAD/polyvasculopathy
Associated significant valve disease	Type 2 diabetes mellitus
COPD	High bleeding risk features
Associated anticoagulant	Previous failed PCI
Previous MI	Hypersensitivity disorders

(CKD: chronic kidney disease; COPD: chronic obstructive pulmonary disease; PAD: peripheral arterial disease; PCI: percutaneous coronary intervention)

TABLE 2: High risk and complex coronary lesions.

Multivessel CAD	Calcified CAD
High thrombus burden lesions	Unprotected LM and LM bifurcation
CTO	Complex true bifurcation lesion
Last remaining vessel lesion	Long and diffuse lesions especially >60 mm
Need for atherectomy usage	Long dwelling time of coronary occlusion by devices

(CAD: coronary artery disease; CTO: chronic total occlusion; LM: left main; PCI: percutaneous coronary intervention)

TABLE 3: Adverse hemodynamic conditions at the baseline in the high-risk PCI subjects.

Elevated LVEDP ≥18 mm Hg	Depressed CO/cardiogenic shock
Lower MAP or impending shock	Large area of myocardium in jeopardy
Recurrent ventricular arrhythmias	Low LV/RV EF

(EF: ejection fraction; LV: left ventricular; LVEDP: left ventricular end-diastolic pressure; MAP: mean arterial pressure; PCI: percutaneous coronary intervention; RV: right ventricular)

The main objective of any hemodynamic support is to aim for mean arterial pressure of 70–80 mm Hg and a mixed venous oxygen saturation of about 65%. Each of the above characteristics adds adversity to the success of the procedure and higher major adverse cardiovascular and cerebrovascular event (MACCE) rates in hospital. More these features in a given subject add greater level of complexities and require to be addressed in a diligent manner to avoid major procedural catastrophe and unfavorable outcome.

A real CHIP SCORE is yet to evolve to guide on the level of risk of complexity and predict the procedural success as well as complications. Protty et al.[4] considered 7 patient factors and 6 procedural factors in a large sample study of 3,00,000 patients undergoing PCI in UK and noted higher the CHIP factor score, greater the incidence of in hospital mortality and bleeding. The patient-related factors considered were age ≥80 years, female gender, prior stroke, prior MI, PAD, left ventricular ejection fraction (LVEF) <30% and CKD, while the procedural factors considered were LM PCI, 3 vessel PCI, dual arterial access, LV mechanical support, lesion length >60 mm and use of rotational atherectomy. A total of 13 CHIP-PCI risk scoring factors were assessed—7 patient-related factors and 6 procedural factors—and distinctly showed cumulative factors in any given CHIP-PCI subject was predictive of in-hospital MACCE as well as bleeding as seen in **Figure 3**.[4]

Operators or the CHIP team need to acquire skills—skillsets proficiency—to address each of these complexities in performing high-risk PCI such as unprotected left main, true bifurcation, CTO lesions, graft occlusions, large bore access, hemodynamic device implantations and monitoring thereafter, etc. The interventional cardiologist also needs to be well versed with the use of atherectomy devices, lithotripsy devices, conservative use of contrast dye and therefore be proficient in ultra-low contrast PCI with systematic application of intracoronary imaging modalities. Interventional cardiologist can also undergo certified courses or fellowship programs to acquire proficiency in CHIP-PCI.

This author also feels that apart from the complexity features being considered universally, any patient characteristics defining high bleeding risk (HBR) significantly will add additional dimension to the existing complexity.

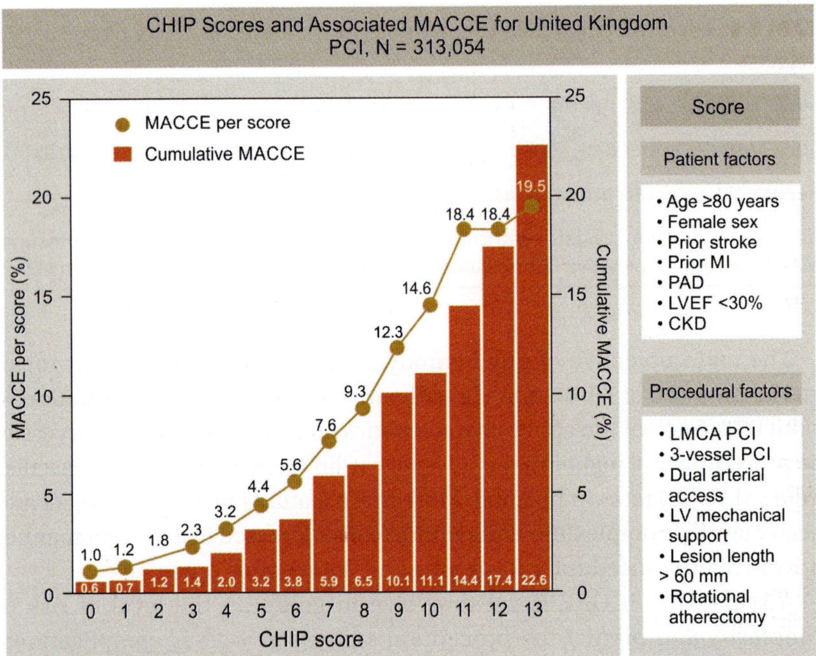

Fig. 3: *CHIP PCI risk score:* As the score increases, cumulative MACCE also increases. (CHIP: complex high-risk indicated; CKD: chronic kidney disease; LMCA: left main coronary artery; LVEF: left ventricular ejection fraction; MACCE: major adverse cardiovascular and cerebrovascular event; PAD: peripheral arterial disease; PCI: percutaneous coronary intervention)

HBR features in CHIP-PCI needs to be actively considered with a view to have optimal PCI results complemented and confirmed by intravascular imaging indices. Achieving optimal PCI results would then allow abbreviating the duration of dual antiplatelet therapy (DAPT) to the shortest period to balance the risk of bleeding and thrombosis.

TOOL KIT FOR CHIP-PCI

In any CHIP-PCI procedure, following the pre-PCI assessment of lesion complexity, CKD status that dictates the volume of contrast usage, LV functional status and hemodynamic conditions, the operator needs to check the tool kit be comprehensive to address the need during the PCI for treating the target lesion.

There is a comprehensive detailing of CHIP-PCI operator skillset and the tool kit as given in **Table 4**[8] that need to be paid attention.

The operator needs to be diligently using intravascular imaging to choose the appropriate tool to modify the plaque to finally allow optimal stent expansion and PCI results thereby. Use of intravascular imaging also shortens the procedural time and reduced the contrast usage. The imaging detailing of

TABLE 4: Tool kit and skill set for CHIP-PCI.

Arterial access	• Large-bore sheaths • Radial access • Bilateral femoral access • Advanced techniques (percutaneous axillary/transcaval)
CTO	• Antegrade wire escalation • Antegrade dissection re-entry • Retrograde
Left main	• One-stent/provisional strategies • Two-stent techniques (double-kissing crush/culotte)
Advanced imaging	• Proficiency with IVUS/OCT
Calcific disease	• Rotational atherectomy/orbital atherectomy
Hemodynamic support	• Impella 2.5/CP for protected PCI treatment of cardiogenic shock • Intra-aortic balloon counterpulsation • Extracorporeal membrane oxygenation
Complication management	• Coronary perforation management techniques (covered stents, coils, embolization) • Access site complications (peripheral skills/covered stent deployment) • Repair of coronary dissection • Emergency pericardiocentesis

[CHIP: complex higher-risk (and indicated) patients; CTO: chronic total occlusion; IVUS: intravascular ultrasound; OCT: optical coherence tomography; PCI: percutaneous coronary intervention]
Source: Adapted from Levisay J.[8]

the target vessel or segment also gives assessment of probable complications that can be anticipated at the beginning of PCI and also have necessary tools to address such events without any delay during complication events.

The contrast volume usage is usually derived from the figure of the estimated glomerular filtration rate (eGFR) value and the interventional cardiologist should apply adequate hydration to maintain euvolemic status and complete the PCI within the restricted volume of the contrast to limit the occurrence of contrast associated acute kidney injury with PCI performed with ultra-low contrast and imaging guidance.

All measures should be exercised to also reduce the radiation exposure both in the case of patient—to prevent radiation burns—as well as to the operator and associated catheterization laboratory staff by utilizing ancillary radiation protection units such as Radpad, Eggnest, or Rampart. Also it is strongly advised to set the fluoroscopy frame rate to 7.5 fps or lower as the case may be.

DEPRESSED LV WITH NEED FOR PROTECTED PCI

The clinical feature of depressed LVEF of <40% distinctly confers high risk of hemodynamic instability and the upfront implant of IABP/Micro-axial IMPELLA pLVAD devices as well as venoarterial extracorporeal membrane oxygenation (VA ECMO) need to be considered to allow safe completion of the CHIP-PCI with least hemodynamic collapse events.

The recent Indian expert consensus arrived at scoring assessment of patient as well as other factors to optimize the appropriateness of the indication of use of IMPELLA or VA ECMO, etc. The hemodynamic support provides maintenance of adequate coronary blood supply and thereby improves the myocardial oxygen delivery with concurrent decreased myocardial oxygen demand facilitating thereby near complete revascularization and decrease the short-term MACCEs.[5] These decision-making flow algorithms for the protected PCI can be made as given in **Flowchart 1**. A score more than 5 makes the hemodynamic support for protected PCI more compelling; while

Flowchart 1: Algorithm for the protected PCI.

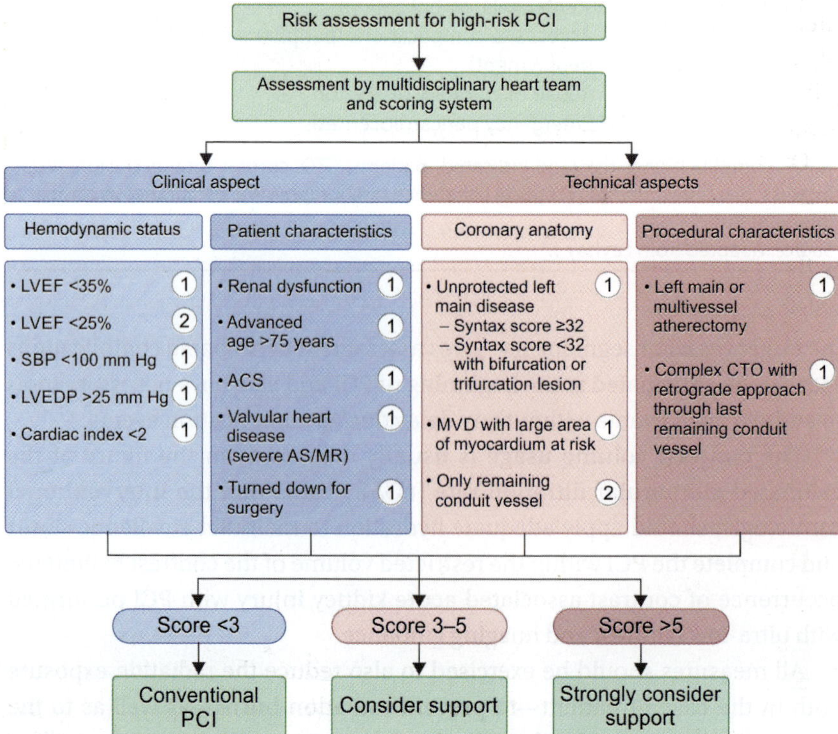

(ACS: acute coronary syndrome; CTO: chronic total occlusion; LVEF: left ventricular ejection fraction; LVEDP: left ventricular end-diastolic pressure; MVD: multivessel disease; PCI: percutaneous coronary intervention; SBP: systolic blood pressure)

Source: Adapted from Tayal, et al.[5]

if the score is 3–5, the need for protected PCI with hemodynamic device support can be considered through a shared decision-making if prevailing conditions are all favorable to have the device support.

The type of hemodynamic support devices to be used would be based on availability of these devices in the cardiac catheterization laboratory, familiarity of the team to implant, and following the postimplant monitoring, understanding the trouble shooting perspectives as well and affordability to the same. When it is anticipated there need to be LV unloading and protection, especially in acute coronary syndrome (ACS) with acute heart failure and with depressed LVEF <35%, it is strongly recommended to use percutaneous axial flow devices such as IMPELLA CP to provide adequate and robust hemodynamic support to tide over many instances of low CO scenarios with uncoupling of LV to aortic pressures during the CHIP-PCI and also to address cardiogenic shock if any. If however CHIP-PCI is envisaged in a patient with recurrent cardiac arrest or with no ROSC or refractory ventricular tachyarrhythmias, VA ECMO would be the choice to provide hemodynamic protection with consideration of LV vent options. IABP is a regularly used hemodynamic device with its versatile availability and familiarity with every interventional cardiologist but with limitation of its augmentation support relying on a reasonable stroke volume and very modest CO enhancement. IABP often fails to provide decent hemodynamic support to maintain adequate MAP if progressive shock ensues.

Once the hemodynamic supported protected PCI is practiced, the next course of decision in weaning the support and removal of the device by de-escalation decision is a natural sequence. This can be reasonably guided by the flowchart algorithm given in **Flowchart 2**[5] arrived through expert consensus. If large bore devices are in place, removal of these devices should

Flowchart 2: Weaning the support.

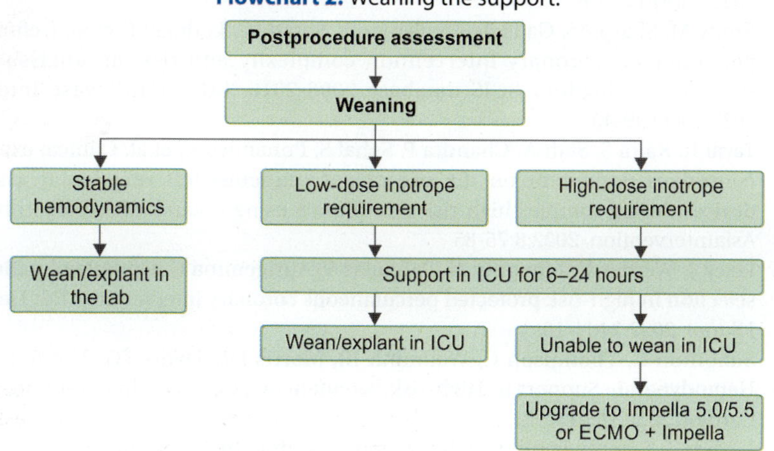

Source: Adapted from Tayal, et al.[5]

be systematically addressed by achieving hemostasis at the access sites by either preclose or postclose methods or through the help extended by vascular surgical colleagues.

CONCLUSION

In any given CHIP-PCI scenario, the flow of decision-making preferably starts with understanding the high-risk PCI features defining the CHIP-PCI as detailed followed by heart team discussion and with significant consideration of the need for protected PCI aiming the best outcome in the most adverse scenario. Therefore, CHIP-PCI envisages multidisciplinary team involving the primary and assistant operator, specialist consultants, experienced cardiac surgery colleague, critical care specialist, well-trained scrub nurse with technical staff experienced in various device usages along with expert perfusionist colleagues to support hemodynamic devices when placed during the CHIP-PCI. Everyone of this MDT makes a vital contribution in the decision-making and execution of the same in patient centric approach.[6]

REFERENCES

1. Ryan TJ, Faxon DP, Gunnar RM, Kennedy JW, King SB, Loop FD, et al. Guidelines for percutaneous transluminal coronary angioplasty. A report of the American College of Cardiology/American Heart Association Task Force on Assessment of Diagnostic and Therapeutic Cardiovascular Procedures (Subcommittee on Percutaneous Transluminal Coronary Angioplasty). Circulation. 1988;78:486-502.
2. Kirtane AJ, Doshi D, Leon MB, Lasala JM, Ohman EM, O'Neill WW, et al. Treatment of Higher-Risk Patients With an Indication for Revascularization. Circulation. 2016;134:422-31.
3. Brener SJ, Cunn GJ, Desai PH, Faroqui M, Ha LD, Handa G, et al. A Novel Risk Score to Predict One-Year Mortality in Patients Undergoing Complex High-Risk Indicated Percutaneous Coronary Intervention (CHIP-PCI). J Invasive Cardiol. 2021;33(4):E253-8.
4. Protty M, Sharp AS, Gallagher S, Farooq V, Spratt JC, Ludman P, et al. Defining percutaneous coronary intervention complexity and risk: an analysis of the United Kingdom BCIS database 2006-2016. JACC Cardiovasc Interv. 2022;15(1):39-49.
5. Tayal R, Kalra S, Seth A, Chandra P, Sohal S, Punamiya K, et al. Clinical expert consensus document on the use of percutaneous left ventricular assist devices during complex high-risk PCI in India using a standardised algorithm. AsiaIntervention. 2022;8:75-85
6. Leick J, Werner N, Mangner N, Panoulas V, Aurigemma C. Optimized patient selection in high-risk protected percutaneous coronary intervention. Eur Heart J Suppl. 2022;24:J4-10.
7. Simonton C, Thompson C, Wollmuth JR, Morris DL, Dahle TG. The Role of Hemodynamic Support in High-risk Percutaneous Coronary Intervention. US Cardiol. 2020;14:e13.
8. Levisay J. Essentials for a CHIP Program. Cardiac Interventions Today. 2018; 12(3):61-4.

CHAPTER 34

Aorto-ostial Stenting: Tips and Tricks

Siva Kumar

INTRODUCTION

Aorto-ostial coronary lesions (AOLs) refer to stenosis exceeding 50% within 3 mm of the orifice in the right coronary artery (RCA), left main coronary artery (LMCA), and aortocoronary bypass grafts.[1] Most AOL cases are associated with diffuse coronary artery disease, with isolated lesions more common in females. Atherosclerotic coronary artery disease is the primary cause of AOL, yet isolated cases may stem from various nonatherosclerotic conditions such as inflammatory or noninflammatory aortic wall issues, prior mediastinal radiation, previous aortic valve surgery, congenital arterial hypoplasia, the presence of circumferential ostial muscle acting as a sphincter, and external compression from a dilated pulmonary artery **(Fig. 1)**.[2]

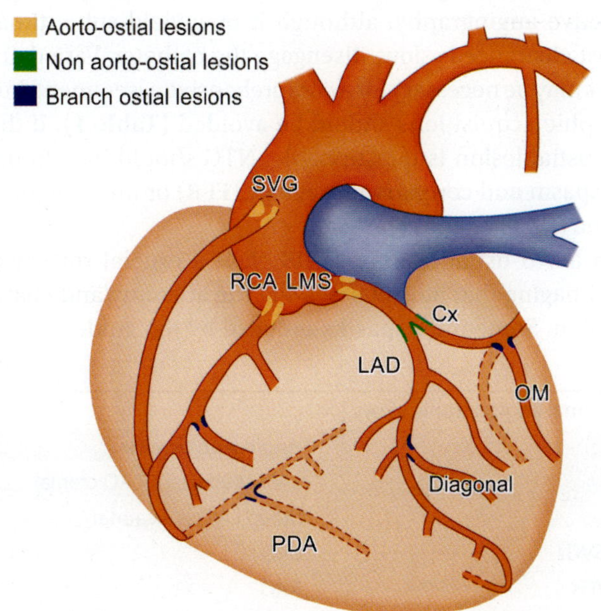

Fig. 1: Aorto-ostial lesions. (LAD: left anterior descending artery; LMS: left main stem; PDA: posterior descending artery; RCA: right coronary artery; SVG: saphenous vein grafts)

ANATOMY OF OSTIUM

Aorto-ostial lesions typically exhibit a distinctive three-dimensional funnel-shaped structure with a variable coronary artery takeoff angle from the aorta. Histologically, these lesions primarily consist of fibrocellular and sclerotic fragments, occasionally containing lipid components. The lesions are characterized as rigid, calcified, eccentric, and burdened with increased plaque.[3] Due to the greater thickness of muscular and elastic tissue in the aortic wall, aorto-ostial lesions resist dilation and are prone to recoil, leading to less favorable outcomes compared to nonostial lesions.

DIAGNOSIS OF AORTO-OSTIAL LESIONS

Diagnosing aorto-ostial lesions involves various methods including:

- *CT coronary angiography (CT CAG):* It clearly defines the anatomy of the coronary ostium, its takeoff, and calcification.[4]
- *Invasive coronary angiogram:* Ensuring precise catheter placement is vital for accurate visualization of the aorto-ostial region. Administering nitroglycerin (NTG) before coronary angiography (CAG) helps rule out spasm. Suspect vasospasm especially if no significant coronary plaque is evident elsewhere. Indicators of aorto-ostial disease include the absence of contrast backflow and pressure waveform dampening. To prevent aortocoronary dissection in patients with dampening, contrast injection should be gentle. In cases of severe dampening, consider nonselective angiography, although it may yield suboptimal images. If contrast clearance is slow, disengage the catheter. Varied angulations and views may be necessary for a comprehensive assessment, but multiple angiographic acquisitions should be avoided **(Table 1)**. If the severity of aorto-ostial lesion is questionable, NTG should be administered to exclude spasm and coronary physiology (FFR) or imaging [intravascular ultrasound (IVUS)] should be used.
- *IVUS:* In aorto-ostial lesions, IVUS plays a crucial role by providing detailed imaging that aids in assessing the anatomy and characteristics of the lesion. Sometimes spasms induced by the guide catheter will be

TABLE 1: Optimal angiographic views.

Vessel	*Angiographic view*
Left margin	LAO caudal and LAO cranial
RCA	Steep LAO +/– caudal
Right-sided SVGs	LAO
Left-sided SVGs	RAO
LIMA or RIMA	AP with shallow cranial

(LAO: left anterior oblique; LIMA: left internal mammary artery; RAO: right anterior oblique; RCA: right coronary artery; RIMA: right internal mammary artery; SVG: saphenous vein graft) easily ruled out with the help of IVUS. Disengaging the catheter during pullback risks, noncoaxial imaging of the ostium, and overestimation of the luminal area is one of the limitations of IVUS.[5]

- *FFR:* In aorto-ostial lesions, pressure measurement across the aorto-ostial disease may be valuable but requires pressure equalization in ascending aorta, guide disengagement during FFR measurement, and intravenous adenosine to induce hyperemia.
- *Optical coherence tomography (OCT):* It has a limited role in ostial lesions since the engagement of guide is required for clearing the blood with contrast, whereas the ostial lesion cannot be adequately visualized if the guide is engaged. The innovative telescope-guiding extension catheter features a soft polymer tip, facilitating the observation of aorto-ostial lesions. Its helical coil design with a wide gap allows the penetration of infrared light through the soft polymer, marking a significant advancement in the realm of OCT-guided ostial stenting.

TREATMENT

In the past, treating AOL with balloon angioplasty before stents was linked to lower success rates and more complications compared to nonostial lesions. This included a high chance of emergency bypass surgery due to sudden vessel closure and restenosis in half of the cases.[6,7] Although drug-eluting stents (DESs) improved restenosis rates in some studies, results vary, and DES placement in AOL still shows poorer outcomes than in nonostial lesions.[8-10]

ACCURACY OF STENT IMPLANTATION

To place a stent optimally in the aorto-ostial area of a coronary artery, it is important to ensure the entire starting edge of the stent is within a specific landing zone. This zone, known as aorto-ostial landing zone (AOLZ), is within 1 mm of the aorto-ostial plane **(Fig. 2)**.[11,12] If the stent's edge is not properly placed in this zone, it is considered a stent geographic miss.[13] Geographic miss is divided into two types. Proximal geographic miss with protrusion of the stent into the aorta may hinder future catheter access to the coronary artery **(Fig. 3)**. Distal geographic miss may leave part of the AOL uncovered by stent struts and increase the likelihood of restenosis **(Fig. 4)**. Factors contributing to this misplacement include limitations of 2D angiography, the angle at which the coronary artery branches from the coronary sinus, catheter instability, and stent designs that do not match the anatomy well.

CHOICE OF HARDWARE

Guide Catheter

Use gentle catheters such as Judkins or extra backup for regular coronary vessels to avoid getting stuck in the lesion and help with easy removal

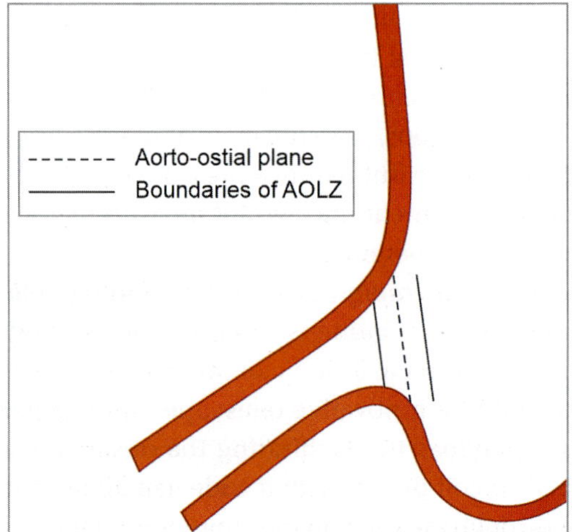

Fig. 2: Aorto-ostial landing zone (AOLZ).

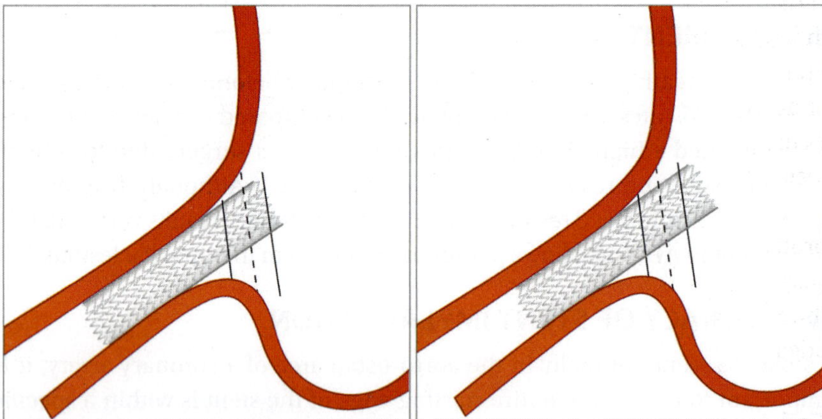

Fig. 3: Proximal geographic miss.

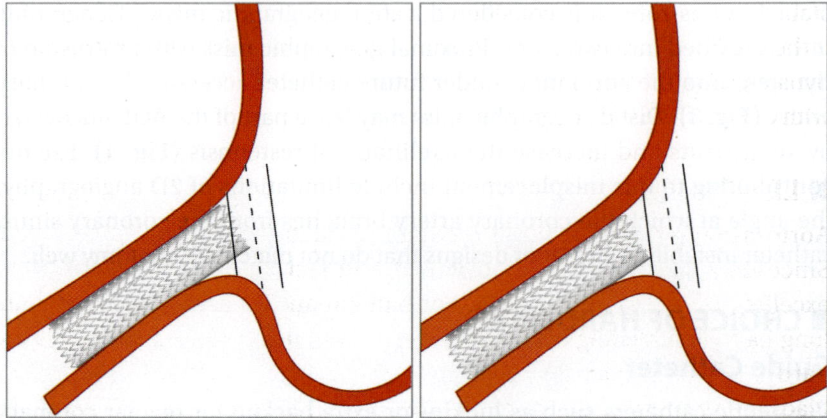

Fig. 4: Distal geographic miss.

during stent placement. Avoid Amplatz-type guides for aorto-ostial lesions. For specific cases, such as right coronary arteries with a high takeoff and RCA vein grafts, a multipurpose guide is ideal.

Aorto-coronary bypass grafts need a guide catheter with sufficient reach and support without going too deep. Commonly used catheters include Judkins right, multipurpose, right coronary bypass (RCB), left coronary bypass (LCB), and Amplatz left.

Use caution with side-hole guide catheters, as they may not accurately show pressure changes and ischemia. Avoid them in an unprotected LMCA due to the large ischemic risk area. However, they can be used in the RCA, bypass grafts, and a protected left main coronary artery. Avoid using them in the RCA if it is the donor vessel for left system. Limitations are contrast exiting through side holes, hindering lesion visibility and potentially requiring more contrast for percutaneous coronary intervention (PCI) completion.

Preload the guide catheter with the guide wire. As soon as the guide catheter selectively engages the ostium, the wire is quickly advanced and the guide catheter is removed from the stenosed aorto coronary ostium. This will avoid ischemia. After positioning the undeployed stent, balloon, or atherectomy blade in a proper place, the guide should be disengaged 1 or 2 cm into the aorta, so that the balloon or the stent is not inflated or deployed inside the guide.

Engaging vessels with prior aorto-ostial stenting can be difficult due to protruding stent struts and may result in stent deformation. In such cases, the vessel can be wired with the guide catheter disengaged and ideally knuckling the wire to avoid wire advancement through stent struts followed by guide engagement over the wire.

Guidewire

Use a standard workhorse wire, placing it in distal most part of vessel for stability during disengagement. Consider wires with extra support, especially if the guide catheter's position is tricky, like in a challenging aortocoronary bypass graft. If a hydrophilic coated guidewire is used in a tough case, swap it with a supportive wire through a microcatheter for better support.

■ LESION PREPARATION

Aorto-ostial lesions are often resistant to dilatation and prone to recoil. Since they are often heavily calcified and resistant to regular balloons, excellent preparation is crucial. For balloon angioplasty, a noncompliant long balloon matching the vessel size (1:1) is used. It should be positioned partly in the vessel and partly in the aorta for effective lesion preparation. Plaque modification balloons (scoreflex, cutting balloon) can facilitate lesion expansion and prevent excessive balloon movement.

Severely calcified vessels may need special devices. Rotational atherectomy should be done with rotawire extra support. Activate the burr at the guide catheter's end without tension to prevent it from jumping through the lesion, which could cause entrapment.[14,15] For orbital atherectomy, if the crown passes the lesion, move it forward and treat while pulling back. If the lesion is too severe, keep the crown close and activate it carefully to avoid vessel injury.[16] Intravascular lithotripsy (IVL) is another choice for expanding heavily calcified lesions.

STENTING

When there is distal lesion in addition to the aorto-ostial lesion, the distal lesion should be stented first as advancing equipment through an ostial stent may damage it. Steps of stenting are:

- Advance the stent into the target vessel.
- Disengage the guide catheter by pushing the wire or rotating the guide catheter not by pulling the catheter.
- Pull the stent back slightly about 1–2 mm into the aorta, and check it with multiple views and stent boost.[17]
- Deploy the stent.
- Partially pull the stent balloon back into the aorta and inflate it with high pressure.
- Advance the guide catheter over the stent balloon to re-engage the vessel.
- Do final assessment.

Challenges in Stent Positioning

- Suboptimal visualization of lesion due to guide catheter disengagement and resultant poor contrast opacification
- Difficulty in using appropriate angiographic views to show the ostium properly and avoid overlap or foreshortening
- Excessive stent movement in relation with cardiac and respiratory motion

Methods to Overcome the Problems of Stent Positioning

- Respiratory motion is minimized by breath holding or gentle shallow breathing.
- Cardiac motion can be minimized by rapid ventricular pacing, intravenous beta blockers or atropine. Intracoronary adenosine can be used, especially for RCA stenting.
- *Floating wire or sepal wire technique:* Keep the second wire in the aorta just below the ostium. It prevents the guide catheter movement into the ostium **(Fig. 5)**.[18]
- *Partial preinflation technique:* After approximate positioning, inflate the stent balloon at 2 atm. This should increase the stent profile and

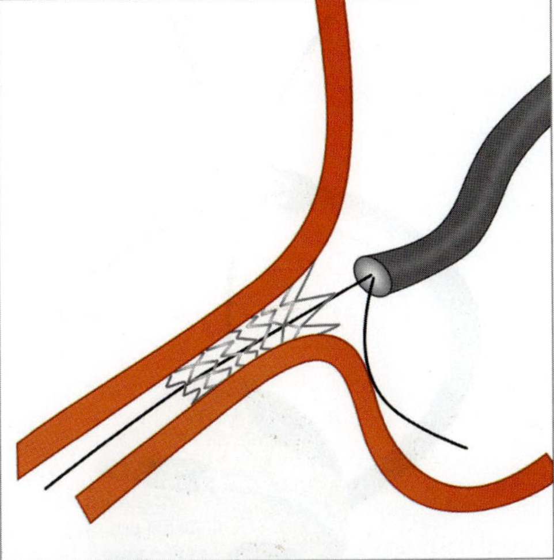

Fig. 5: Floating wire technique.

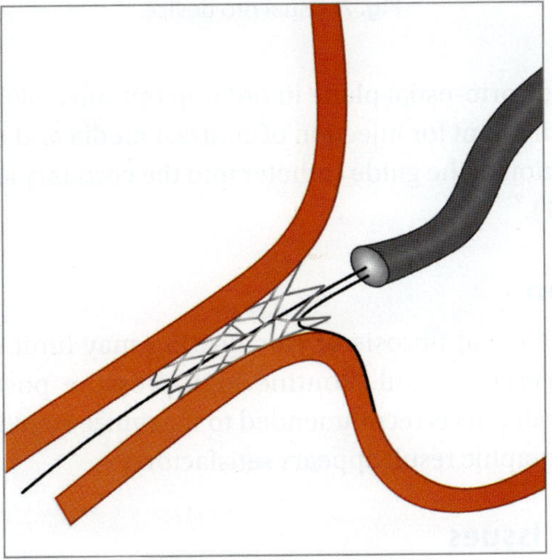

Fig. 6: Szabo technique.

reduce oscillation while still allowing positional adjustment before full deployment.

- *Szabo technique:* Szabo proposed a method whereby the second guidewire was passed through the most proximal stent cell and placed within the aorta, thereby preventing deep insertion of the stent into the vessel beyond the aorto-ostial plane.[19,20] Sometimes, it may lead to stent deformation and dislodgement **(Fig. 6)**.[21]
- *Ostial pro device:* The ostial pro device has self-expanding nitinol legs that protrude laterally from the distal catheter end. This device is designed to

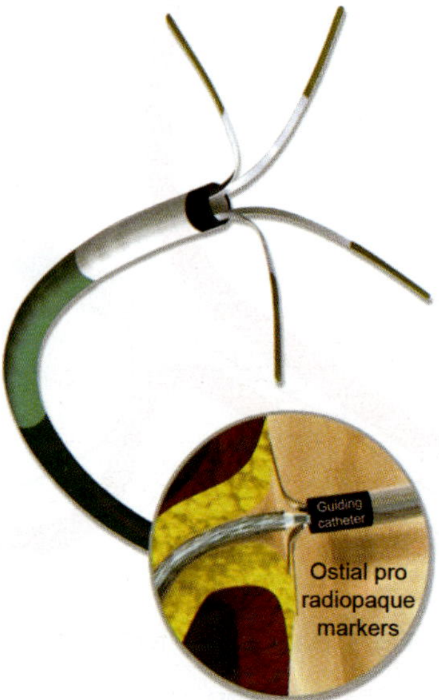

Fig. 7: Ostial pro device.

delineate the aorto-ostial plane in order to optimize AOL stenting and to reduce requirement for injection of contrast media and may also prevent deep intubation of the guide catheter into the coronary artery beyond the AOLZ **(Fig. 7)**.[22]

Postdilatation

The presence of ostial fibrosis or calcification may limit stent expansion or result in excessive recoil. Routine high-pressure postdilatation with noncompliant balloons is recommended to maximize stent lumen area even when the angiographic result appears satisfactory.

Poststenting Issues

- *Pressure still damped after PCI:* Deploy another stent to cover the ostium.
- *Unable to re-engage the vessel after stenting due to stent protruding too far into the aorta:* Inflate a short oversized balloon to flare the overhanging portion of the stent. If >50% of the stent protrudes outside the ostium, it is possible to snare and remove it.
- *Failure to expand the stent:* It should be treated as balloon undilatable lesion.
- *Acute stent recoil*: Postdilate again. If recoil recurs, deploy another stent having high radial strength.
- *Stent deformity due to guide catheter advancement:* Additional balloon dilatation or implantation of an additional stent may be required.

FINAL ASSESSMENT

- Absence of pressure dampening, brisk contrast clearance, and adequate contrast back flow in check angiogram are markers of good result.
- IVUS can confirm full ostium coverage and adequate stent expansion.

CONCLUSION

Ostial lesions in coronary arteries pose challenges for interventional cardiologists. Success in dealing with this complex issue involves understanding coronary anatomy, hardware, and intervention techniques. By carefully addressing the anatomy and challenges during ostial stenting, this challenging subset of coronary artery disease can be effectively managed.

REFERENCES

1. Zampieri P, Colombo A, Almagor Y, Maiello L, Finci L. Results of coronary stenting of ostial lesions. Am J Cardiol. 1994;73(12):901-3.
2. Rissanen V. Occurrence of coronary ostial stenosis in a necropsy series of myocardial infarction, sudden death, and violent death. Heart. 1975;37(2):182-91.
3. Jaffe R, Halon DA, Shiran A, Rubinshtein R. Percutaneous treatment of aorto-ostial coronary lesions: Current challenges and future directions. Int J Cardiol. 2015;186:61-6.
4. Pesenti-Rossi D, Chouli M, Gharbi M, Ghostine S, Habib Y, Brenot P, et al. Coronary aorto-ostial stenosis analysed by multislice computed tomography: a new tool for percutaneous coronary intervention? EuroIntervention. 2011;6(6):717-21.
5. Kim SW, Mintz GS, Ohlmann P, Hassani SE, Michalek A, Escolar E, et al. Comparative intravascular ultrasound analysis of ostial disease in the left main versus the right coronary artery. J Invasive Cardiol. 2007;19(9):377-80.
6. Ellis SG, Vandormael M, Cowley MA, DiSciascio G, Deligonul U, Topol EJ, et al. Coronary morphologic and clinical determinants of procedural outcome with angioplasty for multivessel coronary disease. Implications for patient selection. Multivessel Angioplasty Prognosis Study Group. Circulation. 1990;82(4):1193-202.
7. Tan KS, Sulke N, Taub N, Sowton E. Percutaneous transluminal coronary angioplasty of aorta ostial, non-aorta ostial, and branch ostial stenoses: acute and long-term outcome. Eur Heart J. 1995;16(5):631-9.
8. Al-Lameé R, Ielasi A, Latib A, Godino C, Mussardo M, Arioli F, et al. Comparison of long-term clinical and angiographic outcomes following implantation of bare metal stents and drug-eluting stents in aorto-ostial lesions. Am J Cardiol. 2011;108(8):1055-60.
9. Park DW, Hong MK, Suh IW, Hwang ES, Lee SW, Jeong YH, et al. Results and predictors of angiographic restenosis and long-term adverse cardiac events after drug-eluting stent implantation for aorto-ostial coronary artery disease. Am J Cardiol. 2007;99(6):760-5.
10. Hsieh I, Chen CC, Chang S, Wang CY, Lee CH, Lin FC. Acute and long-term outcomes of drug-eluting stent implantations in aorto-ostial, left anterior

descending artery-ostial, and nonostial lesions. Catheter Cardiovasc Interv. 2013;82(5):727-34.

11. Dishmon DA, Elhaddi A, Packard K, Gupta V, Fischell TA. High incidence of inaccurate stent placement in the treatment of coronary aorto-ostial disease. J Invasive Cardiol. 2011;23(8):322-6.
12. Rubinshtein R, Ben-Dov N, Halon DA, Lavi I, Finkelstein A, Lewis BS. Geographic miss with aorto-ostial coronary stent implantation: insights from high-resolution coronary computed tomography angiography. EuroIntervention. 2015;11(3):301-7.
13. Veeranna V, Pradhan J, Ali M, Afonso L. Complex intervention of an in-stent restenosis of ostial right coronary artery stent protruding into aortic sinus of Valsalva: a case report and brief review of the literature. J Invasive Cardiol. 2009;21(11):E226-8.
14. Popma JJ, Brogan WC, Pichard AD, Satler LF, Kent KM, Mintz GS, et al. Rotational coronary atherectomy of ostial stenoses. Am J Cardiol. 1993;71(5):436-8.
15. Motwani JG, Raymond R, Franco I, Ellis SG, Whitlow PL. Effectiveness of rotational atherectomy of right coronary artery ostial stenosis. Am J Cardiol. 2000;85(5):563-7.
16. Shlofmitz E, Martinsen BJ, Lee M, Rao SV, Généreux P, Higgins J, et al. Orbital atherectomy for the treatment of severely calcified coronary lesions: evidence, technique, and best practices. Expert Rev Med Devices. 2017;14(11):867-79.
17. Vuurmans T, Patterson MS, Laarman GJ. StentBoost used to guide management of a critical ostial right coronary artery lesion. J Invasive Cardiol. 2009;21(2):E19-21.
18. Puri R, Kapadia SR, Nicholls SJ, Harvey JE, Kataoka Y, Tuzcu EM. Optimizing Outcomes During Left Main Percutaneous Coronary Intervention With Intravascular Ultrasound and Fractional Flow Reserve. JACC: Cardiovasc Interv. 2012;5(7):697-707.
19. Szabo BA, PT V. New Technique of Aorto-Ostial Stent Placement. Am J Cardiol. 2005;96:212H.
20. Kern MJ, Ouellette D, Frianeza T. A new technique to anchor stents for exact placement in ostial stenoses: the stent tail wire or Szabo technique. Catheter Cardiovasc Interv. 2006;68(6):901-6.
21. Vaquerizo B, Serra A, Ormiston JA, Miranda-Guardiola F, Webber B, Fantuzzi A, et al. Bench top evaluation and clinical experience with the szabo technique. Catheter Cardiovasc Interv. 2011;79(3):378-89.
22. Fischell TA, Malhotra S, Khan S. A new ostial stent positioning system (Ostial ProTM) for the accurate placement of stents to treat aorto-ostial lesions. Catheter Cardiovasc Interv. 2008;71(3):353-7.

CHAPTER 35

Zero-contrast Percutaneous Coronary Intervention: Step-by-Step Approach

Prathap Kumar, Blessvin Jino, Manu Rajendran

INTRODUCTION

Contrast-induced acute kidney injury (CI-AKI) is a common complication of percutaneous coronary intervention (PCI). Kidney Disease: Improving Global Outcomes (KDIGO) defines it as an increase in serum creatinine by ≥0.3 mg% within 48 hours of contrast administration or ≥50% increase within 7 days.[1] The National Cardiovascular Data Registry (NCDR) Cath PCI registry data suggests that the overall incidence of CI-AKI in patients undergoing PCI is 7.1%.[2] ST-elevation myocardial infarction (STEMI), cardiogenic shock, and an estimated glomerular filtration rate (eGFR) <30 mL/min/1.73 m^2 are the common risk factors for CI-AKI requiring dialysis. CI-AKI increases the hospitalization cost and the short-term and long-term mortality rates.[3] Data from the NCDR Cath-PCI registry showed that the CI-AKI risk had increased by 42% for every 75 mL of incremental contrast used.[4] The MOZART trial concluded that the use of intravascular ultrasound (IVUS) during PCI decreased the contrast volume (CV) requirement.[5] Moreover, recent studies have shown that ultra-low CV <eGFR reduces the CI-AKI risk. Zero-contrast PCI is a newer technique that has a high potential to prevent CI-AKI and to improve survival after PCI.

HOW TO SELECT CASES FOR ZERO-CONTRAST PCI?

Both IVUS and optical coherence tomography (OCT) may be used to guide zero-contrast PCI. Zero-contrast PCI under OCT guidance may also be done using dextran 40 or hydroxyethyl starch.[6] However, the IVUS is commonly used due to the availability of longer pullback, easier pushability, and the ability to do without contrast clearance. Injecting a large amount of saline may precipitate heart failure symptoms in patients with moderate-to-severe left ventricular systolic dysfunction. Currently, there are not many studies on zero-contrast PCI to guide us in selecting patients for whom it is clearly beneficial, and there are no universally accepted criteria for selecting patients for zero-contrast PCI. We follow a simplified criterion at our institution to select patients for zero-contrast PCI. When a patient needs PCI as per the standard guidelines, we consider zero-contrast PCI if they have any of the following:[7]

- eGFR <30 mL/min/1.73 m^2
- Serum creatinine >1.5 mg% or eGFR 30–45 mL/min/1.73 m^2, *and* any of the following:
  - Age >75 years
  - Left ventricular ejection fraction (LVEF) <35%
  - Diabetes mellitus
  - Recent hypotension or shock

Though the zero-contrast PCI is more beneficial in patients with chronic kidney disease (CKD) and not on maintenance dialysis, it is also useful for patients who are already on hemodialysis as it preserves the residual renal function. Residual renal function is an important predictor of long-term quality of life in CKD patients. The BMC2 risk score is an important and reliable tool to predict CI-AKI, death, and transfusion in patients undergoing PCI. It can be calculated before PCI, and an online calculator is available for easier calculation. The predicted risks of <1%, 1–7%, and >7% are considered low risk, intermediate risk, and high risk, respectively.[8] Patients with a predicted risk >7% may be considered for zero-contrast PCI.

TIMING OF THE PROCEDURE

The initial coronary angiogram is mandatory in all cases, and the PCI can be done as a staged PCI in stable patients. The interval between the coronary angiogram and the zero-contrast PCI is variable, and it depends on the patient's clinical condition. There are no standard recommendations for the time interval. However, most of the studies have an average time interval of 1 week.[9,10] Most of the low osmolar contrast media have a half-life of around 2 hours, and it takes 20 hours for the contrast to be eliminated in patients with normal renal function. Hence, it is logical to give an interval of at least 24 hours after the coronary angiogram. However, this interval is not recommended by the ACR committee on contrast media,[11] and this interval may vary according to the patient's renal status. Additionally, patients with an acute coronary syndrome and ongoing angina may require urgent revascularization. Hence, a personalized decision should be taken regarding the time interval between the coronary angiogram and zero-contrast PCI. In general, PCI can be done on an ad-hoc basis in most cases. However, when the coronary angiogram is done at another center, it is better to delay PCI for 1 day because of the unreliability of the volume of contrast used.

PREPARATION OF THE PATIENT

Though PCI may be planned as a zero-contrast procedure, all patients must be given adequate hydration with isotonic saline before the procedure. The POSEIDON trial concluded that left ventricular end-diastolic pressure

(LVEDP)-based intravenous fluid administration prevents CI-AKI effectively. All patients need to undergo routine baseline electrocardiogram (ECG) and echocardiographic examinations before the procedure so that any new changes during the procedure may be easily identified.

CORONARY ANGIOGRAM

Femoral access is generally preferred in zero-contrast PCI as it allows preservation of the radial arteries for future dialysis. Additionally, larger catheters may be used in the femoral approach. Larger catheters provide a larger lumen for multiple wires and IVUS runs. Moreover, aggressive lesion preparation using atherectomy devices may be required in CKD patients who have heavily calcified vessels. Hence, femoral access is commonly used by many operators. The coronary angiogram must be done with ultra-low CV <eGFR. Totally, three angiographic projections are sufficient in most of the cases. That is, right anterior oblique (RAO) caudal and AP/RAO cranial projections for the left system and left anterior oblique (LAO) cranial for the right system. 5F catheters and catheters without side holes are preferred for angiograms to minimize contrast use. Higher frame rates improve the image quality so that diluted contrast can be used. Frequent contrast puffing in between catheter engagements should be avoided.

CATHETER ENGAGEMENT AND WIRING THE VESSEL

When a guide catheter is used for a coronary angiogram, the contrast in the guide catheter should be removed before inserting the guidewires. Frequent flushing of the catheter with saline is essential during zero-contrast PCI. Thrombus formation inside the catheter is common even when the activated clotting time is >250 seconds due to the stagnation of blood inside the catheter when multiple wires and an imaging catheter are used. Catheter engagement is easier for experienced operators. Before engagement, it is essential to have previous coronary angiographic views as a roadmap. If the coronary angiogram is done at another center, keeping a separate display for the angiographic views is needed inside the catheterization laboratory. Guidewire crossing, lesion preparation, and stent deployment should be done in the same fluoroscopic projections such as coronary angiogram **(Flowchart 1)**. Calcified ostium allows easy identification and engagement. Once catheter engagement is done, it can be confirmed by inserting the guidewire into the coronary. Similarly, repolarization changes in the ECG from injecting saline into coronaries also suggest catheter engagement.

METALLIC SILHOUETTE

After catheter engagement and lesion crossing, the main operating wire may be parked as distal as possible. Creating a loop in the distal tip of the

Flowchart 1: Step-by-step zero-contrast percutaneous coronary intervention (PCI).

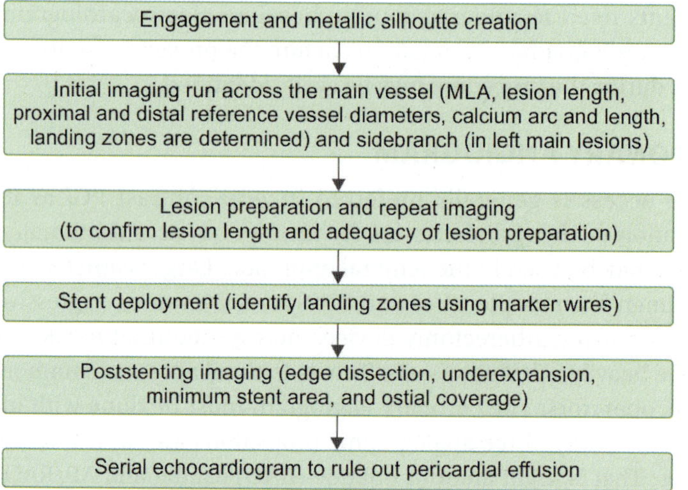

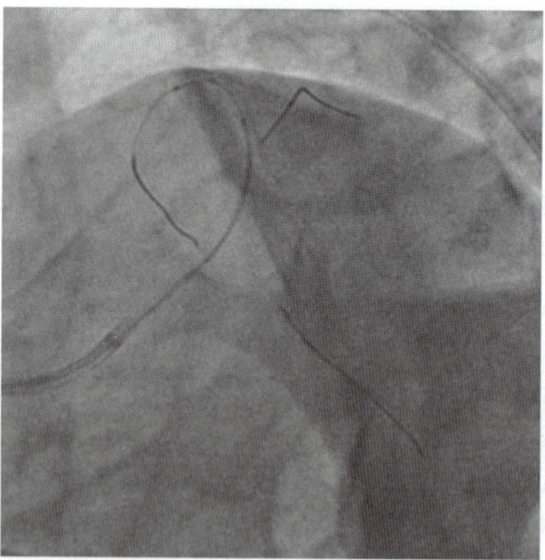

Fig. 1: Intravascular ultrasound (IVUS) imaging across left anterior descending artery (LAD) after creating a metallic silhouette.

guidewire is helpful, as the looped wire usually goes inside the lumen of the vessel. Extra guidewires are placed in the major branches of the main vessel (marker wires), using the roadmap as guidance. The left circumflex artery (LCX), major septal artery, and major diagonal are the preferred branches for marker wire in left anterior descending artery (LAD) stenting **(Fig. 1)**. Similarly, the obtuse marginal (OM) and LAD are wired for LCX stenting. The conus branch, right ventricular (RV) branch, posterior descending branch (RPDA), and posterolateral branch (RPLB) are the preferred marker branches for right coronary artery (RCA) stenting.

LESION PREPARATION AND INTRACORONARY IMAGING

After inserting marker wires, it is essential to keep the wires separate to avoid wire wrap. Then intracoronary imaging using IVUS or OCT is done. Pushability of IVUS is better than OCT in complex lesions. However, some lesions are hard to cross with the imaging catheter, and predilatation may be needed. Operator experience is needed for predilatation before imaging, as subintimal tracking of wire is possible in difficult wiring. It is advisable to use smaller diameter balloons, such as 1.25–1.5 mm, to predilate before imaging. Then an imaging catheter is inserted as distal as possible, as angiographically normal areas may have significant disease on intracoronary imaging. Commercially available IVUS imaging systems have a 100–150 mm pullback length, which is sufficient for most cases. IVUS has the advantage of a longer pullback length compared to OCT. During the initial run, it is essential to confirm the wire position in true lumen. Then minimal luminal area, proximal and distal reference vessel diameters, lesion length, and calcium arc and length are measured, along with the identification of proximal and distal landing zones. During IVUS pullback, whenever good landing zones are seen, "cine" storage may be done. Later, this position may help in stent placement.

REPEAT IMAGING AND STENT SIZING

Whenever possible, repeat imaging after the initial lesion preparation is done. This helps to identify the adequacy of lesion preparation and confirm the lesion length again. When two stents are selected, the stent overlap length is considered before selecting the stent length. Similarly, in aorto-ostial stenting, stent protrusion into the aorta should also be considered. During image analysis, the distance from the distal landing zone to the most distal marker wire and the proximal landing zone to the most proximal marker wire should be measured clearly. This helps in positioning the stent fluoroscopically **(Fig. 2)**. In cases in which two stents are required, repeat imaging may be done after the first stent deployment. This repeat pullback helps to select the second stent length more accurately, which is measured from the first stent edge to the proximal or distal landing zones. "Stent boost" and "clear stent" technologies help us to position the second stent fluoroscopically.

IMAGING AFTER STENTING AND STENT OPTIMIZATION

After stenting, imaging is done to identify the adequacy of stent expansion, malapposition, edge dissection, minimal stent area (MSA), and ostial coverage. Stent optimization is done as per the operator's discretion, and a final run is done to confirm the optimization. In general, the achievement of MSA >80% of average reference lumen area, or MSA >5.5 mm^2 in non-left main coronary artery (LMCA) and >8 mm^2 in LMCA without significant edge

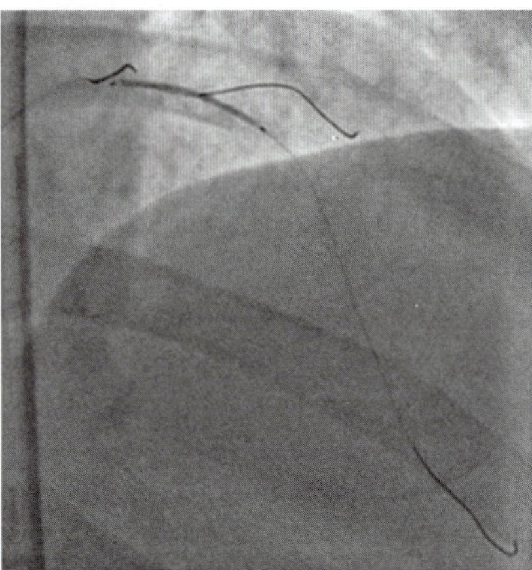

Fig. 2: Stent positioning using marker wires in left circumflex artery (LCX) and diagonal.

dissection or malapposition, is considered an optimized procedure. Final angiographic TIMI flow is a strong predictor of long-term outcome after PCI. However, the final flow in the vessel cannot be graded using intracoronary imaging. The long-term outcome of zero-contrast PCI is still not known, and it needs further large-scale studies.

CONCLUSION

The most common cause of death in stage 4 and stage 5 CKD is cardiovascular diseases. In spite of the available evidence, PCI remains underutilized in CKD patients. Fear of precipitating AKI and dialysis is the major reason for denying PCI. Zero-contrast PCI is a major boon for these patients. Meticulous analysis of IVUS imaging and operator experience play major role in the widespread usage of this technique.

REFERENCES

1. Kellum JA, Lameire N, Aspelin P, Barsoum RS, Burdmann EA, Goldstein SL, et al. Kidney Disease: Improving Global Outcomes (KDIGO) Acute Kidney Injury Work Group. KDIGO clinical practice guideline for acute kidney injury. Kidney Int Suppl. 2012;2:1-138.
2. Tsai TT, Patel UD, Chang TI, Kennedy KF, Masoudi FA, Matheny ME, et al. Contemporary incidence, predictors, and outcomes of acute kidney injury in patients undergoing percutaneous coronary interventions: Insights from the NCDR Cath-PCI Registry. JACC Cardiovasc Interv. 2014;7:1-9.
3. Finn WF. The clinical and renal consequences of contrast-induced nephropathy. Nephrol Dial Transplant. 2006;21:i2-10.
4. Amin AP, Bach RG, Caruso ML, Kennedy KF, Spertus JA. Association of variation in contrast volume with acute kidney injury in patients undergoing percutaneous coronary intervention. JAMA Cardiol. 2017;2(9):1007-12.

5. Mariani J Jr, Guedes C, Soares P, Zalc S, Campos CM, Lopes AC, et al. Intravascular ultrasound guidance to minimize the use of iodine contrast in percutaneous coronary intervention: the MOZART (Minimizing cOntrast utiliZation with IVUS Guidance in coRonary angioplasTy) randomized controlled trial. JACC Cardiovasc Interv. 2014;7(11):1287-93.
6. Vasu N, Subban V, Ajit Mullasari S. Zero contrast optical coherence tomography-guided percutaneous coronary intervention for in-stent restenosis of the saphenous vein graft using a non-contrast flush medium. Indian Heart J. 2018;70(Suppl 3):S492-5.
7. Kumar P, Blessvin J, Manu R. Zero contrast percutaneous coronary intervention: a novel approach to reduce contrast induced acute kidney injury. Medical Research Archives, [S.l.], v. 10, n. 12, Dec. 2022.
8. Gurm HS, Seth M, Kooiman J, Share D. A novel tool for reliable and accurate prediction of renal complications in patients undergoing percutaneous coronary intervention. J Am Coll Cardiol. 2013;61:2242-8.
9. Ali ZA, Karimi Galougahi K, Nazif T, Maehara A, Hardy MA, Cohen DJ, et al. Imaging- and physiology-guided percutaneous coronary intervention without contrast administration in advanced renal failure: a feasibility, safety, and outcome study. Eur Heart J. 2016;37(40):3090-5.
10. Sacha J, Gierlotka M, Lipski P, Feusette P, Dudek D. Zero-contrast percutaneous coronary interventions to preserve kidney function in patients with severe renal impairment and hemodialysis subjects. Postepy Kardiol Interwencyjnej. 2019;15(2):137-42.
11. Davenport MS, Asch D, Cavallo J, Cohan R, Dillman JR, Ellis JH, et al. (2020). ACR Manual on Contrast Media 2020: ACR Committee on Drugs and Contrast Media. [online] Available from https://xray.ufl.edu/wordpress/files/2020/05/2020_ACR_Manual_Contrast_Media.pdf [Last accessed October, 2024].

CHAPTER 36

Interventional Management of Coronary Aneurysms

Arun Gopi

INTRODUCTION

Coronary artery aneurysms (CAAs) are defined as dilation of coronary arteries more than 1.5 times that of adjacent normal segment. Its angiographic prevalence is 0.3–5.3%.[1] CAA was first described by Dr Charles Bougon in 1812.[2] Saccular CAA is spherical in shape having transverse diameter more than longitudinal and fusiform aneurysms are spindle shaped with bigger longitudinal diameter. Giant CAA is defined as those with diameter more than 8 mm in children and more than 20 mm or more than 4 times the reference normal segment in adults.[3] Majority of time it is an incidental finding on angiogram. Coronary artery ectasia (CAE) is defined as dilation of more than one-third of the entire coronary length at least 1.5 times the normal reference segment **(Table 1)**.

Most do not have any symptoms. Effort angina is the most common symptom arising from reduced flow from the dilated coronary segment. Only when the CAA gets complicated by thrombus formation causing acute coronary syndrome does it manifest clinically. Fistula formation, thrombus formation, compression of surrounding structures and rupture are rare fatal complications of CAAs. Acute cardiac tamponade, albeit rare, is a fatal complication of giant CAAs particularly resulting from Kawasaki disease with ongoing vasculitis. The major concerns are always about rupture of giant CAA, causing sudden cardiac death.

Coronary artery aneurysms are more common in men than women. Similarly, right coronary is affected more than the left coronary and proximal or mid segments are more affected than the distal segments.[1] Most common cause of CAA in adults is atherosclerosis and in children Kawasaki disease. The other uncommon causes are congenital, traumatic, infectious mycotic aneurysm, vasculitis, and trauma.

DIAGNOSIS

Coronary angiogram (CAG) remains the gold standard and most used test for diagnosis and devising treatment plan for CAA. But CAG underestimates the size of the aneurysm or neglects CAA when it is occluded or contains substantial thrombus. In such scenarios, intravascular imaging, especially intravascular ultrasound (IVUS), is very useful in such scenario and it

TABLE 1: Definitions and classifications of CAA.

Types and classifications	*Descriptions*
Coronary artery aneurysm (CAA)	
Definition of CAA	Focal dilation of at least 1.5 times the adjacent normal segment
Morphology:	
Saccular aneurysm	Transverse > longitudinal diameter
Fusiform aneurysm	Transverse < longitudinal diameter
Vessel wall composition by intravascular ultrasound (IVUS):	
True aneurysm	Vessel wall composed of three layers: Adventitia, media, and intima
Pseudoaneurysm	Loss of vessel wall integrity and damage to the adventitia
Size:	
Giant aneurysm (adults)	Size reached about 4× dilation when compared with the reference vessel or >20 mm in diameter
Giant aneurysm (children)	Diameter >8 mm
Coronary artery ectasia (CAE)	
Definition of CAE	Diffuse dilation of at least 1.5 times the adjacent normal segment exceeds more than a third of the artery length
Extent of involvement:	
Type I	Diffuse ectasia of two or three vessels
Type II	Diffuse ectasia in one vessel and localized disease in another
Type III	Diffuse ectasia of one vessel only
Type IV	Localized or segmental ectasia

also helps to differentiate among true aneurysm and pseudoaneurysm. Computed tomography coronary angiography (CTCA) is also very useful in evaluation of CAA by providing aneurysm size, thrombus, calcification, and early detection of complications. In pediatric population especially with Kawasaki disease (KD), echocardiography also helps in diagnosing CAA involving proximal vessel segments.

MANAGEMENT

Management strategy is controversial and there are no appropriate guidelines. So, the treatment must be individualized. The Coronary Artery Aneurysm Registry (CAAR) was a multicenter registry (32 hospitals across 9 countries,

Flowchart 1: Proposed algorithm for management of CAA.

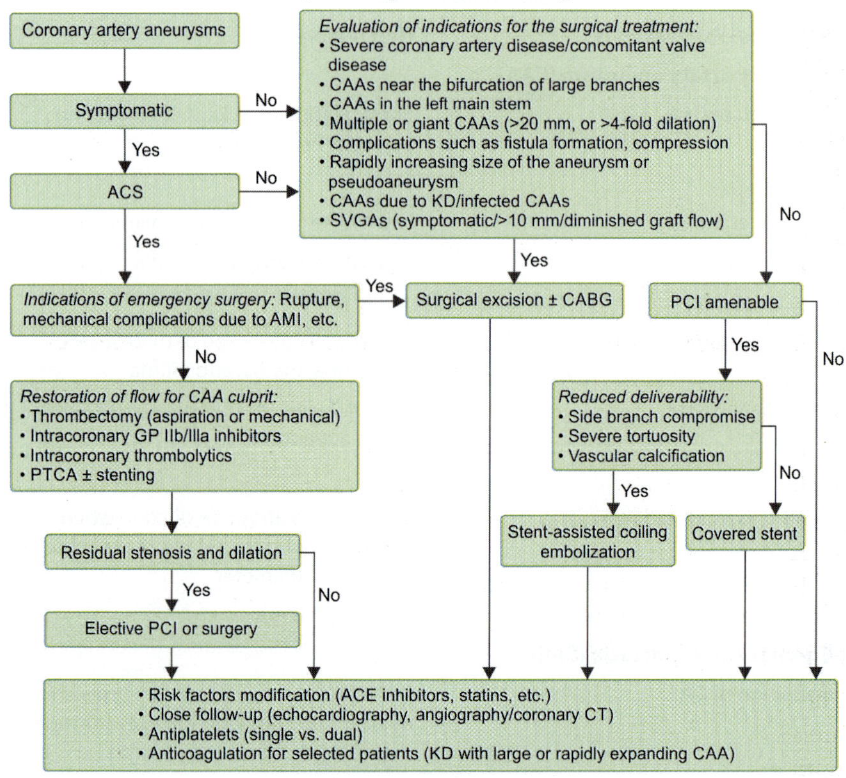

(ACE: angiotensin-converting enzyme; CAA: coronary artery aneurysm; CABG: coronary artery bypass grafting; CT: computed tomography; KD: Kawasaki disease; PCI: percutaneous coronary intervention; PTCA: percutaneous transluminal coronary angioplasty; SVGA: saphenous vein graft aneurysm)

1,565 patients with CAAs) that investigated the short- and long-term results of a variety of management strategies of CAA.[4] The proposed strategy has been explained in **Flowchart 1**.

Medical Management

Antiplatelets and anticoagulant medications to prevent thromboembolic complications and risk factor modification form the basic therapy of CAA. This approach has been studied in the CAAR study with a median follow-up of 37 months. Oral anticoagulants (vitamin K antagonist) maintaining INR between 2 and 3 has been a standard of care for CAE. Consequently, the current guidelines recommend warfarin just for KD patients with current or persistent large and giant CAA, achieving a target international normalized ratio of 2 to 3 for thromboprophylaxis (Class IIa recommendation).[10]

- Unjailing of side branches
- Formation of a cap (neomedia) over lipid rich plaque
- Plaque regression

Advantages of Vascular Bioresorbable Scaffolds

- Unjails covered side branches, restoring access
- Avoids full metal jacket, restoring late bypass surgery options
- Allows treatment of in-stent restenosis without necessitating a permanent additional metal layer
- Facilitates noninvasive imaging follow-up without artifacts
- Addresses physician's and patient's desires to avoid a permanent implant

Disadvantages of First-generation Vascular Bioresorbable Scaffolds

- Some devices require cold storage and specific deployment techniques
- Thicker/wider struts with larger crossing profile (more difficult to deliver)
- Greater attention to procedural technique required
- Greater risks of acute strut fracture compared with metallic DES
- Intraluminal scaffold dismantling
- Higher early rates of scaffold thrombosis (ScT) and target vessel-related myocardial infarction (TVMI), particularly in small vessels

The vascular healing of bare-metal stent is different from bioresorbable vascular scaffold (BVS) **(Fig. 1)**. Optical coherence tomography (OCT) at 6–12 months and 2–5 years after absorb implantation shows absorption of

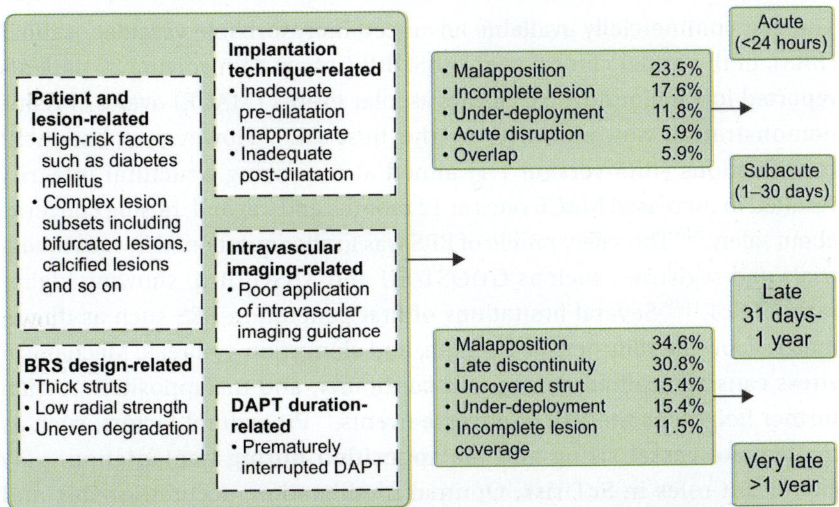

Fig. 1: Differences in vascular healing between metal stents and absorb BRSs.[8]
(BRS: bioresorbable scaffold; DAPT: dual antiplatelet therapy)

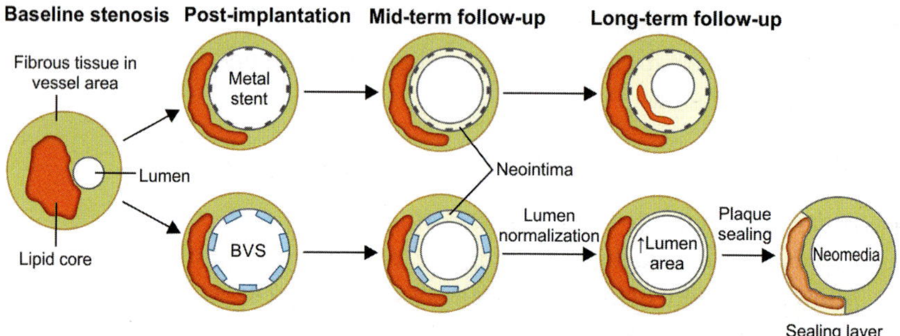

Fig. 2: Mid-term and long-term follow-up of bare metal stent and bioresorbable vascular scaffold.[7]

struts and endothelial layer formation and by formation of a connective tissue neo media after strut resorption. BMS leads to constraint of vessel leading to neoatherosclerosis **(Fig. 2)**.[7]

PHASES OF BIORESORBABLE SCAFFOLD FUNCTIONALITY

The three phases of BRS functionality are: (1) Mechanical support and drug delivery immediate phase at ≈6 months, (2) the restoration phase where struts begin to disappear and cyclic pulsatility and vasomotion return at 12 months, and (3) total resorption leading to return of adaptive vascular remodeling responses by 24 months **(Fig. 3)**.[7]

LESSONS FROM FIRST-GENERATION BIORESORBABLE SCAFFOLD

The first commercially available advanced bioresorbable vascular scaffold (BRS), in the initial clinical trial (ABSORB Cohort A) involving 30 patients reported low major adverse cardiovascular events (MACE) over 2–5 years, demonstrating noninferiority to the best DES. However, subsequent modifications (BRS version 1.1) aimed at improving structural integrity resulted in increased MACE rates at 12 months and beyond, raising concerns about safety.[9,10] The safety profile of BRS was further questioned in subsequent trials and registries, such as GHOST-EU and ABSORB-II, showing higher rates of ScT.[11,12] Several limitations of first-generation BRS such as due to material low ductility, tensile strength, and elongation-to-break. Mechanical stress causing scaffold damage, discontinuity, and malapposition, which further heightens the risk of adverse events.[13] Procedural factors, such as inadequate vessel sizing and malapposition during implantation, play significant roles in ScT risk. Optimal predilatation, accurate sizing, and postdilatation (PSP) strategies have been suggested to reduce adverse events, with imaging guidance crucial for precise implantation and follow-up

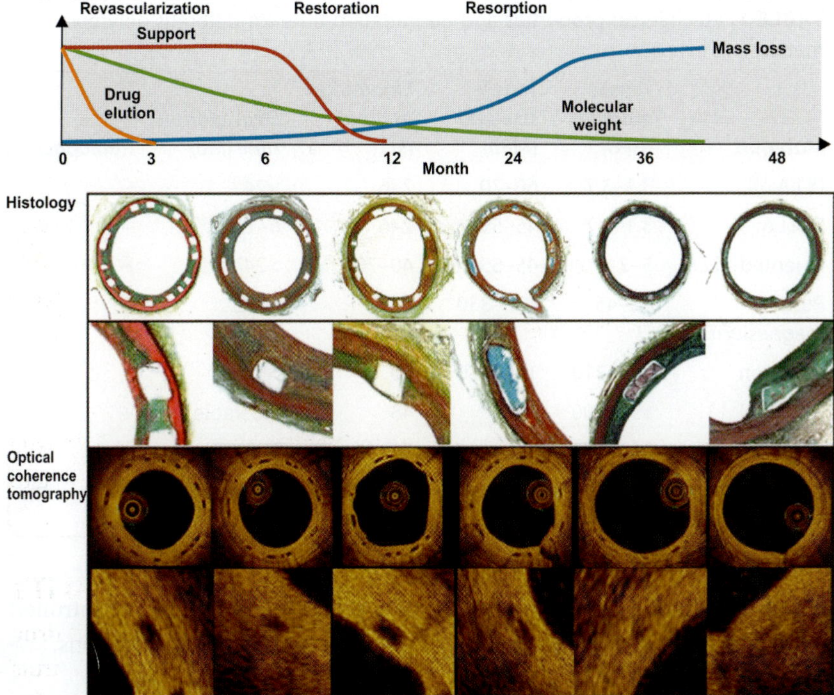

Fig. 3: Post BVS implantation follow up with OCT and histopathology.[7]

assessment.[14] Diabetic patients may have increased scaffold restenosis rates, and specific lesion types like bifurcation or heavily calcified lesions may require more aggressive preparation.[15] Advanced imaging techniques like optical coherence tomography help in assessing vessel injury and neointimal hyperplasia, influencing strut embedment. Understanding these factors is vital for optimizing BRS implantation strategies and monitoring patient outcomes effectively.[16]

IMPROVEMENT OF THE MECHANICAL PROPERTIES (TABLE 1)

The next generation of BRSs ArterioSorb BRS from Arterius Ltd. has decreased strut thickness to 95 μm.[17] HARTSORBTM by HARTLON is another innovative BRS with 90 m struts.[18] Magnesium, a promising bioresorbable material, outperforms poly-L-l actic acid (PLLA) and poly-D-L-lactic acid (PDLLA) in terms of tensile strength and elongation at break. These magnesium alloy-based BRS begin to degrade after around 3 months, eventually changing into an amorphous calcium phosphate phase during the resorption process.[19,20] STENTiT, a new BRS incorporates polymeric microfibers into its support grafts.[17] Each of these developments indicates continuous attempts to develop

TABLE 1: Mechanical properties and degradation time for different polymers and metals.[19]

Materials	*Tensile modulus (GPa)*	*Tensile strength (MPa)*	*Elongation at break (%)*	*Degradation time (Mo)*	*Radiopacity*
PLLA	3.1–3.7	60–70	2-6	>24	–
PDLLA	3.1–3.7	45–55	2-6	6–12	–
Oriented-PLLA	5–7	45–55	40–70	>24	–
Pure magnesium	40–45	220–330	2–20	3–12	+
Pure iron	200–210	170–270	50	>9	+
316 steel	190–200	668	48	Biostable	+
CoCr	210–235	820–1,200	35–55	Biostable	+

(CoCr: cobalt chromium; PDLLA: poly-D-L-lactic acid; PLLA: poly-L-l actic acid; –: the material is lack sufficient radiopacity; +: better radiopacity)

BRS with enhanced mechanical qualities, biocompatibility, and controlled degradation, improving the field of BRSs for cardiovascular applications.

CURRENT STATUS

The fundamental distinction between BRS and DES is their bioresorbability. **Table 2** offers an overview of the key characteristics of both currently available and upcoming BRSs, highlighting the most important qualities to consider.

What we learned from the past is that ScT is the Achilles heel of BRS.

SCAFFOLD THROMBOSIS ETIOLOGY AND PREVENTION

Bioresorbable scaffold was designed to gradually degrade thus restoring vasoreactivity and prevent late stent thrombosis (ST) due residual metallic stent. But the incidence of ScT led to ultimately withdrawn from the global market on September 14, 2017.

PATIENT AND LESION CHARACTERISTICS AND INFLUENCE ON OUTCOME

Patient Related

For early ST, acute myocardial infarction (MI) and heart failure where the significant contributing factors. Cardiogenic shock causes insufficient coronary perfusion which leads to liver dysfunction and limited drug absorption. Late ST is predisposed by diabetes mellitus and renal failure, with history of malignancy being the strongest predictor [odds ratio (OR) 17.5, 95%

TABLE 2: Key characteristics of various Biovascular resorbable scaffolds (BRS).

	Device	*Manufacturer*	*Backbone*	*Coating*	*Strut thickness (μm)*	*Antiproliferative drug*	*Drug dose*	*Resorption time (months)*
Biodegradable	Absorb BRS	Abbott Vascular	PLLA	PDLLA	157	Everolimus	100 μg/mm^2	24–48
Polymer scaffold	DESolve Nx	Elixir Medical	PLLA	Polylactide-based polymer	150	Novolimus	5 μg/mm	24
	Fantom	REVA Medical	PTD-PC	PTD-PC	125	Sirolimus	115 μg (3.0 × 18 mm)	36
	ART 18AZ	Arterial Remodeling Technologies	PDLLA	N/A	170	None	None	6
	FAST	Boston Scientific	PLLA	N/A	<99	Everolimus	N/A	12–24
	MeRes-100	Meril Life Sciences	PLLA	PDLLA	100	Sirolimus	1.25 μg/mm^2	24
	Firesorb	MicroPort Medical	PLLA	PDLLA	100–125	Sirolimus	4 μg/mm	36
	NeoVas	Lepu Medical	PLLA	PDLLA	170	Sirolimus	15.3 μg/mm	36
	IDEAL BioStent	Xenogenics	PAE salicylic acid	Adipic acid	200	Sirolimus	NA	6–9
Metal bioabsorbable	DREAMS 1G	Biotronik	Magnesium alloy	PLGA	125	Paclitaxel	7.4 μg/cm^2	9–12
Scaffold	Magmaris (DREAMS 2G)	Biotronik	Magnesium alloy	PLLA	150	Sirolimus	140 mg/cm^2	9–12
	IBS	LifeTech Scientific	Iron alloy	PDLLA	70	Sirolimus	235 μg/cm^2	12–24

[PAE: poly (anhydride-esters); PDLLA: poly-D-L-lactic acid; PLGA: poly(lactic-co-glycolic acid); PLLA: poly-L-l actic acid].

confidence interval (CI) 4.7–65.3] due to prothrombotic phenotype bleeding under dual antiplatelet therapy (DAPT) treatment.[8]

Lesion Related

Type B and C lesions, vessel diameters of <2.25 mm and >3.75 mm due high risk of ScT is in small vessels (<2.25 mm) and scaffold dislocation larger diameter vessels; however, it is safe to implant in well-prepared calcified lesions.

Bioresorbable Scaffold Design on Outcome

Bioresorbable scaffolds have thicker struts than contemporary DES 100–150 µm versus 50–80 µm. This hinders endothelialization. In the future, the thickness of scaffolds needs to be reduced thus minimizing coronary flow disturbance and better mechanical properties.

IMPLANTATION TECHNIQUE AND INFLUENCE ON OUTCOME

A meta-analysis of five ABSORB prospective studies showed that the factors which reduced ScT were predilation with a ≥1:1 balloon-to-artery ratio and optimal postdilation.[8]

SIZING OF SCAFFOLD

It is preferred to use intravascular imaging (IVI) for BRS implantation. We need to select the appropriate scaffold size. Undersized and malapposed scaffold may collapse into the lumen and hastening the formation of ScT. 1 year MACE and MI rates also increase when oversized scaffolds in a relatively small vessel.

Postdilation of Scaffold

Postdilation is also preferably done under IVI with a noncompliant balloon at 16–25 atm, with a nominal diameter up to 0.25–0.50 mm larger than that of the scaffold.

INTRAVASCULAR IMAGING

Intravascular imaging is mandatory for implantation and follow-up. OCT is the preferred modality.

DUAL ANTIPLATELET THERAPY DURATION

Duration of DAPT should be for 6–12 months, may be longer in complicated lesions.

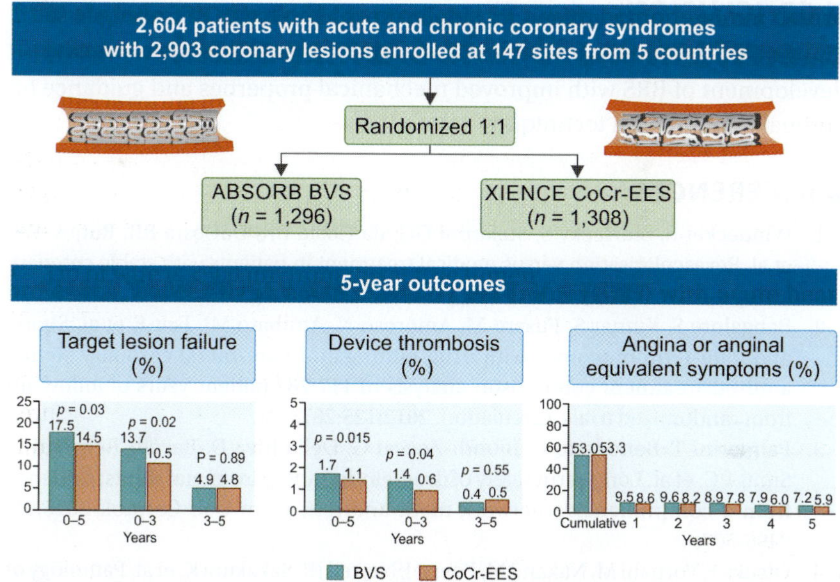

Fig. 4: 5-year result from the ABSORB-IV trial. (BVS: bioresorbable vascular scaffold; CoCr-EES: cobalt chromium everolimus-eluting stents)

Five-year results from ABSORB IV trial:

- Comparison of BRS to metallic DES showed that 5-year rates of target lesion failure were higher with BRS than DES (17.5% vs. 14.5%, $p = 0.03$) **(Fig. 4)**.
- Device thrombosis rates were also higher with BRS than DES at 3-year follow-up and between 3 and 5 years.
- However, rates of angina were at nearly 50% of patients within 5 years and were similar with both devices.[21,22]

INDIAN SCENARIO

The MeRes 100 PLLA sirolimus-eluting scaffold, 100 μm thick, features a hybrid cell design and is expected to degrade over 2–3 years. Its structure enables optimal vessel wall conformity, high radial strength, and includes platinum markers for better positioning. Initial MeRes-1 study[23] findings ($n = 108$) showed promising results at 6 and 12 months, reporting low late lumen loss (LLL) and no restenosis. Intravascular ultrasound (IVUS) revealed minimal neointimal hyperplasia, while OCT displayed robust scaffold coverage. Extended outcomes confirmed its efficacy and safety up to 3 years with maintained lumen patency and no very late scaffold thrombosis. The MeRes-1 Extend study (64 patients) reported a 1.61% MACE rate at 2 years with minimal target lesion revascularization (TLR) and no ScT. OCT imaging showed consistent flow and excellent strut coverage at 6 months with a low LLL.[24]

CONCLUSION

The role of BRS in clinical practice remains investigational and will need development of BRS with improved mechanical properties and guidance on optimal implantation techniques.

REFERENCES

1. Windecker S, Stortecky S, Stefanini GG, da Costa BR, DaCosta BR, Rutjes AW, et al. Revascularisation versus medical treatment in patients with stable coronary artery disease: network meta-analysis. BMJ. 2014;348:g3859.
2. Bangalore S, Kumar S, Fusaro M, Amoroso N, Attubato MJ, Feit F, et al. Short- and long-term outcomes with drug-eluting and bare-metal coronary stents: a mixed-treatment comparison analysis of 117 762 patient-years of follow-up from randomized trials. Circulation. 2012;125:2873-91.
3. Palmerini T, Benedetto U, Biondi-Zoccai G, Della Riva D, Bacchi-Reggiani L, Smits PC, et al. Long-term safety of drug-eluting and bare-metal stents: evidence from a comprehensive network meta-analysis. J Am Coll Cardiol. 2015;65: 2496-507.
4. Otsuka F, Vorpahl M, Nakano M, Foerst J, Newell JB, Sakakura K, et al. Pathology of second-generation everolimus-eluting stents versus first-generation sirolimus- and paclitaxel-eluting stents in humans. Circulation. 2014;129:211-23.
5. Iqbal J, Serruys PW, Silber S, Kelbaek H, Richardt G, Morel MA, et al. Comparison of zotarolimus- and everolimus-eluting coronary stents: final 5-year report of the RESOLUTE all-comers trial. Circ Cardiovasc Interv. 2015;8:e002230.
6. Yamaji K, Kimura T, Morimoto T, Nakagawa Y, Inoue K, Soga Y, et al. Very long-term (15 to 20 years) clinical and angiographic outcome after coronary bare metal stent implantation. Circ Cardiovasc Interv. 2010;3:468-75.
7. Kereiakes DJ, Onuma Y, Serruys PW, Stone GW. Bioresorbable Vascular Scaffolds for Coronary Revascularization. Circulation. 2016;134:168-82.
8. Peng X, Qu W, Jia Y, Wang Y, Yu B, Tian J. Bioresorbable Scaffolds: Contemporary Status and Future Directions. Front Cardiovasc Med. 2020;7:589571.
9. Onuma Y, Dudek D, Thuesen L, Webster M, Nieman K, Garcia-Garcia HM, et al. Five-year clinical and functional multislice computed tomography angiographic results after coronary implantation of the fully resorbable polymeric everolimus-eluting scaffold in patients with de novo coronary artery disease: the ABSORB cohort A trial. JACC Cardiovasc Interv. 2013;6(10):999-1009.
10. Serruys PW, Ormiston J, van Geuns RJ, de Bruyne B, Dudek D, Christiansen E, et al. A polylactide bioresorbable scaffold eluting everolimus for treatment of coronary stenosis: 5-year follow-up. J Am Coll Cardiol. 2016;67(7):766-76.
11. Capodanno D, Gori T, Nef H, Latib A, Mehilli J, Lesiak M, et al. Percutaneous coronary intervention with everolimus-eluting bioresorbable vascular scaffolds in routine clinical practice: early and midterm outcomes from the European multicentre GHOST-EU registry. EuroIntervention. 2015;10(10):1144-53.
12. Serruys PW, Chevalier B, Sotomi Y, Cequier A, Carrié D, Piek JJ, et al. Comparison of an everolimus-eluting bioresorbable scaffold with an everolimus-eluting metallic stent for the treatment of coronary artery stenosis (ABSORB II): a 3 year, randomised, controlled, single-blind, multicentre clinical trial. Lancet. 2016;388(10059):2479-91.

13. Sotomi Y, Onuma Y, Collet C, Tenekecioglu E, Virmani R, Kleiman NS, et al. Bioresorbable scaffold: the emerging reality and future directions. Circ Res. 2017;120(8):1341-52.
14. Byrne RA, Stefanini GG, Capodanno D, Onuma Y, Baumbach A, Escaned J, et al. Report of an ESC-EAPCI Task Force on the evaluation and use of bioresorbable scaffolds for percutaneous coronary intervention: executive summary. Eur Heart J. 2018;39(18):1591-601.
15. Anadol R, Schnitzler K, Lorenz L, Weissner M, Ullrich H, Polimeni A, et al. Three-years outcomes of diabetic patients treated with coronary bioresorbable scaffolds. BMC Cardiovasc Disord. 2018;18(1):92.
16. Sotomi Y, Tateishi H, Suwannasom P, Dijkstra J, Eggermont J, Liu S, et al. Quantitative assessment of the stent/scaffold strut embedment analysis by optical coherence tomography. Int J Cardiovasc Imaging. 2016;32:871-83.
17. Kawashima H, Ono M, Kogame N, Takahashi K, Chang CC, Hara H, et al. Drug-eluting bioresorbable scaffolds in cardiovascular disease, peripheral artery and gastrointestinal fields: a clinical update. Expert Opin Drug Deliv. 2020;17(7):931-45.
18. Wu X, Wu S, Kawashima H, Hara H, Ono M, Gao C, et al. Current perspectives on bioresorbable scaffolds in coronary intervention and other fields. Expert Rev Med Devices. 2021;18(4):351-66.
19. Barkholt TØ, Webber B, Holm NR, Ormiston JA. Mechanical properties of the drug-eluting bioresorbable magnesium scaffold compared with polymeric scaffolds and a permanent metallic drug-eluting stent. Catheter Cardiovasc Interv. 2020;96(7):E674-82.
20. Ang HY, Huang YY, Lim ST, Wong P, Joner M, Foin N. Mechanical behavior of polymer-based vs. metallic-based bioresorbable stents. J Thorac Dis. 2017;9(Suppl 9):S923.
21. Stone GW, Abizaid A, Onuma Y, Seth A, Gao R, Ormiston J, et al. Effect of technique on outcomes following bioresorbable vascular scaffold implantation: analysis from the ABSORB trials. J Am Coll Cardiol. 2017;70:2863-74.
22. Stone G, Kereiakes D, Gori T, Metzger DC, Stein B, Erickson M, et al. 5-year outcomes after bioresorbable coronary scaffolds implanted with improved technique. J Am Coll Cardiol. 2023;82(3):183-95.
23. Seth A, Onuma Y, Chandra P, Bahl VK, Manjunath CN, Mahajan AU, et al. Three-year clinical and two-year multimodality imaging outcomes of a thin-strut sirolimus-eluting bioresorbable vascular scaffold: MeRes-1 trial. EuroIntervention. 2019;15:607-14.
24. Abizaid A, Kedev S, Ali RBM, Santoso T, Cequier A, van Geuns RVG, et al. Imaging and 2-year clinical outcomes of thin strut sirolimus-eluting bioresorbable vascular scaffold: The MeRes-1 extend trial. Catheter Cardiovasc Interv. 2021;98(6):1102-10.

CHAPTER 38

How to Treat Coronary Perforations: Large Vessels, Distal Vessels, and Collaterals?

Sharath Reddy Annam

INTRODUCTION

Percutaneous coronary artery intervention (PCI) has become the mainstay of treatment for coronary artery disease (CAD). Although major complications rarely occur during PCI, they can be associated with high in hospital mortality and major adverse cardiac events (MACE).[1] Coronary artery perforation (CAP) is a rare complication of PCI with a reported incidence of 0.3–0.5% but unfortunately carries high mortality burden if not recognized and treated promptly.[2] With the increasing experience of interventional cardiologists, evolving technologies, more and more complex PCIs are performed in calcific lesions and chronic total occlusions. Plaque modification methods in these lesions increase the incidence of perforations with reported incidence as high as 8.9% and in hospital mortality of 10–15%.[3,4] Thus, the risk of coronary perforations is directly proportional to the complexity of the procedure, tortuosity, and calcification in the coronaries and the use of newer hardware.

CLASSIFICATION

Coronary artery perforation can be classified based on location and severity since the causes for perforation and the management strategy to seal it vary.

Types of coronary perforation based on location **(Fig. 1)**:

- Large vessel perforation
- Distal vessel perforation
- Collateral vessel perforation either epicardial or septal

Types of coronary perforation based on severity: Assessment of severity of perforation is important to prepare for swift response to seal it and also to plan pericardiocentesis. Severity is graded based on fluoroscopic features at the site of vessel injury as mentioned in **Table 1**.

Type V has been reclassified as:

- *Definite:* Myocardial contrast infiltration/blush detectable by angiography
- *Probable:* Cause of pericardial effusion/tamponade without angiography detection (ghost perforation)[6]

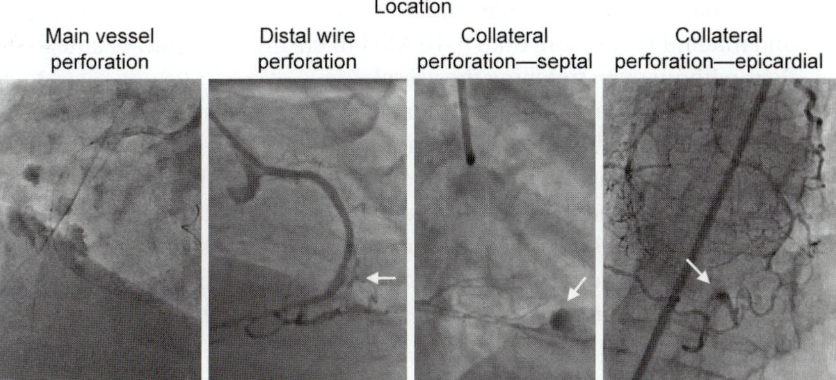

Fig. 1: Types of coronary perforation as per location.

TABLE 1: Modified Ellis classification of coronary perforations.[5-7]

Types	*Description*	*Pericardial tamponade*	*Mortality*
I	Extraluminal crater without jet extravasation	0.4%	0.3%
II	Pericardial or myocardial blush without contrast jet extravasation	3.3%	0.4%
III	Active jet extravasation with exit >1 mm	45.7%	21.2%
IV (also called cavity spilling III-CS)	Perforation with drainage into an anatomic cavity chamber (coronary sinus, right or left ventricle except pericardium)	0.2%	0.6%
V	Distal vessel or side branch perforation usually caused by guidewire *Type Va:* Definite *Type Vb:* Probable	10.2%	6.8%

MANAGEMENT OF CORONARY PERFORATIONS

Coronary artery perforation carries high mortality risk. Hence, prompt recognition and treatment initiation is of utmost importance. The treatment strategy is best guided by the specific angiographic location, type of CAP and the hemodynamic status of the patient. The main intention of the operator should be directed toward preventing further blood leakage to avoid hemodynamic instability and to gain time until definitive treatment can be delivered.

The following general measures should be implemented first in all CAPs to gain time:[8,9]

- *Prolonged balloon inflation:* Balloon inflation proximal to or at the site of the perforation should be performed immediately to prevent accelerated accumulation of blood in the pericardial space and cardiac tamponade.

The balloon to artery ratio should be 1:1 and must be semicompliant and inflated to no more than 8–10 ATM to ensure occlusion of antegrade flow, without overstretching the vessel.

Balloon inflation should be prolonged, lasting at least for 10–15 minutes. The duration of balloon inflation is guided by development of chest pain or hemodynamic instability due to ischemia. Hence, intermittent deflation is needed to allow antegrade flow to the distal vessel. Perfusion balloon if available would allow prolonged inflations with preservation of distal flow. In some cases, balloon inflation alone may be sufficient to achieve sealing of the perforation (particularly if the perforation is less severe, such as Ellis class I or II).

- Patient hemodynamic monitoring to recognize blood pressure drop promptly
- Administration of intravenous fluids and vasopressors (atropine in case of vasovagal reaction)
- 2D echocardiography monitoring immediately to check for pericardial effusion, presence of ongoing leak and to look for clues of early tamponade such as right ventricle early diastolic collapse and late diastolic right atrial collapse. These signs on 2D-ECHO precede the onset of hypotension. Of note, as little as 100 mL of collection in pericardial cavity in an acute setting can lead to hemodynamic instability.
- *Heparin reversal:* Reversal of anticoagulation may be considered but needs to be balanced with the risk of clotting in catheters till the perforation sealing is achieved. Protamine dose for heparin reversal is 1 mg per 100 units of heparin (maximum: 50 mg), administered at a rate not exceeding 5 mg per minute.
- Glycoprotein IIb/IIIa or Cangrelor infusion should be stopped immediately as soon as CAP is detected regardless of the type of CAP.
- *Timing of emergency pericardiocentesis:* In case of hemodynamic instability, emergency pericardiocentesis has to be performed. Pericardiocentesis can be performed under fluoroscopic guidance due to contrast exit into the pericardial space or under 2D Echo guidance.

  Smaller size pericardial effusions may be best managed conservatively, as the elevated pericardial pressure due to the entrance of blood into the pericardial space may help "tamponade the perforation site" and minimize the risk of further bleeding.
- *Call for cardiac surgical team:* Cardiac surgical team should be notified immediately to expedite the surgical management in case all the percutaneous treatment strategies fail to seal the perforation.

MANAGEMENT OF LARGE VESSEL PERFORATIONS

Large vessel perforations include perforation in vessel ≥2.5 mm in size. **Flowchart 1** depicts the algorithmic approach to large vessel perforations. Covered stent plays a major role in arresting large vessel perforations.

Flowchart 1: Algorithm for management of large vessel perforation.[11]

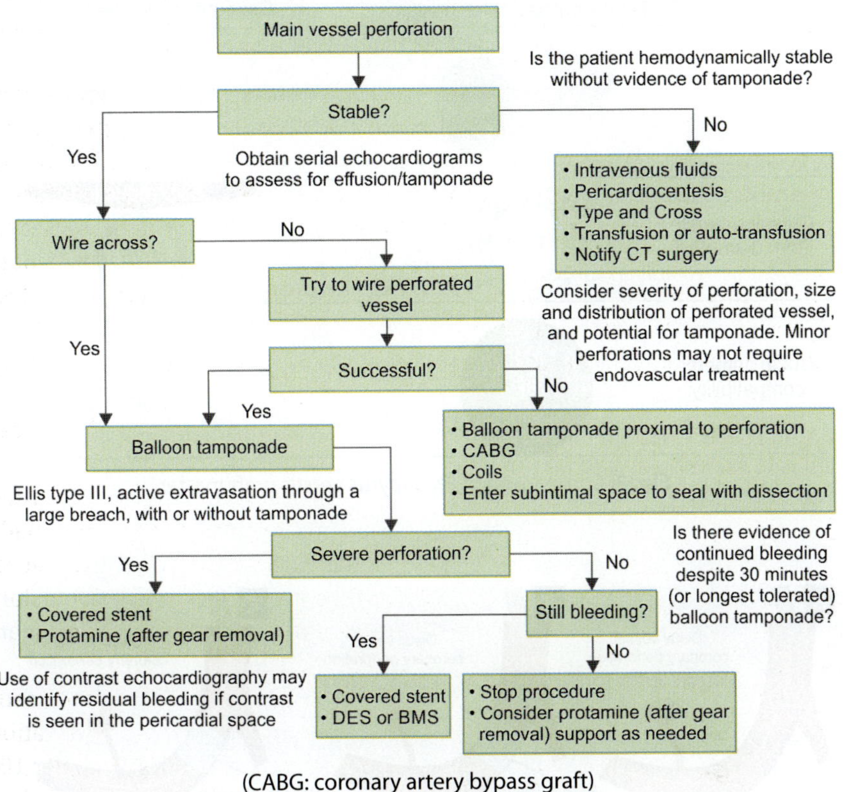

(CABG: coronary artery bypass graft)

Use of covered stents:[10] Covered stents **(Fig. 2)** offer an effective bailout treatment in CAP representing a potentially lifesaving treatment strategy. These are metallic stent platforms covered with a synthetic or biological membrane. A variety of covered stents are available across the globe. The Graft Master (Abbott Vascular, CA, USA) is the commercially available covered stent available in India. PK Papyrus is the new generation covered stent mostly commonly used worldwide.

Covered stents are bulky devices with limited flexibility. Hence, difficulties are routinely encountered while delivering the stent to the desired location especially in presence of tortuosity or calcific lesions. Depending on the size of the guide catheter being used and the size of the covered stent, delivery of the covered stent can be achieved using:

- Single guide catheter (also called "*block and deliver*" technique) **(Figs. 3A to G)**
- Two guide catheters (dual guide catheter, also called "ping pong" guide catheter, or "duelling" guide catheter technique)

The goals of both techniques is to minimize bleeding into the pericardium while preparing for covered stent delivery and deployment. If the balloon

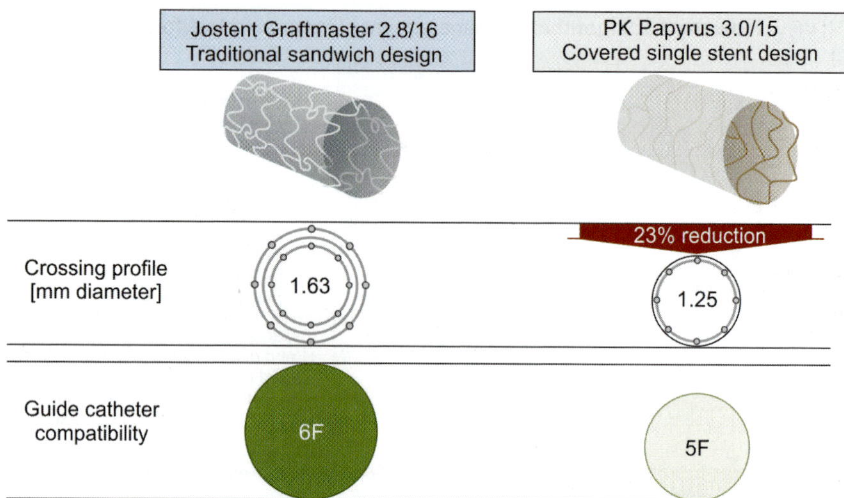

Fig. 2: Comparison of PK papyrus versus graft master.

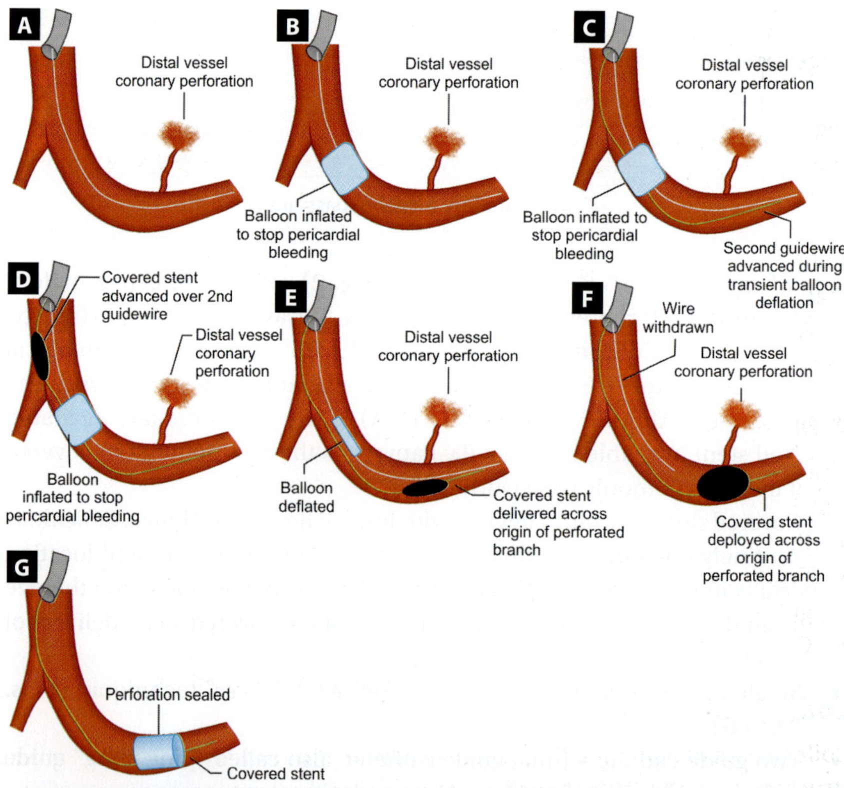

Figs. 3A to G: Covered stent for distal vessel perforation to seal the ostium of side branch with perforation (block and deliver technique using single 8 French guide).[15]

used for hemostasis and the covered stent can fit through a single (usually 8 Fr for graft master covered stents) guide catheter, then the single guide catheter technique is used, otherwise two guide catheters are required.[12-14]

Practical tips and tricks for use of covered stents:[12-14]

- These are bulky devices with lower deliverability.
- Stiff wires or buddy wires might be useful.
- Anchoring balloons or guide catheter extensions are alternatives.
- Stent size selection should be done at 1:1 basis.
- Covered stents usually require higher inflation pressures but care should be taken not to tear the covering membrane due to higher pressures (pericardial CS).
- Graft master can be used in vessels more than ≥2.75 mm and PK Papyrus in vessels ≥2.5 mm
- The length of the ePTFE foil is shorter than the reported strut length.
- After expansion of the stent, the ePTFE foil may be up to 1.6 mm shorter from each end of the stent graft.
- The covered length of the stented area may be up to 3.2 mm shorter than the stent length. Hence, the stent length should be selected accordingly.

The CRACK registry studied procedural and 1-year outcomes following large vessel coronary artery perforation treated by covered stents implantation in 119 patients and concluded that such patients should remain under regular follow-up due to relatively higher MACE rates especially attributed to stent thrombosis and target lesion revascularization (TLR) and target vessel revascularization (TVR).[16]

The CRACK-II registry compared Graft Master with PK Papyrus covered stents in patients with large vessel perforation in 106 patients and concluded that PK Papyrus had shorter delivery time and lower rates of TLR and TVR at 30 days, but no significant difference was seen between the two covered stents at 1 year follow-up.[17]

MANAGEMENT OF DISTAL VESSEL PERFORATIONS

The existing treatment options available for distal vessel perforation **(Table 2)** consist of:

- Prolonged balloon inflation as previously described
- Embolization with coils, microspheres, thrombin injection, particles of guidewire, and suture material
- Covered stent

Coil Embolization

Coils are permanent metallic (stainless steel or platinum) agents with a wired structure of synthetic wool or Dacron fibers and thrombogenic properties. Coils can be delivered through microcatheters for distal and more precise placement. The chosen coil size should be larger than the target vessel size to

TABLE 2: Management strategies for distal vessel perforation.[20,21]

Modality	*Description*	*Delivery*	*Implications*
Coils: • Detachable coils (predictable positioning) • Pushable coils (unpredictable and irreversible delivery) • The size of these coils should be larger than the size of the treated vessel • The choice of microcatheter is crucial	*Commonly available coils:* • Interlock (Boston Scientific) • Azur (Terumo) • Micronester (Cook) *Neurovascular coils (detachable):* • Axium (Medtronic) • Smart coil (Penumbra)	*Microcatheters*: 0.018 inch 0.018 inch 0.018 inch 0.014 inch	*0.018 Microcatheters:* • Prograat (Terumo), Transit (Cordis), and Renegade (Boston scientific); can use only a 0.014 inch FineCross (Terumo) instead of a 0.018 inch microcatheter • All neurovascular coils are compatible with 0.014 inch microcatheters
Autologous subcutaneous adipose tissue[7]	• Refers to fat from the abdominal or femoral (next to the puncture point) site • Can be dipped in contrast for a minute to render it radiopaque	Small fat globules are delivered through a microcatheter or over-the-wire balloon pushed by a guidewire/saline/contrast	The catheter should be positioned close to the perforation to avoid a large periprocedural MI
Microspheres	Spherical, hydrophilic, and nonabsorbable particles that come in sizes ranging from 1 to 1,500 microns	Delivered through microcatheters to occlude and cause precise sealing of perforations	
Thrombin	Helps sealing by assisting in the formation of fibrin clots	It is delivered precisely through an inflated over-the-wire balloon or microcatheter	
Clotted autologous blood	Can provide adequate sealing when suspended in contrast/saline		
Covered stents	Deploys covered stents in the main branch to occlude the side branch if other measures have failed to seal small branch perforations		The disadvantages are thrombogenicity and the occlusion of side branches

ensure complete vessel adherence and embolization. Coils that are too large may inadvertently be deployed too proximally, and coils that are too small may migrate too distally. Coils are generally used for CAPs in more distal and smaller caliber segments.[18]

The most important characteristics of coils are:

- Microcatheter compatibility (0.018 vs. 0.014 inch)
- Mechanism of release (pushable vs. detachable)

It is ideal to have 0.014' compatible coils (which can be deployed through the standard CTO microcatheter) that are also detachable (which allows for accurate delivery to the desired location) **(Figs. 4A to L)**.

Covered Stent for Distal Vessel Perforation

When the perforated vessel is too small or too tortuous, advancing a guidewire into it may not be feasible. Such cases could be treated with coiling of a more proximal larger branch, but if the perforated vessel is originating from a large vessel, occlusion of that vessel can be undesirable. An alternative solution is implantation of a covered stent over the origin of the perforated branch.

Novel Techniques to Treat Distal Vessel Perforation

Recently, a case reported by Al-Omary et al.[22] and Alavi et al.[23] reports a less familiar technique to treat distal coronary perforation. In this case, a distal posterior descending artery perforation was successfully sealed with 2 distal balloon fragments. Owing to the lack of availability of more common materials, the authors innovatively snipped the distal end of a used balloon and loaded it on the guidewire. The balloon fragment was then advanced with another balloon loaded on the wire, proximal to the balloon fragment. Once the fragment reached the distal portion of the vessel, the guidewire was withdrawn, leaving the balloon fragment in place and successfully sealing the perforation **(Figs. 5A to E)**.[24]

In another case series of distal vessel perforations, these CAPs were successfully treated with embolized absorbable suture. An absorbable Vicryl suture was cut into small fragments 5–6 mm long, followed by insertion of these fragments into a microcatheter. The suture fragments were then advanced by inserting a workhorse wire into a microcatheter and pushing the fragments out to the desired location to successfully seal the perforation.[22] Both techniques were effective in treating the distal vessel perforation, can be cheaper alternatives to other well-known strategies, and are available to operators when more.

■ MANAGEMENT OF COLLATERAL PERFORATIONS

Retrograde PCI through septals, epicardial vessels or bypass graft conduits are routinely being performed by CTO operators worldwide. These procedures may be complicated by perforation of these collateral channels during

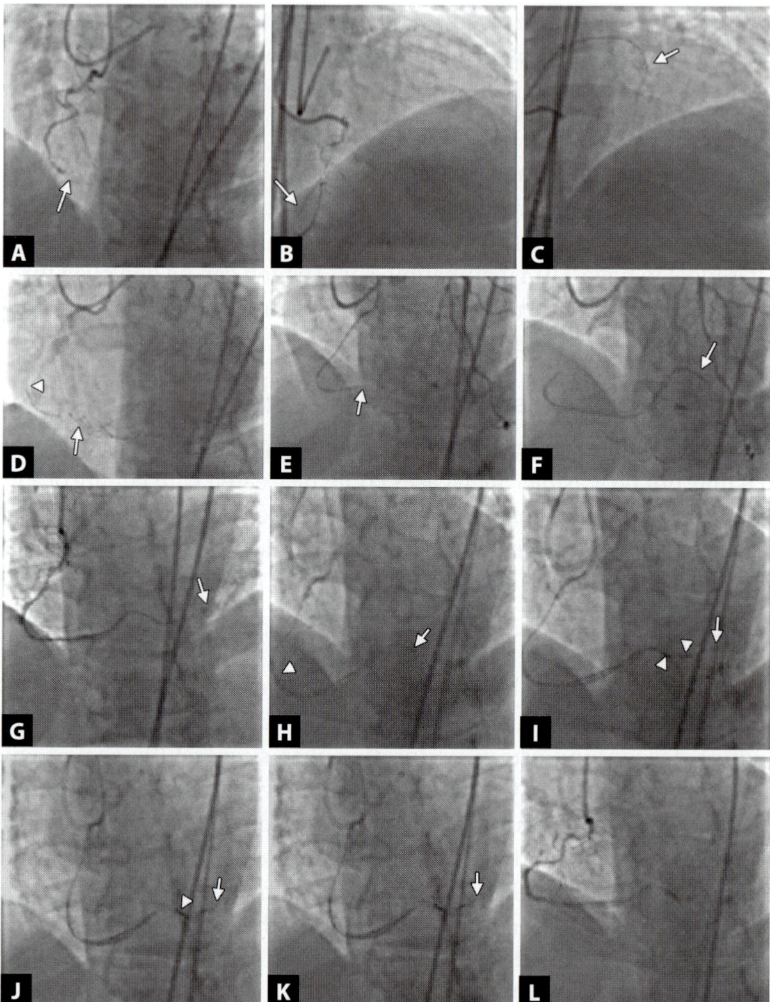

Figs. 4A to L: Example of distal vessel perforation treated with coil embolization. Coronary angiography using dual injection demonstrating a chronic total occlusion of the right coronary artery (arrow, A). Antegrade crossing attempts with a guidewire failed (arrow, B). Retrograde crossing attempts through a septal collateral (arrow, C) also failed. Repeat antegrade crossing with a CrossBoss catheter (arrowhead, D) and a knuckled Fielder XT guidewire (arrow, D) achieved subintimal crossing. Re-entry attempts with a stingray balloon and guidewire (arrow, E) failed, but distal true lumen entry was achieved advancing the knuckled guidewire (arrow, F) (subintimal tracking and re-entry—STAR technique). Coronary angiography after balloon predilation demonstrated distal vessel perforation (arrow, G). A balloon (arrowhead, H) was inflated, stopping pericardial bleeding, and a Progreat microcatheter (arrow, H) was delivered to the perforation site. Bleeding (arrow, I) continued after deployment of two 2 × 5 mm coils (arrowheads, I). Bleeding (arrow, J) slowed after deployment of a 2 mm × 2 cm detachable helical hydro coil (arrowhead, J) and stopped 15 minutes later (arrow, K). Final angiography (L) revealed complete occlusion of the perforation site.[19]

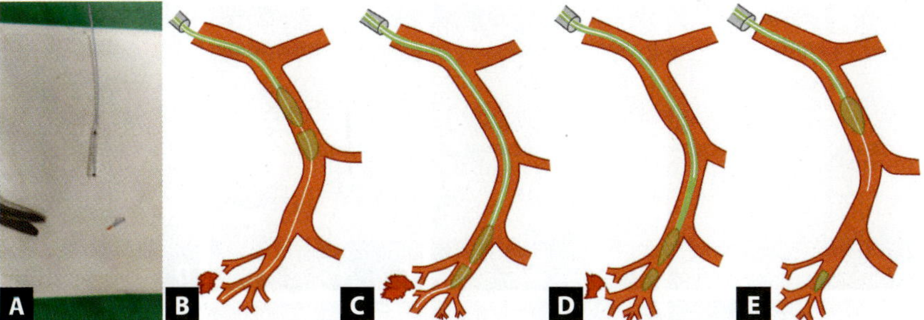

Figs. 5A to E: Schematic steps for sealing distal wire perforation using balloon remnant. (A) Distal half of already used balloon is cut by scissors; (B and C) The remnant piece is mounted on to the wire in the perforated vessel and pushed with another intact balloon to the distal vessel before the perforation; (D and E) Withdrawal of the wire and the intact pushing balloon with the remnant part left distally as embolization materials.

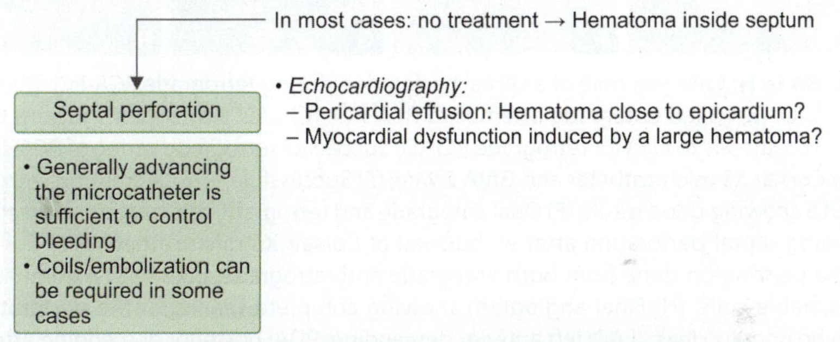

Fig. 6: Management of septal collateral perforation.[20]

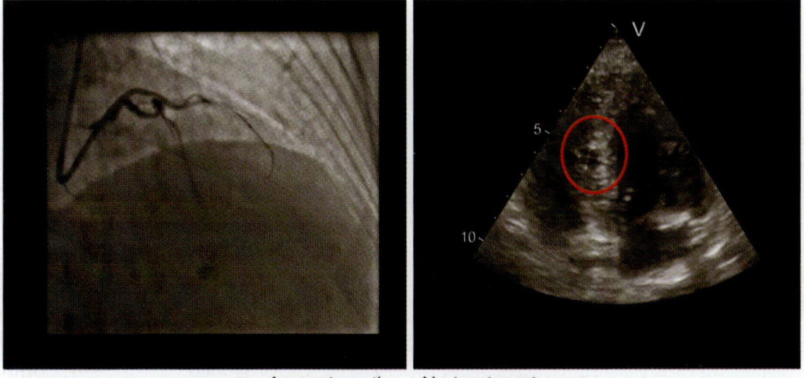

Fig. 7: Example of contained septal perforation with small interventricular septal hematoma.[20]

hardware manipulation. Most common perforations are seen in septals (29%) followed by epicardial collaterals (16%).[25] The most common cause being wire induced followed by microcatheter advancement in most cases **(Figs. 6 to 8)**.

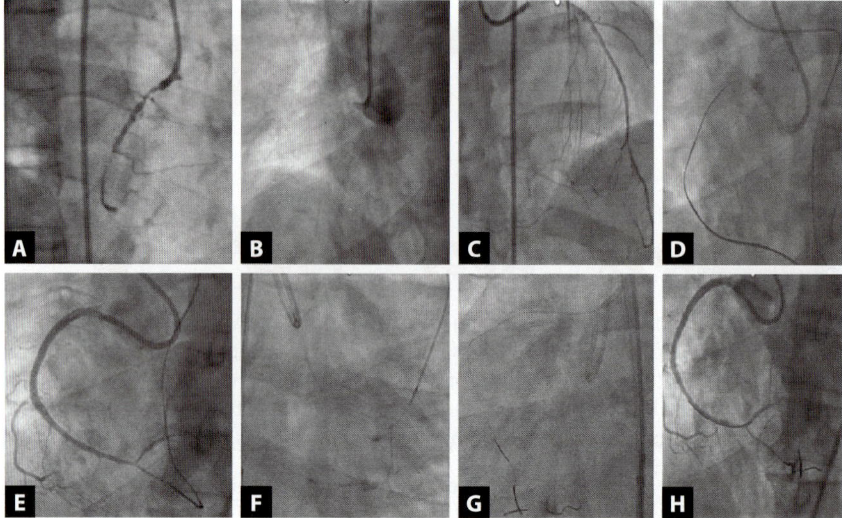

Figs. 8A to H: Case example of a septal perforation during retrograde RCA-PCI. (A) Mid RCA-CTO; (B) Failed antegrade attempt to RCA-PCI; (C) LAD angiogram showing CC2 septal collaterals to PDA for retrograde PCI; (D) Successful retrograde wiring of RCA-CTO with Corsair XS microcatheter and GAIA 2 wire; (E) Successful mid RCA stenting with 3 × 28 DES showing good result; (F) Dual antegrade and retrograde microcatheter injection showing septal perforation after withdrawal of Corsair XS microcatheter; (G) Coiling of the perforation done from both antegrade and retrograde sides with Axium 0.014 detachable coils; (H) Final angiogram showing complete sealing of the perforation with no ongoing leak. (LAD: left anterior descending; PDA: posterior descending artery; PCI: percutaneous coronary intervention; RCA: right coronary artery)

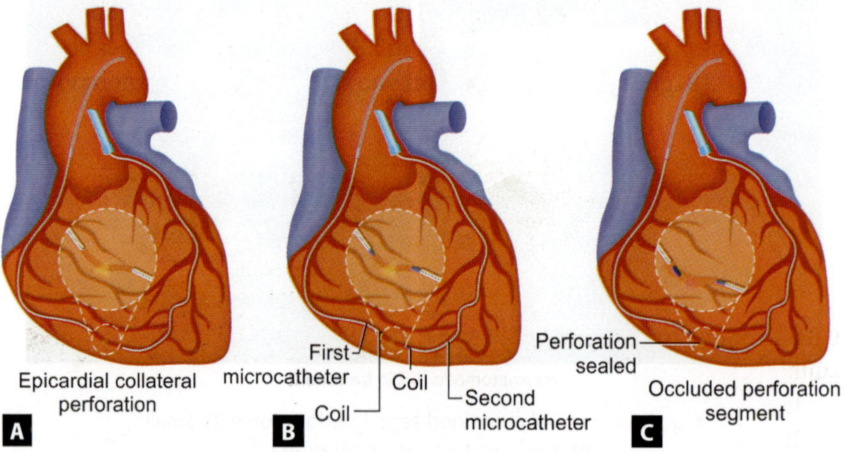

Figs. 9A to C: Management of epicardial collateral perforation.[20]

COILING IN EPICARDIAL COLLATERALS

A microcatheter is usually already in place for CTO PCI procedure. Hence, coils compatible to same microcatheter should be used **(Figs. 9A to C)**.

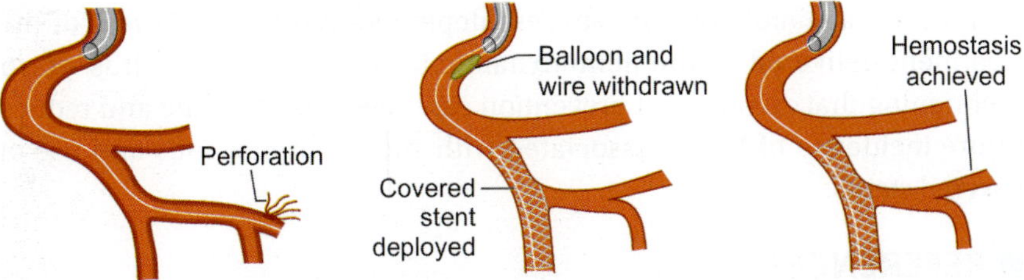

Fig. 10: Covered stent in epicardial perforation.[20]

Flowchart 2: Algorithm for management of distal vessel/coronary perforation.[11]

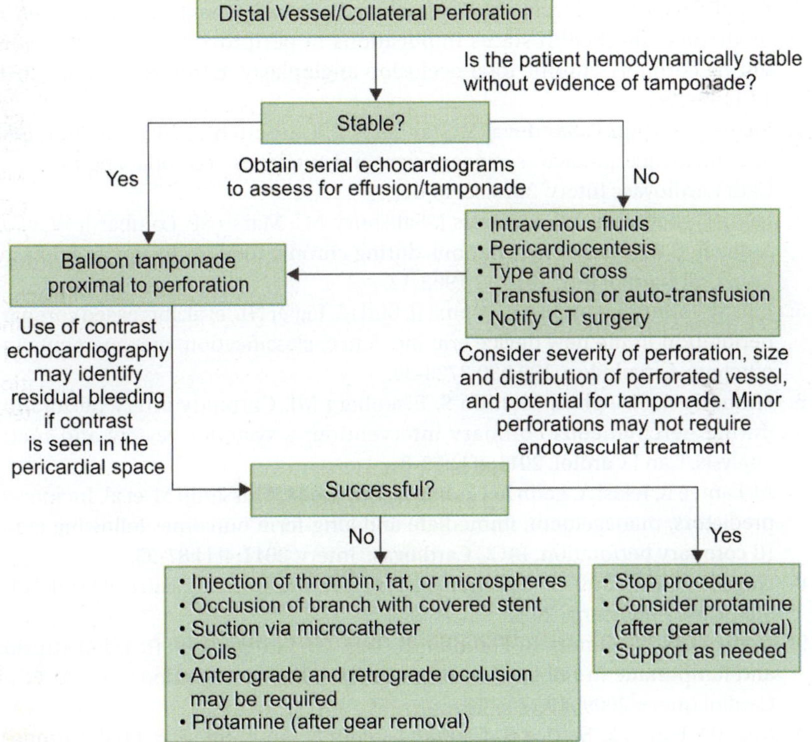

0.014' coils usually helical coils and microvention Terumo coils are more suitable (L 20 mm, r 2 mm).[26]

If coiling fails, fat embolization or thrombin injection can be tried.

If all measures fail, then covered stent across the origin of epicardial collateral can be placed **(Fig. 10 and Flowchart 2)**.

CONCLUSION

Though, CAP is an infrequent complication of PCI, but carries high mortality burden. Hence, it needs to be addressed immediately. A number of treatment options are available but the success depends on the promptness of the treatment delivered before hemodynamic instability develops. It is worth mentioning that an ounce of prevention can save a patient's life and reduce future incidence of MACE associated with such complications and use of covered stents.

REFERENCES

1. Bauer T, Boeder N, Nef HM, Möllmann H, Hochadel M, Marco J, et al. Fate of patients with coronary perforation complicating percutaneous coronary intervention (from the Euro Heart Survey Percutaneous Coronary Intervention Registry). Am J Cardiol. 2015;116:1363-7.
2. Riley RF, Sapontis J, Kirtane AJ, Karmpaliotis D, Kalra S, Jones PG, et al. Prevalence, predictors, and health status implications of periprocedural complications during coronary chronic total occlusion angioplasty. EuroIntervention. 2018; 14:1199-206.
3. Shaukat A, Tajti P, Sandoval Y, Stanberry L, Garberich R, Nicholas Burke M, et al. Incidence, predictors, management and outcomes of coronary perforations. Cath Cardiovasc Interv. 2019;93:48-56.
4. Hirai T, Nicholson WJ, Sapontis J, Salisbury AC, Marso SP, Lombardi W, et al. A detailed analysis of perforations during chronic total occlusion angioplasty. J Am Coll Cardiol Intv. 2019;12:1902-12.
5. Ellis SG, Ajluni S, Arnold AZ, Popma JJ, Bittl JA, Eigler NL, et al. Increased coronary perforation in the new device era: incidence, classification, management, and outcome. Circulation. 1994;90:2725-30.
6. Shimony A, Joseph L, Mottillo S, Eisenberg MJ. Coronary artery perforation during percutaneous coronary intervention: a systemic review and meta-analysis. Can J Cardiol. 2011;4(1):79-86.
7. Al-Lamee R, Ielasi A, Latib A, Godino C, Ferraro M, Mussardo M, et al. Incidence, predictors, management, immediate and long-term outcomes following grade III coronary perforation. JACC Cardiovasc Interv. 2011;4(1):87-95.
8. Nagalli S, Hajaouli S. Coronary artery perforation. Treasure Island (FL): Statpearls Publishing; 2020.
9. Homes DR, Nishimura R, Fountain R, Turi ZG. Iatrogenic pericardial effusion and tamponade in the percutaneous intracardiac intervention era. J Am Coll Cardiol Interv. 2009;2(8):705-17.
10. Kilic ID, Fabris E, Serdoz R, Caiazzo G, Foin N, Abou-Sherif S, et al. Coronary covered stents. EuroIntervention. 2016;12(10):1288-95.
11. Kearney K, Tremmel JA. Management and prevention of perforations Chronic Total Occlusion Percutaneous Coronary Intervention. In: Rinfret S (Ed). Percutaneous Coronary Intervention for Chronic Total Occlusion. Cham: Springer; 2015.
12. Barbero U, Cerrato E, Secco GG, Tedeschi D, Belliggiano D, Pavani M, et al. PK Papurus coronary stent system: the ultrathin struts polyurethane covered stent. Future Cardiol. 2020;16(5):405-11.
13. Kufner S, Schacher N, Ferenc M, Schlundt C, Hoppmann P, Abdel-Wahab M, et al. Outcomes after new generation single layer polytetrafluoroethylene covered stent implantation for the treatment of coronary artery perforation. Catheter Cardiovasc Interv. 2019;93(5):912-20.

14. Hernandez-Enriquez M, Lairez O, Campelo-Parada F, Lhermusier T, Bouisset F, Roncalli J, et al. Outcomes after use of covered stents to treat coronary artery perforations. Comparison of old and new generation covered stents. J Interv Cardiol. 2018;31(5):617-23.
15. Sandoval Y, Lobo AS, Brilakis EA. Covered stent implantation through a single 8-french guide catheter for the management of a distal coronary perforation. Catheter Cardiovasc Interv. 2017;90(4):584-8.
16. Wnna W, Januszek R, Kołodziejczak M, Kuźma Ł, Tajstra M, Figatowski T, et al. Procedural and 1-year outcomes following large vessel coronary artery perforation treated by covered stents implantation: Multicenter CRACK Registry. PLoS One. 2021;16(5):e0249698.
17. Bartus J, Januszek R, Hudziak D, Kołodziejczak M, Kuźma Ł, Tajstra M, et al. Clinical outcomes following large vessel coronary artery perforation treated with covered stent implantation: Comparison between polytetrafluoroethylene- and polyurethane-covered stents (CRACK-II REGISTRY). J Clin Med. 2021;10(22): 5441.
18. Pershad A, Yarkoni A, Biglari D. Management of distal coronary perforations. J Invasive Cardiol. 2008;20:187-91.
19. Tarar MN, Christakopoulos GE, Brilakis ES. Successful management of a distal vessel perforation through a single 8-French guide catheter: combining balloon inflation for bleeding control with coil embolization. Catheter Cardiovasc Interv. 2015;86:412-6.
20. Brilakis ES. Manual of Percutaneous Coronary Interventions: A Step-by-Step Approach. London: Academic Press; 2021.
21. Jacob D, Savage MP, Fischman DL. Novel Approaches to Coronary Perforations: Everything but the Kitchen Sink. JACC Case Rep. 2022;4(3):142-4.
22. Al-Omary MS, Collins NJ, Sung JG, Bhagwandeen R, Ho KH, Yam PW, et al. Absorbable suture embolization in distal coronary perforation. J Am Coll Cardiol Case Rep. 2022;4:133-6.
23. Alavi SH, Hassanzadeh M, Dehghani P, Namdar ZM, Aslani A. A novel technique for managing guidewire-induced distal coronary perforation using coronary balloon pieces. J Am Coll Cardiol Case Rep. 2022;4:137-41.
24. Abdalwahab A, McQuillan C, Farag M, Egred M. Novel economic treatment for coronary wire perforation: A case report. World J Cardiol. 2021;13(6):177-82.
25. Azzalini L, Polleti E, Ayoub M, Ojeda S, Zivelonghi C, La Manna A, et al. Coronary artery perforation during chronic total occlusion percutaneous coronary intervention: epidemiology, mechanisms, management and outcomes. EuroIntervention. 2019;15(9):804-11.
26. Shemisa K, Karatasakis A, Brilakis ES. Management of guidewire induced distal coronary perforation using autologous fat particles versus coil embolization. Catheter Cardiovasc Interv. 2017;89(2):253-8.

CHAPTER 39

Stent and Wire Loss during Percutaneous Intervention

Ajay J Swamy

INTRODUCTION

The widespread use of percutaneous coronary interventions (PCIs) in the last three decades along with the rise in the complexity of procedures performed, has led to higher number of complications associated. One of these complications, although it is quite rare, is stent loss. It can have malignant outcomes such as myocardial infarction, emergency coronary bypass surgery, and mortality, but if detected early and managed well, can result in a safe outcome. It can also increase morbidity by embolizing into any artery, e.g., into the intracranial circulation. In previous studies, the reported incidence of stent loss was between 0.21 and 8.4%.[1,2] Although stent loss was common before the 21st century due to manual handling of the stent, its incidence has decreased in the last two decades.[2]

MECHANISM OF STENT LOSS

Stent loss can occur by essentially three mechanisms. First, stent loss may occur at the balloon catheter when advancing it to a diseased coronary artery segment. Secondly, a stent may become trapped within the lesion while advancing through the coronary lesion and may detach from the balloon when pulling it back. The third, and by far the most common mechanism, is that the stent may be stuck at the distal part of the guide catheter when attempting to retrieve it into the catheter and so get stripped off the balloon.[3] A stent can be stripped off its delivery balloon at the lesion or, not uncommonly, a deformed stent strut can prevent reentry into the guide catheter. If not anticipated and detected, inadvertent pulling on the stent catheter at this stage will cause the mouth of the guide to displace the stent off the delivery balloon.

FACTORS CAUSING STENT LOSS

Factors affecting stent loss during percutaneous intervention may depend on the patient, the material used, and the operator. Among the factors related to the patient (or lesion), coronary calcification, acute angulation and tortuosity make it difficult for the stent to pass through the coronary artery lesion.[4-6] In the presence of tortuosity and acute angulation, the vessel can be straightened using double wires or stiff wires in order to facilitate the passage of the stent. In the presence of calcification, however, calcified protrusions do not allow the passage of the stent and may cause stent deformation. This makes both forward and backward movement of the catheter difficult and predisposes to stent loss.

The factors related to the materials used can be due to stent characteristics, guide catheter characteristics, or wire characteristics. Stent retrieval may also depend on the structural characteristics of the stents used. It was once reported that the incidence of stent loss and embolization with the older generation of paclitaxel-coated stents was greater than in sirolimus-eluting stents and bare metal stents.[7,8] Although it is not common nowadays, manual handling of the stent also increases the risk of stent loss.[2,9] Because poor guide catheter support can reduce the stent's reach to the coronary lesion, stent loss can occur at the balloon while retrieving the stent with the catheter. It may additionally make delivery of the stent to the lesion challenging due to the poor support it offers. If a poorly supportive wire is used in combination, it could additionally make stent delivery difficult.

An important stent loss factor related to the operator is direct stenting, especially without predilating calcified vessels. In addition, trying to cross the acute angle and tortuous segment with the stent without using a double wire or stiff wire in the tortuous vessels is another operator-induced factor that can cause stent loss. Implanting the first stent proximally is also among the operator-induced factor. Care must be taken when two stents need to be implanted. This is especially so when the proximal stent will need to be a long one. Because stent loss may occur in an attempt to implant a stent distal to the lesion after implanting a stent proximal to the lesion, the stent must ideally be implanted in the distal lesion first, especially in tortuous anatomy. Accidental inflation of the stent balloon can also cause stent loss. In most patients, stent loss occurs while retrieving the guide into the catheter, while the other important contributor was due to lesion calcification.

Stent losses may be more likely during percutaneous interventions performed on the left circumflex (LCx) artery. This may be particularly related to the lack of coaxial insertion of the catheter as well as the sharp or narrow angle between the circumflex artery and the left main coronary artery. Coaxial insertion of the catheter to prevent the proximal stent from being trapped in the tip of the guide catheter during stent retrieval will reduce the likelihood of stent loss. Retrospective analysis[10] of over 4,000 stent implantations has revealed higher embolization rate for manually crimped stents [1% versus 0.3% ($p < 0.01$)] than factory crimped devices. There appears to be no association with different target vessels in this situation.

PREVENTION OF STENT LOSS

Prevention of stent loss is an important concept to have during PCI: Coaxiality of the guide catheter is important, especially in LCx PCI and calcified and tortuous vessel PCI. Adequate predilation and calcium modification as par standard protocols must be undertaken prior to attempting stent delivery in calcified lesions. Cases considered suitable for direct stenting must be carefully reviewed to look for calcium and tortuosity and risk factors for calcium (age, hypertension, calcium in other vessels, and mitral annular calcification). Careful attention to the feel of the stent shaft while delivering or withdrawing the catheter cannot be overemphasized and force must always be tempered with judgment and tactile feedback during stent delivery.

APPROACH TO STENT LOSS

Approach to a situation of stent loss depends on location of stent loss, experience of operator in dealing with stent loss, whether the wire is still across the stent and support and hardware available. In the event of a loss of stent from the balloon, the first goal is to move the stent to a point where it will not cause vital or other serious hazards. Patient hemodynamic stability is the first question to be answered in this situation. Once stent loss has occurred, the options are to remove the stent percutaneously (snare, multiple wires, and forceps), deploy the stent (in a suitable areas in the coronary vasculature) if it is possible. If that is not possible, the next option is to crush it with another stent **(Flowchart 1)**. And if none of these is possible, or all of the mentioned options fail, surgery remains an option. Medical methods are rarely preferred for coronary arteries and are preferred only in cases of embolism in the peripheral arteries except cranial arteries.[11-13]

REMOVAL OF THE STENT

If the lost stent is on the guidewire, multiple methods can be used. The best is to use a coronary microsnare of 2 mm over the wire across. The use of a

Flowchart 1: Algorithm to approach stent loss without wire.

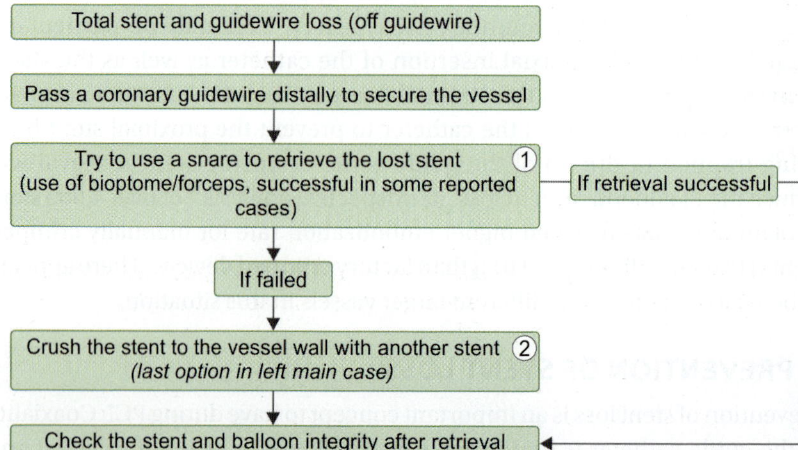

guide extension catheter (GEC) may facilitate this process. The GEC is taken over the wire and left in the guide catheter. The microsnare can then be taken over the wire and used to snare the stent preferably about 10 mm distal to proximal edge. The GEC can be threaded over the microsnare and the entire assembly can be removed as a single unit. Where microsnares are not available, a balloon inflated inside a GEC can be used to fashion a microsnare. Technical tips for snare use are summarized in **Box 1**. The snare can also be attempted if the guidewire is inadvertently pulled off the stripped stent, but this will need to be rewired at least proximally so that the snare can be delivered.

When the stent is secured by the snare, the whole assembly is pulled back and extracted through the sheath. Sometimes, even an undeployed stent cannot be retrieved through a 6 Fr sheath, which may therefore need to be upsized to 9 Fr. A potential caveat when snaring the distal part of the stent concerns the potential for the stent to be bent at the proximal part when it is withdrawn into the femoral sheath. At that level, the force is applied to the distal end and if the proximal end catches on the edge of the sheath, stent

BOX 1: Snare technique tips.

Snare technique in the event of total stent loss—using a loop snare or Goose Neck snare:

- Retrieval of the stent by a snare is an approach which will be favored in the case of inadvertent loss of guidewire position
- Commercially available snares, sometimes referred to as "Goose Neck" snares, have shaft diameters of 0.018 inch and are tipped by a closed wire loop of 2 mm diameter, angulated 90° to the shaft axis **(Fig. 1)**
- This right angle of the loop facilitates the grasping of the target object. Successful capture will depend on a correct alignment of the loop to the free end of the stent. There are two main commercially available snares: The Amplatz Goose Neck snare (ev3, Plymouth, Minnesota) and the En Snare (Merit Medical Systems Inc, South Jordan, Utah). The former consists of a single loop and the latter has three loops, which provides a larger area for capture. Alternatively a "bespoke" snare can be fashioned using an 0.014 inch angioplasty wire threaded through a guide-extension catheter looped back on itself and trapped inside the guide extension catheter (GEC) with an inflated balloon so that both proximal and distal ends exit the hub
- *The following technical tips are recommended:*
  - Careful localization under fluoroscopy of the free end of the stent
  - The plane of the snare must be held at right angles to the estimated plane of the stent. For that purpose, the full length of the stent should be seen under fluoroscopy. To confirm the perpendicular position of the snare loop in relation to the stent, it must appear as a straight line or a close loop. Only this position allows correct ensnarement of the free stent
  - Securing the free stent. The operator must be sure that the snare has correctly encircled the stent. The exchange catheter is then advanced and the embolized stent will bend when the snare is engaged. Withdrawing first the snare loop to capture the stent is not recommended because it can cause disengagement

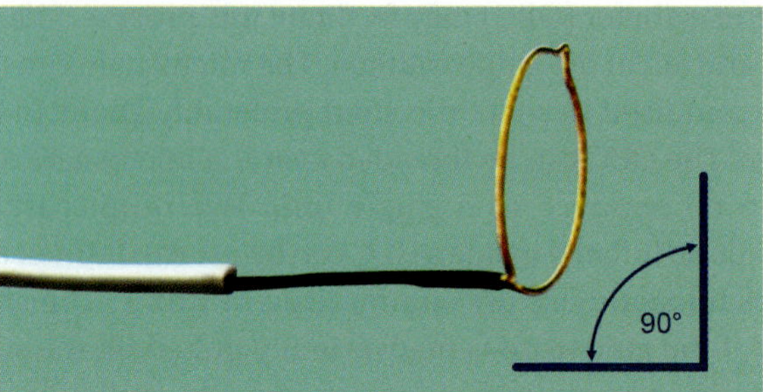

Fig. 1: Distal portion of a Goose Neck snare.

deformation may result. If this occurs, the stent may not be withdrawn even into a large sheath. This can be avoided by snaring the proximal end of the stent so that is crushed. The resulting reduced profile will then be the first element to contact the distal end of the sheath. Cutting or flaring the distal end of the sheath can also be performed in order to facilitate material extraction.

A second method described is to take multiple wires through the stent and entwine them by spinning them to entangle them and then withdraw the wire stent complex into the guide. However, this method is fraught with the danger of losing the wire or embolizing the stent if the stent is not securely entangled. This requires a second wire to be carefully advanced through a strut of the stent, the first wire being still in place. The two wires outside the guiding catheter are bound together by a torquing device which is rotated about 15–20 times, until the wires are observed twisting together near the proximal end of the stent. Then, the twisted wires are pulled back together and the guiding catheter advanced. The whole assembly consisting of the stent trapped between the twisted wires and the guiding catheter is pulled out gently. If the stent has been captured properly the guiding catheter should engage deeper into the ostium during initial removal. Once the stent is brought to the level of the common iliac artery, it can be removed by conventional methods after the wires are untwisted.

The major step in this technique is to ensure that the second wire is placed through the struts of the stent and not through the central lumen. Once the stent is brought to the level of the introducer it can be pulled out gently through the introducer sheath.

FORCEPS RETRIEVAL

Biopsy forceps have been attempted to be used, but may traumatize the coronary vasculature. Retrieval using this is feasible if the stent is present within the most proximal part of the left main or right coronary arteries but cannot be recommended as a first line option as it is aggressive. If employed then use of small French (pediatric sized) myocardial bioptomes is best (3 Fr 1.3 mm). Alternatively, a biliary forceps can be employed. Forceps can also be used from the homolateral or contralateral femoral sheath once the retained material is brought down to the level of the iliac artery.

STENT DEPLOYMENT TECHNIQUE

If the wire is still across the stent and the stent is in a safe location where it is feasible to deploy it, it may be decided to deploy it where it is. This is often a strategy employed in the distal LCx or mid-distal left anterior descending (LAD) and the distal right coronary artery (RCA). Sequential dilatation of progressively larger balloons will usually accomplish this easily and the stent can finally be postdilated with an appropriate-sized balloon.

STENT CRUSH TECHNIQUE

If it is not possible or feasible to remove the stent, then it can be crushed by a second stent at the same location. Often this is the final path after attempts at retrieving it have resulted in deformation of the stent and loss of the wire within the stent. It is important to predilate vessel well and crush the stent adequately prior to delivery of the second stent. The use of a GEC to deliver the second stent after crushing the first stent is a useful tip. This is also the principal bailout technique if the wire gets pulled out of the stent during manipulation after stent dislodgement.

GUIDEWIRE FRAGMENT EMBOLIZATION

Embolization of a guidewire fragment is even rarer and is due inadequate attention to handling technique. Equipment knots and wire fractures occur as a result of pushing the structural integrity of equipment beyond its limit. Knowledge of wire characteristics, improved proficiency, and training are the only means to prevent these occurrences. This is usually related to fragments breaking behind jailed stents. Care should be taken to avoid jailing reuse wires and wire entrapment in calcified vessels or between two stent layers in two-stent bifurcation techniques [e.g., double-kissing (DK) crush or culotte). Rarely, wire may get pulled out

CONCLUSION

- Always ensure adequate anticoagulation.
- In case of stent loss in the left main stem, favor use of retrieval technique instead of crushing.
- Align the guiding catheter during the retrieving of the lost stent.
- Check the stent and balloon integrity after retrieval.
- Difficulties increase from LAD-RCA-LCx.
- Identify lost stent/scaffold by fluoroscopy.
- Multiwire and recrossing technique is not recommended as low successful rate and potentially dangerous.

- Bioptome technique has been discouraged, delicate to implement but it has been used successfully.
- If diagnosed early and a step-by step approach followed, most cases have a successful outcome with percutaneous solutions.

REFERENCES

1. Iturbe JM, Abdel-Karim AR, Papayannis A, Mahmood A, Rangan BV, Banerjee S, et al. Frequency, treatment, and consequences of device loss and entrapment in contemporary percutaneous coronary interventions. J Invasive Cardiol. 2012;24:215-21.
2. Alomar ME, Michael TT, Patel VG, Altomare CG, Rangan BV, Cipher D, et al. Stent loss and retrieval during percutaneous coronary interventions: a systematic review and meta-analysis. J Invasive Cardiol. 2013;25:637-41.
3. Brilakis ES, Garratt KN. Device loss during percutaneous coronary intervention: incidence, complications, and retrieval methods. In: Ellis SG, Holmes DR Jr (Eds). Strategic Approaches in Coronary Intervention, 3rd edition. Philadelphia, USA: Lippincott Williams & Wilkins; 2005. pp. 434-3.
4. Brilakis ES, Best PJ, Elesber AA, Barsness GW, Lennon RJ, Holmes DR Jr, et al. Incidence, Retrieval Methods, and Outcomes of Stent Loss During Percutaneous Coronary Intervention: A Large Single-Center Experience. Catheter Cardiovasc Interv. 2005;66:333-40.
5. Colkesen AY, Baltali M, Acil T, Tekin G, Tekin A, Erol T, et al. Coronary and systemic stent embolization during percutaneous coronary interventions: a single center experience. Int Heart J. 2007;48:129-36.
6. Bolte J, Neumann U, Pfafferott C, Vogt A, Engel HJ, Mehmel HC, et al. Incidence, management, and outcome of stent loss during intracoronary stenting. Am J Cardiol. 2001;88:565-7.
7. Yurtdas M. Aladag N. Yaylali YT. Successful Transcatheter Retrieval of the Embolized Coronary Stent During Primary Percutaneous Coronary Intervention. J Med Cases. 2016;7:417-9.
8. Singh V, Khare R, Chandra S, Dwivedi SK, Saran RK. Dislodgement of a sirolimus-eluting stent in the right coronary artery and its successful deployment with a small-balloon technique. J Indian Coll Cardiol. 2014;4:44-6.
9. Schatz RA, Baim DS, Leon M, Ellis SG, Goldberg S, Hirshfeld JW, et al. Clinical experience with the Palmaz-Schatz coronary stent. Initial results of a multicenter study. Circulation. 1991;83:148-61.
10. Eggbrecht H, Haude M, Von Birgelen C, von Birgelen C, Oldenburg O, Baumgart D, et al. Nonsurgical retrieval of embolized coronary stents. Cath Cardiovasc Intervent. 2000;51:432-40.
11. Saleh L, Movahed MR. Successful Conservative Treatment of an Undeployed Embolized Intracoronary Stent With Dual Antiplatelet and Warfarin Therapy. Exp Clin Cardiol. 2010;15:e70-2.
12. Kammler J, Leisch F, Kerschner K, Kypta A, Steinwender C, Kratochwill H, et al. Long-term follow-up in patients with lost coronary stents during interventional procedures. Am J Cardiol. 2006;98:367-9.
13. Kocayigit I, Can Y, Yılmaz S, Kılıç H. Undeployed and uncrushed coronary stent in the proximal region of the normal left anterior descending artery revealed four years after intervention. Postepy Kardiol Interwencyjnej. 2015;11:256-57.

CHAPTER 40

Entrapped Balloon and Balloon Fracture during PCI Management

Placid Sebastian

"Good judgment comes from experience and experience comes from bad judgment"

INTRODUCTION

Percutaneous coronary intervention (PCI) of complex lesions is becoming more and more frequent and complications related to material manipulation such as loss of stent, entrapment of guidewires, entrapment of balloon or balloon shaft rupture have become more frequent (up to 0.8% of procedures). This kind of complication could turn into a life-threatening condition. Every interventional cardiologist should be acquainted with the different techniques of material retrieval and develop competence to tackle complications. Surgery should be a means of last resort.

UNDEFLATABLE BALLOON

Undeflatable balloon occurs due to:[1]

- Invisible kink in metal hypotube of stent balloon at metal and plastic junction, which produces unidirectional valve like action for dye flow
- Excessive twisting and force on the balloon in order to cross a distal lesion
- Entrapment in the distal portion of tight lesion
- Using undiluted contrast
- Reused balloon
- Poor balloon preparation with organized contrast remaining in the balloon from previous use
- The balloon inflated above the burst pressure may contribute trouble deflating it

Balloon malfunction can be suspected by inability to inflate balloon at nominal pressure.

Management Options (Flowchart 1)

- Deflate the balloon with 50 mL syringe connected directly at the inflation port of the balloon.
- Dilute the contrast material in the deflator with saline, resulting in decrease in fluid viscosity within the balloon. Inflate the balloon further

Flowchart 1: Management strategies for an undeflated balloon.

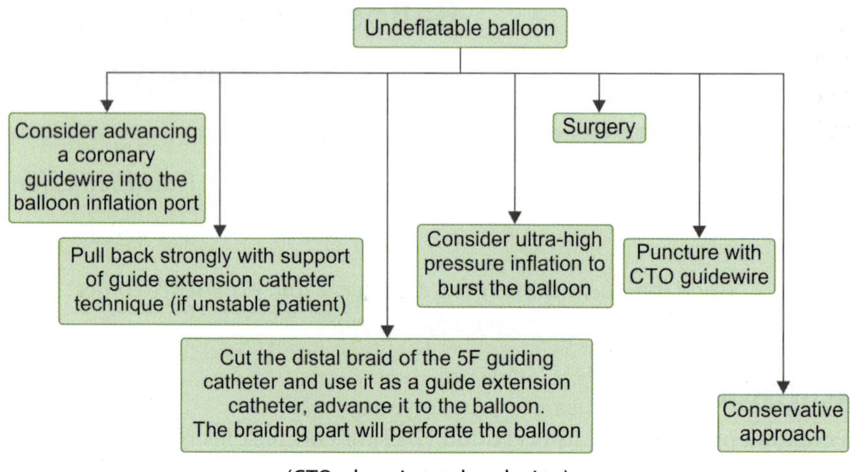

(CTO: chronic total occlusion)

with saline and try to deflate. This will help to dislodge any particles in the balloon which prevents deflation.

- Consider advancing a coronary guidewire in to the balloon through the inflation port to dislodge any obstruction in the balloon which prevents deflation.
- Pull back the balloon and the entire system as one piece keeping the negative pressure in the balloon.
- If the patient is unstable pull back strongly with support of guide extension catheter. Cut the hub of balloon, advance a GuideLiner on the balloon, take it distally till the stuck balloon and pull it back with counter traction on GuideLiner. If the undeflated balloon is located in the proximal part of the coronary, the guide catheter can be advanced gently over the balloon shaft till the balloon. While pulling the balloon apply a counter force with the guide catheter.
- Inflate the balloon to rupture it. Be prepared for damage control from dissection or coronary perforation.
- Puncture the balloon with a hard wire or back end of a coronary wire. Advance a microcatheter till the undeflated balloon, through the microcatheter advance the wire and puncture the balloon. Although there is a risk of coronary perforation, the wire-induced perforations would be quite small and unlikely to cause any significant complications.
- Cut the distal braid of 5F guide catheter and use it as a guide extension catheter. Advance the cut end of the 5F guide to the balloon. The braiding part will perforate the balloon.
- Surgical removal of the balloon is the final option.

If the undeflated balloon is managed to pull out of the coronary artery to aorta, the entire system can be pulled back to the radial or femoral sheath. If the balloon could not have pulled out through the sheath use a 21-gauge needle to puncture the balloon under fluoroscopic guidance or ultrasound guidance.

Prevention of the Complication

- Always use diluted contrast to fill the balloon. Use half contrast half saline in balloons and stent balloons for PCI.
- Wait full deflation before pulling the balloon, especially for longer balloon, usually seen with air bubbles coming back quickly in the inflator after deflation.
- Careful retrieval of the device should be performed, especially if you feel abnormal resistance when retrieving the device.
- Always pull the deflated balloon under fluoroscopy till it enters the guide catheter.
- When reused balloons are used, inflate and deflate outside before advancing in to coronary artery.

BALLOON SHAFT FRACTURE

Balloon shaft fracture is a rare complication but could be life-threatening. The predictors of device fracture within the coronary artery are well-known, especially calcified lesions and tortuous arteries.[2] That is why we should well prepare complex lesions before placing the stents, using predilatation as well as rotablator.

The fractured shaft of the balloon can be still in the guiding catheter or outside the guiding catheter.[3]

Management Options (Flowchart 2)

Balloon Trapping Technique

If a part of the fractured balloon shaft is in the guiding catheter, it could be removed by entrapping it between inflated balloons in the guiding catheter. If the fragment inside the guiding catheter is shorter, it is possible to advance a guiding catheter extension and trap it with a balloon. It is preferable to use at least 2 mm noncompliant (NC) balloon for 6F guide and 2.5 mm NC balloon for 7F guide. Once the proximal end of the balloon is well trapped it can be pulled out gently en masse **(Fig. 1)**.

When retrieving the shaft balloon fractured within the aorta outside the guiding catheter, the snare technique is feasible with a Trifold En snare system **(Fig. 2)**. When retrieving the shaft balloon fractured within the coronary artery, the snare technique is feasible with a Gooseneck snare **(Fig. 3)**. It is easier when the fragment is located proximally in the coronary artery.

Flowchart 2: Management strategies for balloon shaft fracture.

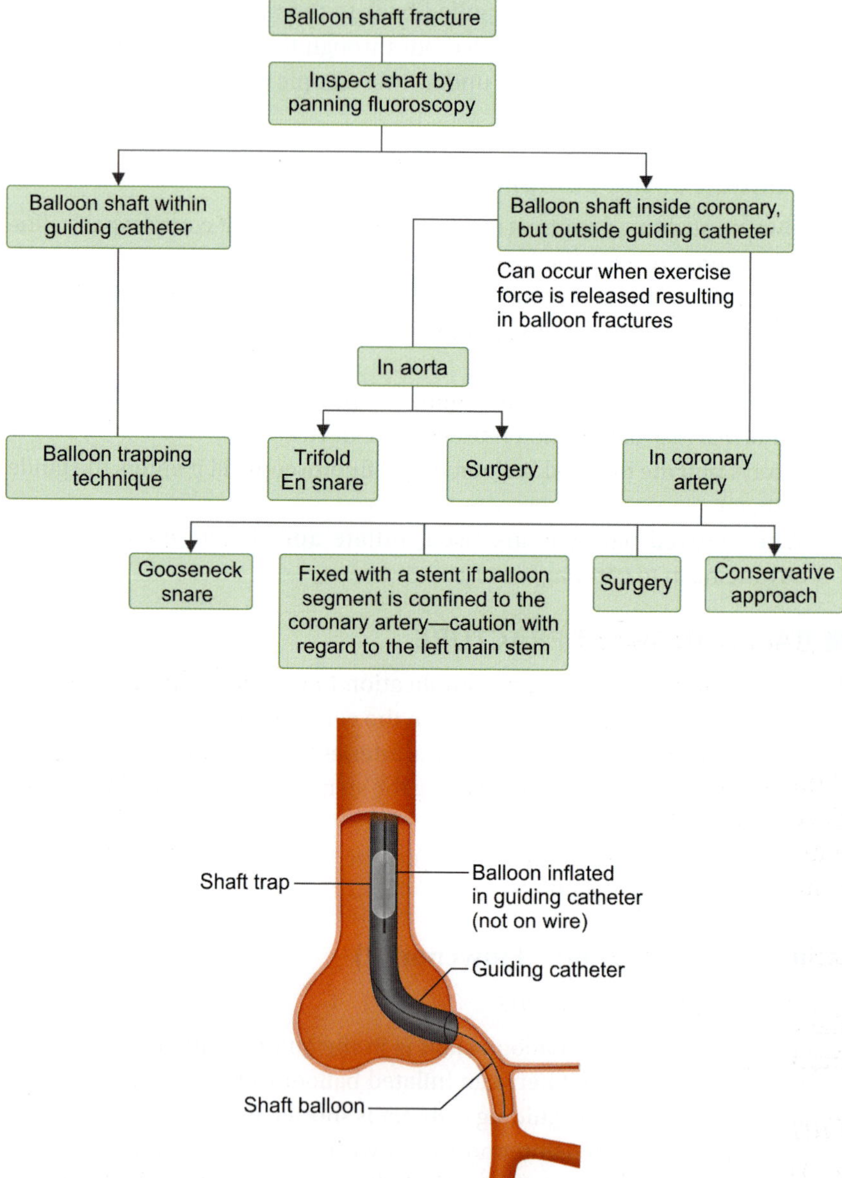

Fig. 1: Trapping the shaft of the fractured balloon with another balloon inside the guide catheter.

We can advance and twist guidewires to entwine the lost device and try to retrieve it. If all the earlier mentioned methods were unsuccessful, a stent can be deployed to crush the balloon against the coronary wall. Disadvantage of this technique is potential thrombus formation and it may be dangerous

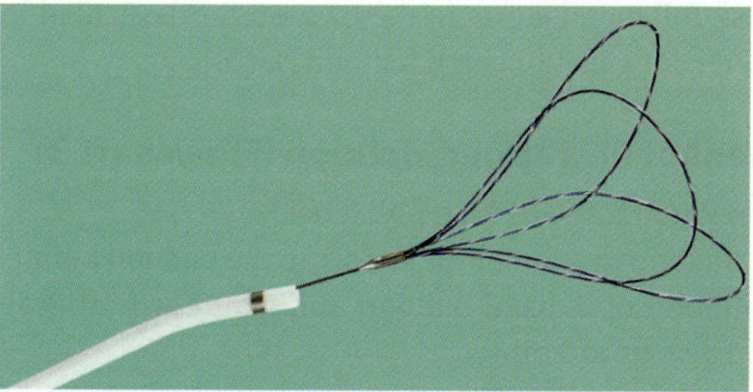

Fig. 2: *Trifold snare:* EN snare system.

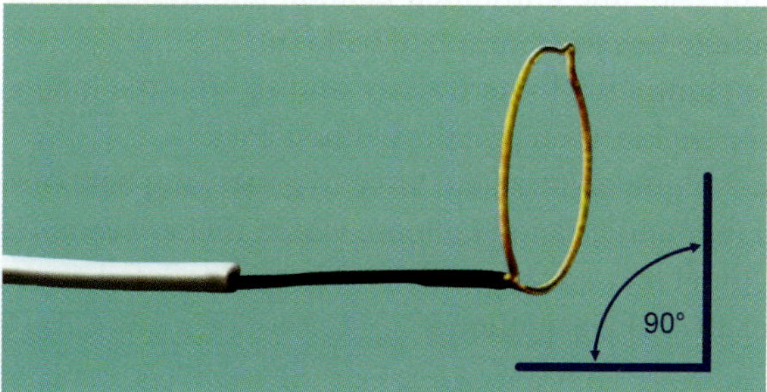

Fig. 3: Goose neck snare.

if the balloon lies in the left main coronary or across a major branch. In the case of suspected fracture of balloon or stent shaft within the catheter, it may be advisable to avoid performing a check angiogram to avoid the rare complication of potential embolization of distal fragments.

When retrieving the shaft balloon fractured within the aorta, the snare technique is feasible with a Trifold snare.

When retrieving the shaft balloon fractured within the coronary artery, the snare technique is feasible with a Gooseneck snare. It is easier when the fragment is located proximally in the coronary artery.

Crush Technique

- Deploy a stent and compress it against the coronary wall **(Fig. 4)**.
- Potential risk with this approach includes thrombosis and if the balloon remains in the left main or across a major branch.

ENTRAPPED DEFLATED CORONARY BALLOON

Entrapment of deflated coronary balloon occurs mainly due to tortuous, calcified, and angulated coronary lesions.[4] Disruption of balloon catheter is extremely rare complication and might occur due to the lesion and device complexity like full metal jacket in the tortuous and calcified lesion, bended guiding catheter, long drug-coated balloon (DCB), etc.

Management of Entrapped Balloon (Flowchart 3)

- Push the balloon forward then pull it back.
- Twist the balloon in an attempt to rewrap the balloon before pulling back.
- Partial inflation of a distal balloon and gentle withdrawal of the entire device can also be attempted.
- Insert a stiffer wire alongside the entrapped balloon before pulling the balloon back.
- Advance a second wire distally, then insert an over-the-wire (OTW) balloon alongside the entrapped balloon and inflate the new balloon at low pressure to free the entrapped balloon.
- Advance a commercial micro snare and tighten the loop as near to the balloon as possible, then pull the balloon back.
- A novel technique of adequate force to grasp long balloon was achieved by GuideLiner and inflated balloon, which theory seemed similar to the way the GuideLiner advanced smoothly with inflated anchoring balloon in "mother-in-child" technique.[5]

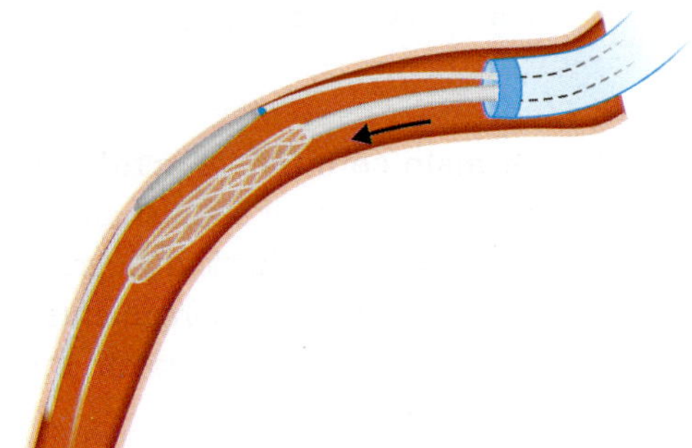

Fig. 4: Deploying a stent and compressing it against the coronary wall.

Flowchart 3: Management of entrapped deflated coronary balloon.

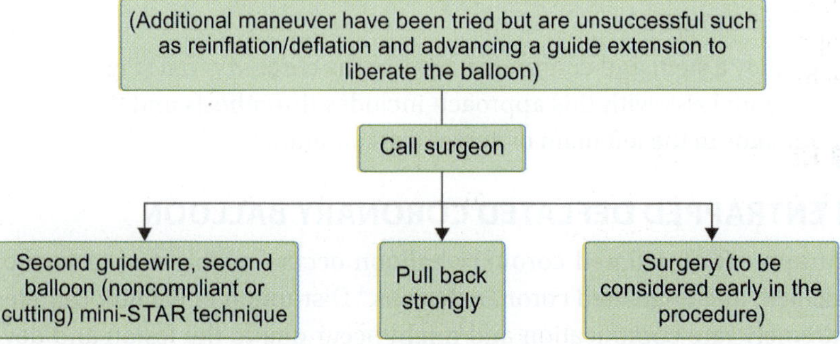

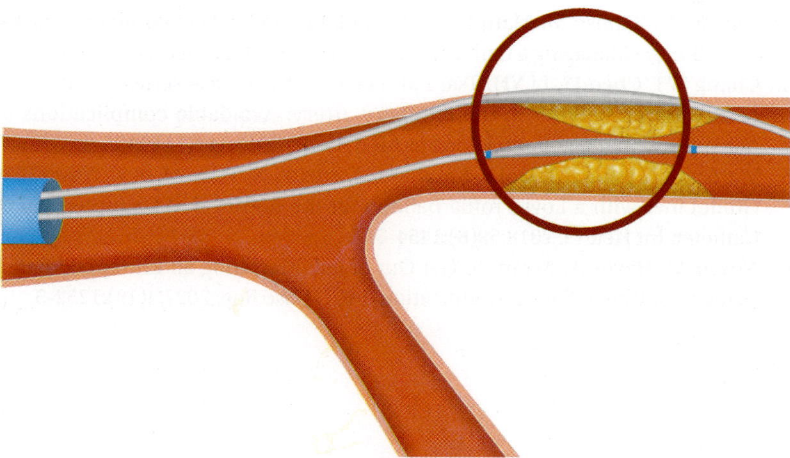

Fig. 5: *Mini-STAR technique:* A second guidewire is advanced in the subintimal space. A second small balloon is advanced on this guidewire and is inflated facing the entrapped balloon zone.

MINI-STAR AS BAIL-OUT STRATEGY FOR PCIs AND COMPLICATIONS

Coronary Balloon Fracture Complications

The mini-STAR technique is a promising bailout strategy for the management of entrapped balloons in the event of complications, achieving a high procedural success rate, and low occurrence of procedural adverse events.[6]

A second guidewire is advanced in the subintimal space upstream from the entrapped balloon zone and reenter downstream from it. A second small balloon is advanced on this guidewire and is inflated facing the entrapped balloon zone. This maneuver can unblock the entrapped balloon.

Mini-STAR technique may be successful for entrapped rotablator burr and entrapped balloon **(Fig. 5)**.

CONCLUSION

Though balloon related complications are relatively rare during PCI, it may happen during complex PCI in calcified lesions. Appropriate use of bail out techniques may result in better clinical outcomes.

REFERENCES

1. Takama T, Ito Y, Ishimori H, Tsukahara R, Muramatsu T. Failure of a balloon to deflate during post dilatation in a coronary artery. Cardiovasc Interv Ther. 2015;30(1):57-60.
2. Hammami R, Ellouze T, Bahloul A, Abid L. A ruptured balloon shaft during an angioplasty. Clin Case Rep. 2022;10(12):e6600.

3. Oliveira C, Raposo M, Marques da Costa J, Pinto FJ, Silva Marques J. When the Shaft Breaks: Managing a Cath Lab Nightmare. JACC Case Rep. 2025;30(3):103123.
4. Chang WT, Chen JY, Li YH, Tsai LM, Lee CH. A two-case series of entrapment of a ruptured balloon in the coronary artery: Avoidable complications and nonsurgical management. J Formos Med Assoc. 2015;114(11):1135-9.
5. Warisawa T, Mitarai T, Doi S, Kasahara M, Suzuki N, Takai M, et al. Novel Use of GuideLiner with a Low-Profile Balloon for the Retrieval of Disrupted Balloon Catheter. Int Heart J. 2018;59(6):1454-7.
6. Nosair M, Hayek A, Avram R. Get Out of Jail: Managing an Entrapped Balloon Using Subintimal Plaque Modification. JACC Case Rep. 2022;4(19):1252-5.

41

CHAPTER

Transseptal Puncture and Balloon Mitral Valvotomy: Technical Tips and Tricks

Harikrishnan S

INTRODUCTION

Transseptal puncture (TSP) is necessary to perform interventions on the left side of the heart. It is needed in balloon mitral valvotomy, MitraClip procedure, left-sided accessory pathway ablation, percutaneous mitral valve repair and replacement, left atrial appendage (LAA) closure, etc. Other procedures requiring TSP are patent foramen oval closure, LAA occlusion, paraprosthetic valve leak repair, atrial fibrillation (AF) ablation, and positioning of left ventricular assist device. It involves creating a small opening in the atrial septum to access the left-sided structure like the mitral valve or the LAA. With the rise of mitral and left atrial procedures, TSP has become a vital technique that ensures accurate and successful interventions.

It is important to have a good understanding of the anatomy of the interatrial septum (IAS) when performing a safe septal puncture. Mitral valve disease results in the enlargement of the left atrium (LA) leading to distortion of the normal anatomy, while distortion can also happen in right heart pathologies such as tricuspid and pulmonary valve disease and right ventricular (RV) cardiomyopathies.

The TSP technique was developed in the late 1950s to allow for left heart catheterization for evaluating valvular heart disease by Ross, Braunwald, and Morrow at the National Heart Institute.[1] Refinements made to the needle and catheter as well as the development of the combined catheter and dilator set by Mullins have made the procedure much safer.

ANATOMY OF THE ATRIAL SEPTUM

It is crucial to have a good understanding of the anatomy of the IAS before describing the TSP procedure. The IAS refers to the entire area between the two atria and should not be confused with the "true" IAS, which only accounts for about 20% of the total septal area and can be crossed without entering the extracardiac space.

The IAS is bounded posteriorly by a fold of pericardium between the left and right atria, superiorly by the superior vena cava (SVC), anterosuperior by the noncoronary sinus of Valsalva, anteriorly by the septal tricuspid annulus, anteroinferior by the coronary sinus os and inferiorly by the inferior vena cava (IVC) **(Fig. 1)**.

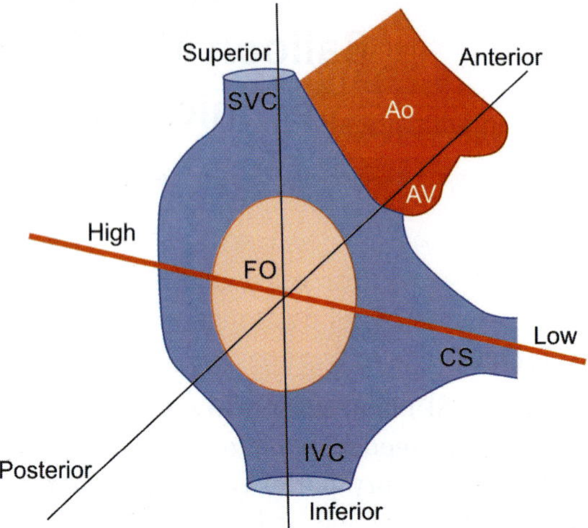

Fig. 1: Anatomy of IAS. (Ao: aorta; AV: atrioventricular; CS: coronary sinus; FO: fossa ovalis; IAS: interatrial septum; IVC: inferior vena cava; SVC: superior vena cava)
Source: Adapted from Vahanian A, Brochet E. Transseptal puncture for structural heart intervention: an old technique with new indications. Heart. 2017;103:1830-7.

The fossa ovalis is a part of the true IAS and is situated in the lower posterior part of the IAS. It is typically an oval or occasionally a circular-shaped depression that consists mainly of thin fibrous tissue. It is considered the safe place to create a puncture for entry into the LA. The limbus is the pronounced anterosuperior margin of the fossa ovalis within the right side of the IAS. It represents the inferior margin of the septum secundum during fetal life. The fossa ovalis appears as a depression in the IAS when viewed from the right atrium (RA). The fossa ovalis is surrounded by the muscular septum, the thick portions of the septum secundum and primum composed primarily of atrial muscle.

Fluoroscopic Landmarks

Fossa ovalis does not have a distinctive appearance in radiographs. However, using fluoroscopic landmarks can help avoid accidental puncture of adjacent structures. Placing a pigtail catheter in the noncoronary sinus of the aortic root can provide a valuable landmark. These landmarks may assist in locating the fossa ovalis and identifying areas where puncturing could be harmful.[1]

The fluoroscopy unit should be placed in a left anterior oblique (LAO) position between 30 and 45° to get a perpendicular view of the IAS. This view will allow you to see the transseptal access device in full profile when the tip is perpendicular to the septum. The right anterior oblique (RAO) view will help you divide the septum into anterior and posterior planes and determine the relative anterior and posterior location of the fossa ovalis.[1]

The septum lies between the two atria. The septum's posterior limit is usually the LA's lateral border. However, in patients with mitral stenosis (MS) and large left atria, the left atrial border may be lateral to the right atrial border, causing "the shadow out of shadow sign" in fluoroscopy. In instances where the septum is not present beyond the right atrial border, the latter serves as the posterior boundary of the septum.

Preprocedural Assessment

It is recommended that all patients undergoing TSP should undergo periprocedural transesophageal echocardiography (TEE) as it provides useful insights into the anatomy of the IAS. For instance, it can detect the presence of a patent foramen ovale or atrial septal defects (ASDs). Additionally, TEE can help identify the presence of left atrial thrombus or an atrial tumor, both of which are contraindications to TSP.

HOW TO PERFORM TRANSSEPTAL PUNCTURE

Catheters/Instruments

- Transseptal sheaths and dilator
- Brockenbrough needle
- Three-way stopcock with saline and contrast

Transseptal Sheaths and Dilator

Several types of sheaths are available for use with Brockenbrough needle. The sheath and dilator serve as a conduit for the transseptal puncture needle to pass across the IAS. These sheaths feature a dilator that extends beyond the tip of the sheath. The most common types of sheaths are the Mullins sheath and the Swartz SL transseptal sheath **(Figs. 2 and 3)** (manufactured by Abbott Vascular). They come in various sizes (8–12 F being the most commonly used) and different curvature versions to accommodate different atrial anatomical features. For Mullins sheath there is a 270° curve which straightens out with the help of the dilator **(Table 1)**. Several manufacturers now produce transseptal kits, although they have only slight variations in design.

Brockenbrough™ curved needles are made of stainless steel and are used for TSP **(Fig. 4)**. They come in both adult and pediatric sizes. The original needle used by Ross had a curved distal end to allow for controlled tip movements, and an arrow-shaped proximal handle to help define needle orientation. It is an 18-gauge hollow tube that tapers distally to 21-gauge **(Table 2)**.

The standard BRK needle, which is a type of Brockenbrough needle manufactured by Abbott Vascular, features a 19° angle between the distal curved portion and the needle shaft. In contrast, the BRK 1 (also manufactured by Abbott Vascular) features a 53° angle curvature.

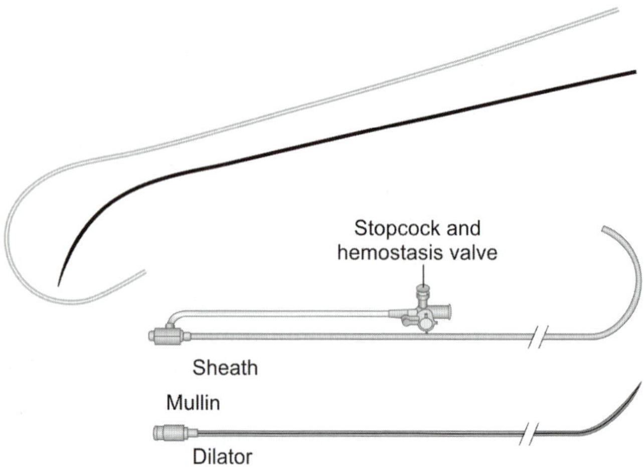

Fig. 2: Mullins sheath and dilator.
Courtesy: Newtech Medical Devices Pvt. Ltd.

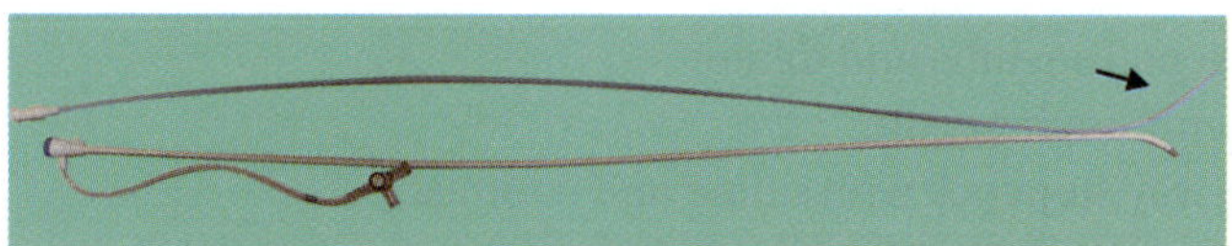

Fig. 3: Swartz SL sheath with dilator (arrow).

TABLE 1: Mullins sheath (specifications).

Type	*Size*	*Sheath length*	*Dilator length*	*Wire size*
Adult	8 Fr with hemostasis valve	59 cm	67 cm	.032″
Adult	8 Fr	59 cm	67 cm	0.032″
Pediatric	8 Fr	44 cm	52 cm	0.025″
Pediatric	6 Fr	44 cm	52 cm	0.024″

Source: https://asiapac.medtronic.com

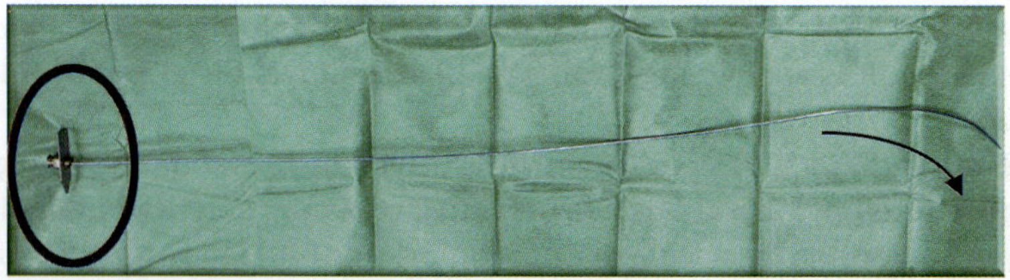

Fig. 4: Transseptal needle (Medtronic) (circle-arrow showing needle orientation).

TABLE 2: Brockenbrough needle (specifications).

Type	*Size*	*Length*
Adult	18 gauge shaft and 21 gauge tip	71 cm
Pediatric	19 gauge shaft and 22 gauge tip	56 cm

Source: https://asiapac.medtronic.com

STEPS IN TRANSSEPTAL PUNCTURE

Step 1: Access the Left Innominate Vein

A multipurpose angiographic (MPA) catheter is inserted into the left innominate vein.

Step 2: Exchange MPA Catheter

To facilitate the easy exchange of the multipurpose catheter with the Mullins dilator/sheath system, a 300 cm exchange length wire is inserted into the left innominate vein **(Fig. 5A)**.

Step 3: Mullins Sheath into the Left Innominate Vein

Mullins sheath or dilator is inserted into the innominate vein using the exchange length wire for guidance. Verify the length of the sheath/dilator and the puncture needle before selecting the sheath **(Fig. 5B)**.

Step 4: Formation of Needle Sheath Assembly

After removing the exchange length wire, insert the TSP needle into the Mullins sheath to form the needle sheath assembly. First, check the length of the needle in relation to the dilator. Ideally, the needle should protrude 3–5 mm from the tip of the dilator when fully inserted **(Fig. 5C)**.

After confirmation, the Brockenbrough needle, which is connected to a three-way stopcock, along with a syringe filled with saline, should be introduced through the Mullin's sheath/dilator. It is recommended to continuously flush saline while tracking the needle, as this will help make the passage smoother.

To ensure the smooth introduction of the needle system, it is important to allow it to rotate freely. This can be done by supporting the needle system with your left palm and slowly pushing the needle with your right hand, allowing for free rotation of the needle as it is introduced. By doing so, the needle system will be able to rotate 270° without any hindrance, enabling a smooth and efficient procedure.

The needle should be placed at least 1 cm (approximately two finger breadths) proximal to the Mullins sheath tip. To prevent the Brockenbrough needle from moving forward and protruding from the catheter tip, the operator should fix their right index finger between the catheter hub and

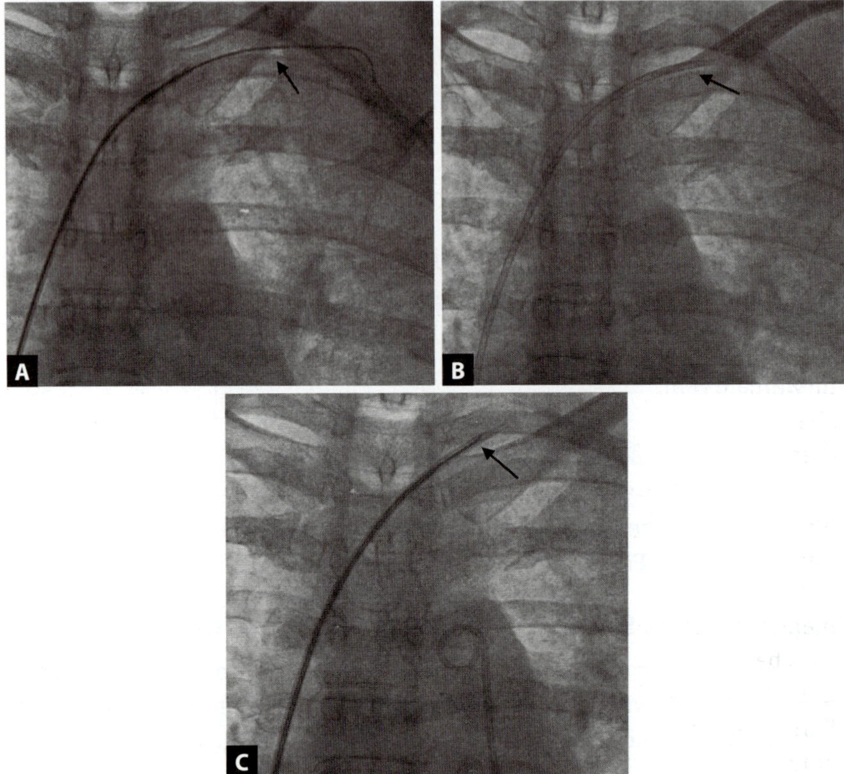

Figs. 5A to C: Placement of Mullins sheath. Arrow indicates (A) exchange length wire parked in left innominate vein (LIV) with the help of multipurpose angiographic catheter; (B) Mullins sheath placed in LIV; (C) Brockenbrough needle placed inside Mullins sheath.

the direction indicator of the needle. Typically, the direction indicator of the needle is positioned between 3 o'clock and 5 o'clock (12 o'clock being the ceiling). The thumb and middle finger should be used to maintain the direction and position of the needle.

After placing the needle, disconnect the saline and attach a three-way stopcock to diluted contrast (1:4 dilution). Inject a small amount of contrast through the needle to confirm flow.

Step 5: Mark the Landmark

Using fluoroscopy, identify the bottom end of the aortic root by placing the pigtail catheter in a nonaortic sinus.

Step 6: Pull Back

To approach the fossa ovalis region, the transseptal needle assembly is lowered. This is best done in the LAO view where the septum is vertical, but it can also be done in the anteroposterior (AP) view. It is important to keep the pointer of the septal puncture needle between the 3 o'clock and 5 o'clock position when viewed from the foot end of the patient. This will ensure that the distal curve of the sheath, dilator, and needle is perpendicular to the IAS. Never lose the position of the dial of the TSP needle while descending—it should be maintained at 3–5 o'clock positions.

When descending in LAO or AP view, it is important to observe the tip of the dilator during the drag for any abrupt medial movement. Slowly drag the entire sheath-dilator-needle assembly downward from the SVC to the RA, making sure that the components of the assembly are not rotating or changing their relative positions to each other. The detection of the "falling forward" motion in the LA may pose a challenge given the atrium's large size and pressure overload. The shallower fossa ovalis further complicates detection.

The first inward/medial movement seen will be the catheter falling into the RA from the SVC. There will then be a second more subtle movement as the catheter falls over the limbic ridge to the fossa ovalis. Occasionally, a third movement indicating the aortic root may be observed between the earlier mentioned two movements, but this is a rare occurrence.

The catheter can appear as if it is "falling forward" if accidentally placed in the coronary sinus os due to the needle being too anterior and inferior. Similarly, it may engage with the membranous septum if it is even more anterior. To determine the AP position of the catheter, check the RAO and lateral view. The pigtail should be lowered until its caudal limit is one-third of the distance from the tip to the diaphragm. If the LA is large, more descent may be necessary.

When the catheter enters the RA, there may be a few atrial ectopic beats visible on the monitor. If the transseptal needle is connected to a pressure transducer, as the assembly is pulled down from the SVC to the RA and into the fossa ovalis, the pressure tracing gradually dampens and then becomes a straight line to indicate the dilator is abutting the septum.

Landmarks for Septal Puncture

Fluoroscopic guidance is typically used to perform the TSP, with specific landmarks used to identify the location. The pigtail catheter indicates the location of the lowermost aortic sinus. When viewed from the AP angle, the tip of the transseptal dilator is seen to contact the inferior and medial fossa ovalis, ultimately reaching the aortic valve. The cardiac silhouette identifies the posterior and lateral borders of the atria.

To choose the best location for a TSP, two imaginary reference lines need to be identified first—the vertical "midline" and the horizontal M-line. The ideal spot for septal puncture is where the vertical "midline" and the horizontal M-line intersect, as shown in **Figures 6A and B**.

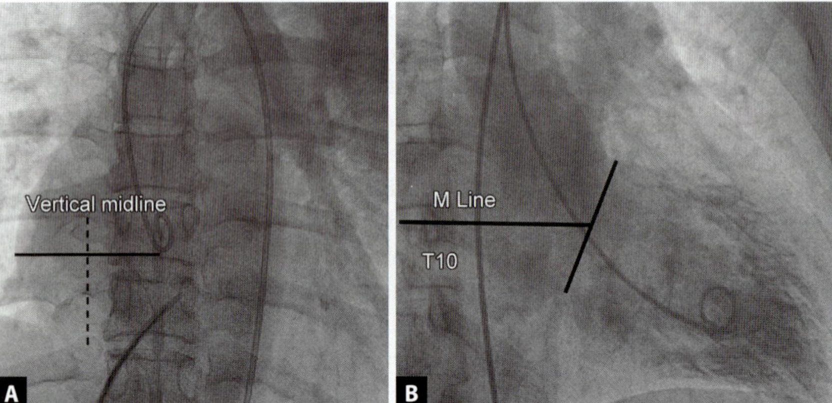

Figs. 6A and B: Fluoroscopic landmark for transseptal puncture (TSP). The M-line is obtained using the left ventriculogram with a stop frame right anterior oblique (RAO) view. This line is memorized in relation to the vertebral body T10, and transcribed in the (A) frontal and (B) RAO views. The vertical "midline" is defined in fluoroscopic frontal view. The target site for septal puncture is located at the intersecting point of the vertical "midline" and the horizontal M-line. (Note: Position of needle sheath assembly does not indicate puncture point here).

In their study, Inoue et al. explained a method for performing septal puncture during percutaneous mitral valvotomy (PMV) using angiography. Later, Hung et al. modified this technique and introduced the "Hung's fluoroscopic method", which relied on two landmarks:[2] The visible LA shadow in most cases of MS and the pigtail catheter placed in the noncoronary sinus of the aortic root.

In **Figures 6A and B**, a horizontal line is drawn from the tip of the pigtail catheter, which is placed in the noncoronary sinus of the aortic root, to the lateral border of the LA. The midpoint of this line is used to draw a vertical line, which is called the "vertical midline".

The next step is to locate the horizontal M-line. The horizontal M-line is the line that passes through the center of the mitral annulus. It is obtained from a diastolic stop frame of diagnostic left ventriculography, which is taken in a 30° RAO projection. The plane of the mitral annulus is determined by joining the fulcrum points of the mitral valve. From the midpoint of this line, a horizontal line is drawn toward the vertebral body, which serves as a reference point. The ideal puncture site is the point where the vertical midline intersects the M-line. Usually, this intersection point will be located half to one vertebral body below the horizontal line drawn from the aortic root in the vertical midline.

It is correct to make the puncture half to one vertebral space below the horizontal plane of the tip of the aortic root catheter if we have a mental picture of the vertical midline **(Figs. 6A and B)**.

How to Adjust Needle Orientation?

When performing a procedure in the atrium, the position of the needle will vary depending on the size of the atrium. If the LA is <4 cm, the needle will naturally orient itself between the 4 and 5 o'clock positions. For a moderately enlarged atrium (40–50 mm), the needle will be found between 5 and 6 o'clock positions. If the LA is grossly enlarged, the needle will be located at the 6 o'clock position.

During the procedure, try to keep the needle oriented correctly as it descends. First, the needle position is checked and altered in RAO 40° and lateral (90°) views. If altered, it is rechecked in RAO 40°, AP, and left lateral views.

When dealing with a large LA, it may be necessary to adjust and orient the needle. This is typically done in the lateral view and then confirmed in other views. While some practitioners puncture in AP, RAO, or LAO views, we typically do so in the lateral view. The approach used may vary depending on the practitioner's experience and preferred practice.

If we are unable to position the needle correctly, we remove it from the catheter and make a fresh attempt. To do this, we pass a guidewire through the Mullins sheath and place it again in the innominate vein. Shaw et al.[3] have described a technique called the "staircase movement" technique, which involves using the same needle assembly to be put back into the SVC.

If you encounter any resistance while inserting the catheter, especially if it hits the right atrial appendage or free wall, it is advisable to remove the needle and reinsert the Mullins sheath in the innominate vein.

Staining of the Septum

After correctly positioning the needle, attempt to flush contrast and stain the septum. If the needle fits tightly against the septum, flushing may not be possible, but the septum will still be stained. A vertical stain on the septum indicates that we are parallel to it and dissecting it. A more horizontal stain indicates a relatively favorable orientation of the needle with the septum. If the puncture site is too low and the needle is facing the thick muscular septum, it will produce a more horizontal septal stain.

If you encounter difficulty in puncturing the LA after creating a horizontal septal stain, it is recommended to reposition the needle more caudally and try again. However, if the stain is visible on the aortic sinus or aortic wall **(Fig. 7)**, the procedure should be discontinued. In such cases, the patient must be monitored for signs of cardiac tamponade, aortic dissection, or aortic regurgitation.

Step 7: Confirmation in Right Anterior Oblique View (Fig. 8)

In this view, the septum should be fully en-face to the operator. The Mullins sheath and puncture should be anterior to the descending aortic catheter.

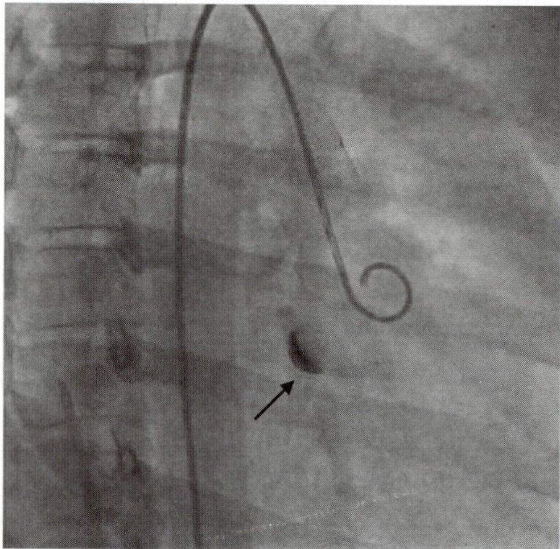

Fig. 7: Staining in transseptal puncture (TSP). Arrow indicates staining aortic sinus while attending TSP.

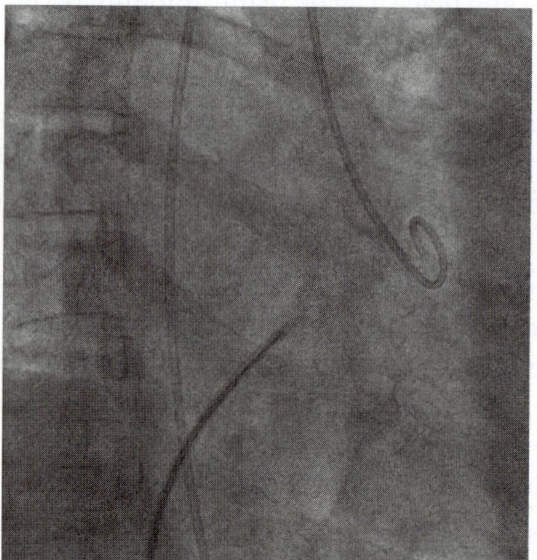

Fig. 8: Transseptal puncture (TSP) in right anterior oblique (RAO) shows needle position in RAO view.

Step 8: Confirmation in Lateral View (Fig. 9)

The position of the needle has been confirmed in the lateral view. Typically, in the lateral projection, the fossa is located halfway along an imaginary line that runs from the tip of the pigtail catheter to the posterior border of the heart. The needle should be placed toward the postero-supero-medial direction.

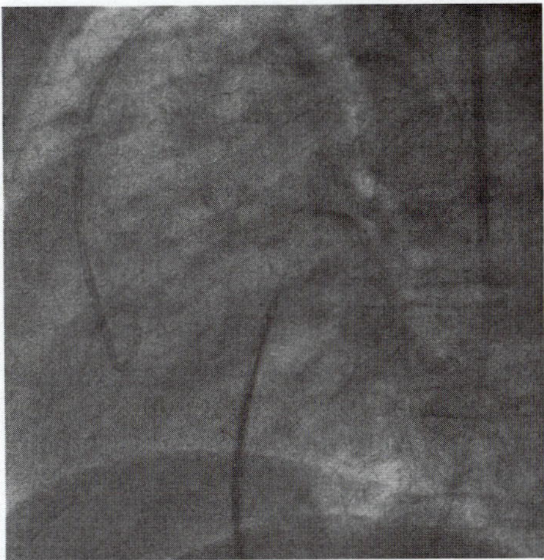

Fig. 9: Needle position in lateral view. Contrast injection depicting left atrium (LA) posterior wall.

Step 9: Aortic Root Angiogram

Although not always mandatory, an aortic root angiogram can help identify the position of aortic sinuses and confirm that the needle is safely away from the aortic root.

Step 10: Septal Puncture

To puncture, you need to abruptly jerk the needle forward inside the Mullins sheath while maintaining the direction of the needle with the right hand. The left hand should be used to hold and fix the sheath. This process should be observed on fluoroscopy, and you will see and feel a "give way" sensation as the needle suddenly jumps across the septum. Needle puncture with connected pressure transducer shows sudden pressure elevation before LA wave.

After confirming the entry of the LA through the fossa ovalis, advance the sheath/dilator assembly into the LA. To ensure better accuracy, it is recommended to keep the needle in a fixed position and advance the sheath alone. While advancing, direct the system posteriorly (3 o'clock position) in the lateral view and give puffs of contrast to see the posterior limit of the left atrial wall.

How can We Confirm the Left Atrium Entry Through Proper Septal Puncture?

We can ensure accurate placement of the catheter in the LA by observing the following cues:

- Left atrial pressure will be displayed.
- Oxygen saturation will show bright blood with a level of over 95%.

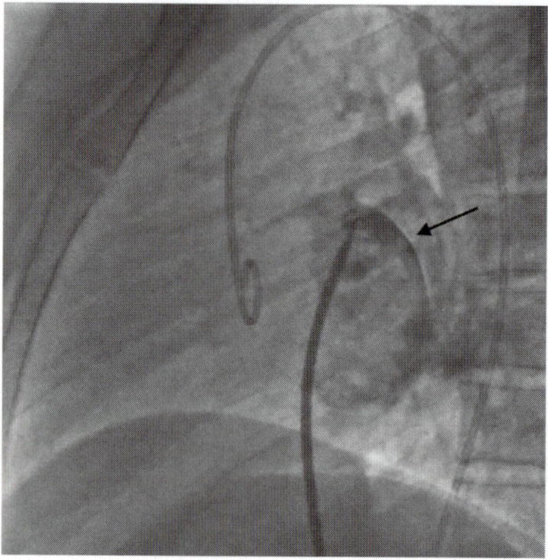

Fig. 10: Confirm left atrium (LA) entry. Lateral view showing transseptal puncture (TSP) needle in LA. Arrow indicates contrast injection delineating posterior extend of LA.

- The catheter tip will be visible in the postero-superior position on a lateral view.
- Contrast injection will help delineate the LA and posterior wall on a lateral view **(Fig. 10)**.
- In the LAO view, the left main bronchus represents the roof of the LA.

SEPTAL PUNCTURE BY TRANSESOPHAGEAL ECHOCARDIOGRAPHY GUIDANCE

Transesophageal echocardiography imaging of the septum requires two views: (1) Bicaval (90°) to delineate superior-inferior extent and (2) short-axis (45°) to delineate AP orientation. The use of X-plane imaging in 3D echo facilitates simultaneous visualization of both views **(Fig. 11A)**.

The needle and sheath should be pulled back caudally until they are visible in the lower part of the SVC. During this process, the tenting should be closely monitored with the help of echocardiography (bicaval view) **(Fig. 11B)**. The operator should avoid moving the image from the membranous portion of the septum while the needle is positioned in the fossa.

Under TEE monitoring (bicaval view), the needle and sheath are pulled back until they fall into the fossa and tenting is obtained. At this point, TEE moves to the short axis (SAX) at the base view and position of the tenting is checked; it should be posterior in most patients undergoing mitral interventions.

Once the transseptal system is in place in the fossa, the operator needs to move in two directions simultaneously to prevent the needle from pivoting when changing positions. An isolated clockwise rotation will result in rotation of the sheath without a change in the contact point. To move posterior, rotate

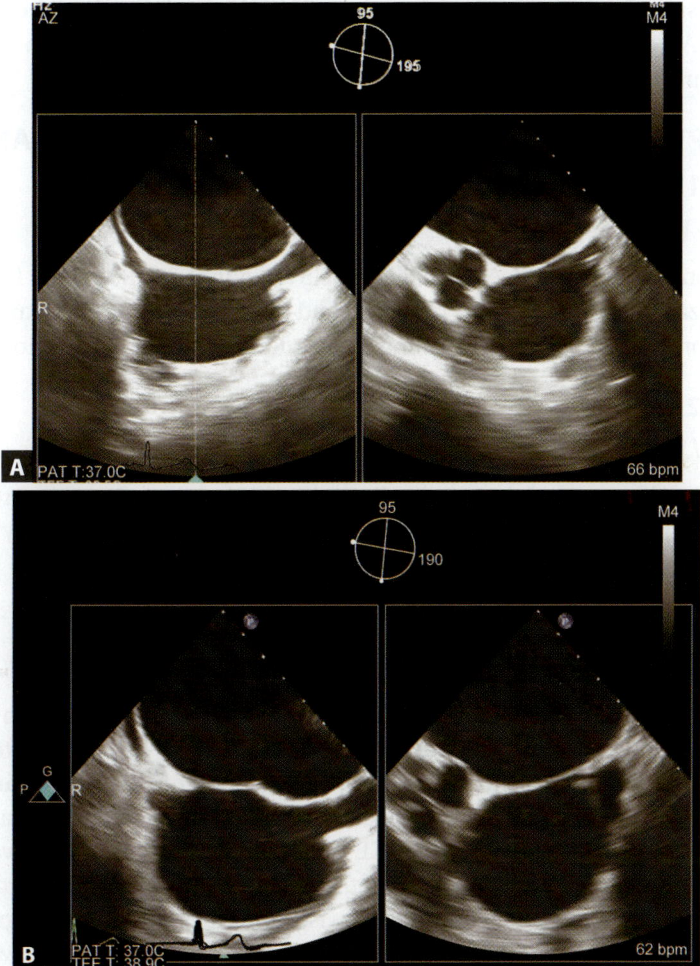

Figs. 11A and B: Transesophageal echocardiography (TEE) image showing interatrial septum (IAS). (A) Indicates bicaval view and shows simultaneous short axis view; (B) Tenting of the septum by transseptal puncture (TSP) needle visible.

the catheter and pull it gently. Clockwise rotation and pullback movement should be applied if too anterior, while counterclockwise rotation and pullback movement should be applied if too posterior.

In the case of MitraClip (Abbott Vascular) procedures, TEE should now switch to the four-chamber view and measure the height of the puncture (the distance between the tenting and the mitral annulus). In patients with degenerative mitral regurgitation, the ideal height is >4 cm, whereas in functional mitral regurgitation, a 3 cm distance is acceptable.[4]

The ideal location for punctures during medical procedures depends on the devices being used and the patient's individual characteristics. For instance, when performing a MitraClip procedure, posterior punctures in the superior-posterior segments are typically used. On the other hand, for a LAA closure procedure TSP is usually performed through an inferior puncture, typically inferior posterior.

SEPTAL PUNCTURE BY INTRACARDIAC ECHO GUIDANCE

Step 1

Home View

Positioning the transducer parallel to the SVC in the mid-RA allows for clear visualization of the RA, right ventricle, and tricuspid valve. This is known as the "home view". Before performing a TSP, rule out pericardial effusion.

Step 2

Septal View

From the "home view", the intracardiac echo (ICE) probe is flexed and rotated 90°, facing the IAS. This displays the IAS, right and left atria, coronary sinus, and pulmonary veins/LAA (depending on the transducer's location).

Step 3

Tenting of Septum

When the sheath and dilator are positioned in the middle of the fossa ovalis (a thin membrane between the atrial chambers of the heart), the "tenting effect" occurs due to the fibroblastic consistency of this membrane. To assess the superior and inferior position of the transseptal needle against the septum, slightly advance the ICE probe along the septum. To evaluate the anterior and posterior position of the needle against the septum, rotate it clockwise (posterior) and counterclockwise (anterior). An anterior alignment of the transseptal needle is required for visualizing the aortic valve, while a posterior alignment is needed for visualizing the far-field pulmonary vein.

Step 4

Transseptal Entry

The needle is advanced into the LA after optimal positioning of the dilator and sheath against the fossa ovalis with tenting sign visualization. Confirmation of successful puncture is done by injecting serum or dye and observing microbubbles in the LA.

Step 5

Catheter in Left Atrium

Intracardiac echo provides essential information on the pulmonary veins such as their number, position, and size, as well as the LAA's size, shape, and spatial relationship with the pulmonary veins.

Step 6

Left Ventricular Long Axis View

Before removing the ICE catheter, it should be bent forward and rotated to pass from the RA through the tricuspid valve inside the right ventricle. This will allow visualization of the left ventricle and exclusion of a pericardial effusion at the end of the ablation procedure.

TRANSSEPTAL CATHETERIZATION WITHOUT NEEDLE PUNCTURE

Krishnamoorthy et al.[5] have reported that in up to 90% of cases, entry of a catheter into the LA can be achieved by probing the fossa ovalis without the need for needle puncture. This is particularly beneficial in conditions such as MS where raised atrial pressure causes the atrial septum to stretch, making it easier to enter the LA by probing. This method reduces the time spent using fluoroscopy and decreases complications related to needle puncture.

TRANSJUGULAR ACCESS FOR SEPTAL PUNCTURE

Transjugular access is a method that is used in rare cases where there are abnormalities in the veins, either due to congenital or acquired conditions, which prevent transfemoral access. To locate the appropriate site for transjugular access, we can use Inoue's angiographic method for transfemoral access. This involves performing transjugular TSP using an LA angiogram. For delineating the LA borders, pulmonary artery (PA) angiography in levophase (RAO 45°) is useful. The appropriate site for puncture is 2 cm (vertebral body height) below the roof of the LA and midway between an imaginary vertical line passing through the pigtail catheter tip located at the aortic valve and the anterior border of the thoracic spine.

Procedure Steps

After Internal jugular vein access, a J-shaped 0.032-inch guidewire is advanced into the IVC. The Mullins sheath and dilator are inserted over the guidewire, and the TSP needle is placed after removing the guidewire. Pediatric TSP needles can be used for convenience. Increase the curvature of the TSP needle here to avoid septal dissection by oblique passage over the septum. The external needle index is placed at 7 and 8 o'clock positions while doing septal puncture, which can turn into a 9 o'clock position after TSP to advance the catheter into the LA cavity. Secure the transseptal access with 0.025 coiled wire placed in LA.

TRANSSEPTAL PUNCTURE IN DEXTROCARDIA

Performing TSP on patients with dextrocardia can be technically challenging due to their distorted anatomy. However, newer cath lab equipment with image inversion capability has made TSP possible without difficulty. As described by Nallet et al.[6] and others,[7] radiographic images can be acquired in inverted positions and used as fluoroscopic guidance for TSP. By using the inverted fluoroscopic settings, the anatomy of the patient can be simulated to appear normal, creating pseudo views that aid in the procedure.

During TSP in situs inversus dextrocardia, the left femoral access is usually preferred to reduce the puncture needle angulation at the point where the iliac veins meet the left-sided IVC. When the C-arm is in the AP position, we get a pseudo-AP view with the image inverted left-right, and when it is in the LAO 30° view, we get a pseudo-RAO 30° view. The needle assembly is descended in a mirror image position with the external needle indicator pointed toward the 7–9 o'clock position. The anterior extent of the septum can be marked by positioning a pigtail catheter in the aortic sinus. Levophase PA angiography is used to delineate LA borders.

TRANSSEPTAL PUNCTURE VIA LEFT FEMORAL VEIN

When performing TSP, two technical challenges are associated with using left femoral venous access. The first challenge is at the IVC and common iliac vein (CIV) junction. This area has an acute angulation, making it difficult to pass the needle sheath assembly through. The second challenge occurs at the IAS, where the broken Brockenbrough needle, with its 15° angulation, remains parallel to the septum.

The telescoping method makes it possible to perform needle passage through the IVC-CIV junction. This involves advancing the needle while simultaneously withdrawing the Mullins dilator, which helps to navigate the IVC-CIV angulation. The patient's head can be slightly tilted toward the right side to improve the relative TSP needle position with IAS. Increasing the angle of the TSP needle to approximately 40° also makes the puncture relatively easy.[8]

COMPLICATIONS

Complications are rare, in the range of 1%.[9] Complications such as pericardial effusion, tamponade, persistent ASD, and accidental aortic puncture can occur after TSP.

Pericardial Tamponade

Pericardial effusion and tamponade are dreaded complications of TSP. These can occur due to needle entry to the pericardial cavity through the superior or posterior walls of RA or anterior/aortic puncture.

How to Manage?

Early recognition is crucial. If only a needle puncture has occurred, we can observe the rate of fluid accumulation and hemodynamic instability after keeping the wire in place. If TSP has been done with prior anticoagulation, consider reversing it. If the sheath has already been advanced, keep it in place until surgical repair.

The TEE/ICE guidance during TSP can help reduce the risk of unintentional pericardial puncture.

Aortic Puncture

Inadvertent aortic puncture is a rare complication that occurs in transcatheter septal procedures (TSP). It has been reported by some studies to occur in only 0.05% of TSP cases. This complication can happen due to difficult septal anatomy, leading to an anterior puncture, or due to an inexperienced operator. There are very few case reports in the literature regarding aortic puncture, but one such report involved a patient who developed tamponade after the TSP needle was removed from the aorta. One practical strategy is to place a guidewire into across the aorta while watching for the development of tamponade and advance a sheath to seal the defect until the patient is taken up for surgery. There have been reports of the development of a persistent aorto-atrial tunnel, and closure of the defect with an Amplatzer device has also been reported in the literature.

How can We Prevent?

At our institution, we occasionally use contrast injection after the needle has been advanced to recognize aortic puncture and avoid inadvertent sheath insertion.

"Stitch" Phenomenon

Stitch is a rare complication that can occur during IAS puncture. It happens when TSP mistakenly enters the pericardial cavity from RA and reenters LA via the LA roof. This complication usually arises when the LA anatomy is distorted, especially in cases of rheumatic heart disease (RHD), where the LA is significantly dilated in comparison to RA. There are two types of pericardial track or stitch path that can occur:

1. RA-pericardial cavity-LA roof
2. IAS-pericardial cavity-LA roof

How to Manage if Stitch Occur?

Early recognition is crucial to prevent further deterioration. Tamponade may occur when we remove the catheter or dilator from the stitched path;

therefore, we attempt to keep it in place and relocate it for surgical repair. If tamponade develops, access the pericardial cavity immediately and perform pericardiocentesis.

Persistent Atrial Septal Defect

During TSP procedure, the use of large-bore sheaths through the septum can lead to the development of persistent or iatrogenic ASDs. According to reports, these defects are detected in most patients (87%) immediately after the procedure. However, the percentage of patients with these defects significantly decreases (to 7%) over the following 12 months.[10] Long-term follow-up studies did not show an increased rate of stroke or systemic embolization or significant shunt across these ASDs.[10]

Conduction Disturbances

Conduction disturbance during TSP is a rare occurrence. The atrioventricular node (AVN) is a subendocardial structure, which means that mechanical collisions with TSP catheters can cause transient conduction blocks. Using a stiff steerable guide catheter while manipulating in transseptal catheterization, especially in anteroinferior punctures, can lead to injury to the AVN and conduction block. There has been a reported case of such conduction disturbance with steerable catheters.[11] Fixed curve catheters are less likely to cause such conduction disturbances.

NEWER TECHNOLOGIES

Transseptal Puncture Crosser

The TSP Crosser™ (Transseptal Solutions Ltd) is an integrated system that combines a sheath, dilator, and a flexible puncturing needle **(Fig. 12)**. It aids in controlled LA access and improving performance during transseptal catheterization procedures. A radiopaque loop wire is positioned at the distal end of the steerable sheath to aid in the localization of the fossa ovalis. The sheath is steerable up to 180° bidirectionally after crossing the fossa ovalis.[12]

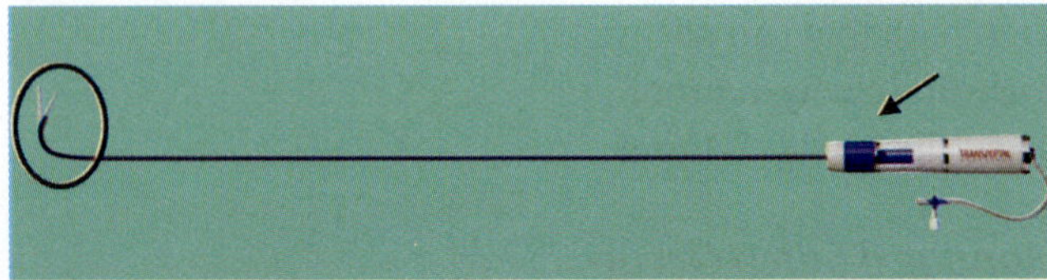

Fig. 12: Transseptal puncture crosser. Arrow indicates bidirectional steering handle and circle shows flexible needle with loop wire.
Courtesy: Transseptal Solutions Ltd.

NRG RF Transseptal Kit

The NRG transseptal needle manufactured by Baylis Medical Company, Inc. can be replaced with the Brockenbrough needle **(Figs. 13A to C)**. The TorFlex transseptal guiding sheath, also produced by Baylis Medical Company, Inc., is used to introduce the dilator-sheath assembly. This RF needle uses 5–10 W energy for 2–5 seconds and can perforate the atrial septum after one to four pulses. This technology may be more beneficial in cases where the atrial septum is thick, scarred, calcified, or patched, as excess force could result in unsuccessful puncture or perforation of the LA free wall.[13]

SafeSept Guidewire

SafeSept™ (Pressure Products Medical Supplies, Inc) is a nitinol guidewire that is especially designed for TSP **(Figs. 14A to C)**. This guidewire is 135 cm long and has a diameter of 0.014 inches. SafeSept™ is carefully designed to perforate the membranous fossa with less force than a standard transseptal needle. After the transseptal dilator has tented the fossa ovalis, the SafeSept tip effortlessly advances through the fossa and perforates the membrane. The tip of the wire takes on a "J" shape, which stops it from penetrating any

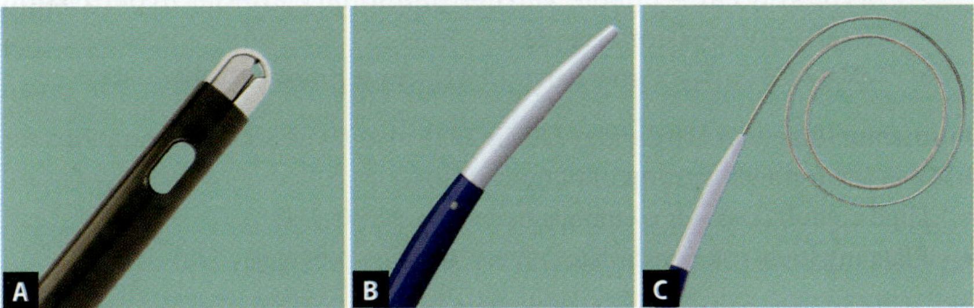

Figs. 13A to C: NRG Transseptal Kit. (A) NRG transseptal needle; (B) TorFlex transseptal guiding sheath; (C) ProTrack Pigtail wire.
Courtesy: Baylis Medical Company, Inc.

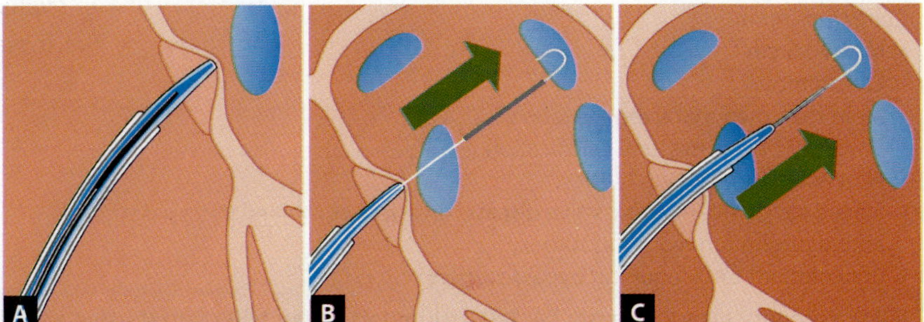

Figs. 14A to C: SafeSept. (A) Tenting the interatrial septum; (B) Advancing SafeSept into the left atrium; (C) Needle and dilator tracking over wire.
Courtesy: Pressure Products Medical Supplies, Inc.

further. The SafeSept™ guidewire is designed to be safe and reliable, making it an excellent choice for medical professionals.[14]

A radiopaque coil along the shaft allows for fluoroscopic visualization of the wire in the LA. Proximal marker bands indicate the location of the SafeSept tip in relation to the needle tip. The needle, dilator, and sheath are advanced over the wire into the LA with minimal risk of perforation.

INDICATIONS FOR BALLOON MITRAL VALVULOPLASTY

Balloon mitral valvuloplasty (BMV) is indicated in patients with symptomatic severe mitral stenosis (MS) with a "pliable valve". Indications for BMV as per different scientific society recommendations are as follows:

American College of Cardiology (ACC) 2021:

- *Symptomatic:*
  - Mitral valve area (MVA) ≤1.5 cm^2—pliable valve, <moderate mitral regurgitation (MR), no left atrial (LA) clot
  - MVA ≤1.5 cm^2—suboptimal valve—not surgical candidate
- *Asymptomatic:*
  - MVA ≤1.5 cm^2—pliable valve + pulmonary arterial hypertension (PAH)—RVP >50 mm Hg (2a)
  - MVA ≤1.5 cm^2—pliable valve + PAH—new onset AF (2b)

European Society of Cardiology (ESC) 2021 also gives recommendations for BMV in the following group of patients also:

- High embolic risk—h/o embolism, dense LASEC (2a)
- Planning high-risk noncardiac surgery, desiring pregnancy (2a)

Contraindications as per ESC 2021 are given in **Box 1**.

BOX 1: Contraindications for percutaneous mitral commissurotomy in rheumatic mitral stenosis[a]

Contraindications:

- MVA >1.5 cm^2[a]
- LA thrombus
- More than mild mitral regurgitation
- Severe or bi-commissural calcification
- Absence of commissural fusion
- Severe concomitant aortic valve disease, or severe combined tricuspid stenosis and regurgitation requiring surgery
- Concomitant CAD requiring bypass surgery

(CAD: coronary artery disease; LA: left atrium/left atrial; MVA: mitral valve area; PMC: percutaneous mitral commissurotomy)

[a]PMC may be considered in patients with valve area >1.5 cm^2 with symptoms that cannot be explained by another cause and if the anatomy is favorable.

PREPROCEDURAL PLANNING

- *Elective admission:* Patients are admitted 1 day before the procedure for detailed assessment.
- *Valve suitability:* Confirm via transthoracic and transesophageal echocardiography (TEE). Transthoracic echo should be used to assess valve morphology and assess MR and LA thrombus and presence of other valve lesions. TEE should be done in all patients which is mandatory to rule out LA clot. TEE also can be used to more accurately assess MR and also assess the interatrial septum for the septal puncture.
- We should use planimetry to measure the MVA, which is more accurate than the pressure half-time (PHT) method.
- Mitral valve gradients depend on the heart rate and that should be considered while interpreting the gradients.
- *Surgical backup:* Preparation for mitral valve replacement (MVR) is crucial, including ensuring the availability of blood and surgical support.

Access

- *Right femoral vein:* 7 F sheath for introducing the balloon catheter.
- *Right femoral artery:* 5 F/6 F sheath for pigtail catheter insertion (to assess LV position and measure LVED pressure)

Hardware

The most important hardware is the mitral valvotomy balloon. All BMV balloons are made of latex and they are dumbbell shaped. On inflation, the distal part gets inflated first and subsequently the proximal part of the balloon gets inflated. The waist at the middle region dilates the valve, leading to splitting of the commissures.

The classical Inoue balloon has three proximal ports. One for the central lumen, one for the vent port, and the third one for the contrast to inflate the balloon. The vent port is incorporated to prevent deflation failure.

The modification of the Inoue balloon is the Accura balloon, which has two ports, one is the central lumen and the other is the contrast port for the balloon inflation.

Another technique developed by Dr George Joseph from CMC Vellore is the JOMIVA balloon which is an over-the-wire technique. Here, the balloon is introduced through a sheath and a wire is parked in LV apex. Over the wire, we will track the balloon across the mitral valve.

Balloon Preparation

This step must be completed under strict aseptic precautions.

Balloon Cleaning

- Check the integrity of the Inoue balloon, transseptal puncture (TSP) needle, and LA guidewire.
- Wash the balloon thoroughly with sterile saline to remove residual Cidex if the hardware is being reused.
- Flush the balloon lumen multiple times with saline.

Air Removal and Inflation

- Prepare a 1:4 contrast-saline mixture manually.
- Connect the balloon hub to a 20-mL syringe via a 10 mm extension tubing with a 3-way stopcock.
- Keep the balloon vertically downward, inject contrast mixture, and tap gently to release air. Repeat 2–3 times until the balloon is air-free.
- Measure the balloon diameter using the provided vernier caliper. Adjust the volume of the contrast mixture to achieve the desired balloon size. *Note:* ~1 mL contrast increases balloon size by 1 mm in a 24 mm balloon (may vary).

Final Preparations

- Lock the contrast mixture in the syringe and seal unused hubs to prevent leakage.
- Insert the straightener to slenderize the balloon. Always the gold and the silver hub should be inserted together. If the gold hub which is connected to the inner plastic tube at the distal end is pushed alone, the inner plastic lumen may kink and the balloon may get damaged.
- Verify all connections and note the total contrast volume to ensure no leaks have occurred.
- The balloon is now ready for introduction into the left atrium.

STEPS OF BALLOON MITRAL VALVULOPLASTY

Hemodynamic Measurement

- *Right atrial (RA) pressure*: Maintain proper hydration to ensure accurate RA mean pressure readings, which are necessary for determining LA mean pressure and the transmitral gradient.
- *Pulmonary artery pressure:* Measure pre- and postprocedure using a Goodale–Lubin (GL) or multipurpose (MPA) catheter. Severe PAH is an indicator of MS severity and fall in pulmonary pressure indicates successful BMV.

Trans-septal Puncture

Septal puncture techniques are described above.

Left Atrium Entry and Balloon Inflation

Step 1: Left Atrial Pressure Measurement

- Following transseptal puncture, measure LA pressure via the Mullins sheath or dilator. Most of the time we use the Mullins dilator. If we plan to use floatation balloon to enter LV for over-the-wire techniques, we need the Mullin's sheath.
- Simultaneously, record LV pressure by advancing the pigtail catheter into the LV (in PA view for ease). Ensure to flush the pigtail in the descending aorta before LV entry.
- Measure simultaneous LA and LV pressures to assess the gradient.
- After measurement, pull the pigtail catheter back into the descending aorta.

Step 2: Introduction of Pigtail-Shaped Left Atrial Guidewire (Figs. 15 and 16)

Introduce the pigtail-shaped guidewire into the left atrium via the Mullins sheath or dilator. Ensure proper positioning by avoiding entry into the LA appendage or pulmonary veins, which can be achieved by adjusting the tip of the Mullins catheter. Once correctly placed, the guidewire will form a freely movable loop within the LA cavity. After confirming its position, carefully remove the Mullins sheath and dilator, leaving the pigtail or coiled LA guidewire securely in place.

Step 3: Septal Dilation

The groin (venous puncture site) is initially dilated using artery forceps to create sufficient space for balloon insertion. A 14 F dilator is then introduced

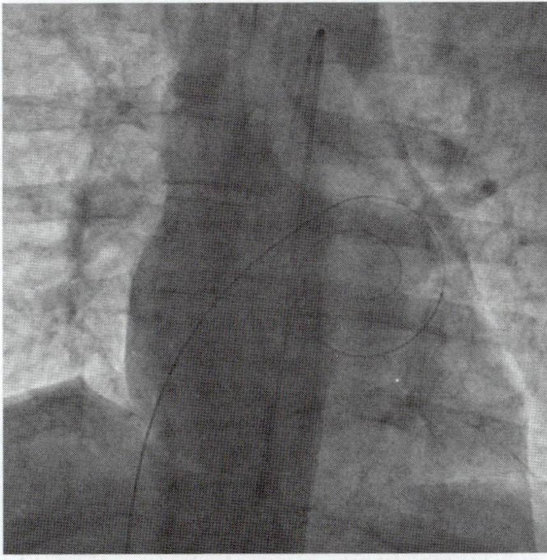

Fig. 15: Coiled wire positioned in the left atrium (LA).

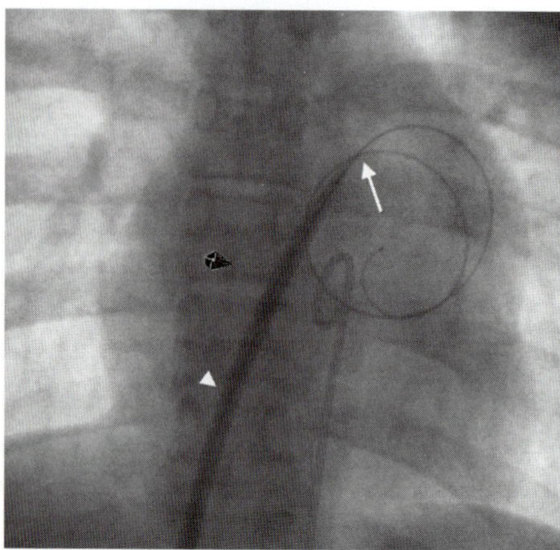

Fig. 16: Dilation of the interatrial septum. The arrow indicates the dilator tip positioned near the left bronchus which is the marker of the roof of left atrium, while the arrowhead marks the catch point at the interatrial septum which is actually much lower in the AP view. (AP: anteroposterior)

over the pigtail wire and used to progressively dilate both the venous access site and the interatrial septum. The dilator should be halted at the shadow of the left bronchus, which defines the superior border of the left atrium. It is important to recognize that the true catch of the septum is lower and corresponds to the double shadow of the left atrium. After completing septal dilation, perform echocardiography to rule out pericardial effusion. If no effusion is detected, administer 100 U/kg of heparin.

Step 4: Balloon Introduction into the Left Atrium

Following septal dilation, the slenderized balloon is introduced into the left atrium. Once the tip of the balloon reaches the bronchus shadow, secure its position in the left atrium. To do so, first remove the gold hub with the silver hub (straightener), allowing the balloon to coil over the wire. A small inflation will prevent balloon slippage into the right atrium. Once the balloon is adequately secured, gently remove the coiled wire, then aspirate and flush the balloon to prepare it for further dilation **(Figs. 17A to D)**.

Step 5: Mitral Valve Crossing and Balloon Dilation

This process is performed in the right anterior oblique (RAO) view. To cross the mitral valve and enter the LV, an LV entry stylet with a slight anterior curve is used. The stylet is rotated 2–3 times counter clockwise to align the balloon toward the LV, indicated by **(Figs. 18A and B)**:

- Bobbing of the balloon
- A drop in aortic pressure due to partial obstruction of the mitral valve
- Ventricular ectopics on the ECG, confirming LV entry

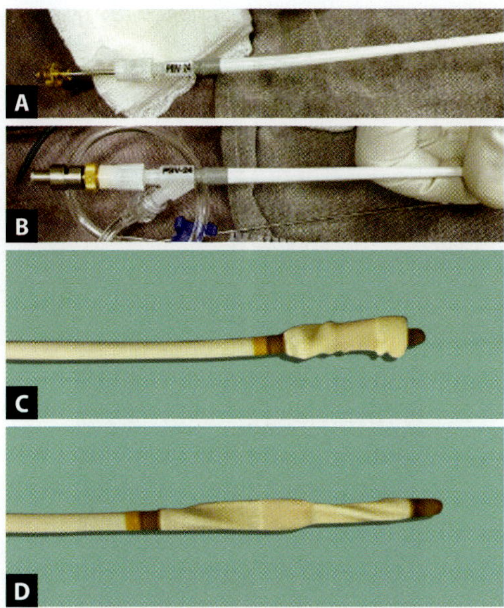

Figs. 17A to D: BMV balloon hub. (A) Accura balloon with a gold-colored hub. (B) Accura balloon displaying a combination of gold and silver hubs attached. (C) BMV balloon in its unslenderized form. (D) Properly slenderized BMV balloon for optimized use. (BMV: balloon mitral valvuloplasty)

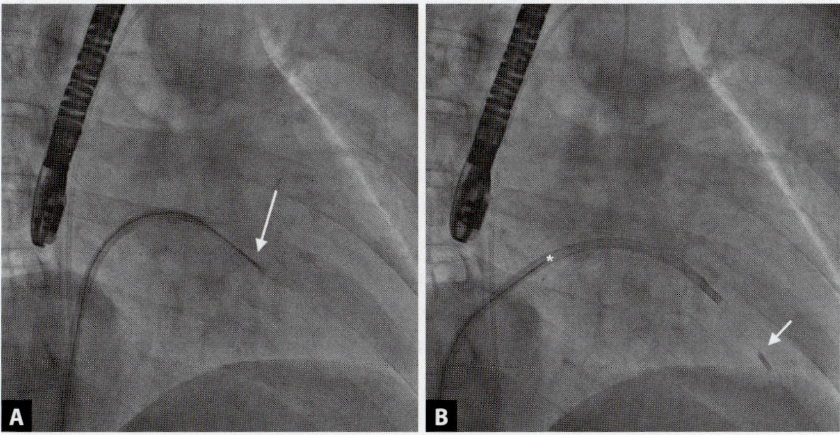

Figs. 18 A and B: Left ventricular (LV) entry. (A) Balloon with the stylet positioned in the left atrium (LA) and aligned across the mitral valve (arrow). (B) Balloon tip advanced into the left ventricle (LV) after crossing the mitral valve, with the stylet withdrawn and visible (*) across the interatrial septum (IAS).

Echocardiography can also confirm proper positioning. Once the balloon reaches the LV apex, inflate the distal balloon. Pull it back to position the waist across the valve orifice and then fully inflate the balloon. This stretches the valve, causing the commissures to give way stages of balloon inflation are given in **(Figs. 19A to C)**.

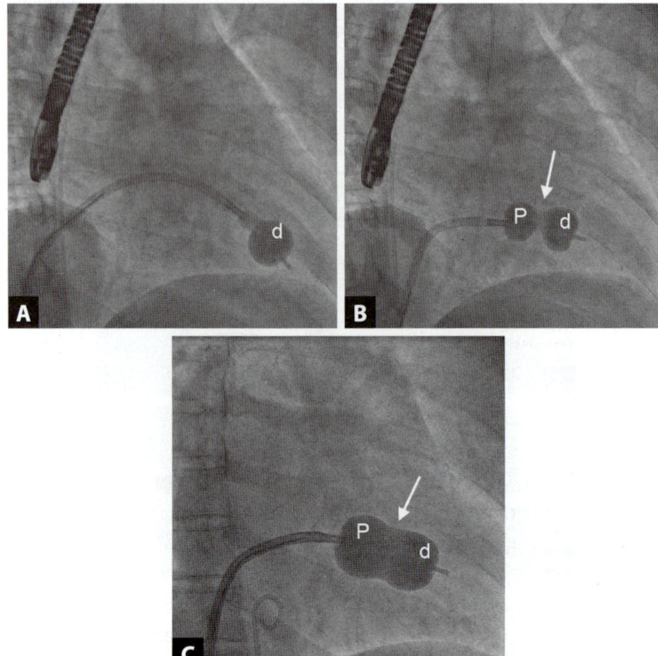

Figs. 19A to C: Stages of balloon inflation during BMV (accura). (A) Initial inflation of the distal segment of the balloon (d) within the left ventricle (LV). (B) Balloon positioned across the mitral commissures, forming a waist (arrow), followed by inflation of the proximal segment (p). (C) Full inflation of the balloon, resulting in near-complete opening of both mitral commissures (arrow).

After dilation, remove the stylet, flush the central balloon port, and check the LA pressure. Use the pigtail catheter to measure left ventricular end-diastolic pressure (LVEDP) and the pressure gradient.

If the LA pressure remains elevated or commissures fail to open on echocardiography, increase the balloon size by adding contrast and repeat dilation. Ensure the initial contrast volume in the syringe is noted, as leakage during the procedure may result in inadequate dilation. If the result is inadequate, we can consider using a higher size balloon like 26 mm when 24 mm balloon is not giving a good result. One fact to be kept in mind is that smaller size balloon at full size (e.g., 24 mm balloon at 24 mm) will give more radial pressure than larger balloon (e.g., 28 mm balloon going to 28 mm) **(Figs. 19 and 20)**.

Step 6: Assessing Procedural Success

Procedure success is evaluated by:

- Echocardiography showing commissural splitting
- Reduced transvalvular gradient on Doppler echocardiography

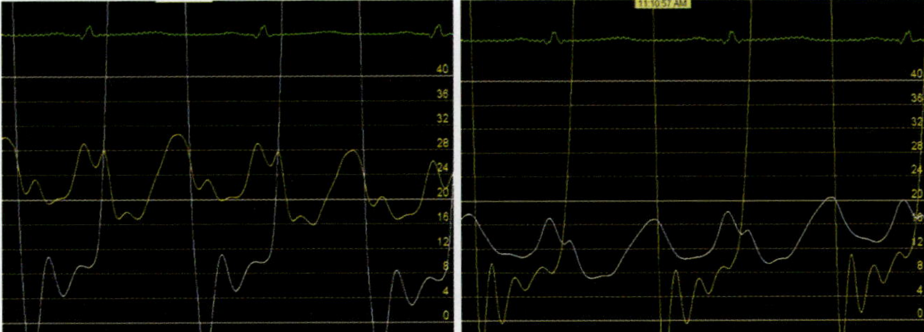

Fig. 20: Simultaneous pressure tracings of the left atrium and left ventricle before (left) and after (right) balloon dilation. Note the significant reduction in LA pressure following the procedure.

- Shortening or resolution of the diastolic murmur of MS
- Significant reduction in LA pressure **(Fig. 20)**.
- Simultaneous LV and LA pressure assessment to account for potential changes in LVEDP due to increased flow or MR

If MR increases by two grades or reaches moderate severity, the procedure should be halted. Indicators of significant MR include an increased LA V wave, lack of LA mean pressure drop, and unchanged PA pressure. If the LA V wave height goes >50% of the systemic pressure, it is an indicator of severe MR and patient may need urgent mitral valve replacement.

Step 7: Balloon and Wire Removal, and Post-Balloon Inflation Steps

After the procedure:

- Reintroduce the pigtail wire into the LA and ensure the balloon is straightened before removal to avoid enlarging the septal puncture. Once straightened, remove the balloon system, leaving the pigtail wire in place. (To straighten the balloon, lock the proximal hub of the straightener to the gold hub, then push the gold and silver tubes together and lock them securely.)
- Insert a 7F sheath and MPA catheter into the LA over the pigtail wire. Remove the pigtail wire carefully, supported by the catheter, to avoid septal damage or ASD enlargement.
- Use the MPA catheter to measure pulmonary artery pressure, collect blood samples for shunt assessment, and calculate the MVA using Gorlin's equation.
- Remove venous and arterial sheaths, achieving hemostasis with manual compression.

Complications of Balloon Mitral Valvuloplasty

- Septal puncture-related cardiac tamponade, aortic root injury
- Mitral regurgitation due to valve tear or excessive commissural split

- *Cerebrovascular accident (CVA) or systemic embolic phenomenon*: If the patient develops CVA, the patient should be referred to a neurointervention and cerebral embolectomy can be done with good recovery.

Postprocedure Management

It will be always better to observe the patient in the ICU for few hours to look for pericardial effusion or stroke or any other vascular complication. Perform a postprocedural echocardiogram to assess the MVA, adequacy of opening of the commissures, gradient across the mitral valve, and severity of MR. If no complications are noted, discharge can typically be planned for the following day.

Patient may be continued on rheumatic prophylaxis, diuretic, and β-blocker if there is residual MS. OAC with warfarin may be continued if patient in AF or those with a history of CVA. Patient should be screened with follow-up echocardiography periodically every 6 months to 1 year.

CONCLUSION

Percutaneous BMV is the preferred treatment option over surgical commissurotomy for severe rheumatic MS. Careful selection of patients and meticulous attention on the procedural steps reduce the complication rates significantly.

REFERENCES

1. Russo G, Taramasso M, Maisano F. (2019). Transseptal Puncture: A Step-by-Step Procedural Guide. [online] Available from https://citoday.com/articles/2019-may-june/transseptal-puncture-a-step-by-step-procedural-guide. [Last accessed October, 2024].
2. Hung JS. Atrial septal puncture technique in percutaneous transvenous mitral commissurotomy: mitral valvuloplasty using the Inoue balloon catheter technique. Cathet Cardiovasc Diagn. 1992;26(4):275-84.
3. Shaw TR. Anterior staircase manoeuvre for atrial transseptal puncture. Br Heart J. 1994;71(3):297-301.
4. Guarracino F, Baldassarri R, Ferro B, Giannini C, Bertini P, Petronio AS, et al. Transesophageal echocardiography during MitraClip® procedure. Anesth Analg. 2014;118(6):1188-96.
5. Krishnamoorthy KM, Dash PK. Transseptal catheterization without needle puncture. Scand Cardiovasc J. 2001;35(3):199-200.
6. Nallet O, Lung B, Cormier B, Porte JM, Garbarz E, Michel PL, et al. Specifics of technique in percutaneous mitral commissurotomy in a case of dextrocardia and situs inversus with mitral stenosis. Cathet Cardiovasc Diagn. 1996;39(1):85-8.
7. Namboodiri N, Harikrishnan SP, Ajitkumar V, Tharakan JA. Percutaneous mitral commissurotomy in a case of mirror-image dextrocardia and rheumatic mitral stenosis. J Invasive Cardiol. 2008;20(1):E33-5.

8. Agarwala MK, Singh M, Grover A, Varma JS. Balloon Mitral Valvotomy in Pregnant Patient with Anomalous Inferior Vena Cava. Asian Cardiovasc Thorac Ann. 1998;6(3):227-8.
9. Salghetti F, Sieira J, Chierchia GB, Curnis A, de Asmundis C. Recognizing and reacting to complications of trans-septal puncture. Expert Rev Cardiovasc Ther. 2017;15(12):905-12.
10. Singh SM, Douglas PS, Reddy VY. The incidence and long-term clinical outcome of iatrogenic atrial septal defects secondary to transseptal catheterization with a 12F transseptal sheath. Circ Arrhythm Electrophysiol. 2011;4(2):166-71.
11. Siroky GP, Bisht D, Huynh H, Yacoub M, Lee S, Keller S, et al. Reversible Mechanical Atrioventricular Block Caused By A Steerable Introducer Sheath During Transseptal Catheterization. J Atr Fibrillation. 2021;13(6):20200469.
12. De Marco F. (2020). TSP Crosser Transseptal access device. Available from https://www.tctmd.com/slide/tsp-crosser-transseptal-access-device. [Last accessed October, 2024].
13. Sherman W, Lee P, Hartley A, Love B. Transatrial septal catheterization using a new radiofrequency probe. Catheter Cardiovasc Interv. 2005;66(1):14-7.
14. Graham AJ, Honarbakhsh S, O'Brien B, Schilling RJ. A Simplified Trans-Septal Puncture Technique using a Needle Free Approach for Cryoablation of Atrial Fibrillation. J Atr Fibrillation. 2017;10(2):1628.

CHAPTER 42

Alternative Sites of Large-bore Access and Devices and Techniques for Large-bore Access Closure

Ashraf SM

INTRODUCTION

Historically, transfemoral arterial access has been the standard of care for large-bore devices given the vessel's size and ease of management with both surgical and percutaneous techniques. However, procedural bleeding complications are common in the setting of large-bore access and are associated with significant increases in mortality, length of stay, and healthcare costs. Peripheral arterial disease, vessel tortuosity, the potential for distal limb ischemia, and limitations related to implant duration occasionally necessitate alternative approaches to large-bore access to limit such complications.

The most common site of large-bore access is femoral artery.

SPECIAL CONSIDERATION FOR LARGE-BORE SHEATH ACCESS

The common femoral artery is used more than any other access site for procedures that require very large sheaths, such as aortic interventions for aneurysms and structural cardiac interventions such as transcatheter aortic valve replacement (TAVR) **(Fig. 1)**. Vascular access site complications remain a major cause of mortality and morbidity during and after these procedures. Even though still used by some, surgical cut-down to explore the vessel for direct access and closure is losing ground; pure percutaneous procedure is the current prevailing technique. Three-dimensional, contrast-enhanced CT images are revolutionizing TAVR screening and procedural planning. This imaging technology is particularly useful for identifying circumferential calcification, excessive tortuosity, and areas of the proximal vessel system that are too narrow to accommodate a large sheath. The access location can be planned and sheath delivery success predicted well before the start of the procedure. During the procedure, micropuncture access with angiography through the microcatheter sheath or ultrasound-guided access seems to be the technique of choice.

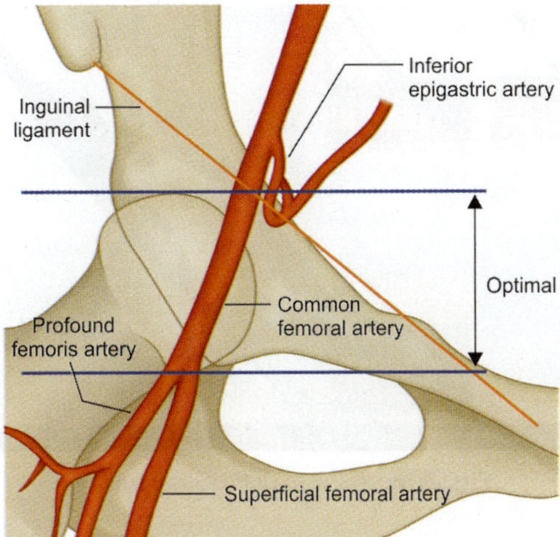

Fig. 1: Anatomy of common femoral artery: Figure shows the area of ideal puncture site for femoral access. Note that puncture should be below the origin of inferior epigastric artery and above the bifurcation of common femoral artery.

Ultrasound-guided Vascular Access

This technique offers multiple advantages over fluoroscopy:[1]

- There is direct visualization of disease in the artery at the access site.
- There is direct visualization of the vessel and its bifurcation, including atherosclerosis, aneurysmal dilatation, dissections, etc.
- The operator can visualize the needle puncturing the anterior wall of the vessel and prevent a posterior wall puncture, as well as prevent a venous puncture.
- After wire insertion through the needle, the operator can again verify the puncture site by following the course of the wire through the artery from the subcutaneous tissues.
- It decreases the amount of fluoroscopy and radiation to both the patient and operators.

TYPES OF VASCULAR CLOSURE DEVICES

Vascular closure devices are divided according to their mechanism of achieving hemostasis.[2] There are three basic types—suture mediated, plug based, and clip based. These can be further subdivided into either extra- or intraluminal devices, depending on the position of the deployed hemostatic closure components. Another way to categorize vascular closure is by how the arteriotomy is approximated to achieve hemostasis. Active approximators physically close the arteriotomy with the use of a suture or a nitinol clip. Passive approximators deploy a plug, sealant, or gel at the arteriotomy site

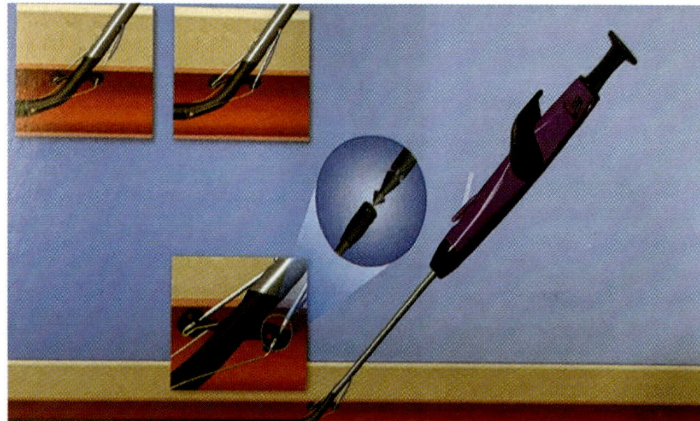

Fig. 2: Mechanism of ProGlide suture.

without actively closing the arteriotomy. External hemostatic devices are placed on top of the skin and provide hemostasis by applying mechanical pressure at the arteriotomy site or by accelerating the in vivo clotting cascade.

The most common active approximator VCD is Proglide (Abbott vascular) **(Fig. 2)**. Puncture size is 5–21 Fr, which is percutaneous deployment of a monofilament polypropylene suture with automatic knot formation. Two devices and a preclose technique are required for sheath size >8 Fr or more. When two Proglides are taken for closure, the direction of closure of one VCD is at 10′0 clock and the other is at 2′0 clock. Alternatively, a Proglide and an Angioseal may be used in combination. The most common passive approximator is Angioseal by St Jude, in two different 6 Fr and 8 Fr devices sizes which deploys an absorbable collagen plug to close arteriotomy site, secured in place by intraluminal anchor and absorbable suture.

Perclose ProGlide suture-mediated closure system uses a plunger and a lever to place the suture across the artery.

ALTERNATE LARGE-BORE ACCESS

- *Transaxillary approach*
- *Transcaval approach*
- *Transcarotid*—needs surgical cut down and distal vessel clamping

Transaxillary Access

Percutaneous access of the axillary artery has traditionally been avoided due to several, largely theoretical concerns **(Table 1)**. First, the media of the subclavian artery has a higher proportion of elastic fibers relative to the thicker media layer of the femoral artery, which consists mostly of smooth muscle cells.

Anatomically, the axillary artery is divided into three segments. The first and most proximal section is between the lateral margin of the first rib and the medial border of the pectoralis minor muscle, the second segment is deep to the pectoralis minor muscle, and the third segment is located between the lateral border of the pectoralis minor muscle and the inferior border of the teres major muscle. Typical percutaneous axillary artery puncture occurs at the distal end of the first segment or proximal end of the second segment with the needle traversing the pectoralis minor muscle **(Fig. 3)**.

TABLE 1: Comparisons between alternative access options.

	Advantages	*Disadvantages*
Transaxillary	No dedicated equipment required	Relatively smaller caliber vessel limits sheath size
	Improved patient mobility while device indwelling	Potential for increased radiation exposure and ergonomic stress compared with standard femoral access, particularly for new operators
	Manual hemostasis possible	
Transcaval	No sheath size restrictions	Cost/dedicated equipment required
	Rare superficial bleeding/ oozing	More difficult remediation of complications due to lack of manual pressure options
	Radiation exposure and ergonomics comparable to standard femoral access	Requirement for patient bed rest, limited mobility with indwelling sheaths

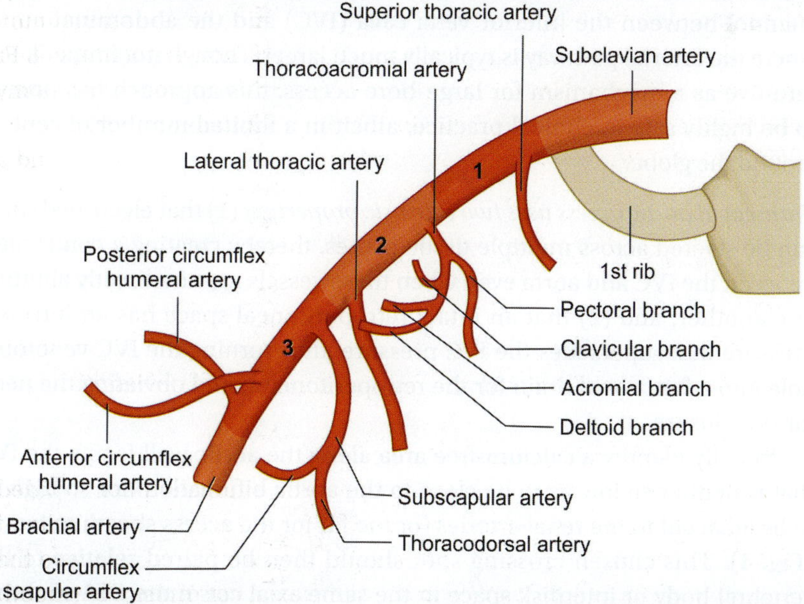

Fig. 3: Anatomy of axillary artery. Axillary artery and its segments are shown here. It starts from the lateral aspect of first rib and ends at the inferior border of teres major muscle.

The typical axillary artery access point is extrathoracic and at the distal end of the first segment or proximal end of the second segment. If bleeding complications occur from this location, they result in hematoma or ecchymosis rather than occult accumulation or hemothorax.

Ultrasound-guided access with a micropuncture system should be considered best practice given adjacent structures, including the brachial plexus, lung, and axillary vein. The axillary artery runs cephalad to the vein as one moves laterally with the ultrasound probe. In scenarios where the vein appears to override the artery, the operator should move more laterally, away from the sternum and clavicle. Once an acceptable position for access has been established, it is key to puncture the vessel with a shallow angle needlestick. There are bony structures both anterior and posterior to the axillary artery (the clavicle and second rib, respectively) that can easily kink an access sheath following a steep entry angle puncture. In practice, the skin puncture at our center is usually close to the inferior aspect of the deltopectoral groove.

Proglide vascular closure device or manual compression are also effective in selected cases of completion of axillary access interventions.

Caval-Aortic Access

Transcaval access facilitates large-bore access by bypassing the iliofemoral arteries in favor of the femoral and iliac veins and creating a sheath-mediated channel between the inferior vena cava (IVC) and the abdominal aorta, where the arterial pathway is typically much larger. Though not immediately intuitive as a mechanism for large-bore access, this approach has proven to be highly safe in clinical practice, albeit in a limited number of centers around the globe.

Transcaval aortic access uses two intrinsic properties: (1) that electrified wires can be steered across multiple tissue planes, thereby creating a connection between the IVC and aorta even when these vessels are not directly abutting one another; and (2) that an intact retroperitoneal space has an intrinsic pressure that supersedes the IVC pressure, thus turning the IVC venotomy hole into a functional drain for the retroperitoneum and obviating the need for IVC closure.

Initially identify a calcium-free area along the aortic wall facing the IVC that is neither so low as to be close to the aortic bifurcation nor so high as to be adjacent to the renal arteries (or too far for the access sheath to reach) **(Fig. 4)**. This chosen crossing spot should then be paired relative to the vertebral body or interdisk space in the same axial cut of the CTA so that it can be identified in the Cath lab. Typically, crossing happens at the level of the third or fourth lumbar spine. The rationale for staying away from the renal arteries and aortic bifurcation is to ensure that use of a covered stent.

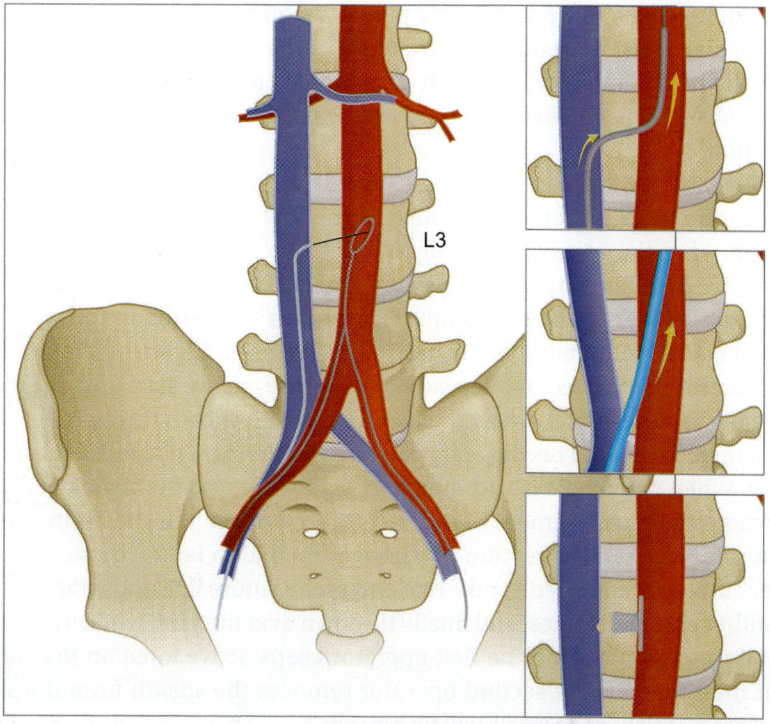

Fig. 4: Steps involved in transcaval access.

The ideal site for puncture in aorta is between renal arteries and aortic bifurcation.

Crossing requires electrifying an insulated 0.014-inch wire via electrosurgery pencil connected to the external/back end. The chosen wire, therefore, needs to be able to transmit the electrical current from the back end of the wire to the tip and to be of reasonably high tip stiffness. Wires with a polymer-jacketed tip should be avoided. Experts typically use an Astato 20 g wire (Asahi Intecc). Telescoping catheters are then used to introduce a 0.035-inch Lunderquist wire (Cook Medical) over which the large-bore catheter is delivered. Occasionally, the aortic wall requires balloon predilation before the telescoping microcatheters will cross. Most operators typically use a 2.0 × 20 mm compliant balloon across the aortic wall, which is well tolerated. Following the intended procedure, transcaval closure usually closed by ADO device.

LARGE-BORE VENOUS SHEATH MANAGEMENT

Currently, the most common indications for using large sheaths in the common femoral vein are shunt closure, left atrial appendage occlusion, paravalvular leak closure, and MitraClip. Some devices such as percutaneous left ventricular assist devices can also require large access to the venous system; however, more frequently patients who require percutaneous left ventricular assist devices may have to leave the catheterization laboratory with the device in place, in which case there is a long delay before sheath removal and closure devices should not be used because of the high risk of infection.

The strategy for managing large sheaths in the venous system is easier than for arterial punctures because of the lower pressure of the venous system. After the access is carefully obtained by a regular 18-gauge needle, place a 7 Fr dilator in the vein. Blunt dissection of subcutaneous tissue facilitates delivery of larger sheaths. The sheath is inserted in the standard manner. After completion of the procedure, we use a "figure of 8" suture for hemostasis. For this technique, use a 0 silk suture and we start from the distal edge of the access site, below the insertion of the sheath through the skin. The orientation of the needle entry can be either from medial to lateral or vice versa. When the needle is withdrawn from the skin, use the same needle on the more proximal segment of the sheath, superior to the sheath insertion, with same the same direction of passage (medial to lateral or vice versa). After cutting off the needle, take one end of the suture line and wrap around the other end three times, and finally tie down over the skin, while the sheath is still through the skin. The first operator keeps active force on the suture over the sheath as the second operator removes the sheath from the skin. Finally, the reinforcing knots will be placed.

COMPLICATIONS OF LARGE-BORE ACCESS

Access site or access-related vascular injury like dissection, stenosis, perforation, rupture, arteriovenous fistula or pseudoaneurysms requiring compression or thrombin injection therapy, or hematomas requiring transfusion of >2 units are major vascular access morbidities.

Distal embolization can be treated with embolectomy and/or thrombectomy and usually not resulting in amputation or irreversible end-organ damage. Vascular closure device failure may result in use of stent graft or surgical correction.

CONCLUSION

The use of large bore access has created a way for the enormous growth of structural heart interventions. Proper puncture site selection and appropriate use of devices are essential for the safety and good clinical outcomes.

REFERENCES

1. Perlowski A, Salinger MH, Levisay JP, Feldman T. Femoral access for TAVR: techniques for prevention and endovascular management of complications. In: Dieter R, Dieter Jr R, Dieter III R, (Eds). Endovascular interventions. New York, NY: Springer New York; 2014:859-73.
2. Hoffer EK, Bloch RD. Percutaneous arterial closure devices. J Vasc Interv Radiol. 2003;14:865-85.

CHAPTER 43

Transcatheter Aortic Valve Replacement: A Step by Step Approach

Ravinder Singh Rao

INTRODUCTION

Transcatheter aortic valve replacement (TAVR) is a minimally invasive procedure used to replace a stenotic aortic valve in patients with severe symptomatic aortic stenosis.[1] It has become the standard of care for suitable patients. The outcomes of the procedure depend on the operator's volume and experience; greater experience leads to safer outcomes. In this chapter, we describe the best practices for the TAVR procedure and provide a detailed step-by-step description with accompanying diagrams.

PREPARATION AND IMAGING

Preoperative Assessment

After selecting a patient for the TAVR procedure, a comprehensive evaluation using echocardiography, CT angiography, electrocardiogram (ECG), hematological assessment, and, if available, cardiac catheterization, helps to determine the optimal approach. A preprocedure heart team meeting to discuss strategy, team member roles, potential complications, and bailout strategies is crucial for a successful outcome. The access site, sheath size, vascular closure device, need for predilatation, postdilatation, and end goals should be planned and discussed with the team before starting the case.

SEDATION AND MONITORING

Anesthesia

Most patients undergo the procedure under conscious sedation. General anesthesia is rarely required and considered only if a transesophageal echo is needed during the procedure. A central line (internal jugular) and radial artery access are advisable. Eutectic mixture of prilocaine and lignocaine is applied to the groins, neck area, and both radial sites 2 hours before the procedure and covered with Tegaderm (occlusive dressing) to numb the areas of vascular access, enhancing patient comfort during conscious sedation.

Monitoring

Continuous monitoring of heart and vital signs is essential throughout the procedure. Cerebral oximetry and bispectral index (BIS) monitoring provide additional information for the cardiac anesthetist regarding the depth of anesthesia.

VASCULAR ACCESS

The femoral artery is most commonly used, but the subclavian artery, carotid artery, and direct aortic access are also considered.[2] In this chapter, we describe the best practices to achieve femoral arterial access. A combination of CT knowledge of bifurcation level, distribution of calcium on the anterior wall of the common femoral artery (CFA), fluoroscopy guidance, ultrasound guidance, and use of micropuncture is vital for safe and successful femoral artery access.[3]

Ultrasound helps identify the CFA in a short-axis view. The superficial femoral artery (SFA), profunda femoris artery (PFA), and femoral vein are identified first **(Fig. 1A)**. The probe is slowly moved cranially to identify where the CFA begins and centered on the ultrasound screen. A micropuncture needle is positioned at a 60–90° angle to the probe and advanced using a jiggle maneuver while watching its advancement on ultrasound, ensuring it enters the center of the CFA at a site free of calcium. This step is crucial for the success of the closure device.

Next, the micropuncture wire is advanced, and a 4F/5F micropuncture sheath is introduced **(Fig. 1B)**. An angiogram confirms the proper site of entry **(Fig. 1C)**. Then, a 0.035-inch 160 cm wire is introduced into the micropuncture sheath, followed by a 6F sheath or a dilator. A small nick is made, and blunt dissection is performed until the artery's top is reached. It is ensured that no skin or subcutaneous tissue tags are on the wire. A single 6 F ProGlide is deployed at the standard 3–9 o'clock position, followed by the delivery of a 9 F sheath. At this point, heparin is administered at 100 U/kg to achieve an activated clotting time (ACT) of >250 seconds.

Initially, femoral arterial access and femoral venous access are preferred on the non-TAVR device side. A 6F arterial sheath and a 6F venous sheath are used, with the 6F sheath connected to the pressure line for continuous hemodynamic measurement.

PIGTAIL CATHETER AND TEMPORARY PACEMAKER WIRE PLACEMENT

A 5 F pigtail catheter is advanced inside a 6 F arterial sheath, allowing continuous blood pressure monitoring. The pigtail is placed in the noncoronary cusp and connected to the injector. An aortic root injection is performed in the coplanar view obtained from the CT scan (15 mL at 15 mL/second). If the view is not coplanar, adjust by following the right cusp rule: If the right cusp is below, go caudal; if above, go cranial; if on the right side, go right anterior oblique (RAO); and if on the left side, go left anterior

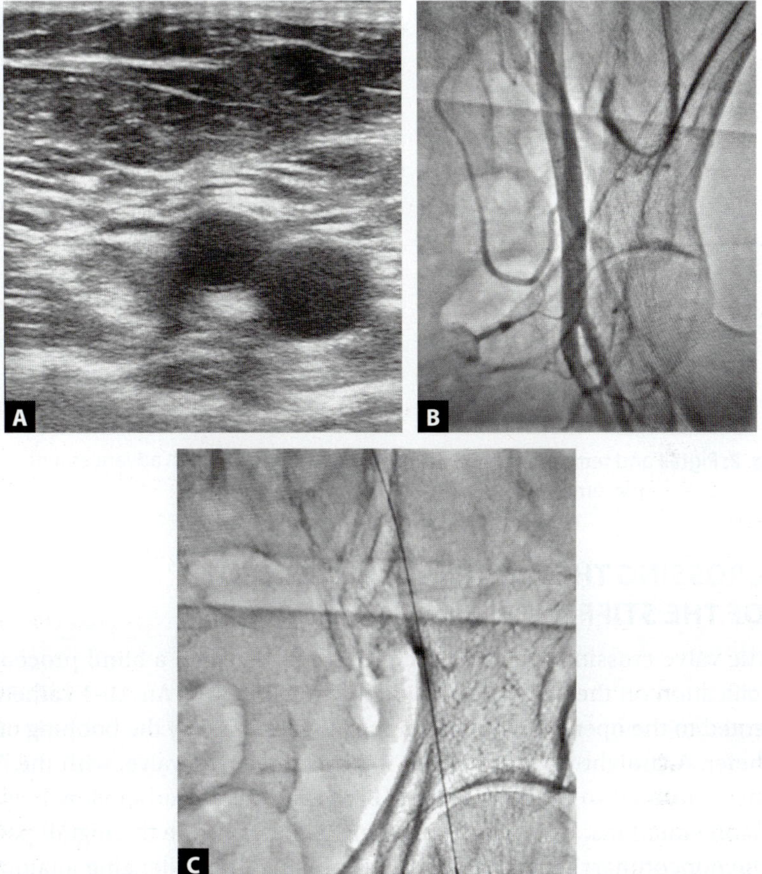

Figs. 1A to C: (A) Ultrasonography (USG) visualization; (B and C) Puncture site in fluoroscopy and angiographically.

oblique (LAO). A 5 F balloon-tipped pacemaker is then placed into the right ventricular (RV) apex and parameters are checked **(Fig. 2)**. It is vital to keep the balloon inflated while positioning to prevent RV injury, allowing the ACT to build up.

TRANSCATHETER AORTIC VALVE REPLACEMENT SHEATH PLACEMENT

A stiff wire is advanced into 9 F sheath. In tortuous anatomies, a JR diagnostic catheter with a guidewire is advanced into the thoracic aorta, and a stiff wire is placed inside it. A 14 F sheath is then advanced under fluoroscopic vision over the stiff wire. Different valves have different requirements and specifications for the sheath, which should be followed **(Fig. 3)**. A 9 F sheath is placed inside the 14 F sheath, allowing better control of the diagnostic catheter used to cross the valve.

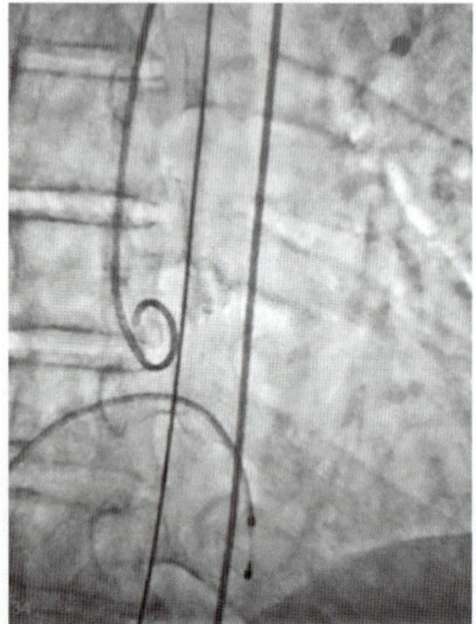

Fig. 2: Pigtail and temporary pacemaker placement.

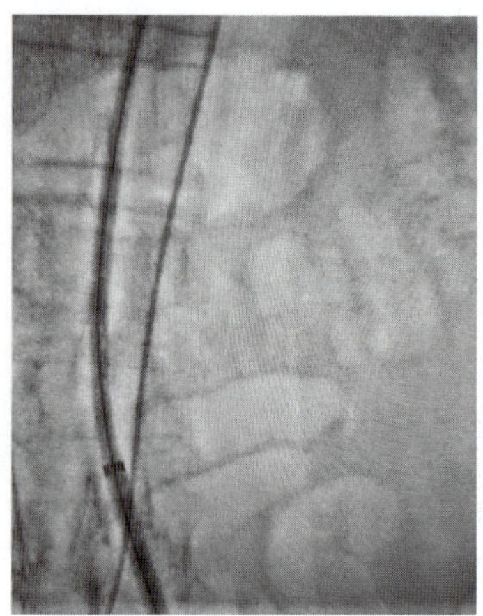

Fig. 3: Sheath advancement.

CROSSING THE VALVE AND PLACEMENT OF THE STIFF WIRE

Aortic valve crossing is a scientific process rather than a blind procedure. Calcification on the leaflets helps identify the opening. An AL-1 catheter is oriented to the opening and path of the jet, identified by the bobbing of the catheter. A straight tip wire is used to cross the aortic valve, with the AL-1 catheter rotated to aid in crossing **(Fig. 4A)**. Cusp overlap view helps in difficult situations. Keeping the crossing catheter inside the pigtail parked in the noncoronary cusp also assists in crossing. In challenging anatomies, changing to an AL-2, AR-1, or rarely JR can be helpful. In extreme situations, one should be prepared to cross integrate after performing a transseptal puncture.

Once the valve is crossed, a 260 cm Teflon wire is placed inside the left ventricular (LV). A 5 F pigtail catheter is advanced over the wire to the apex of the LV, ensuring the catheter is not behind the submitral apparatus **(Fig. 4B)**. A hemodynamic study is performed, and a pre-shaped stiff wire is safely placed inside the LV cavity **(Fig. 4C)**.

PREDILATATION

Not all valves require predilatation. Predilatation is advisable for self-expandable valves, horizontal aorta, bicuspid aortic valves, critical aortic stenosis, to determine the interaction of the leaflets with the coronary arteries, and to assess the size in bicuspid aortic stenosis. The balloon is sized based on the short-axis diameter of the annulus. The aim of predilatation is to make the valve entry inside the annulus smooth and to allow the self-expandable valve to deploy smoothly. A large balloon is used for accurate

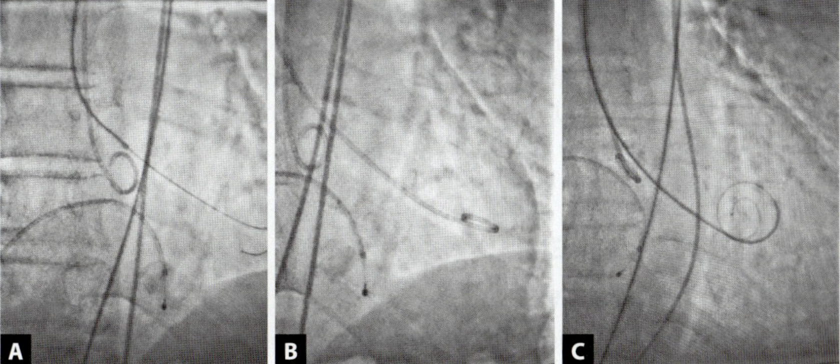

Figs. 4A to C: (A) AL-1 straight tip wire and valve crossing; (B) Pigtail placement in left ventricular (LV); C) Pre-shaped stiff wire placed.

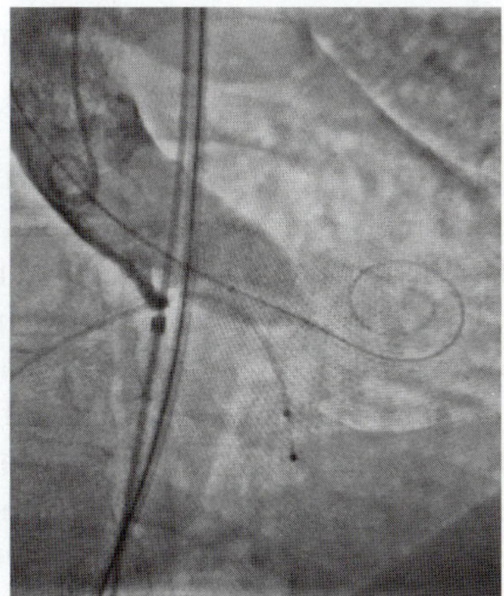

Fig. 5: Predilatation with fluoroscopic image.

neo platform valve deployment. Inject contrast at the peak of balloon expansion to assess sizing and coronary occlusion **(Fig. 5)**.

VALVE ADVANCEMENT

Different valves have different specifications. Most self-expandable valves have inline sheaths. The 14 F sheath is removed, and the self-expandable valve is advanced using its inline sheath. At this point, focus on the wire in the left ventricle, not the valve advancement, unless there is resistance in the valve system advancement. Advance the valve, keeping in mind the commissural alignment.

For the balloon-expandable valve, mounted directly on the balloon, advance with the utilization of a flexion handle as it crosses the arch. The Edwards valve, where the balloon and the valve are separate, is advanced into the straight portion of the thoracic aorta. Remove the parallax in the valve frame by going cranial. Pull the balloon inside the valve frame using the knobs. Align the proximal, middle, and distal markers on the balloon to the top, middle, and distal end of the valve frame correctly. Advance the valve across the arch using the flexion handle in the LAO view (keeping the arch and the wire in the LV in the same field of view).

VALVE DEPLOYMENT

Self-expandable Valves

Advance the valve across the annulus. Confirm pigtail position at the annulus level with an aortogram. Incorrect pigtail position leads to improper deployment. Current generation self-expandable valves are stable during deployment with minimal movement. Markers 3 mm from the lower end of the valve frame are placed at the level of the annulus **(Figs. 6A and B)**. Deploy the valve slowly to open the lower end and make small adjustments to balance valve movement inside or outside.[4]

Once the valve is opened to the third node for the Evolut platform, initiate rapid pacing (at 140 bpm). Open the valve further. The lower end of the frame contacts the annulus. Blood pressure drops as the supra-annular TAVR valve is still constrained inside the frame. Open the valve further until blood pressure normalizes and there is a gap between the capsule marker and the black knob. Stop pacing and remove parallax at the lower end of the valve frame. Perform an aortogram to assess the depth on the noncoronary side, then in the LAO view to assess the depth on the left coronary side. If depth is unsatisfactory (good depth is 3–5 mm), recapture and reposition the valve. Once the position is correct, release the valve. Ensure the delivery system is centered in the aorta. The first operator maintains a forward push while the second operator performs a slow release. Ensure all paddles are released. Pull back the stiff wire to centralize the nose cone, pull the nose cone inside the valve, and push the wire back into the ventricle. Pull the system back into the thoracic aorta and recapture the nose cone. Remove the device and reintroduce the 14 F sheath. Perform hemodynamic

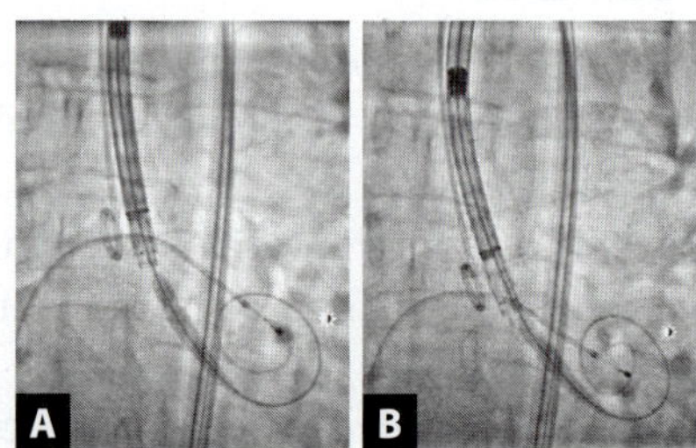

Figs. 6A and B: Pigtail in noncoronary cusp, valve deployment initiated in cusp overlap, and markers aligned with pigtail.

assessment and aortogram. Consider postdilatation in the presence of more than trivial aortic regurgitation (AR) and residual gradient after waiting for 10 minutes. Reintroduce the reshaped wire and select a postdilatation balloon size based on the perimeter-derived diameter. Choose a 6 cm long balloon for stability. Extend the balloon into the left ventricular outflow tract (LVOT) and initiate rapid pacing at 180–200 bpm for postdilatation. Remove the balloon and perform repeat hemodynamics and aortogram.

BALLOON-EXPANDABLE VALVES

Advance the balloon-expandable valve into the annular plane. Confirm pigtail position. For the Edwards valve, pull the pusher proximal to the second marker level.[5] For Myval, directly mounted on the balloon, no such maneuver is required. Identify the first light band on the Myval and the faint line on the Edwards valve, and place them at the pigtail level **(Figs. 7A and B)**. Initiate rapid pacing at 180–200 bpm. Notice a drop in mean arterial pressure (MAP) below 70 and deploy the valve with slow inflation. Complete the inflation if there is no movement in valve position and hold for 3–5 seconds at peak inflation. Deflate and remove the balloon. When the balloon is no longer in contact with the valve frame, stop pacing. The balloon delivery system can be pulled out or kept in the ascending aorta with the wire centralized to assess the need for post-dilatation. If postdilatation is required, add additional volume to the balloon and inflate inside the valve. Remove the valve delivery system. Advance the pigtail inside the left ventricle and remove the stiff wire. Perform hemodynamic assessment. Conduct a final aortogram after removing the parallax of the valve frame. Sometimes, perform an aortogram in the LAO-cranial view to assess the left main coronary artery.

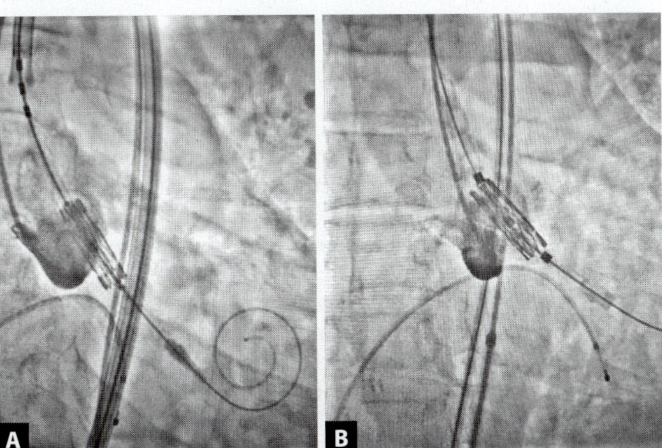

Figs. 7A and B: (A) Edward sapiens valve position based on faint line; (B) Myval placed based on first light band.

VASCULAR CLOSURE

A dilator is placed inside the sheath. Identify the ProGlide threads. Gently pull the blue thread to deliver the knot onto the sheath. Pull out the sheath with the wire in place. Pull the ProGlide thread to deliver the knot onto the wire. Perform a digital subtraction angiography (DSA) from the pigtail on the other side to assess the pelvic and femoral vasculature. Pull the wire, tighten, and cut the knot. Administer protamine according to heparin administered and ACT and apply manual pressure. Depending on the residual flow after deploying the first ProGlide and absence of vascular pinching, a second vascular closure device can be used.

MANAGEMENT OF HOSTILE ACCESS

A crossover 0.018 inch 260 cm wire placed from the contralateral side can be tracked in the SFA. Alternatively, ipsilateral SFA access can be obtained with a micropuncture and micropuncture sheath placed in situ for managing vascular access complications.

FINAL ASSESSMENT

Perform an echo in the cath laboratory at the end of the procedure to assess the pericardial space, valve hemodynamics, and ejection fraction. Remove the temporary pacemaker (TMP) on the table for most patients. However, in patients with the right bundle branch block (RBBB), left bundle branch block (LBBB), complete heart block (CHB) following TAVR, or deep implantation, the TPM should be left in place and removed as per the clinical situation.

CONCLUSION

TAVR has revolutionized the management of native and bioprosthetic aortic stenosis. Proper techniques and skills can produce better outcomes of this procedure.

REFERENCES

1. Cribier A, Eltchaninoff H, Bash A, Borenstein N, Tron C, Bauer F, et al. Percutaneous transcatheter implantation of an aortic valve prosthesis for calcific aortic stenosis: First human case description. Circulation 2002;106:3006-8.
2. Wenaweser P, Stortecky S, Heg D, et al. Short-term clinical outcomes among patients undergoing transcatheter aortic valve implantation in Switzerland: the Swiss TAVI registry. EuroIntervention. 2014;10(8):982-9.
3. Biasco L, Ferrari E, Pedrazzini G, et al. Access sites for TAVI: patient selection criteria, technical aspects, and outcomes. Front Cardiovasc Med. 2018;5:88.
4. Zaid S, Attizzani GF, Krishnamoorthy P, Yoon SH, Dallan LAP, Chetcuti S, et al. First-in-Human Multicenter Experience of the Newest Generation Supra-Annular Self-Expanding Evolut FX TAVR System. JACC Cardiovasc. Interv. 2023;16:1626-35.
5. Zaid S, Atkins MD, Kleiman NS, Reardon MJ, Tang GHL. What's New with TAVR? An Update on Device Technology. Methodist DeBakey Cardiovasc J. 2023;19:4-14.

CHAPTER 44

Transcatheter Aortic Valve Replacement: Complications and Management

Bagirath Raghuraman, Sabarish Sankaran

INTRODUCTION

Earlier surgical aortic valve replacement (SAVR) was the only definitive treatment available for patients with severe aortic stenosis (AS). Since its inception in 2002 transcatheter aortic valve implantation (TAVI) has grown leaps and bounds in offering remarkable hemodynamic improvement and symptomatic relief in suitable patients with AS. With the ever-advancing field of TAVI, it becomes important to promptly recognize and treat the procedural complications associated with it.

MORTALITY RATES

Based on data collected from various TAVI registries, the periprocedural mortality for TAVI varies between 1.1% and 4.2%. Complications warranting conversion of TAVI to open heart surgery is up to 1.4%. However, emergency conversion to open heart surgery has a 30-day mortality rate as high as 45.8%.[1-5]

PARAVALVULAR LEAK

It can be due to under expansion of the valve, malposition of the valve, or error in sizing of the valve. Moderate-to-severe paravalvular leak (PVL) warrants intervention since it is associated with increased mortality. Based on recent trials and registry data, in newer generation valves the incidence of significant PVL varies from 0.8% to 3.4%. Incidence of mild PVL can be as high as 40%, which may be of importance in younger patients with a longer life expectancy. However, more research is needed to provide definitive evidence regarding this.[2,6-8]

Paravalvular leak is typically assessed during postprocedure aortic root angiography or by echocardiography. Retraction of the guidewire or pigtail can help avoid spurious overestimation of PVL. Aortic regurgitation index (ARI) inversely correlates with severity of PVL. ARI less than 25 is a predictor of 1-year mortality in case of PVL. Diastolic pressure can roughly indicate the degree of AR [ARI = 100 × diastolic blood pressure (DBP) – left ventricular end-diastolic pressure (LVEDP)/systolic blood pressure (SBP)].[9,10]

Paravalvular leak from under expansion of valve is managed by postdilatation. If PVL is due to malposition of the valve, a valve in valve procedure is considered.[11]

ANNULAR RUPTURE

It is a life-threatening complication, which can occur after implantation of a balloon expandable valve or during aggressive pre- or postdilatation.

Four types of rupture can occur—(i) intra-annular, (2) subannular, (3) supra-annular, and (4) combined. Risk factors for rupture include a small annulus size (<20 mm) or Sino tubular junction, heavily calcified valve, asymmetric subaortic LV hypertrophy, device oversizing (>20%), and bicuspid valve. Annular rupture can lead to formation of hematoma, which in turn can compress a coronary artery.

Management includes conversion to an open procedure with aortic valve replacement and root reconstruction. Emergency pericardial drainage with autotransfusion should be initiated. In case of high-risk anatomic features, a self-expandable valve is preferred.

Subtle signs of aortic injury such as effusion in the transverse sinus, subepicardial hematoma at the base of the heart, periaortic hematoma, contained or extending aortic dissection should be looked for. Very rarely percutaneous bail out measures such as use of vascular plugs, embolization coils, vascular occlusion device, and implantation of second valve can be considered in cases with prohibitive surgical risk.[12,13]

CORONARY ARTERY OBSTRUCTION

It occurs in less than 1% of TAVI procedures and the incidence increases up to 3.5% for valve in valve procedures. It is more common with low coronary ostial heights (<10 mm), heavy asymmetric valve calcification, and narrow sinus of Valsalva. The left main coronary artery is more commonly involved than the right coronary artery. It is caused by native leaflets or device material. It mainly depends on the final position of displaced bioprosthetic leaflets after the valve in valve implantation **(Fig. 1)**. It presents with hypotension and electrocardiogram (ECG) changes.[14]

In patients with high risk for coronary obstruction, the use of a partially or fully recapturable valve (Evolut-R/PRO, Portico, Lotus) or valve with open cell design (ACURATE neo or NAVITOR) may be advantageous. Immediate angiographic assessment followed by percutaneous coronary intervention (PCI) or coronary artery bypass grafting (CABG) might be required.

Prophylactic placement of a coronary guidewire with or without undeployed stent can be considered in high-risk cases **(Fig. 2)**. Undeployed stent is placed distally in the coronary artery and can be retracted and implanted halfway between the TAVI valve and proximal coronary

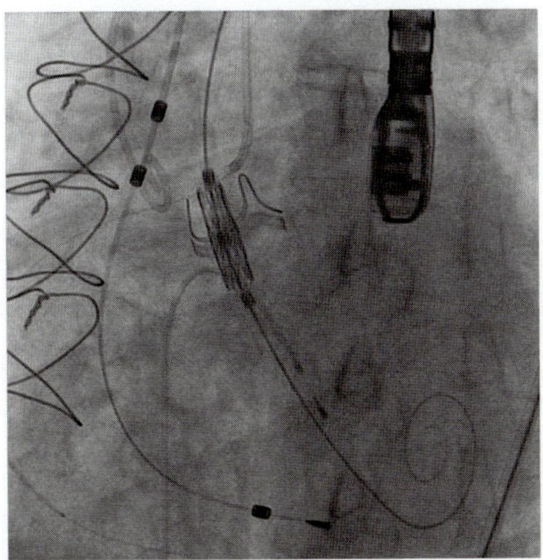

Fig. 1: Valve-in-valve transcatheter heart valve (THV) implantation.

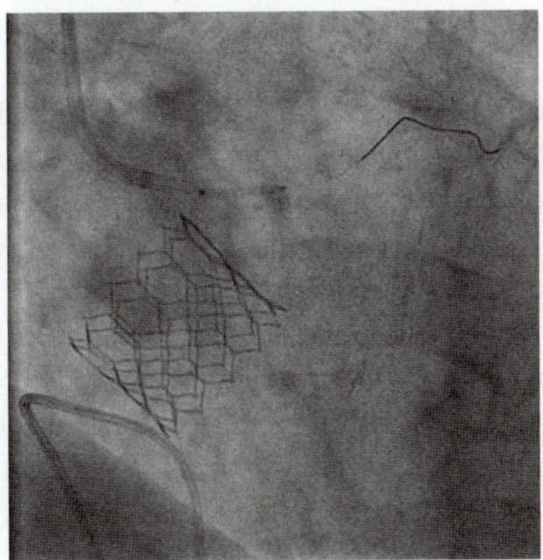

Fig. 2: Coronary protection with left main coronary artery (LMCA) stenting post-transcatheter aortic valve implantation (TAVI).

artery—CHIMNEY or SNORKEL technique. Adequate stent expansion could be a problem in this case. If post-dilatation is required simultaneous kissing balloon inflation of TAVI valve and stent is done. Since the stent protrudes into the aorta, prolonged dual antiplatelet therapy (DAPT) is required.

BASILICA technique is another prophylactic strategy to prevent coronary artery obstruction. Recent reports from BASILICA registry show promising outcomes with this technique.[15]

VALVE EMBOLIZATION

It occurs in approximately 1% of cases. Valve can embolize either toward the aorta or into the LV cavity **(Fig. 3)**. It usually occurs during or immediately

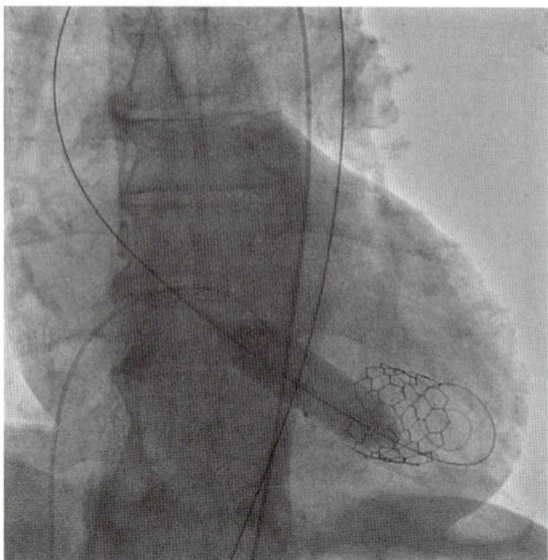

Fig. 3: Valve embolized into the left ventricle (LV) during deployment.

after valve deployment. Late device migration (up to 1 year) has also been reported.[16]

Factors related to valve embolization includes noncalcified native leaflets, eccentric or asymmetric leaflet calcification, preexisting aortic regurgitation, and acute aortic angulation. Technical factors such as failure of rapid ventricular pacing during valve deployment can cause valve embolization. After deployment, caution should be advised while retracting the nose cone or the jailed pigtail, which should be removed with the aid of a 0.035″ wire.[17]

Embolization into the LV requires open surgical repair. In case of low position in left ventricular outflow tract (LVOT) of a self-expanding valve worsening of preexisting mitral regurgitation (MR) can be observed. In case of heavy calcifications of anterior mitral leaflet such as in rheumatic heart disease, there can be worsening of mitral stenosis.

In case of aortic embolization, the first valve can be fixed by a second valve implanted in an appropriate location. In case of embolization with coronary obstruction, immediate proximal retraction of the device should be done.

In case of extensive embolization, repositioning can be attempted using snares or an inflated balloon to move and deploy the valve in an ectopic location preferably in the descending aorta distal to the left subclavian artery **(Fig. 4)**. A covered or uncovered stent within the embolized valve leaflets can be done to fix the valve against the aortic wall.[18]

ATRIOVENTRICULAR CONDUCTION DISTURBANCE AND ARRHYTHMIAS

Individualized risk stratification can identify patients at high risk for developing atrioventricular (AV) block during TAVI. Patient-related factors include preexisting right bundle branch block and prolonged PR interval.

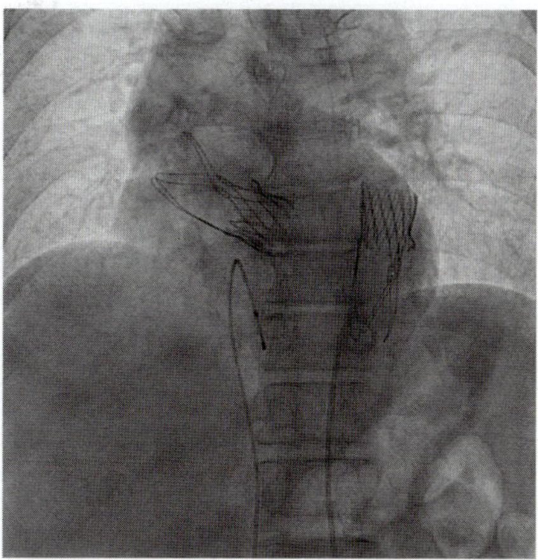

Fig. 4: Embolized valve during transcatheter aortic valve implantation (TAVI) pulled down and deployed in descending aorta with second valve deployed across the annulus.

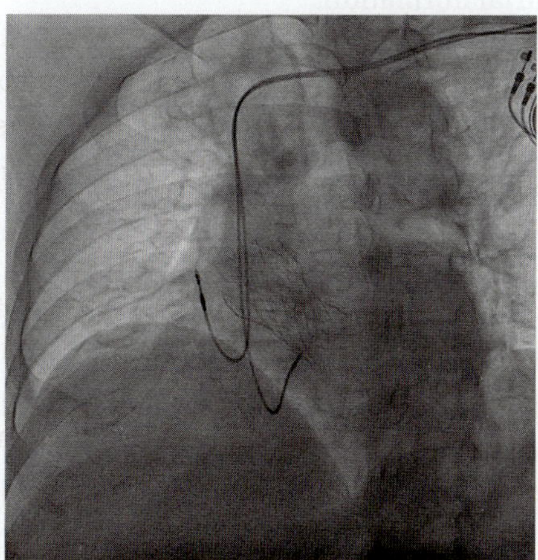

Fig. 5: Transcatheter aortic valve implantation (TAVI) and permanent pacemaker implantation (PPI) due to complete heart block (CHB) postprocedure.

Anatomical factors include increased calcium burden particularly in the device landing zone and LVOT. Procedural factors include deep implantation of the valve.[19]

The overall incidence is higher for self-expanding valves (up to 17.4%) compared to balloon expandable valves (up to 6.5%). It tends to occur within 24 hours of valve deployment. It can develop later than 48 hours or even during postdischarge follow-up. High degree AV block requires permanent pacemaker implantation **(Fig. 5)**.[20]

New onset atrial fibrillation is seen in up to 7.2% of patients undergoing TAVR. Patients with enlarged left atrium, transapical route, and aggressive

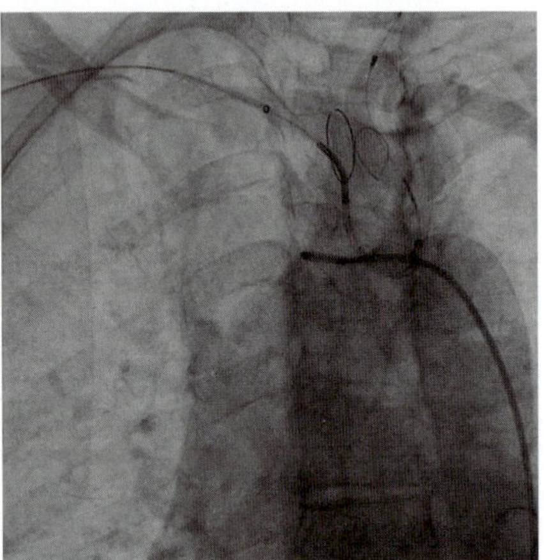

Fig. 6: Cerebral protection with sentinel device.

balloon postdilatation tend to be at increased risk. There is no correlation between PVL and atrial fibrillation.

STROKE

It most commonly occurs during the procedure or within 24–48 hours following the procedure.

The rate of post-TAVI stroke can be up to 2%. Silent ischemic events can be detected in up to 80% of patients undergoing TAVI.[21,22]

Procedural factors include embolization of debris, prolonged hypotension, postdilatation, and inadequate anticoagulation during the procedure. Patient factors include presence of atrial fibrillation, prior history of stroke, and chronic kidney disease. Anatomic factors include heavily calcified aortic valve and severe mitral stenosis.[23]

Role of cerebral embolic protection devices is controversial **(Fig. 6)**. Based on a meta-analysis of multiple large randomized trials, the rates of stroke tend to be similar in groups with and without embolic protection devices. However, in selected subgroups such as younger individuals, bicuspid aortic valve, and valve in valve, it might prove to be of benefit.

ACCESS SITE AND VASCULAR COMPLICATIONS

Risk for bleeding from access site or other access site-related complications include larger sheath to artery ratio, circumferential calcification, excessive tortuosity, and failure of vascular access closure devices.[24]

At the end of the procedure, angiography of access site from contralateral side is done to confirm hemostasis. Continuous access to the punctured artery is essential. This is ensured either via contralateral access or by maintaining antegrade access with wire. In case of perforation, contralateral access allows

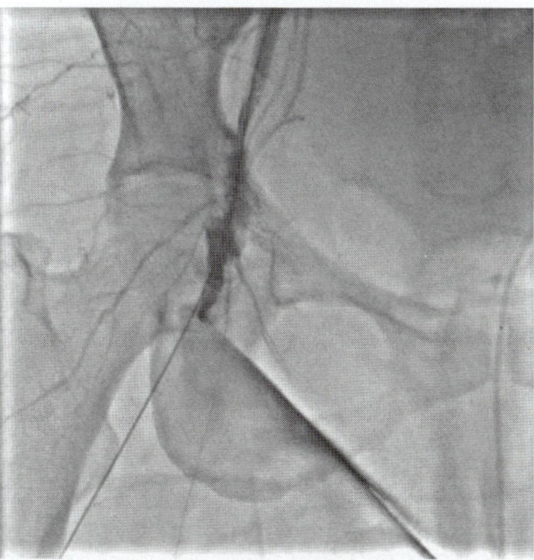

Fig. 7: Femoral artery perforation from transcatheter aortic valve implantation (TAVI) access site.

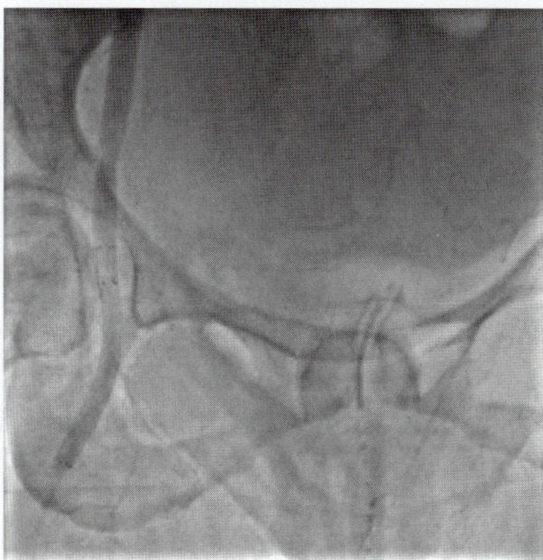

Fig. 8: Femoral artery perforation treated with covered stent.

balloon tamponade followed by deployment of a covered stent for the same **(Figs.7 and 8)**.[25]

Aortic dissection or perforation is a life-threatening complication **(Fig. 9)**. It can be caused by manipulation of guidewire or delivery system, valve recapture, and repositioning. It requires conversion to open heart surgery.

■ ACUTE KIDNEY INJURY

It is classified as stage 1 to stage 3 depending on relative or absolute elevation of serum creatinine up to 7 days following TAVI. Patients requiring dialysis are classified as stage 3 irrespective of the creatinine value. Transapical TAVI

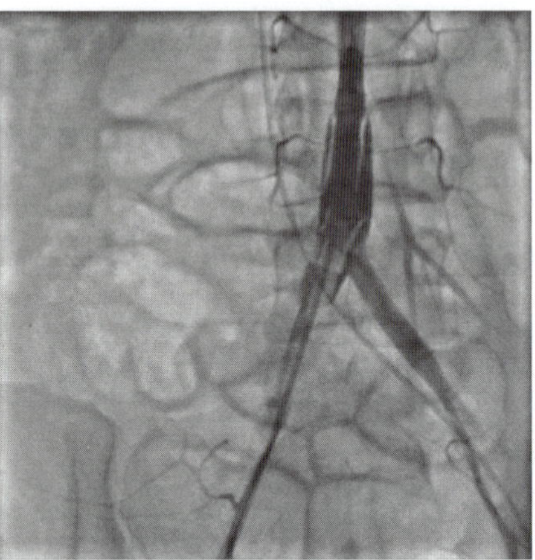

Fig. 9: Aorto iliac dissection during transcatheter aortic valve implantation (TAVI) probably due to the manipulation of guidewire or delivery system.

tends to have slightly higher incidence of acute kidney injury (AKI) compared to transfemoral route (8% vs. 3%).[26]

Acute kidney injury tends to be associated with up to fivefold increase in mortality at 30 days and 1 year following TAVI. Cause tends to be multifactorial namely diabetes mellitus, chronic kidney disease, peripheral vascular disease, embolization of debris, hypotension during rapid ventricular pacing, and multiple blood transfusions.

Ensuring adequate hydration, minimizing contrast, avoiding nephrotoxic drugs, allowing adequate time between preprocedural work-up and procedure can help reduce incidence of AKI. Alternative imaging modalities such as magnetic resonance imaging (MRI) can be utilized in patients with known kidney disease.[27]

SHOCK

It frequently occurs during the procedure or immediately following the procedure. The causes can be grouped as follows:

- Volume loss—secondary to vascular complication
- Mechanical causes—cardiac tamponade, severe MR, severe AR, and suicidal left ventricle
- Arrhythmias—asystole, high degree AV block, and VT/VF
- Reflexes—vagal response and reduced sympathetic tone from anesthesia

Suicidal left ventricle occurs due to the dynamic intraventricular gradient (DIG). In case of chronically increased afterload, the LV adapts by increase in the wall thickness. When the obstruction at the level of aortic valve gets suddenly relieved, the hypercontractile LV creates a dynamic intraventricular gradient, leading to circulatory collapse. This is prevented by ensuring adequate hydration and use of beta-blockers.

Treatment is done by administering vasoconstrictors such as phenylephrine, avoiding inotropes, and RV pacing which relieves the dynamic LVOT obstruction. In refractory cases, intra-arterial balloon counterpulsation, alcohol septal ablation, and extracorporeal membrane oxygenation (ECMO) can be done to buy time for the LV to adapt and recover.[28,29]

VALVE THROMBOSIS AND OBSTRUCTION

Symptomatic valve thrombosis is very rare and can occur in up to 1% of patients undergoing TAVI. It presents with dyspnea on exertion and increased gradient across the valve. Thrombus is usually not visualized on echocardiography.[30]

Post procedure Aortic valve gradient more than 20 mm Hg or increase in gradient by 10 mm Hg can herald valve thrombosis. Subclinical thrombosis is associated with an increased rate of stroke or transient ischemic attack. The valve leaflet thickening detected in computed tomography (CT) is referred to as hypoattenuating leaflet thickening (HALT).[31-33]

Valve hemodynamic deterioration (VHD) is characterized by an increase in mean transvalvular gradient by more than 10 mm Hg between discharge and follow-up. Absence of anticoagulation at discharge, valve in valve procedure, valve size ≤23 mm, increased body mass index (BMI), female sex, younger age, low ejection fraction, atrial fibrillation, severe MR, or tricuspid regurgitation (TR) can all predispose to valve deterioration.

PROSTHETIC VALVE ENDOCARDITIS

Endocarditis after TAVI can be early (within 60 days), intermediate (between 60 and 365 days), or late (after 365 days). It can result in aortic root or paravalvular abscess, valve stenosis, embolic event, valvular or paravalvular regurgitation, and concomitant mitral valve insufficiency. It can result in heart failure.[34]

Rates of early PVE can vary between 0.3% and 3.4%. In-hospital mortality for patients with PVE can be as high as 47.2%. Prosthetic valve endocarditis (PVE) requires antibiotic treatment, valve in valve implantation, or surgical intervention. Antibiotic prophylaxis for endocarditis is suggested for high-risk procedures after TAVI.[35]

REFERENCES

1. Carroll JD, Mack MJ, Vemulapalli S, Herrmann HC, Gleason TG, Hanzel G, et al. STS-ACC TVT Registry of Transcatheter Aortic Valve Replacement. J Am Coll Cardiol. 2020;76(21):2492-516.
2. Kim W-K, Möllmann H, Liebetrau C, Renker M, Rolf A, Simon P, et al. The ACURATE neo Transcatheter Heart Valve: A Comprehensive Analysis of Predictors of Procedural Outcome. JACC Cardiovasc Interv. 2018;11(17):1721-9.

3. Leon MB, Smith CR, Mack MJ, Makkar RR, Svensson LG, Kodali SK, et al.; PARTNER 2 Investigators. Transcatheter or Surgical Aortic-Valve Replacement in Intermediate-Risk Patients. N Engl J Med. 2016;374(17):1609-20.
4. Reardon MJ, Van Mieghem NM, Popma JJ, Kleiman NS, Søndergaard L, Mumtaz M, et al.; SURTAVI Investigators. Surgical or transcatheter aortic-valve replacement in intermediate-risk patients. N Engl J Med. 2017;376(14): 1321-31.
5. Smith CR, Leon MB, Mack MJ, Miller DC, Moses JW, Svensson LG, et al.; PARTNER Trial Investigators. Transcatheter versus surgical aortic-valve replacement in high-risk patients. N Engl J Med. 2011;364(23):2187-98.
6. Athappan G, Patvardhan E, Tuzcu EM, Svensson LG, Lemos PA, Fraccaro C, et al. Incidence, predictors, and outcomes of aortic regurgitation after transcatheter aortic valve replacement: meta-analysis and systematic review of literature. J Am Coll Cardiol. 2013;61(15):1585-95.
7. Binder RK, Webb JG, Toggweiler S, Freeman M, Barbanti M, Willson AB, et al. Impact of post-implant SAPIEN XT geometry and position on conduction disturbances, hemodynamic performance, and paravalvular regurgitation. JACC. Cardiovascular Interventions. 2013;6(5):462-8.
8. Dworakowski R, Wendler O, Halliday B, Ludman P, DeBelder M, Ray S, et al. Device-dependent association between paravalvar aortic regurgitation and outcome after TAVI. Heart (British Cardiac Society). 2014;100(24):1939-45.
9. Kodali S, Pibarot P, Douglas PS, Williams M, Xu K, Thourani V, et al. Paravalvular regurgitation after transcatheter aortic valve replacement with the Edwards sapien valve in the PARTNER trial: characterizing patients and impact on outcomes. Eur Heart J. 2015;36(7):449-56.
10. Pibarot P, Hahn RT, Weissman NJ, Monaghan MJ. Assessment of paravalvular regurgitation following TAVR: a proposal of unifying grading scheme. JACC Cardiovasc Imaging. 2015;8(3):340-60.
11. Van Belle E, Juthier F, Susen S, Vincentelli A, Iung B, Dallongeville J, et al.; FRANCE 2 Investigators. Postprocedural aortic regurgitation in balloon-expandable and self-expandable transcatheter aortic valve replacement procedures: analysis of predictors and impact on long-term mortality: insights from the FRANCE2 Registry. Circulation. 2014;129(13):15-1427.
12. Aminian A, Lalmand J, Dolatabadi D. Late contained aortic root rupture and ventricular septal defect after transcatheter aortic valve implantation. Catheter Cardiovasc Interv. 2013;81(1):E72-5.
13. Pasic M, Unbehaun A, Buz S, Drews T, Hetzer R. Annular rupture during transcatheter aortic valve replacement: classification, pathophysiology, diagnostics, treatment approaches, and prevention. JACC Cardiovasc Interv. 2015;8(1 Pt A):1-9.
14. Dvir D, Leipsic J, Blanke P, Ribeiro HB, Kornowski R, Pichard A, et al. Coronary obstruction in transcatheter aortic valve-in-valve implantation: preprocedural evaluation, device selection, protection, and treatment. Circ Cardiovasc Interv. 2015;8(1):e002079.
15. Ribeiro HB, Nombela-Franco L, Urena M, Mok M, Pasian S, Doyle D, et al. Coronary obstruction following transcatheter aortic valve implantation: a systematic review. JACC Cardiovasc Interv. 2013;6(5):452-61.

16. Clavel M-A, Dumont E, Pibarot P, Doyle D, De Larochellière R, Villeneuve J, et al. Severe valvular regurgitation and late prosthesis embolization after percutaneous aortic valve implantation. Ann Thorac Surg. 2009;87(2):618-21.
17. Meredith Am IT, Walters DL, Dumonteil N, Worthley SG, Tchétché D, Manoharan G, et al. Transcatheter aortic valve replacement for severe symptomatic aortic stenosis using a repositionable valve system: 30-day primary endpoint results from the REPRISE II study. J Am Coll Cardiol. 2014: 64(13):1339-48.
18. Pang PYK, Chiam PTL, Chua YL, Sin YK. A survivor of late prosthesis migration and rotation following percutaneous transcatheter aortic valve implantation. Eur J Cardiothorac Surg. 2012;41(5):1195-96.
19. Koos R, Mahnken AH, Aktug O, Dohmen G, Autschbach R, Marx N, et al. Electrocardiographic and imaging predictors for permanent pacemaker requirement after transcatheter aortic valve implantation. J Heart Valve Disease. 2011;20(1):83-90.
20. Mouillet G, Lellouche N, Yamamoto M, Oguri A, Dubois-Rande J-L, Van Belle E, et al. Outcomes following pacemaker implantation after transcatheter aortic valve implantation with CoreValve(®) devices: Results from the FRANCE 2 Registry. Catheter Cardiovasc Interv. 2015;86(3):E158-166.
21. Daneault B, Kirtane AJ, Kodali SK, Williams MR, Genereux P, Reiss GR, et al. Stroke associated with surgical and transcatheter treatment of aortic stenosis: a comprehensive review. J Am Coll Cardiol. 2011;58(21):2143-50.
22. Kahlert P, Knipp SC, Schlamann M, Thielmann M, Al-Rashid F, Weber M, et al. Silent and apparent cerebral ischemia after percutaneous transfemoral aortic valve implantation: a diffusion-weighted magnetic resonance imaging study. Circulation. 2010;121(7):870-8.
23. Athappan G, Gajulapalli RD, Sengodan P, Bhardwaj A, Ellis SG, Svensson L, et al. Influence of transcatheter aortic valve replacement strategy and valve design on stroke after transcatheter aortic valve replacement: a meta-analysis and systematic review of literature. J Am Coll Cardiol. 2014;63(20):2101-10.
24. Généreux P, Cohen DJ, Mack M, Rodes-Cabau J, Yadav M, Xu K, et al. Incidence, predictors, and prognostic impact of late bleeding complications after transcatheter aortic valve replacement. J Am Coll Cardiol. 2014;64(24):2605-15.
25. Sedaghat A, Neumann N, Schahab N, Sinning J-M, Hammerstingl C, Pingel S, et al. Routine endovascular treatment with a stent graft for access-site and access-related vascular injury in transfemoral transcatheter aortic valve implantation. Circ Cardiovasc Interv. 2016;9(8):e003834.
26. Bagur R, Webb JG, Nietlispach F, Dumont E, De Larochellière R, Doyle D, et al. Acute kidney injury following transcatheter aortic valve implantation: predictive factors, prognostic value, and comparison with surgical aortic valve replacement. Eur Heart J. 2010;31(7):865-74.
27. Barbanti M, Gulino S, Capranzano P, Immè S, Sgroi C, Tamburino C, et al. Acute kidney injury with the renalguard system in patients undergoing transcatheter aortic valve replacement: The PROTECT-TAVI Trial (PROphylactic effecT of furosEmide-induCed diuresis with matched isotonic intravenous hydraTion in Transcatheter Aortic Valve Implantation). JACC Cardiovasc Interv. 2015;8(12):1595-604.

28. Sobczyk D. Dynamic left ventricular outflow tract obstruction: underestimated cause of hypotension and hemodynamic instability. J Ultrason. 2014;14(59): 421-7.
29. Koliastasis L, Drakopoulou M, Latsios G, Apostolos A, Ktenopoulos N, Katsaros O, et al. Overcoming the obstacle of suicide left ventricle after transcatheter aortic valve replacement phenomenon. JACC Case Rep. 2023; 26:102065.
30. De Marchena E, Mesa J, Pomenti S, Marin Y Kall C, Marincic X, Yahagi K, et al. Thrombus formation following transcatheter aortic valve replacement. JACC Cardiovasc Interv. 2015;8(5):728-39.
31. Jose J, Sulimov DS, El-Mawardy M, Sato T, Allali A, Holy EW, et al. Clinical bioprosthetic heart valve thrombosis after transcatheter aortic valve replacement: incidence, Characteristics, and Treatment Outcomes. JACC Cardiovasc Interv. 2017;10(7):686-97.
32. Latib A, Naganuma T, Abdel-Wahab M, Danenberg H, Cota L, Barbanti M, et al. Treatment and clinical outcomes of transcatheter heart valve thrombosis. Circ Cardiovasc Interv. 2015;8(4):e001779.
33. Sondergaard L, Sigitas C, Chopra M, Bieliauskas G, De Backer O. Leaflet Thrombosis after TAVI. European Heart Journal. 2017;38(36):2702-3.
34. Amat-Santos IJ, Messika-Zeitoun D, Eltchaninoff H, Kapadia S, Lerakis S, Cheema AN, et al. Infective endocarditis after transcatheter aortic valve implantation: results from a large multicenter registry. Circulation. 2015; 131(18):1566-74.
35. Latib A, Naim C, De Bonis M, Sinning JM, Maisano F, Barbanti M, et al. TAVR-associated prosthetic valve infective endocarditis: Results of a large, multicenter registry. J Am Coll Cardiol. 2014;64(20):2176-8.

CHAPTER 45

Transcatheter Mitral Valve Replacement: Step-by-Step Approach

Haresh Mehta

INTRODUCTION

Mitral valve disease is the most common cardiac valve condition, with the prevalence of stenosis or regurgitation increasing with age and estimated to be 9.5% in the general population above the age of 75.[1] Treatment for severe mitral valve disease includes surgical mitral valve repair with or without annuloplasty ring, or replacement with either tissue or mechanical prosthesis. Patients receiving mitral bioprosthesis are older compared to mechanical prosthesis due to age and comorbidities that make lifelong anticoagulation high risk. However, the estimated lifespan of a bioprosthetic valve is 10–12 years, and thus this population may require repeat intervention.[2] Mechanisms of prosthesis failure may include degeneration of leaflet tissue, thrombosis, pannus formation, and endocarditis. Repeat mitral valve replacement is associated with increased morbidity and mortality, with highest risk in those over 75 or having multiple repeat replacements. Because of the risks in this population, percutaneous mitral valve-in-valve or valve-in-ring interventions are being increasingly done for patients at prohibitive surgical risk with prosthetic valve or annuloplasty dysfunction.

Compared to transcatheter aortic valve replacement (TAVR), transcatheter mitral valve replacement (TMVR) is more challenging, since the mitral valve is larger, less calcific, and experiences more hemodynamic stress than aortic valve. This renders the principle of passive fixation of the transcatheter heart valve (THV) by radial strength used in TAVR, insufficient for use at mitral valve and creates need for active fixation mechanisms to prevent embolization. TMVR is of four types: valve-in-valve (ViV), valve-in-ring (ViR), valve-in-MAC (ViMAC), and valve in native annulus. ViV TMVR is technically easier, more frequently performed, and has shown the most favorable results till now. The degenerated bioprosthetic valve acts as an anchoring point for the transcatheter valve. This helps in avoiding any complications associated with TMVR in native mitral annulus position.[3] The Food and Drug Administration (FDA) approved the SAPIEN valve for the treatment of bioprosthetic mitral valve failure in 2017. ViR TMVR is much more complex due to varying types of rings. It is not easy to identify each ring directly from its fluoroscopic appearance. Incomplete rings/bands and rigid rings cannot become circular whereas semirigid and flexible rings can become circular. When a ring cannot become circular, the THV is either going to be under expanded or become deformed, resulting in suboptimal result. Apart from the ability to become circular, the ring should also be able to provide a secure anchor otherwise the THV will embolize. Incomplete rings cannot provide a good anchor. Semirigid rings are best of both and provide a good anchor as well as having the ability to become circular or near circular. ViR TMVR remains a more investigational procedure involving off-label use of transcatheter aortic valves. Patients with symptomatic severe mitral valve disease due to severe mitral annular calcification (MAC) are often elderly with multiple comorbidities and are at high surgical risk due to technical challenges secondary to severe calcification. ViMAC TMVR provides an alternative for this subgroup, but at least 270° circumferential calcium and computed tomography (CT)-based MAC score ≥7 is required for procedural success and lower embolization risk. This criterion is met in only about 1% of these patients rendering majority of cases of severe MAC anatomically unsuitable for TMVR.

Although other valves have been used in the past, currently balloon expandable transaortic valves, Edwards SAPIEN (Edwards LifeSciences Corp., Irvine, CA, USA), and Myval (Meril Life) are being primarily used as repurposed THVs for ViV, ViR, and ViMAC cases. Dedicated transcatheter mitral valve devices such as AltaValve (AltaValve early feasibility study), Cardiovalve (AHEAD EU and AHEAD US EFS trials), Evoque (Edwards EVOQUE TMVR early feasibility study), Tiara (TIARA II extended early feasibility study), Tendyne (SUMMIT trial), M3 (ENCIRCLE trial), and intrepid (APOLLO study) are in study for TMVR in native annulus for ≥3+ MR. The tendyne device received the CE mark approval in 2020 (first TMVR system approved for clinical use in Europe). The ongoing SUMMIT trial is aiming to compare TMVR using the tendyne system versus TEER with the mitraclip device. It is also being evaluated in a single arm study for use in patients with severe MAC.

The Intrepid TMVR system consists of a bioprosthesis and transapical delivery system. The bioprosthesis is a trileaflet bovine pericardial valve contained in a self-expanding nitinol frame consisting of a circular inner stent housing the valve and a conformable outer fixation ring to engage the mitral annular anatomy. It is built around a 27-mm inner valve with effective orifice area (EOA) of 2.4 cm^2 and is being investigated in 43 mm, 46 mm, and 50 mm outer diameters.

The prosthesis is designed to preserve the native leaflets and chordae and leverage them to seal around the device. The delivery system is designed for transapical access only and consists of a introducer sheath and hydraulically actuated delivery catheter. Importantly, the system does not require rotational alignment, tethering or capture of native leaflets before or during device deployment.

The Evoque transcatheter mitral valve is self-expanding trileaflet bovine prosthesis with a nitinol frame and a symmetric design that does not require rotational alignment to the mitral annulus. The polyurethane foam covered left ventricular anchors are designed to engage and preserve the subvalvular MV apparatus. The device can be delivered either via transfemoral/ transseptal or transapical route using 33F delivery system.

The Tendyne valve has the trileaflet valve sewn within two self-expanding nitinol stents, and EOA is >3.0 cm^2. The outer stent is D-shaped to conform to the native annulus. Atrial flange offers atrial sealing and anchoring. Left ventricular apical tethering system with apical pad reduces paravalvular insufficiency and assists with apical closure. The D-shaped outer stent needs to be oriented such that the straight side and atrial cuff align with the aortomitral continuity and aorta. A tension gauge tool is used to adjust the tether tension from the valve to the left ventricular apex. The valve can be fully repositioned and retrieved even after full deployment.

The Tiara TMVR prosthesis is D shaped to geometrically fit the native MV annulus, and the device is fixated radially by expansion of the tiara valve and axially by the ventricular tabs (two anterior and one posterior). It has two sizes 35 mm and 40 mm and is implanted via transapical approach using 32 Fr delivery system.

The AltaValve has recently received the FDA breakthrough device designation for severe mitral regurgitation (MR) and severe MR in MAC. It uses the atrial fixation TMVR technology to treat patients at risk of left ventricular outflow tract (LVOT) obstruction. The device is oversized to the left atrium for anchoring and marginally anchored to the mitral annulus for sealing. Since it is not rigidly anchored to the native valve, it may be beneficial in patients with moderate or severe MAC. Anatomical inclusion criteria for AltaValve includes, left atrium (LA) size in systole <85 mm, mitral annulus >29 mm, and <51 mm in diameter and volume change in LA <20% between systole and diastole. It is deployed via transseptal approach.

Currently two systems are approved for transcatheter edge to edge repair (TEER), MitraClip (Abbott), and PASCAL (Edwards lifesciences) and have been used in both symptomatic severe primary MR (PMR) and secondary MR (SMR). The EVEREST trial and EXPAND registry looked at anatomic suitability criteria for M-TEER using the mitraclip system. The CLASP study evaluated the use of PASCAL system for M-TEER. The COAPT study had previously evaluated suitability criteria and benefit in severe SMR with M-TEER and came up with the simplified COAPT criteria.

The initial experiences with ViV-TMVR were conducted via a transapical and transatrial approach offering direct access.[4] However, with improvement in the technology with smaller and steerable delivery systems, now transseptal has emerged as the preferred option for ViV and ViR TMVR. This allows for fully percutaneous approach via the femoral vein avoiding mini thoracotomy. It has also been shown to be advantageous in terms of clinical outcomes resulting in less morbidity and less recovery time compared to the surgical valve replacement and when compared with transapical approach for TMVR.[4-6]

Herein, we discuss important aspects of transseptal ViV-TMVR with a balloon expandable transcatheter system such as the Edwards SAPIEN 3 Transcatheter Heart Valve System or the MyVal System.

The following steps are being briefly covered: (1) Selecting the right patient, (2) Planning (imaging), (3) access, (4) transseptal puncture, (5) valve deployment, and (6) final steps.

SELECTING THE RIGHT PATIENT

This is a very critical step to perform a successful transseptal ViV/ViR TMVR. A trained and experienced heart team must be involved and consider if the patient with a degenerated mitral valve bioprosthesis at high-risk for repeat open-heart surgery is suitable for percutaneous approach of treatment. There may be factors that may not allow patients for a ViV TMVR. For example, any previously done atrial septal defect repair. Small LVOT and a long, calcified anterior mitral valve leaflet may not be good candidates as they are at increased risk for LVOT obstruction. This is the most life-threatening complication associated with TMVR [7]. Presence of endocarditis, severe paravalvular leak (PVL), and thrombosis of the bioprosthesis may also be a contraindication.[7,8]

PLANNING

Preoperative CT is mandatory for planning a TMVR procedure to evaluate the risk like of LVOT obstruction. CT can give an estimate of neo-LVOT area after ViV-TMVR by adding a virtual valve. Projected neo-LVOT area ≤1.7 cm^2 carries high sensitivity for LVOT obstruction.[7] CT can also be used to measure the internal diameter of the preexisting bioprosthesis helping in deciding the transcatheter valve size.[8] It can also estimate the MAC score and extent of circumferential calcium in valve-in-MAC cases. Transesophageal echocardiography (TEE) can be used to evaluate the etiology of bioprosthetic failure.

ACCESS

A 6-French (Fr) sheath under Doppler guidance is used to access the bilateral common femoral veins via the Seldinger technique. A Perclose Proglide (Abbott Laboratories, Chicago, IL, USA) device is preemptively placed in the right femoral vein for suture-mediated closure of the venotomy that will be used for insertion of the large-bore sheath. After this, a steerable vascular access sheath such as the Agilis NxT Steerable Introducer

(Abbott Laboratories, Lake Bluff, IL, USA) is advanced into the right femoral vein. Under fluoroscopy, the Agilis NxT Steerable Introducer is floated up the inferior vena cava (IVC) and positioned at the junction of the IVC and right atrium (RA).

A temporary pacemaker wire is inserted through the left femoral venous sheath into the right ventricle.

TRANSSEPTAL PUNCTURE

The patient needs to be heparinized based on the body weight. A Mullins sheath (Cook Group, Bloomington, IN, USA) is inserted into the right femoral vein and advanced into the RA. An NRG transseptal needle (Baylis Medical, Burlington, MA, USA) or a BRK transseptal needle is advanced through this sheath and directed toward the fossa ovalis under TEE and fluoroscopic guidance **(Figs. 1 and 2)**. The atrial septum is punctured through the transseptal needle, and the Agilis sheath is advanced into the LA **(Fig. 3)**. The introduction of the sheath into the LA should be confirmed by transduction of LA pressures. The transseptal needle is withdrawn and an Inoue wire (Toray Medical Co., Ltd., Tokyo, Japan) is advanced through the sheath into the LA. The wires must be maintained in the LA, and the Agilis sheath is advanced further into the LA. The activated clotting time (ACT) must be maintained at 250–350 seconds, the Agilis sheath is steered toward the left ventricular apex, and a standard J-wire is passed toward the left ventricle (LV). In case there is any chordal entanglement, a pulmonary artery catheter can be advanced across the wire with the balloon inflated to confirm the lack of entanglement. Advance pigtail catheter into the LV over the J-wire.

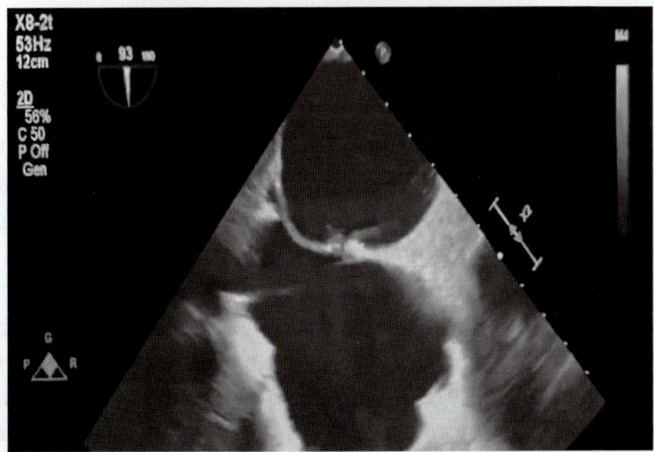

Fig. 1: Transesophageal echocardiography (TEE)-guided septal needle directed toward the fossa ovalis.

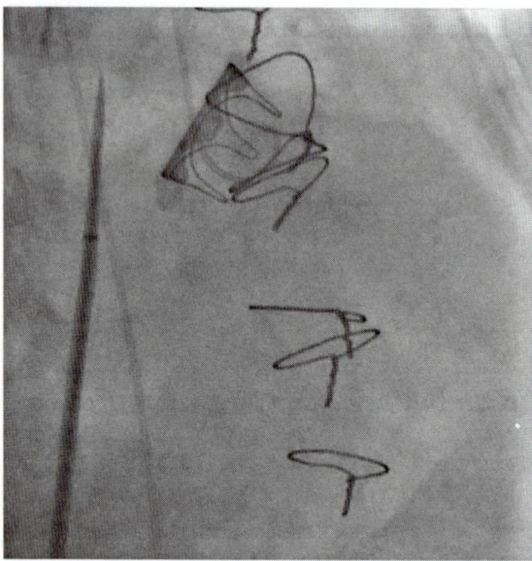

Fig. 2: Fluoroscopic-guided septal needle directed toward the fossa ovalis.

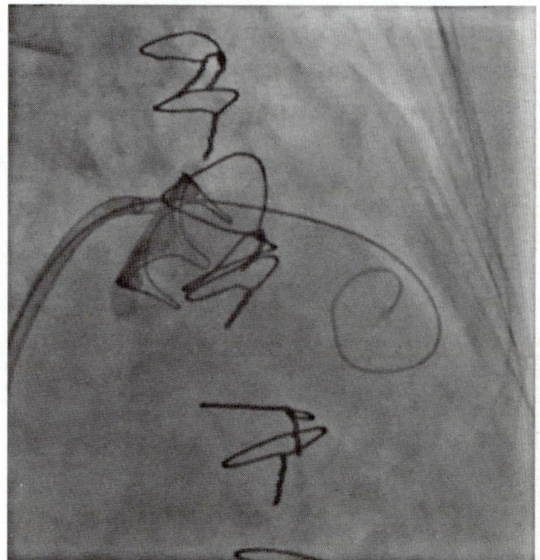

Fig. 3: Agilis sheath advanced into the left atrium.

VALVE DEPLOYMENT

A Safari wire (Boston Scientific Corp., Marlborough, MA, USA) is advanced through the pigtail catheter, across the mitral valve, and placed into the apex of the LV. Over this wire, the interatrial septum is dilated using a 14-mm balloon **(Fig. 4)**, and the mitral valve is flossed. Then the transcatheter valve is advanced into the IVC. Ensure the mounted valve is correctly oriented with the skirt away from the LV side (opposite direction to that when loaded for TAVR). Advance the system across the atrial septum and into the LA. Position the valve satisfactorily and deploy the valve under rapid pacing with slow inflation; ViV **(Fig. 5A)**, ViR **(Fig. 5B)**. Use TEE to assess valve position, motion of the leaflets, gradients, and the presence of any leak. In case there

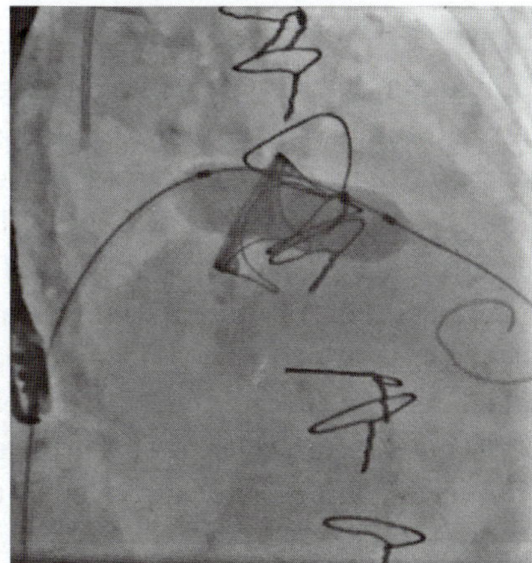

Fig. 4: Dilation of the interatrial septum and flossing of mitral valve using a 14-mm balloon.

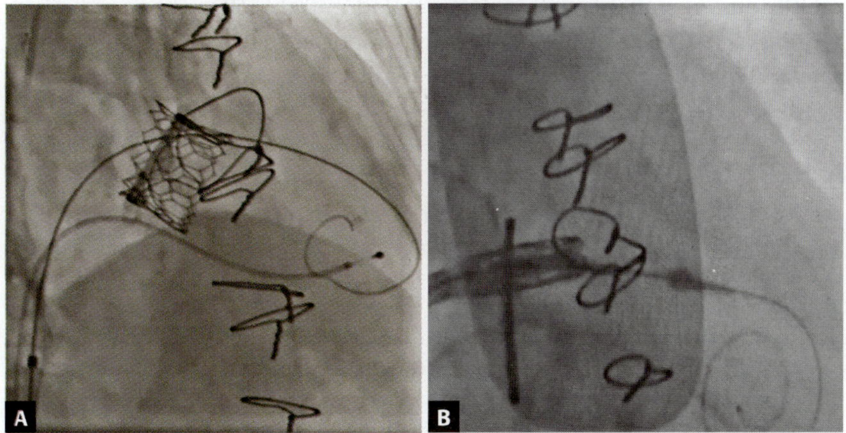

Figs. 5A and B: (A) Valve-in-valve (ViV) and (B) Valve-in-ring (ViR). Positioning the valve satisfactorily and deployment under rapid pacing with slow inflation.

is any PVL seen, a postdilation can be considered by adding contrast to the delivery system.

FINAL STEPS

The septal puncture is not routinely closed. In case there is a presence of a significant right-to-left interatrial shunt or desaturation, the septostomy can be closed with a percutaneous closure device. Next step is the withdrawal of the temporary pacer, delivery system, and sheaths. The heparin is reversed by administering protamine. The closure device in the right femoral vein is tied down. Over the left venous access manual compression is applied which helps in achieving hemostasis.

DISCUSSION

ViV-TMVR, in spite of being in its early stages, is a fast-growing technology offering an option of treatment for patients with preexisting bioprosthetic valve in the mitral position which has degenerated and are at a high risk for surgical redo procedure.[9-11] One of the major risks is LVOT obstruction. Some techniques have been described to overcome the risk of LVOT obstruction, such as the intentional laceration of the anterior mitral leaflet to prevent left ventricular outflow tract obstruction (LAMPOON) technique, antegrade LAMPOON, retrograde LAMPOON, or rescue LAMPOON, which utilizes the radiofrequency energy to lacerate the anterior mitral leaflet so that it does not obstruct the LVOT.[12-14] This technique is not approved by the FDA.

CONCLUSION

Advancements in TMVR technologies and preference for a less invasive approach have allowed the application of transseptal ViV-TMVR to grow rapidly among patients with a degenerated mitral bioprosthesis at high or prohibitive surgical risk. The outcomes reported have shown this to be a safe and feasible procedure. Further studies with long-term outcomes are needed.

REFERENCES

1. Nkomo VT, Gardin JM, Skelton TN, Gottdiener JS, Scott CG, Enriquez-Sarano M. Burden of valvular heart disease: a population-based studu. Lancet. 2006;368:1005-11.
2. Ruel M, Chan V, Bedard P, Kulik A, Ressler L, Lam BK, et al. Very long-term survival implications of heart valve replacement with tissue vs mechanical prosthesis in adults <60 years of age. Circulation. 2007;116:I294-300.
3. Yoon SH, Whisenant BK, Bleiziffer S, Delgado V, Schofer N, Eschenbach L, et al. Transcatheter mitral valve replacement for degenerated bioprosthetic valves and failed annuloplasty rings. J Am Coll Cardiol. 2017;70:1121-31.
4. Regueiro A, Granada JF, Dagenais F, Rodés-Cabau J. Transcatheter mitral valve replacement: insights from early clinical experience and future challenges. J Am Coll Cardiol. 2017;69:2175-92.
5. Webb JG, Wood DA, Ye J, Gurvitch R, Masson JB, Rodés-Cabau J, et al. Transcatheter valve-in-valve implantation for failed bioprosthetic heart valves. Circulation. 2010;121:1848-57.
6. Webb JG, Murdoch DJ, Boone RH, Moss R, Attinger-Toller A, Blanke P, et al. Percutaneous transcatheter mitral valve replacement. J Am Coll Cardiol. 2019;73:1239-46.
7. Yoon SH, Bleiziffer S, Latib A, Eschenbach L, Ancona M, Vincent F, et al. Predictors of left ventricular outflow tract obstruction after transcatheter mitral valve replacement. JACC Cardiovasc Interv. 2019;12:182-93.
8. Urena M, Himbert D, Brochet E, Carrasco JL, Iung B, Nataf P, et al. Transseptal transcatheter mitral valve replacement using balloon-expandable transcatheter heart valves: a step-by-step approach. JACC Cardiovasc Interv. 2017;10:1905-19.

9. Alkhouli M, Rihal CS, Holmes DR. Transseptal techniques for emerging structural heart interventions. JACC Cardiovasc Interv. 2016;9:2465-80.
10. Bapat VN, Attia R, Thomas M. Effect of valve design on the stent internal diameter of a bioprosthetic valve: a concept of true internal diameter and its implications for the valve-in-valve procedure. JACC Cardiovasc Interv. 2014;7:115-27.
11. Wang DD, Guerrero M, Eng MH, Eleid MF, Meduri CU, Rajagopal V, et al. Alcohol septal ablation to prevent left ventricular outflow tract obstruction during transcatheter mitral valve replacement: first-in-man study. JACC Cardiovasc Interv. 2019;12:1268-79.
12. Mack MJ, Leon MB, Thourani VH, Makkar R, Kodali SK, Russo M, et al. Transcatheter aortic-valve replacement with a balloon-expandable valve in low-risk patients. N Engl J Med. 2019;380:1695-705.
13. Popma JJ, Michael Deeb G, Yakubov SJ, Mumtaz M, Gada H, O'Hair D, et al. Transcatheter aortic-valve replacement with a self-expanding valve in low-risk patients. N Engl J Med. 2019;380:1706-15.
14. Babaliaros VC, Greenbaum AB, Khan JM, Rogers T, Wang DD, Eng MH, et al. Intentional percutaneous laceration of the anterior mitral leaflet to prevent outflow obstruction during transcatheter mitral valve replacement: first-in-human experience. JACC Cardiovasc Interv. 2017;10:798-809.

CHAPTER 46

Transcatheter Edge-to-Edge Repair: Current Devices and Techniques

Praveen Chandra

INTRODUCTION

Mitral regurgitation (MR) results from anatomic or functional changes in the complex mitral valve apparatus. Around 10% of individuals aged 75 years or more have clinically significant MR.[1] MR leads to left ventricular dysfunction, resulting in heart failure (HF), increased morbidity, and mortality.[2] Many patients with severe MR are at high surgical risk or are inoperable; to address treatment of this patient population, transcatheter therapies were developed. The concept of transcatheter edge-to-edge repair (TEER) is a percutaneous replication of the surgical Alfieri method[3] instead of suturing the free edge of the leaflets (commonly A2-P2 scallops), clip with grasping arms is deployed to secure the mitral leaflets, creating a valve with two orifices.

TIMELINE OF ADVANCEMENTS IN TRANSCATHETER EDGE-TO-EDGE REPAIR SINCE FIRST IN HUMAN PROCEDURE

The first in-human mitral valve transcatheter edge-to-edge repair (M-TEER) using MitraClip was done in 2003,[4] subsequently CE (European Conformity) mark in 2008. Based on EVEREST II trial, US Food and Drug Administration (FDA) approval for primary MR (PMR) came in 2013 and for secondary MR (SMR) in 2019 based on COAPT trial. Based on retrospective studies and case studies, TEER was found safe and effective even in atrial secondary MR, severe mitral annular calcification (MAC), in ring, and commissural MR. The PASCAL transcatheter MV repair system was first used in 2016 and got FDA approval in 2022.

COAPT trial, a randomized, multicenter trial of MitraClip in symptomatic HF patients despite OMT with moderate to severe or severe MR with LVEF 20–50%. COAPT trial demonstrated a benefit of MitraClip with a reduction in HFH over 24 months from 67.9% (GDMT alone) to 35.8% in patients treated with MitraClip ($p < 0.001$). There was also a reduction in all-cause death observed over 24 months from 46.1 to 29.1% in patients treated with MitraClip ($p < 0.001$). COAPT trial 5-year follow-up showed that 57.3% mortality in device group compared to 67.2% in control group (CI: 0.58–0.89). Only four patients (1.4%) in the device group had device specific complications over period of 5 years.

EVEREST II trial is a multicenter, randomized, nonblinded trial of the MitraClip compared with conventional surgery in moderate-to-severe degenerative MR at 1 year showed M-TEER was less effective at reducing MR but was associated with superior safety and similar clinical outcomes compared to surgery. 2-year follow-up showed no device failure and stability in outcomes. At 5-year follow-up, reduction in MR severity to <2 +in 75% patients, postprocedural adverse events were stable through 5 years.

GUIDELINES

AHA/ACC Valve Guidelines 2020

Class IIa for patients with high or prohibitive surgical risk with anatomy favorable for transcatheter approach and life expectancy >1 year for either primary (PMR) or secondary (SMR) etiology.[5]

ESC Valve Guidelines 2021

Primary MR

Class IIb for symptomatic patients who fulfill echocardiographic criteria of eligibility, are judged inoperable or at high risk by heart team and for whom the procedure is not considered futile.

Secondary MR

Class IIa for symptomatic patients, who are judged not appropriate for surgery by heart team with or without concomitant CAD.

Class IIb in high-risk symptomatic patients not eligible for surgery and are not fulfilling criteria, suggesting an increased chance of responding to TEER.

BASELINE EVALUATION

Transthoracic echocardiography (TTE) is the initial test to confirm the diagnosis and severity of MR, mechanism of MR, mitral valve area, pulmonary vein flow pattern, septal morphology, left atrial/left atrial appendage (LA/LAA) clot, estimate pulmonary artery pressures, and evaluate other valvular disease and assess left ventricle (LV) and right ventricle (RV) functions. Transesophageal echocardiography (TOE) is required in all M-TEER candidates to assess leaflet target and major MR jet, guide septal puncture, guide safe steering of steerable guide catheter (SGC) in LA, proper alignment of clip, confirm leaflet capture, assessment of MR reduction after clip deployment, exclusion of significant MS, and assessment of residual atrial septal defect (ASD).

MITRAL VALVE TRANSCATHETER EDGE-TO-EDGE REPAIR SYSTEMS

Two M-TEER devices are currently approved: The MitraClip (Abbott) and PASCAL (Edwards Lifesciences) systems. **Figure 1** shows the comparison between two types of M-TEER devices.

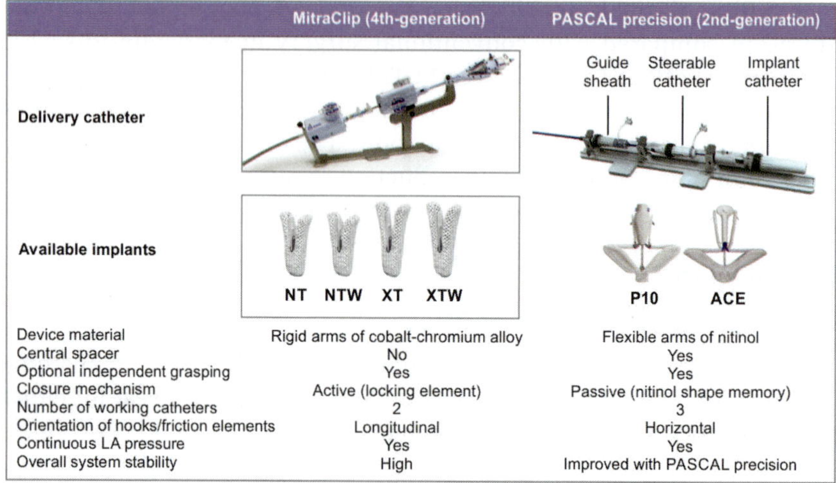

	MitraClip (4th-generation)	PASCAL precision (2nd-generation)
Delivery catheter		
Available implants	NT NTW XT XTW	P10 ACE
Device material	Rigid arms of cobalt-chromium alloy	Flexible arms of nitinol
Central spacer	No	Yes
Optional independent grasping	Yes	Yes
Closure mechanism	Active (locking element)	Passive (nitinol shape memory)
Number of working catheters	2	3
Orientation of hooks/friction elements	Longitudinal	Horizontal
Continuous LA pressure	Yes	Yes
Overall system stability	High	Improved with PASCAL precision

Fig. 1: Comparison of MitraClip and PASCAL device.

Mitraclip

The fourth-generation MitraClip has four implant sizes, "classic" NT and XT clip sizes [4 mm width; 9 (NT) and 12 (XT) mm arm length], NTW and XTW [6 mm width; 9 (NTW) and 12 (XTW) mm arm length]. The MitraClip has two rigid arms made of cobalt-chromium alloy with flexible "grippers" (nitinol), which have longitudinally arranged small hooks ("frictional elements"). For the treatment of larger coaptation gaps and flail gap, the longer clip arms (XT/XTW) are preferred. The fourth-generation MitraClip system (G4) provides a 50% wider grasping area, allows for independent and controlled gripper actuation (CGA) to optimize leaflet grasping, and enhances continuous left atrial pressure monitoring, helping in treating patients with complex anatomy with reduced number of clips without much leaflet stress. **Figure 2** shows the MitraClip system.

PASCAL System

PASCAL system (second generation) consists of three catheters: A 22 Fr steerable guide sheath and catheter, with an implant catheter to which the device is attached at the distal end, allowing for a high range of motion and maneuverability in the left atrium. PASCAL P10 (nitinol based) consists of two spring-loaded, curved paddles with grasping length of 26 mm when open to 180°, two clasps (10 mm each), which can be controlled individually, helping in independent leaflet capture and a central spacer to fill the regurgitant orifice as well as coaptation gap within the main MR jet area, reducing the forces on the MV leaflets. PASCAL Ace has similar grasping width with 6 mm wide paddles to accommodate smaller anatomies and facilitate multiple

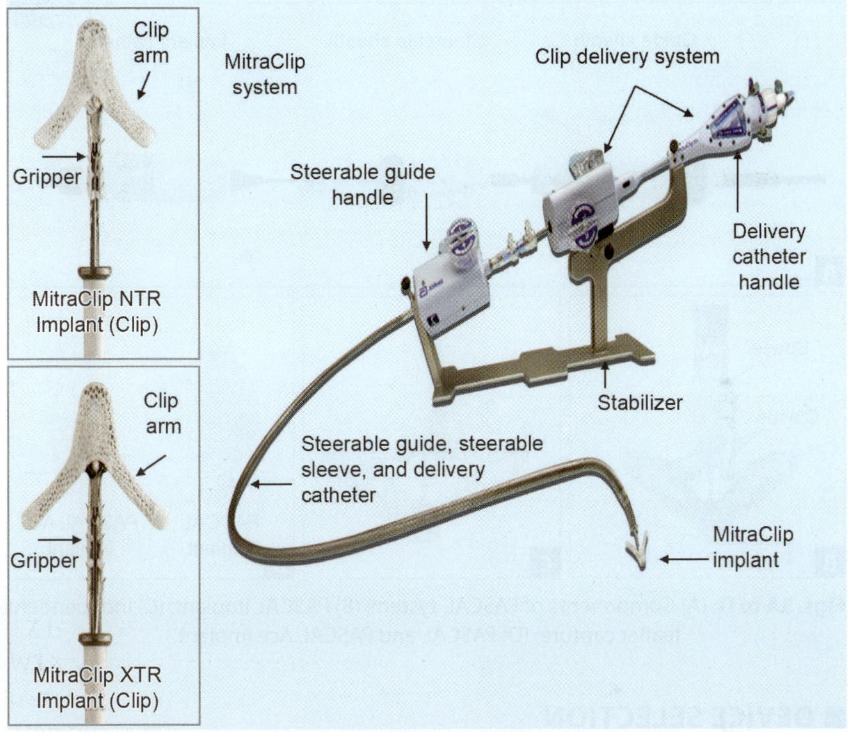

Fig. 2: MitraClip system.

implant strategies. The second-generation PASCAL Precision platform was introduced with changes in the catheter system for improving device stability and steerability. **Figures 3A to D** show the PASCAL system.

ANATOMICAL SUITABILITY

EVEREST MV criteria for optimal M-TEER in case of functional MR: Mitral valve area (MVA) >4 cm^2, minimal leaflet calcification in grasping area, coaptation length >2 mm and coaptation depth of <11 mm and for primary MR flail gap of <10 mm and width < 15 mm, outside of these criteria, there is a lower likelihood of an excellent and durable valve repair.[6] Complex anatomy includes wide coaptation gap (≥15 mm), large flail gap (≥10 mm), grasping area leaflet calcification, transmitral gradient >5 mm Hg, jet outside anterior 2/posterior 2 (A2/P2), and small MVA <4 cm^2, which are predictors for an increased transmitral gradient (≥5 mm Hg) after M-TEER.[7,8] Grasping area severe calcification, active endocarditis, and significant mitral stenosis are contraindications for M-TEER. **Table 1** shows the anatomic suitability for M-TEER.

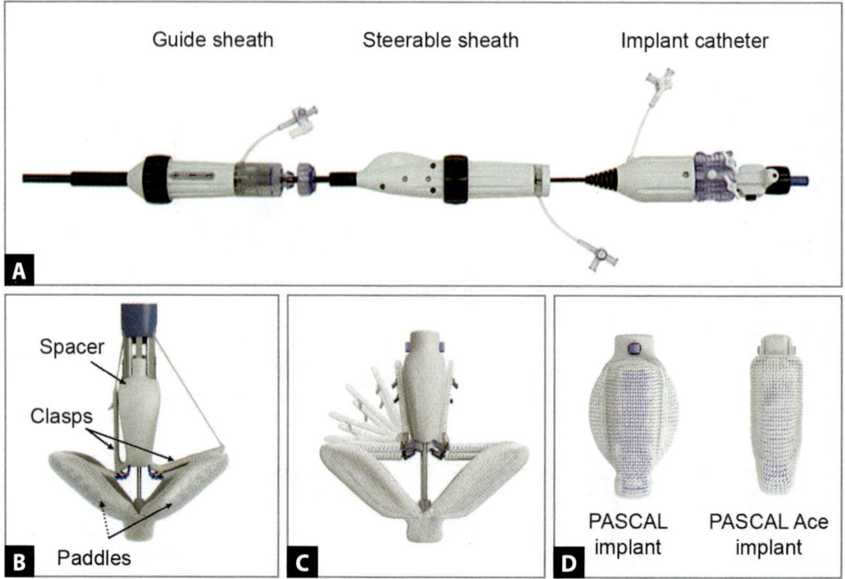

Figs. 3A to D: (A) Components of PASCAL system; (B) PASCAL implant; (C) Independent leaflet capture; (D) PASCAL and PASCAL Ace implant.

DEVICE SELECTION

Mitral valve area reduction following M-TEER depends on the type of device (47% in PASCAL p10, 52% NTR, 57% XTR), location of device, and commissural placement results in minimum reduction whereas A2P2 position results in maximal reduction. Devices with extended arms (XT, XTW, or PASCAL) are preferred in patients with large flail gaps or wide prolapses. PASCAL P10 should be avoided in case where multiple clips are required. For commissural lesions, devices with small arms (e.g., NT/NTW) and stable steering are preferred. In case of annular calcifications with leaflet infiltration, the use of smaller/more flexible devices is preferred. Devices with extended arms, such as MitraClip XT and XTW, should be avoided and PASCAL devices (nitinol design and horizontal orientation of the grasping elements) preferred in patients with short and tethered posterior leaflet to prevent single leaflet device attachment (SLDA) or leaflet injury.

PROCEDURE

Transseptal puncture: Posterosuperior aspect of fossa ovalis about 4–5 cm above mitral annulus is ideal for transseptal puncture. Higher transseptal puncture is preferred in medial pathologies and primary MR. Superior and inferior aspect of septum is identified in bicaval view, and anterior aspect of the septum is the part that is closest to the aortic valve in short-axis view at aortic valve level. Final confirmation of septal puncture is to be done in biplane

TABLE 1: Anatomic suitability for M-TEER.

Noncomplex Ideal for M-TEER	*Complex Suitable for M-TEER*	*Very complex Challenging for M-TEER*	*Criteria favoring replacement M-TEER hard or impossible*
Central pathology: • No calcification • MVA >4.0 cm^2 • Posterior leaflet >10 mm • Tenting height <10 mm • Flail gap <10 mm • Flail width <15 mm	• Isolated commissural lesion (A1/P1 or A3/P3) • Annular calcification without leaflet involvement • MVA 3.5–4.0 cm^2 • Posterior leaflet length 7–10 mm • Tenting height >10 mm • Asymmetric tethering • Coaptation reserve <3 mm • Leaflet-to-anulus index <1.2 • Flail width >15 mm • Flail gap >10 mm • Two jets from leaflet indentations	*Commissural lesion with multiple jets:* • Annular calcification with leaflet involvement • Fibrotic leaflets • Wide jet involving the whole coaptation • MVA 3.0–3.5 cm^2 • Posterior leaflet length 5–7 mm • Barlow's disease • Cleft • Failed surgical annuloplasty	• Concentric MAC with stenosis • MVA <3.0 cm^2 • Relevant mitral valve stenosis (mean gradient >5 mm Hg) • Posterior leaflet <5 mm • Calcification in the grasping zone • Deep regurgitant cleft • Leaflet perforation • Multiple/wide jets • Rheumatic mitral stenosis

(MAC: mitral annular calcification; MVA: mitral valve area; M-TEER: mitral valve transcatheter edge-to-edge repair)

imaging that simultaneously confirms the superior and posterior locations of the puncture. In case of distorted anatomy of fossa ovalis, bending (or, more rarely, straightening) the needle helps. In the case of thickened or floppy septum electrocautery applied directly on the conventional needle may be used, or the stiff end of a coronary percutaneous coronary intervention wire can be used to cross the septum. **Figure 4** shows transesophageal echocardiography (TEE)-guided transseptal puncture.

Advancement of the steerable guide catheter: The curved tip stiff wire is passed across the septum into the left upper pulmonary vein followed by dilating the septum. The SGC is then advanced into the left atrium under 2D and 3D transesophageal echocardiography (TEE) guidance to avoid interaction with left pulmonary vein and left atrial appendage. **Figure 5** shows SGC advancement into LA.

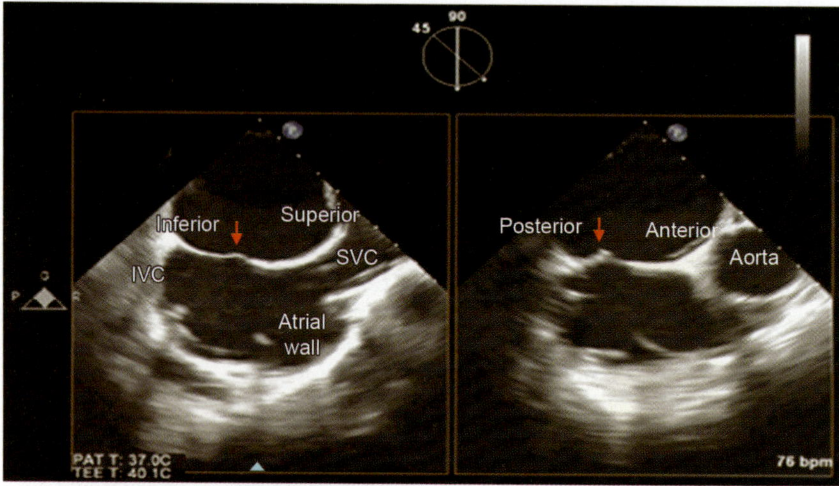

Fig. 4: Transesophageal echocardiography (TEE)-guided transseptal puncture.

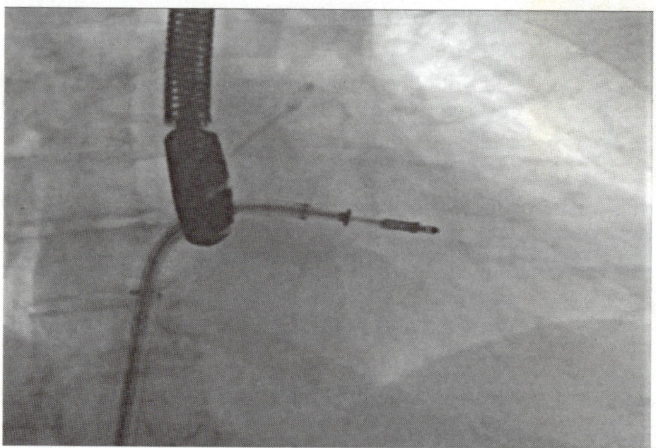

Fig. 5: Steerable guide catheter (SGC) advancement.

Device positioning: Simultaneous visualization of both planes, an intercommissural view (50–70°) and a left ventricular outflow tract (LVOT) view (140–160°), allows for the correction of the trajectory of the catheter, to facilitate leaflet grasping and avoid valve distortion **(Fig. 6)**. Clip arms are oriented perpendicular to coaptation line **(Figs. 7A and B)**. Pulling/pushing the whole assembly, as well as flexing/unflexing, will displace the catheter toward the medial and lateral, respectively. Clockwise rotation of the catheter will result in posterior movement and a counterclockwise rotation in anterior movement of the device. Flexing the guide sheath will lead to lose of height, while a posterior rotation will help to gain height.

Leaflet grasping: After confirmation of the device position and trajectory in the left atrium, the device is advanced into the left ventricle. Clear visualization of

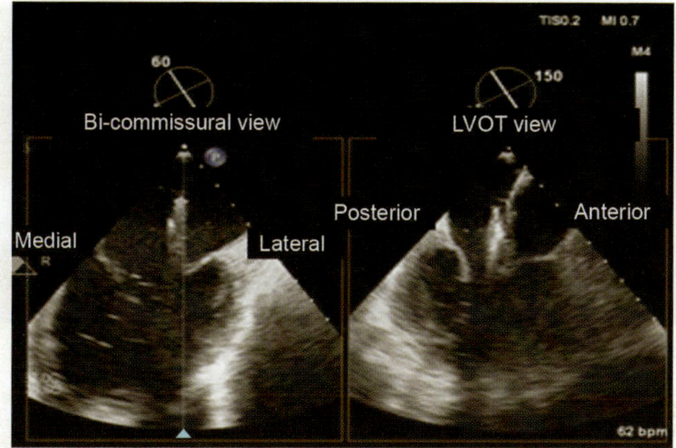

Fig. 6: Device positioning. (LVOT: left ventricular outflow tract)

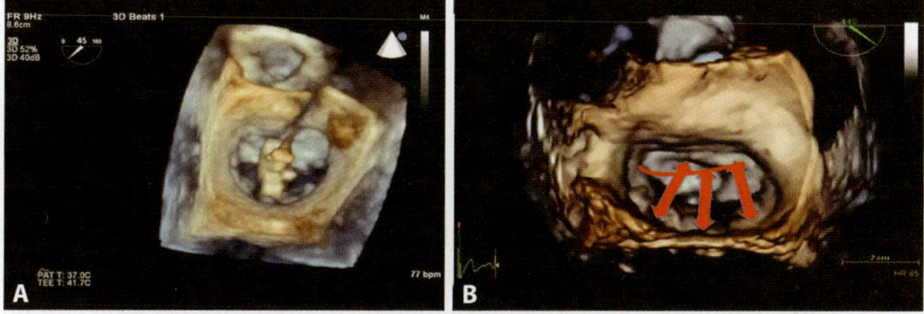

Figs. 7A and B: Clip orientation perpendicular to coaptation line.

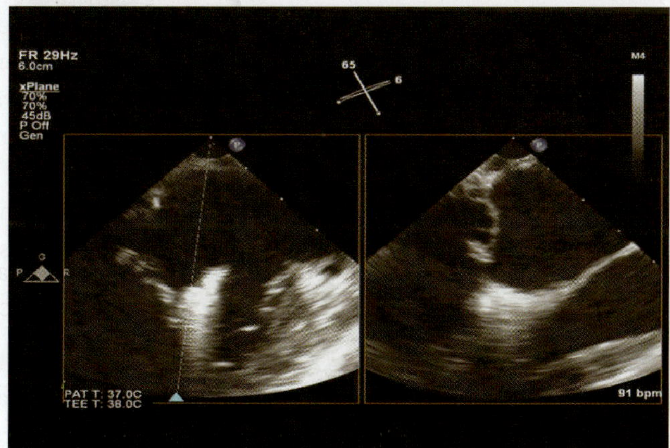

Fig. 8: Adequate leaflet grasping.

the leaflets is important to make sure enough tissue is being grasped **(Fig. 8)**. Leaflet insertion should be carefully assessed and quantified before device release.

Hemodynamic assessment: Assessment of residual MR by size of regurgitant jet, pulmonary vein flow **(Figs. 9A and B)**, and left atrial pressure. If there is

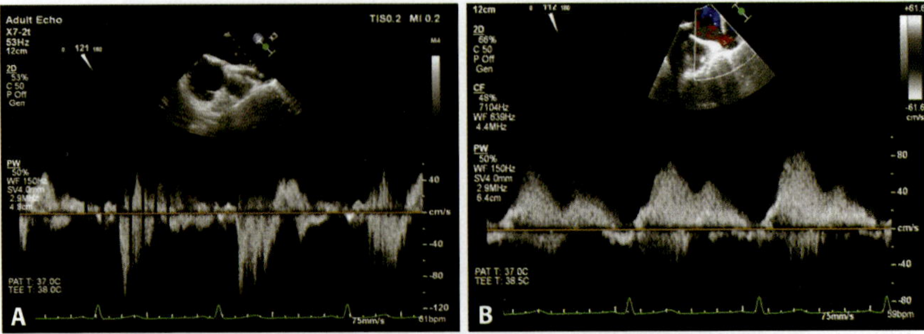

Figs. 9A and B: Pulmonary vein flow before and after mitral valve transcatheter edge-to-edge repair (M-TEER) device.

significant residual MR, then reposition the device or add a second device, in the absence of mitral stenosis. In case of multiple clips, first device is usually positioned more medially.

COMPLICATIONS

- *Device-related complications:*
  - *Residual MR:* Amplatzer vascular plug (Abbott) can be implanted for treatment of significant interclip or paraclip residual MR.[9] Even expanded polytetrafluoroethylene double-disk occlude can be implanted for residual MR.[10]
  - *SLDA:* It is seen in 2–5% cases, when there is disengagement of insertion of one of the leaflets from the device, during the procedure or follow-up. SLDA can be avoided by ensuring a good grasp with both leaflets tucked in the closed device. SLDA can be managed by deployment of additional clips if feasible.
  - *Clip embolization:* Device detachment from both leaflets, occurring in less than 1%. In case clip embolization to distal arteries causing ischemia, surgical removal is required.
  - Leaflet perforation, leaflet tear, and chordal rupture
- *Transseptal puncture* complications are usually seen in patients that have large atria, thick or redundant septum, and prior septal surgery. Iatrogenic ASD, cardiac tamponade, pericardial effusion, and aortic perforation are some reported complications.
- *Systemic* infective endocarditis, stroke
- *Vascular* dissection, thrombosis, pseudoaneurysm, and bleeding

Follow-up transthoracic echocardiogram should be performed on the first postprocedural day to assess residual MR and any complication, at 30 days and at 6–12 months to assess long-term hemodynamic effect of MR reduction.

SINGLE CENTER EXPERIENCE IN INDIA

At our center, we have performed over 68 MitraClip procedures (M-TEER) in a span of 4 years with only one patient experiencing SLD, indicating proficiency and efficacy of the procedure. Residual MR was not more than mild in nearly all patients, indicating successful mitigation of regurgitant flow. There were no mortalities intraprocedure or during hospital stay.

CONCLUSION

TEER has evolved rapidly as an important therapeutic option in patients with MR. Most of the data show good safety profile and better clinical outcomes. Proper case selection and operator experience remain the key to success.

REFERENCES

1. Nkomo VT, Gardin JM, Skelton TN, Gottdiener JS, Scott CG, Enriquez-Sarano M. Burden of valvular heart diseases: a population-based study. Lancet. 2006;368:1005-11.
2. Goel SS, Bajaj N, Aggarwal B, Gupta S, Poddar KL, Ige M, et al. Prevalence and outcomes of unoperated patients with severe symptomatic mitral regurgitation and heartfailure: comprehensive analysis to determine the potential role of MitraClip for this unmet need. J Am Coll Cardiol. 2014;63:185-6.
3. Alfieri O, Maisano F, De Bonis M, Stefano PL, Torracca L, Oppizzi M, et al. The double-orifice technique in mitral valve repair: a simple solution for complex problems. J Thorac Cardiovasc Surg. 2001;122:674-81.
4. Feldman T, Wasserman HS, Herrmann HC, Gray W, Block PC, Whitlow P, et al. Percutaneous mitral valve repair using the edge-to-edge technique: six-month resultsof the EVEREST Phase I Clinical Trial. J Am Coll Cardiol. 2005;46:2134-40.
5. Otto CM, Nishimura RA, Bonow RO, Carabello BA, Erwin JP 3rd, Gentile F, et al. 2020 ACC/AHA Guideline for the Management of Patients With Valvular Heart Disease: A Report of the American College of Cardiology/American Heart Association Joint Committee on Clinical Practice Guidelines. Circulation. 2021;143(5):e72-227.
6. Lesevic H, Karl M, Braun D, Barthel P, Orban M, Pache J, et al. Long-Term Outcomes After MitraClip Implantation According to the Presence or Absence of EVEREST Inclusion Criteria. Am J Cardiol. 2017;119:1255-61.
7. Thaden JJ, Malouf JF, Nkomo VT, Pislaru SV, Holmes DR Jr, Reeder GS, et al. Mitral Valve Anatomic Predictors of Hemodynamic Success With Transcatheter Mitral Valve Repair. J Am Heart Assoc. 2018;7:e007315.
8. Oguz D, Padang R, Rashedi N, Pislaru SV, Nkomo VT, Mankad SV, et al. Risk for Increased Mean Diastolic Gradient after Transcatheter Edge-to-Edge Mitral Valve Repair: A Quantitative Three-Dimensional Transesophageal Echocardiographic Analysis. J Am Soc Echocardiogr. 2021;34:595-603.
9. Niikura H, Bae R, Gössl M, Lin D, Jay D, Sorajja P. Transcatheter therapy for residual mitral regurgitation after MitraClip therapy. EuroIntervention. 2019;15:e491-9.
10. Nakajima Y, Kar S. First experience of the usage of a GORE CARDIOFORM Septal Occluder device for treatment of a significant residual commissural mitral regurgitation jet following a MitraClip procedure. Catheter Cardiovasc Interv. 2018;92:607-10.

CHAPTER 47

Endovascular Aortic Aneurysm Repair: Basics and Techniques

NN Khanna, Saurabh Bhardwaj, Kritika Arora

INTRODUCTION

An aortic aneurysm is a focal dilation of the aorta to more than two times the normal size. Usually, a focal segment of abdominal aorta with a diameter of >3.0 cm is considered an aortic aneurysm.[1,2] It is an increasingly recognized condition, and its incidence has tripled over the past 30 years, probably due to improvement in diagnostic methods and mass screening programs, and also the increase in aged population. Rupture of the aneurysm is the most dangerous complication, which is usually fatal in >75% cases. The size of aneurysm and the presence of inflammation in the aneurysm predict the risk of rupture.

Aneurysms are classified based on the site, anatomy, and pathology **(Figs. 1A to F)**. Abdominal aortic aneurysms (AAA) can involve only few walls (pseudoaneurysm) or all the walls (true aneurysm). AAA is classically divided

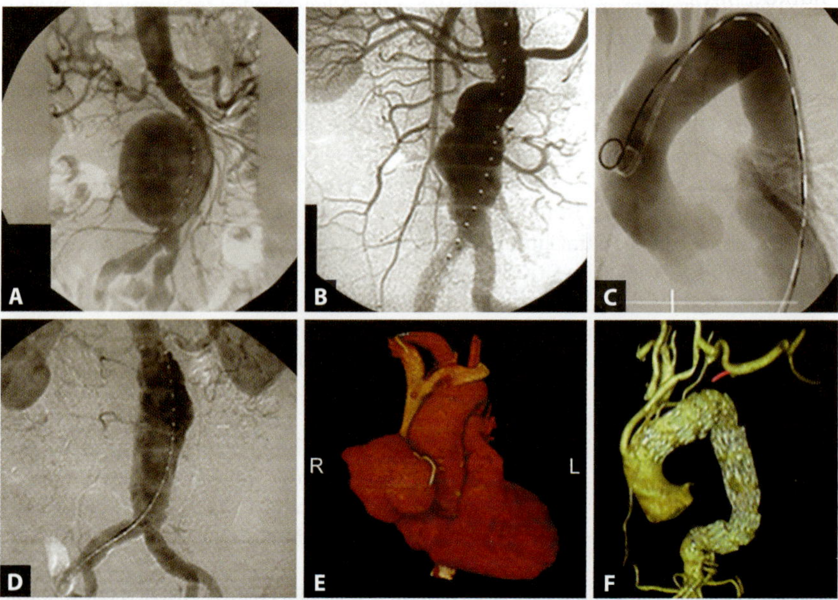

Figs. 1A to F: Types of aneurysm: (A) Saccular aneurysm; (B) Abdominal aneurysm; (C) Thoracic aneurysm; (D) Fusiform aneurysm; (E) Pseudoaneurysm of ascending aorta; (F) Poststenting for arch aneurysm.

into infrarenal, juxtarenal, and suprarenal and may have extension upward to thoracic aorta or below to bilateral iliac arteries. These anatomical features are important in planning of endovascular aortic aneurysm repair (EVAR).[3]

ENDOVASCULAR AORTIC ANEURYSM REPAIR

Before the development of EVAR technique, surgical resection was the mainstay of AAA management. Charles Dubost first described surgical resection in 1950.[4] Open surgical repair is now superseded by the deployment of a covered stent (stent-graft) for elective cases.[5]

Surgical or endovascular treatment is indicated to prevent rupture of aneurysms when the size of AAA exceeds 5.5 cm or when it is rapidly expanding (>5 mm in 6 months). Saccular aneurysms and penetrating ulcers of any size should be treated. Urgent treatment is warranted if there is a contained rupture or a threatening rupture, clinically manifested by abdominal pain or tenderness.

Endovascular aortic aneurysm repair is a treatment option for aneurysm patients who are at high risk for surgery.[3] Over the past few years, the availability of aortic stent-grafts has radically changed the management of AAA. There have been significant developments in stent-graft technology. However, the basic EVAR technique remains the same—delivering a two-piece or a three-piece device into the abdominal aorta and the common iliac arteries to seal and exclude the aneurysm via femoral artery access.

The world's first EVAR was performed in 1987 by Nicholas Volodos in Kharkov, Soviet Union.[5] In 1991, Juan Parodi introduced it in Argentina and in the same year it was introduced in the USA by Michael Dake.[6]

The short-term technical success rate for endovascular aortic aneurysm repair ranges from 83% to >95%.[7-9] Trials have shown that the short-term morbidity and mortality rates of endovascular therapy were found to be better than those of open surgical repair.[10,11] In high-risk candidates for surgery, the short-term mortality rate is significantly lower with endovascular repair.[12] Large randomized controlled trials (RCTs) are evaluating efficacy of EVAR in those with rupture.[13,14]

Advantages of EVAR over surgical repair include decreased anesthesia time, reduced hospital stay, reduced blood loss, and the absence of trauma associated with major abdominal surgery.[15] DREAM,[16] and OVER,[17] are three RCTs which compared EVAR with open surgery for AAA, and showed significant reductions in perioperative morbidity and mortality with EVAR.

Trials such as EUROSTAR,[18] a large multicenter-registry, highlighted the drawbacks of first-generation aortic endografts, which subsequently helped to technically improve the next generations of endografts, EVAR1.[19]

Who can Perform Endovascular Aortic Aneurysm Repair?

Professionals from three main specialties are involved in performing EVAR—interventional cardiology, vascular surgery, and interventional radiology.

The advantage of interventional cardiologists over other specialists in performing EVAR is that they have a good knowledge of managing patients with cardiovascular diseases, cardiovascular pharmacology, and are familiar with catheterization procedures, percutaneous access management, and catheter-wire handling. Moreover, they can also detect and manage coexisting coronary artery disease which is the leading cause of early and late mortality after EVAR. In terms of hardware, there is vast overlap in those used in coronary, structural heart and peripheral interventions which favors the interventional cardiologist to solve problems relating to EVAR. Interventions such as valvuloplasty, device closure, and transcatheter aortic valve replacement involve large diameter vascular access and manipulation of large devices within the vascular system. Experience in peripheral interventions is useful before performing EVAR.

AORTIC ANEURYSMS

Etiology and Pathogenesis

There are multiple etiological factors for development of aortic aneurysm. These include atherosclerosis, arteritis (Takayasu, viral, SLE, and syphilitic), aortic dissection, and cystic medial necrosis (as seen in Marfan syndrome, Ehler-Danlos syndrome, and aortic annular ectasia).

Aneurysms of the ascending thoracic aorta most often result from cystic medial degeneration, which leads to weakening of the aortic wall, resulting in aortic dilatation and aneurysm formation. Cystic medial degeneration occurs normally to some extent with aging, but the process is accelerated by hypertension.[20]

Familial thoracic aortic aneurysm syndrome occurs due mutation on 3p24.2–25, with histological evidence of cystic medial degeneration.[21,22]

Many cases of ascending thoracic aortic aneurysms are associated with an underlying bicuspid aortic valve.

Natural History

Rupture is the most dreaded complication of aortic aneurysm. The natural course of an AAA is continued expansion of 2–3 mm per year and a rupture risk which is exponentially related to AAA diameter.[23,24] The 5-year risk of rupture is approximately 5% for AAAs 3.0–4.0 cm in diameter, 10–20% for AAAs 4.0–5.5 cm in diameter, and 30–40% for AAAs 5.5–6.0 cm in diameter.[25] The likelihood that an aneurysm will rupture is influenced by factors including aneurysm size, expansion rate, and sex. The risk of rupture for AAAs larger than 6.0 cm in diameter rises even more rapidly, exceeding 80% for AAAs larger than 7.0 cm. 60% of thoracic aortic aneurysms involve the aortic root and/or ascending aorta, 40% involve the descending aorta, 10% involve the arch, and 10% involve the thoracoabdominal aorta (with some involving >1 segment).

Clinical Manifestations

Most patients with aortic aneurysms are asymptomatic at the time of diagnosis, and the aneurysms are typically discovered incidentally on imaging studies (chest X-ray, CT scan, or echocardiogram) ordered for other indications. Symptomatic patients present with pain, usually located in the hypogastrium or lower back, which is typically steady and gnawing, lasting for hours to days. Secondary aortic regurgitation may be produced by aneurysms of the root or ascending aorta. Large thoracic aortic aneurysms may cause local mass effect, such as compression of the trachea or main bronchus (causing cough, dyspnea, wheezing, or recurrent pneumonitis), compression of the esophagus (causing dysphagia), or compression of the recurrent laryngeal nerve (causing hoarseness). A potentially lethal consequence of aneurysms is aortic dissection or rupture (referred to as an acute aortic syndrome), presenting as abrupt onset of severe pain in the chest, neck, back, and/or abdomen.

Management

The management of aortic aneurysm depends on the size of the aneurysm, complications, arch vessel involvement, presence or absence of penetrating aortic ulcers/dissections and the rate of expansion of aneurysm. Management options for patients with an asymptomatic AAA include observation with follow-up, medical therapy, surgery, and endovascular stenting.

Risk factor modification is imperative: hypercholesterolemia and hypertension should be controlled and cigarette smoking discontinued. Aneurysms too small to be considered for surgery should be followed up with periodic surveillance imaging to monitor their size. If the aneurysm is expanding more than 1 cm in a year or more than 0.5 cm in 6 months, it needs urgent attention. Usually, asymptomatic aneurysms more than 5 cm in diameter, symptomatic aneurysms, ruptured or saccular aneurysms and aneurysms which are rapidly expanding need surgical or endovascular treatment.

The cornerstone of primary therapy is proper control of blood pressure. The aim of medical therapy is to reduce dP/dt and to control blood pressure. Beta-blocker therapy is considered important for reducing the risk of AAA expansion[26] and rupture. Once beta-blocker therapy is maximized, any persistent hypertension should be treated with other antihypertensive agents to bring the blood pressure down to a low-normal range, e.g., a systolic pressure of 105–120 mm Hg.

With regard to aneurysm size and the risk of rupture or dissection, in their series Davies et al.[27] found an annual rate of 2% for aneurysms >5 cm, 3% for aneurysms 5–5.9 cm, and 7% for aneurysms >6 cm in diameter. The risk appears to rise abruptly as thoracic aneurysms reach a size of 6 cm. For most ascending thoracic aortic aneurysms, surgery is indicated at a diameter of

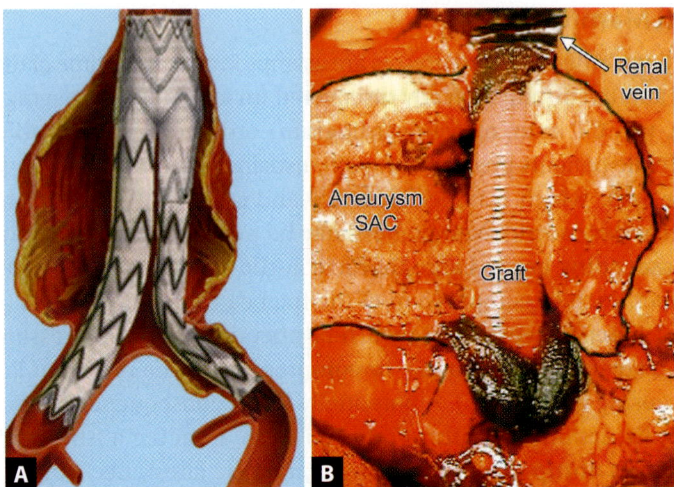

Figs. 2A and B: Types of aortic aneurysm repair. (A) Endovascular aortic aneurysm repair; (B) Surgical repair for aortic aneurysm.

>5.5 cm, and when aortic valve or coronary arteries are involved. Among those with an increased operative risk (e.g., the elderly or those with comorbidities), the threshold is raised to 6 cm or more before recommending surgery. Conversely, among patients at increased risk of aortic dissection or rupture (e.g., Marfan syndrome or bicuspid aortic valve), ascending aortic repair is recommended when aneurysms reach only 5 cm and in selected cases (those at especially high risk), at even smaller diameters. However, surgery carries a much higher mortality and morbidity as compared to endovascular repair.

Surgical procedure involves opening up of the aneurysmal sac and replacing the aneurysm with a synthetic Dacron or polytetrafluoroethylene (PTFE) graft. Surgery carries significant mortality and morbidity (10–20%), especially in elderly patients with other comorbid conditions. It also involves longer hospital stay and use of general anesthesia. Because of this, EVAR came into being and has seen lot of refinement in terms of techniques and hardware **(Figs. 2A and B)**.

Open surgical repair remains the standard approach to treating most large aortic aneurysms. As of today, EVAR is reserved for high-risk surgical patients or in patients with short life expectancy. However, with the advancement in techniques and refinement of hardware, it is likely that endovascular stent-grafting will assume an increasingly important role.

ENDOVASCULAR AORTIC ANEURYSM REPAIR

Imaging

Aneurysms may be detected on physical examination as a pulsatile mass extending from the xiphoid to the umbilicus. Thoracic aortic aneurysms may be seen on chest X-ray films as widening of the mediastinal silhouette, enlargement of the aortic knob, or tracheal deviation. Transesophageal echocardiography is quite useful for imaging the aortic root and is often used to evaluate patients with Marfan syndrome. The arch and descending thoracic aorta are better evaluated by MR and CECT using 1-mm cuts.

Abdominal ultrasonography (USG) is considered the screening modality of choice for diagnosis of an AAA before the development of clinical symptoms to prevent rupture. Some advantages of USG are its high sensitivity of 95–100% and a specificity of nearly 100%, as well as its safety, relatively low cost,[28,29] wide availability, and no use of contrast agent.

Compared with ultrasonography, CECT has an advantage of better visualization of the aneurysm with regards to the neck, aortic bifurcation, tortuosity, calcification, and access vessels (femoral and iliac) **(Figs. 3A to D)**. It is very useful in planning the endovascular treatment. Narrow slice thickness (1–2 mm cuts) is important in the endograft landing zones where precise measurement of vessel diameter, angulation and taper is crucial. Precise information on aortic side-branch location, diameter, and

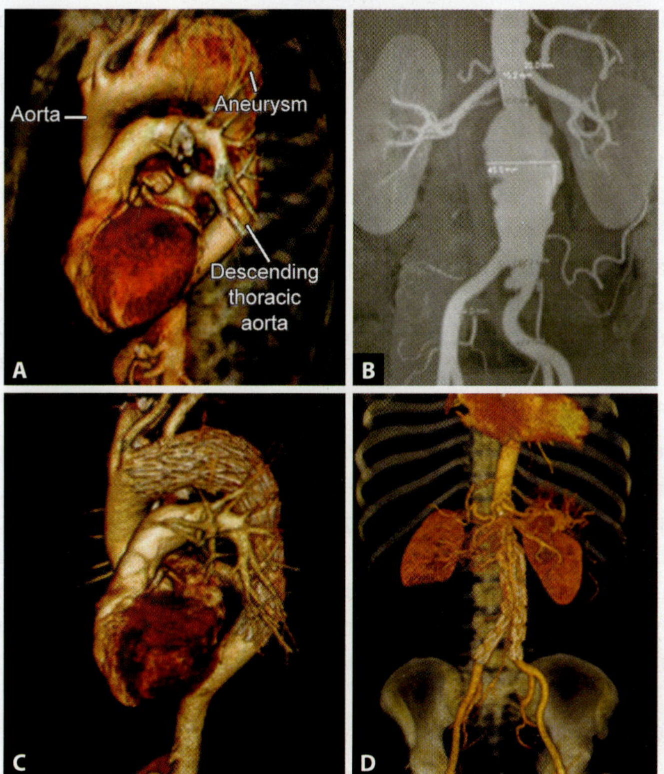

Figs. 3A to D: Aortic aneurysms (arch and infrarenal aorta) status pre- and poststenting.

take-off angulation is required when chimney grafts or fenestrations are planned. A thorough knowledge of vascular anatomy and the ability to study this in individual patients using computed tomography angiography (CTA) and digital subtraction angiography (DSA) is essential. The study should provide anatomic information of the entire aorta, its main branches, and the access vessels. The operator should read the CTA images first hand and integrate information obtained from axial, coronal, and sagittal slices with 3D reconstructions. MR angiography is an alternative for the comprehensive evaluation of aortic aneurysms. As a practice, the volume data is acquired and is loaded on special imaging software, e.g., Terarecon and Osirix. This is especially useful in planning the treatment and sizing the devices in cases of complex aortic anatomies. DSA studies should be done with marker pigtail catheters, power injector, adequate contrast volume, and rapid rate of injection. Use of end-hole catheters, hand injections, and conventional (nonsubtracted) angiography results in poor-quality images and should be avoided.

CT angiograms depicting aneurysms as well as stents in prestenting and poststenting.

Angiography is an essential diagnostic tool for EVAR. The following information is required on CT angiography for planning EVAR for abdominal aortic aneurysm:

- Distance from lowest renal to bifurcation, taking into account any tortuosity
- Distance from lowest renal to main body iliac bifurcation/hypogastric origin
- Distance from the aortic bifurcation to both iliacs

For endovascular repair of thoracic aneurysm, we need to assess the diameter, length, and angulation of proximal length and distal landing zone.

Case Selection

It is essential to determine whether an individual patient has a good life expectancy and quality of life before taking up the patient for EVAR. Patients with terminal illnesses should not be subjected to EVAR procedures, especially in third world countries where the cost of EVAR may place a huge financial burden on the family. Before planning the procedure, any coexisting coronary artery disease and cerebrovascular disease needs to be assessed and treated. It is also important to ensure that an indication exists to perform EVAR.

If the aneurysm is expanding >1 cm in a year or >0.5 cm in 6 months, it needs urgent attention. Usually, asymptomatic aneurysms >5 cm in diameter, symptomatic aneurysms, ruptured or saccular aneurysms and aneurysms which are rapidly expanding need endovascular treatment.

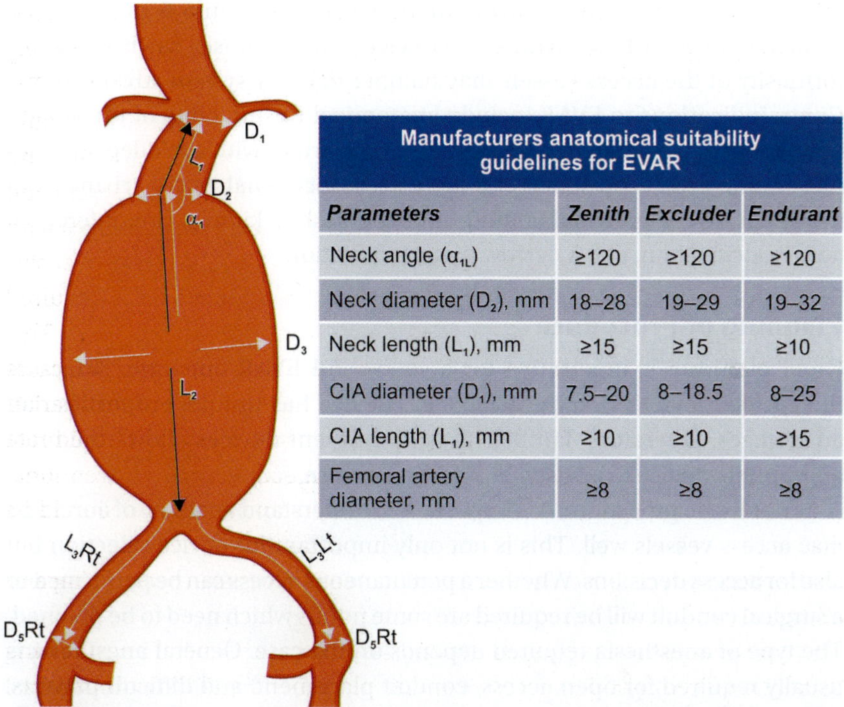

Manufacturers anatomical suitability guidelines for EVAR			
Parameters	***Zenith***	***Excluder***	***Endurant***
Neck angle (α_{1L})	≥120	≥120	≥120
Neck diameter (D_2), mm	18–28	19–29	19–32
Neck length (L_1), mm	≥15	≥15	≥10
CIA diameter (D_1), mm	7.5–20	8–18.5	8–25
CIA length (L_1), mm	≥10	≥10	≥15
Femoral artery diameter, mm	≥8	≥8	≥8

Fig. 4: Criteria used to assess anatomical suitability for EVAR. (EVAR: endovascular aortic aneurysm repair)

Sources:

1. England A, Mc Williams R. Endovascular aortic aneurysm repair (EVAR). Ulster Med J. 2013;82(1):3-10.
2. The Ulster Medical Society, 2013.

Anatomic suitability for EVAR needs to be assessed before planning the procedure **(Fig. 4)**. For infrarenal AAAs, the most important anatomic criterion is the proximal aortic neck, where the length needs to be adequate to provide proximal sealing; varying between devices from 10 to 15 mm. The diameter and angulation of proximal aortic neck and presence of thrombus and/or calcification need to be carefully assessed. Significant thrombus, calcification, conical shape, or severe angulation (>60°) in the neck can lead to device migration and proximal endoleak.

Tortuosity, calcification, stenosis, occlusion, or aneurysmal enlargement of iliac arteries can limit device delivery and distal sealing. As far as possible, flow into the internal iliac arteries should be preserved. In case the common iliac artery is ectatic or aneurysmal, flared iliac endograft limbs or a branched iliac device may be used to preserve the flow.

Anatomy of the access vessels (common femoral and iliac arteries) is important. A minimum diameter of 7–8 mm is required for devices used in thoracic endovascular aortic aneurysm repair, while 6 mm may be sufficient for AAA EVAR with some devices. Any stenosis, calcification, or tortuosity of the access vessels may hamper delivery system advancement. Contraindications to EVAR include anatomical unsuitability of the vessels or aneurysm, large patent inferior mesenteric artery with occluded superior mesenteric artery, presence of a large accessory renal artery arising from the aneurysm or proximal landing zone, horseshoe kidney, circumferential aortic calcification, and a narrow aortic bifurcation.

Planning of Procedure

Good planning is imperative for a successful EVAR outcome. Selecting the correct device is very crucial; each device has unique properties and advantages. Operators' familiarity with different devices allows the most appropriate device to be used in a particular case.

Prior to the procedure, it is important to understand anatomy of aorta and iliac access vessels well. This is not only important for device selection but also for access decisions. Whether a percutaneous access can be performed or a surgical conduit will be required are some points which need to be planned. The type of anesthesia required depends on the case. General anesthesia is usually required for open access, conduit placement, and difficult patients. Standby general anesthesia is kept for percutaneous access and for conscious sedation after initial imaging so patient can cooperate with breath-hold for DSA.

After diagnosis of AAA, further assessment of aneurysm morphology is done by a CT scan. The CT data is displayed as a series of virtual 3D aortic models. The diameter and length of the infrarenal aorta is assessed together with the suitability of the distal landing zones. Vessel length measurement is an essential step and stent-grafts are planned to be of adequate length while allowing sufficient overlap of the modular components **(Fig. 5)**.

Suitability for EVAR may be determined by the relevant stent-graft manufacturer's eligibility criteria set down in their "*Instructions for Use*". One of the strictest criteria surrounds the aortic neck which, for the majority of devices, must be parallel for 15 mm below the lowest renal artery, free from thrombus and excessive angulation.[30]

The three configurations of stent-graft currently available are: tube, bifurcated and Aorto-Uni-Iliac (AUI) **(Fig. 6)**. Bifurcated systems are used in the majority (90%) of cases[31-33] as it has an advantage of being more stable within the aorta.

Oversizing the diameter of the endograft in the region of the proximal aortic neck by 15–20% is generally recommended for aneurysms. It is important to ensure that the contralateral limb gate will open into the sac of the aneurysm so that it can be easily cannulated from the contralateral

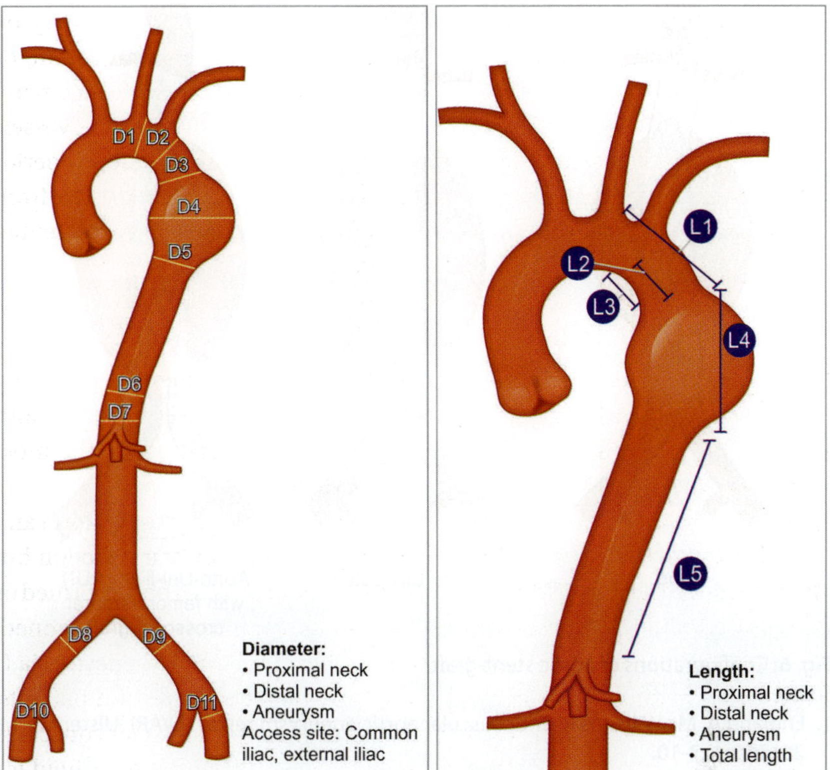

Fig. 5: Planning of procedure by measurement of diameter and length of aorta and vessels.

iliac artery when using bifurcated endografts. The endograft delivery system should be introduced from the side where the access vessels are larger and less tortuous. Once this side is decided, the required distal diameter and total length of the main body can be determined with an aim to land as close to the iliac bifurcation as possible to maximize the distal seal. Extra devices of length and diameter above and below that required should be kept as standby during the procedure. Apart from this, all equipment required during the procedure, including equipment (such as snares) that may be required in unexpected situations, should be procured before the procedure.

Vascular Access

Access: Traditionally, femoral access has been obtained by common femoral artery puncture under direct visualization after surgical femoral cut-down. Vertical or oblique skin incisions may be employed to expose the common femoral artery. While both incisions allow optimal selection of the arterial puncture site, the former allows easy extension of the incision for urgent iliac artery or infrainguinal revascularization. Surgical femoral cut-down is

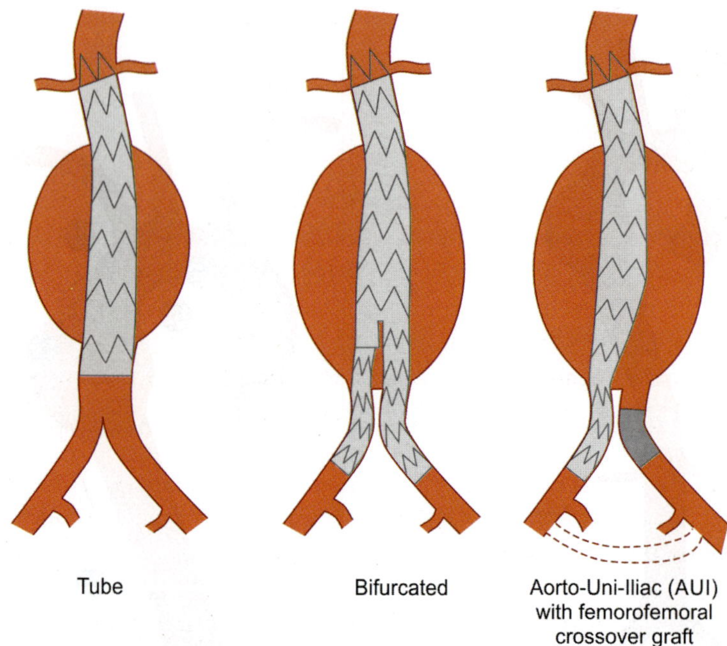

Fig. 6: Configurations of aortic stent-graft.
Sources:
1. England A, Mc Williams R. Endovascular aortic aneurysm repair (EVAR). Ulster Med J. 2013;82(1):3-10.
2. The Ulster Medical Society, 2013.

gradually being replaced by percutaneous access, which is associated with shorter time to hemostasis, less blood loss, and less groin pain.

Percutaneous access (PEVAR): Percutaneous femoral access has been reported with two suture-mediated "preclose" techniques, using either the Abbott ProStar XL or Abbott Perclose ProGlide. Both techniques involve blind or ultrasound-guided percutaneous access using micropuncture or standard access needles. It is very important that access point is optimized and in the anterior wall of common femoral artery (CFA). Percutaneous needle access is done under fluoroscopy to avoid calcium, and angiogram through needle to assess location in CFA. Alternatives include US-guided access of CFA. After access, 5F sheaths are placed on both sides. Two Proglide closure devices are placed in each vessel and angled to 45° off the centerline, so that their axes are 90° apart. It has to be made sure to follow wires and device tips on fluoroscopy as you work so that AAA is not disturbed. Amplatz wire is placed into the last closure device and 10F sheath placed in each CFA.

Closure: The access site is closed over a soft J-wire. Another Proglide should be available in case of failure. The wire is removed once it appears and hemostasis will be secured (before cinching knot). If hemostasis fails, a 14–16F sheath is placed and surgical repair must be done.

Steps of Device Deployment

After obtaining vascular access and the patient heparinized, landmarks for deployment of the upper end of the AAA endograft are obtained by angiography. The marker pigtail or Omniflush catheter is placed at the level of the renal arteries, and DSA is performed. The non-main body CFA for is used for the initial angiogram so the catheter can be left in place for device deployment. Alternatively, in patients with renal failure, a 6F IM renal guide can be placed in the lowest renal, and secured with a BMW wire, which is then used to locate the renal during deployment.

In cases where access is limited or difficult, it is dilated with a 14F dilator prior to introducing >18F EVAR device. Contralateral gate is lined up on fluoroscopy outside the body. The placement of the gate will be done to:

- Optimize gate access after main body deployment
- Stabilize device
- Carefully advance device under fluoroscopic guidance through the iliacs, minimize rotation

Proximal markers are lined up at the renal artery. Some cranial angulation is required in order to remove parallax and infrarenal neck is taken as much as possible. Small (5–10 cc) injections of contrast will identify the renal arteries. The sheath is pulled back to appropriate position to allow full deployment. The graft is then deployed till contralateral gate is out.

Contralateral gate access: A J-wire is placed into the pigtail and the trapped catheter is carefully removed from behind the graft, without losing the position within the aneurysm below the gate. Reaccessing the aneurysm sac after equipment is in can be difficult. Using an angled Glidewire and angled catheter or Omniflush, and multiple fluoroscopic views, the contralateral gate is accessed. Once in, a pigtail or Omniflush is placed into graft neck and rotated to assure intragraft position.

Hemodynamic monitoring is important, especially when the endograft delivery system is removed from the groin—it is at this point that an iliac rupture becomes evident; this can usually be effectively managed by deploying a covered stent.

Contralateral limb: An Amplatz wire is placed into the marker pigtail used to spin in the graft, but the catheter is not removed. The markers at the bottom of the gate are lined up and it is made sure markers extend well into the iliac arteries. The fluoroscope is angled to contralateral caudal 20–20 position. Contrast is injected through the contralateral sheath to identify the hypogastric, so that distance can be measured. A limb long enough to take as much of the iliac as possible is chosen and deployed carefully in gate. A Coda or Reliant balloon is used to dilate the proximal infrarenal attachment site, all graft overlap sites, and distal iliac attachment sites. The stent limbs are postdilated only for persistent external compression or twisting.

Role of Intravascular Ultrasound

Intravascular ultrasonography (IVUS) can be a helpful adjunct for graft selection, deployment, and further interrogation during EVAR. Usually for aortic procedures, 8–15 MHz transducers are selected. Lower frequencies offer the ability to view the entire artery. The IVUS catheter is inserted after obtaining access to both groins and is used to mark the location of the renal arteries aortic bifurcation, and hypogastric arteries, and measure the diameters of the proximal aorta, aortic bifurcation, and iliac arteries. With this, contrast angiography and significant fluoroscopy can be avoided until the main body is positioned for deployment. The contralateral gate can then be cannulated with IVUS, further reducing radiation exposure and contrast administration. The entire endograft can be examined for endoleaks.[34]

Endograft Surveillance

Frequent and life-long surveillance is mandatory for all patients who undergo EVAR in order to minimize risk of aneurysm rupture, though the frequency can be progressively reduced if the outcome is satisfactory. The modality most commonly used is CTA, although duplex ultrasonography and magnetic resonance imaging can also be used. CTA is typically performed at 1, 6, and 12 months and then annually thereafter. The primary aim for surveillance includes evaluation of residual aneurysm sac size and presence of endoleak, as well as potential adverse device specific events, such as endograft migration and separation of its components.

Endoleak

One of the major technical difficulties associated with the stent-graft technique that has yet to be overcome is the frequent occurrence of endoleaks, which occur in 10% of cases[35] and are seen angiographically as persistent contrast flow into the aneurysm sac because of failure to completely exclude the aneurysm from the aortic circulation. If left untreated, these endoleaks may potentially leave the patient at continued risk for aneurysm expansion or rupture **(Figs. 7A to D)**.

Endoleaks are of different types (Type I–Type V) **(Fig. 8)**. They can arise from the stent edges, overlap points, or retrograde filling from translumbar collaterals or inferior mesenteric or internal iliac arteries or from graft porosity. The first two types have to be treated on table to prevent aneurysm expansion and rupture. The retrograde filling is better avoided by proper

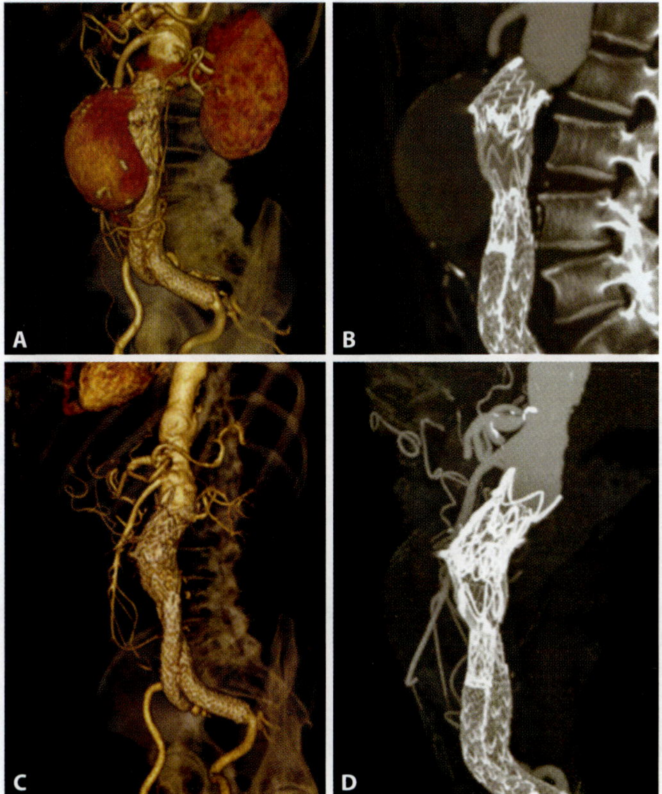

Figs. 7A to D: Endovascular aortic aneurysm repair (EVAR) for infrarenal aortic aneurysm. Patient developed pulsating swelling in abdomen after 2 weeks of stenting. CT angiogram revealed major endoleak. (A and B) Major endoleak; (C and D) After restenting.

preoperative planning and pre-graft embolization of the feeding vessel or can be treated later by CT-guided translumbar or transmesenteric embolization using a glue or a coil.

Recent innovations and stent design to tackle endoleak have come in the form of Nellix sac sealing devices, which aim at filling the aneurysmal sac with a sealing so that there is no space for an endoleak or stent migration. This device is currently undergoing FDA-IDE trial.

Ruptured Aneurysm

Ruptured AAAs are being treated by endovascular aortic aneurysm repair (EVAR) and other endovascular techniques with increasing frequency.

The minimally invasive nature of EVAR makes it an option in critically ill patients with ruptured or symptomatic AAA. Emergency EVAR is associated with a significant reduction in mortality, ICU and hospital stay, blood loss

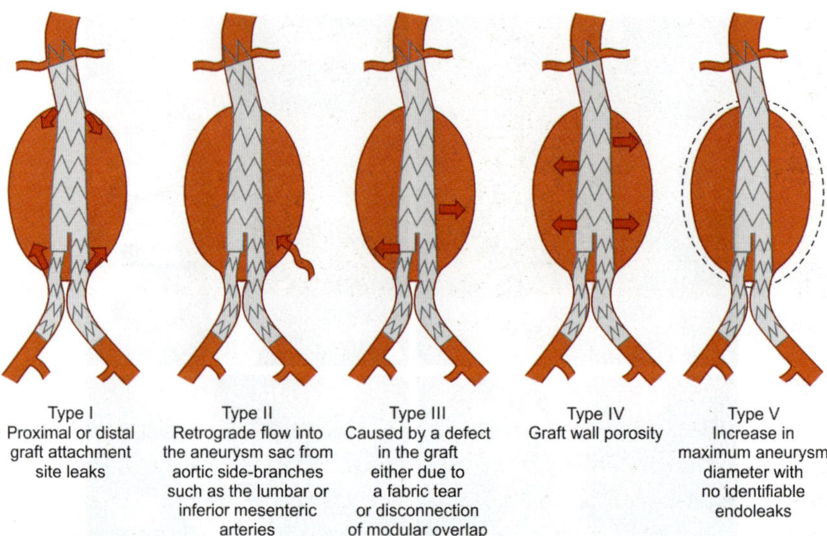

Fig. 8: Endoleak classification system.

Sources:

1. England A, Mc Williams R. Endovascular aortic aneurysm repair (EVAR). Ulster Med J. 2013;82(1):3-10.
2. The Ulster Medical Society, 2013.

and procedure time compared to open repair. Proper use of aortic balloon control (techniques have been developed to maintenance of continuous aortic control until the endograft has sealed the leak using multiple balloons to minimize renal and visceral ischemia by placing secondary balloons within the endograft while the supraceliac balloon is deflated and removed through its supporting sheath), adequate recognition and treatment of abdominal compartment syndrome, and the establishment of a structured system and protocol for the treatment all contribute to improved survival outcomes in patients with ruptured aneurysms.

Rarely ascending aorta may develop postoperative pseudoaneurysm which may rupture and cause fatal bleeding and surgery may not be an option at this stage. We report such a case which was probably the first reported case in literature of treating ruptured pseudoaneurysms of ascending aorta (Zone 0) by atrial septal defect (ASD) closure device (AMPLATZER Inc., USA) **(Figs. 9A to C)**.

Mycotic Aneurysm

These are usually saccular aneurysms with mold like appearance as result of bacterial infection in the aortic wall. They usually have high risk of rupture and are associated with sepsis. Unlike their name, they are not of fungal origin but are associated with bacterial infections which is usually salmonella,

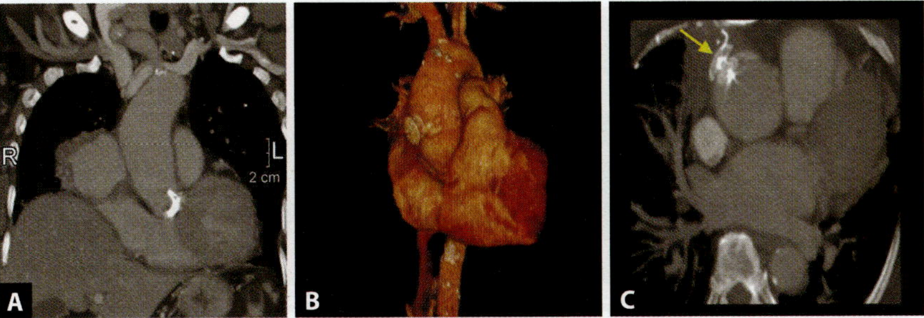

Figs. 9A to C: (A) Large ruptured Zone 0 pseudoaneurysm, (B) successfully treated by ASD closure device, (C) follow-up CT angio confirming complete closure. (ASD: atrial septal defect)

streptococci, or mycobacterium tuberculosis. Untreated mycotic aneurysms are associated with almost 90–95% mortality. Surgery is the mainstay of treatment but carries a high perioperative mortality. Patients require high dose of long-term parenteral antibiotic therapy. In rare situations, if surgery is turned down because of very high perioperative risk and severe comorbidities, EVAR may be offered, usually as a bail out procedure or sometimes even as definitive procedures. However, it does carry a high risk of graft infection. Long-term parenteral antibiotic therapy is a rule in these cases.

We report two cases of large mycotic aneurysm with rupture leading to aortoesophageal fistula **(Figs. 10A to E)** and another one with rupture of large infrarenal aortic aneurysm **(Figs. 11A to E)**.

Recent Advances in EVAR: Fenestrated, Chimney, Multilayered Flow Modulator

Recent advances in technology have allowed complex thoracic and AAAs to be treated via the endovascular approach. Patients considered for treatment include those with bilateral common iliac artery aneurysms, short infrarenal necks, thoracoabdominal aneurysms and those with tortuous iliac vessels. Newer techniques are progressively pushing the limits of EVAR into territories hitherto considered unsuitable for EVAR such as juxtarenal (aneurysm originating at the level of the renal arteries) and suprarenal (aneurysm originating above the renal arteries) AAAs. Some of these techniques are described below:

Fenestrated endografts: These are endografts which have holes made in the fabric to permit flow into aortic branches which would otherwise be occluded by the endograft **(Fig. 12)**. Fenestrated stent-grafts are not well suited if the fabric of the stent-graft cannot abut the aortic wall at the level of the visceral arteries. The intermediate-term results with this technology have been encouraging.[36] However "off-the-shelf" fenestrated endografts may become

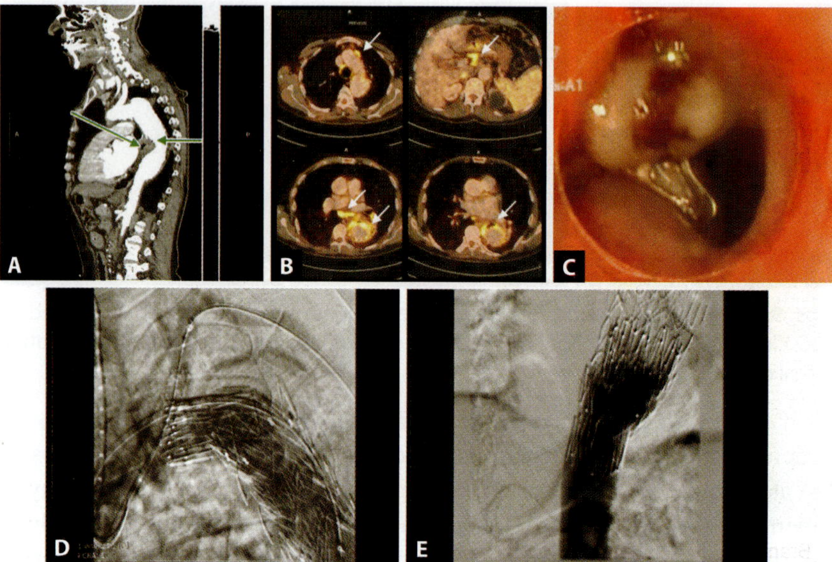

Figs. 10A to E: (A and B) Depicts a case of perioperative thoracic mycotic aneurysm with high fluorodeoxyglucose (FDG) uptake on PET scan leading to rupture into the esophagus presenting with hematemesis. Patient underwent an upper gastrointestinal endoscopy which confirmed (C) aortoesophageal fistula (AEF) and stent struts visible through the fistula in the esophagus. Patient underwent long-term parenteral antibiotic therapy and antitubercular treatment followed by successful (D) chimney procedure along with (E) thoracic endovascular aortic repair (C-TEVAR). (PET: positron emission tomography)

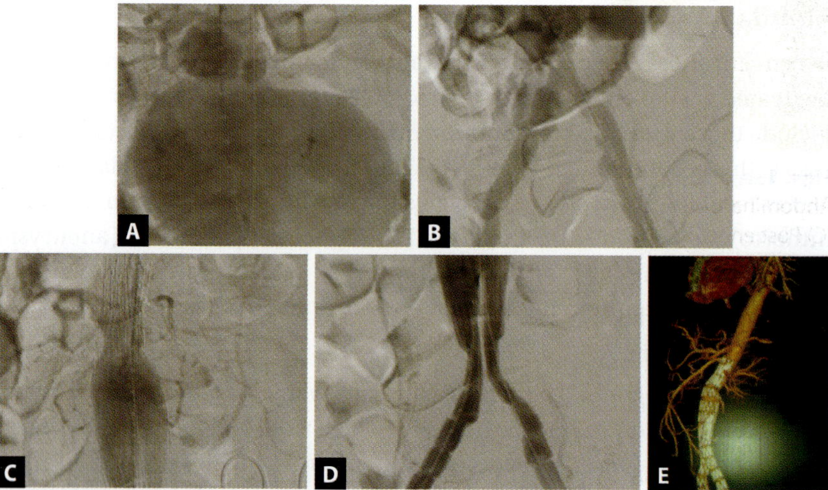

Figs. 11A to E: Another patient with (A and B) multiple large infrarenal mycotic aneurysms and contained ruptured underwent (C and D) successful EVAR as at definitive therapy with (E) 2-year follow-up. (EVAR: endovascular aortic aneurysm repair)

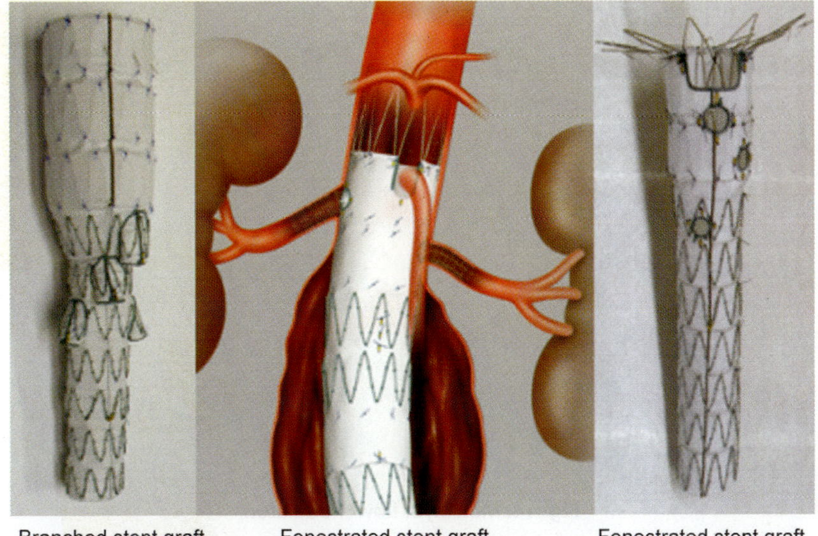

Fig. 12: Fenestrated stent grafts.

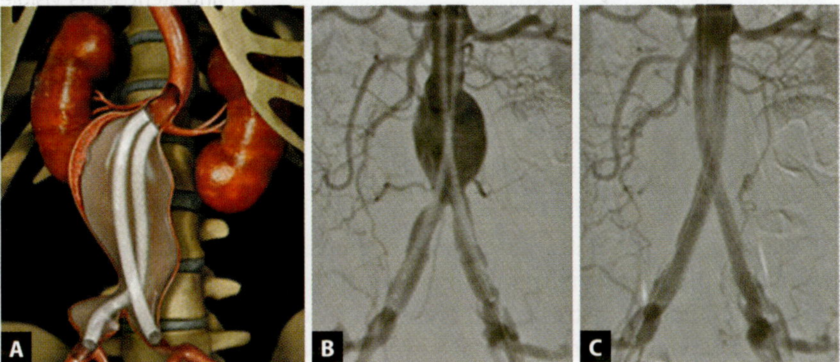

Figs. 13A to C: Nellix sac sealing device. (A) Principle of Nellix sac sealing device; (B) Abdominal aortic aneurysm—endovascular aortic aneurysm repair using Nellix device; (C) Post endovascular aortic aneurysm repair using Nellix device.

commercially available in the near future such as the Endologix Ventana fenestrated system.[37]

Nellix endovascular aneurysm sealing system: The Nellix Sac-Anchoring Endoprosthesis Dual balloon expandable endoframes provide flow lumens **(Figs. 13A to C)**. Polymer-filled endobags obliterate aneurysm sac, provide support and eliminate endoleak space. Fixation is not dependent on proximal neck and iliac arteries. Common iliac aneurysms are treated with preservation of internal iliac. The 30-day results of the Nellix system

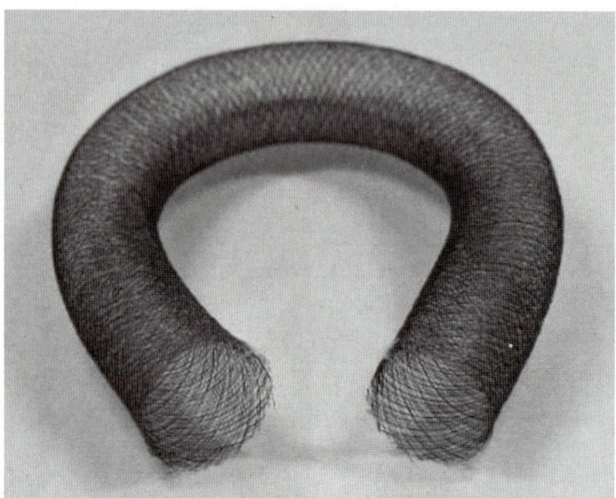

Fig. 14: Multilayer flow modulator.

investigational device exemption pivotal trial for endovascular aneurysm sealing were published recently and showed encouraging results with very low morbidity and mortality.[38]

Cardiatis multilayer flow modulator: Multilayered flow modulators (MFMs) are the in-thing for complex aortic arch aneurysms and are undergoing an FDA trial **(Fig. 14)**.

They work on the principle of directing the flow to the central lumen and stopping Eddy currents and vortex in the aneurysmal sac and increasing the flow in the involved branches arising from the aneurysm.

Chimney grafts: The chimney or snorkel graft is a covered stent deployed parallel to the aortic endograft into a side branch covered by the aortic endograft; it points upstream and preserves flow to the side branch covered by the aortic endograft. A similar covered stent pointing downstream is called a periscope graft. Use of the chimney graft makes it possible to use standard endografts to treat aneurysms with inadequate proximal sealing zones. Chimney grafts have been used in the abdominal aorta and in the aortic arch[39] and are generally reserved for high-risk patients and bail-out situations **(Fig. 10)**.

THORACIC ENDOVASCULAR AORTIC REPAIR

Thoracic endovascular aortic repair (TEVAR) is an emerging treatment modality, which has been rapidly embraced by clinicians treating thoracic aortic disease—chronic aneurysm and acute aortic syndromes. Acute aortic syndromes are a group of acute aortic pathologies, viz., acute dissection, ruptured TAA, penetrating ulcer, intramural hematoma, traumatic injuries **(Fig. 15)**.

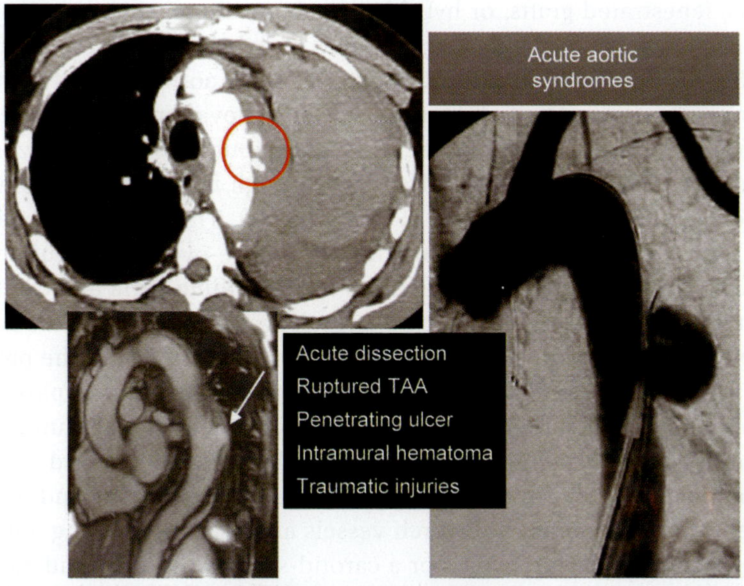

Fig. 15: Acute aortic syndrome.

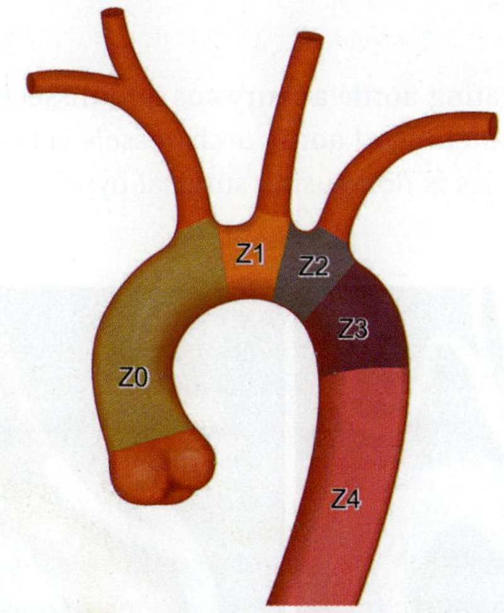

Fig. 16: Zone wise classification of aorta.

For treatment purposes, the aortic arch is divided into five zones (Z0–Z4). Z0 is from aortic root to end of innominate artery; Z1 from end of innominate to end of left common carotid artery; Z2 is from end of left common carotid to end of left subclavian artery; Z3 is from left subclavian artery to end of aortic arch, and Z4 is descending thoracic aorta **(Fig. 16)**.

The TEVAR is the standard of care for aneurysms involving zone 3 and zone 4 and has extended to zone 2 and zone 1 with the help of chimney grafts, fenestrated grafts, or hybrid procedures. Zone 0 aneurysms are a real challenge but are being managed now by hybrid procedures involving total aortic debranching and graft from ascending aorta or use of multiple chimneys or fenestrated endografts. Recent innovations include the use of multilayered flow modulator (MFM) for aneurysms involving zone 0 to zone 2. TEVAR is usually performed through femoral arteriotomy as the device is bulky (usually 20–24 F diameter). The procedure is done in a standard manner by advancing the device over a stiff guidewire passed through the femoral artery into the ascending aorta and carefully desheathing the device, taking care not to cover the arch vessels. Many a times, we may have to cover the left subclavian artery, and if the patient gets symptomatic, to do a left carotid to left subclavian artery bypass. This complication can sometimes be avoided by putting in a chimney graft or doing a fenestrated graft procedure. The left common carotid and the innominate arteries can also be covered to get proper landing and sealing zones, after we debranch the arch vessels and do an ascending aorta to carotid and subclavian bypass or a carotid-subclavian or carotid-carotid bypass. MFMs are the in-thing for complex aortic arch aneurysms and are undergoing an FDA trial **(Fig. 14)**.

HYBRID

Hybrid repair for treating aortic aneurysms and dissections is a technique where surgical debranching of aortic arch vessels **(Figs. 17 and 18)**, renal and mesenteric arteries is done using surgical bypass grafts and ligation of

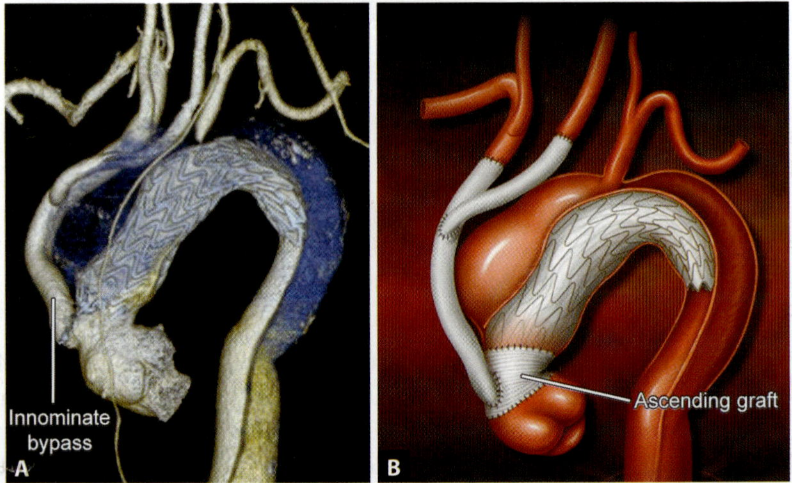

Figs. 17A and B: DeBakey I dissecting aneurysm of aorta. Treatment by hybrid aortic endovascular repair using a conduit to debranch right innominate artery and left common carotid artery.

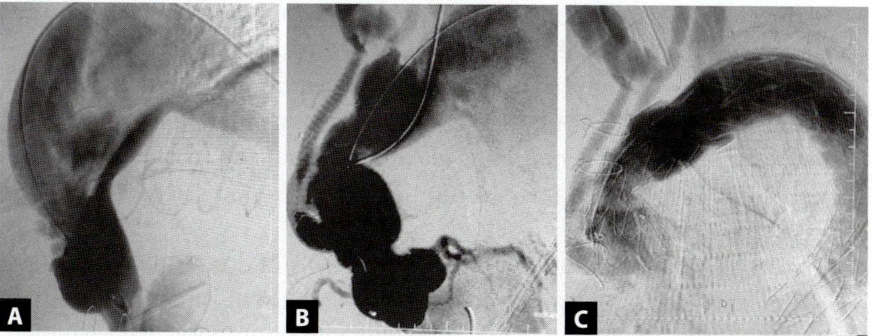

Figs. 18A to C: (A) DeBakey I dissecting aneurysm of aorta. Treatment by hybrid aortic endovascular repair using; (B) a conduit to debranch right innominate artery and left common carotid and subclavian artery; (C) stent grafts from ascending aorta to descending thoracic aorta.

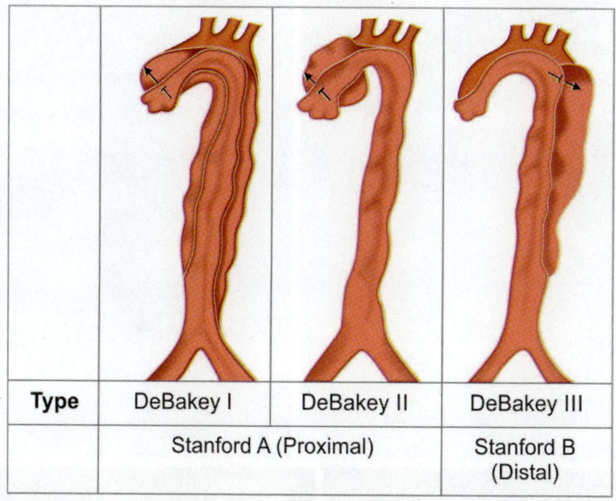

Fig. 19: DeBakey and Stanford classification of aortic dissections.

these vessels near the origin of these arteries. This allows extra anatomical perfusion to brain, arm, kidney and gut and allows extra landing space for the graft to adequately seal the aneurysm or treat the entry tear in aorta. This allows us to conquer zone 0. Zone 1 and zone 2 of thoracic aorta and suprarenal and juxta mesenteric thoracoabdominal aneurysms. This procedure reduces the operating time, cardiopulmonary bypass time, need for prolonged hypothermia and excessive blood loss can significantly reduce the mortality and morbidity for treatment.

DISSECTION OF AORTA

Dissection of aorta can involve both thoracic and abdominal aorta but thoracic aorta is more commonly involved. Thoracic aortic dissection is classically classified as DeBakey 1, 2, and 3 or Stanford A and B **(Fig. 19)**.

Stanford A is dissection of ascending aorta which traditionally requires surgery and Stanford B is dissection of descending aorta which may require EVAR as first-line therapy. In acute type B dissection if the patient presents with renal, mesenteric, or lower limb ischemia, the indication of treatment is emergency-in-situ fenestration. This allows equalization of pressure and perfusion for in true and false lumen leading to reperfusion of ischemic organs **(Figs. 20A to D)**.

Type B aortic dissections which are <2 months of duration or where the false lumen is enlarging can be treated by TEVAR. This allows immediate expansion of true lumen and depressurization and thrombosis of false lumen. Sometimes, the true lumen may be expanded in entire length by putting

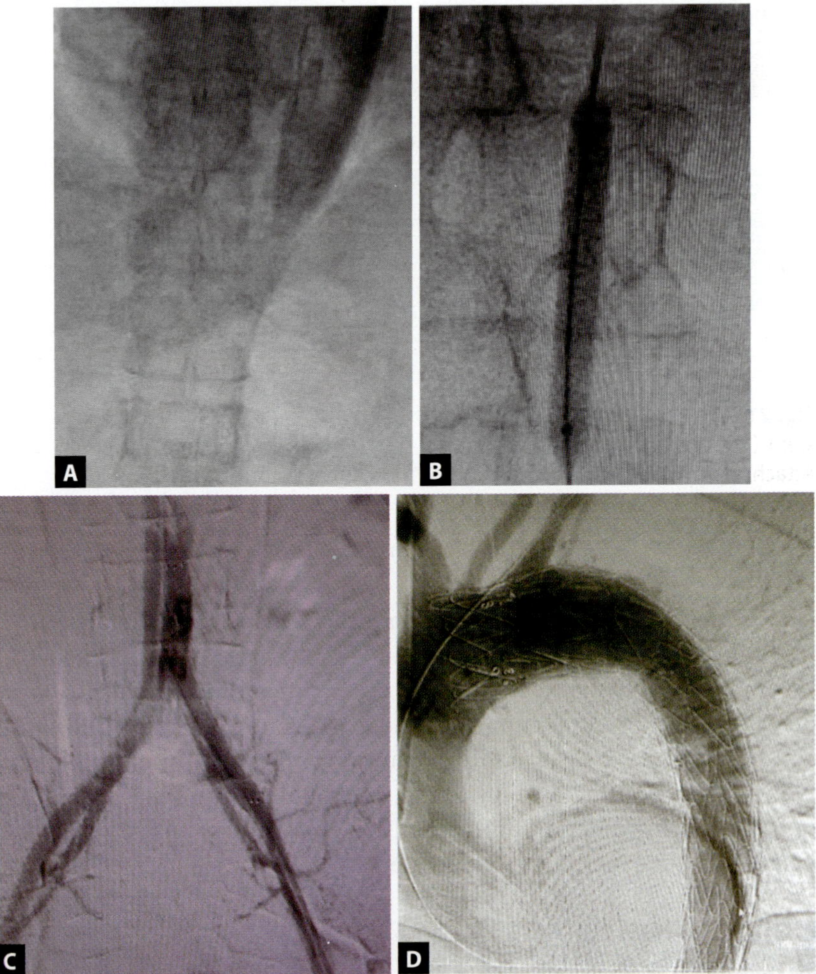

Figs. 20A to D: (A) Stanford type B aortic dissection with severe mesenteric and lower limb ischemia treated by (B and C) in-situ fenestration and (D) chimney TEVAR. (TEVAR: thoracic endovascular aortic repair)

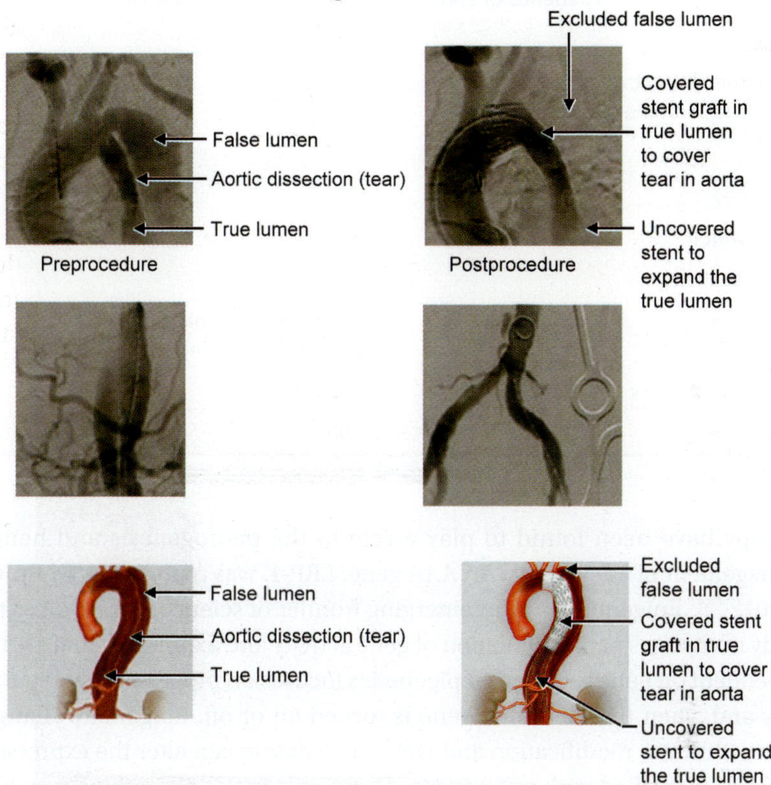

Fig. 21: TEVAR for type B dissection using stent graft and uncovered self-expanding stent (PETTICOAT technique). (PETTICOAT: Provisional Extension To Induce Complete Attachment; TEVAR: thoracic endovascular aortic repair)

additional noncovered self-expanding stents Provisional Extension To Induce Complete Attachment (PETTICOAT) technique **(Fig. 21)**.

However, type B dissections if they are >2 months of duration and are stable they can be followed up on optimal medical therapy and may not require endovascular or surgical repair.

Stanford A dissections or DeBakey III can be treated by hybrid TEVARs using trifurcated synthetic PTFE grafts from ascending aorta to right innominate, left common carotid and left subclavian artery and putting in aortic endograft from ascending aorta (Zone 0) to aortic arch and descending thoracic aorta. We are reporting our experience of EVAR and TEVAR over a period of last 24 years in **Table 1**.

GENOMICS, PROTEOMICS, AND CELLULAR THERAPY IN AORTIC ANEURYSMS

Device development has been and will continue to be the key component in the management of AAAs. However, genomics, proteomics, and cellular

TABLE 1: Personal experience of endovascular aortic aneurysm repair.

Number	901
Abdominal aortic aneurysm/ thoracoabdominal aortic aneurysm	580/321
Hybrid	63
Chimney	127
CIE/conduit	26
Embolization	51
Endoleak	33 (no type I endoleak was left untreated on table)
Technical success	899/901
Mortality	2/901

therapy have been found to play a role in the pathogenesis and hence, management of aneurysms. An *AAA* gene, LRP-1, was reported by M Brown in 2012.[40,41] Epigenomics is an emerging frontier of science that involves the study of changes in the regulation of gene activity and expression that are not dependent on gene sequence. Epigenetics focuses on processes that regulate how and when the identified gene is turned on or off. Epigenetic changes such as histone modification and DNA methylation can alter the expression of genes identified with aneurysms. These epigenetic alterations may also stem from known AAA risk factors such as smoking, aging, and inflammation. Understanding the human genome and the science of epigenomics and influencing it will make fundamental changes in healthcare delivery by detecting, treating, reversing, and preventing AAAs.

CONCLUSION

Endovascular aortic aneurysm repair requires extensive preoperative preparation not only for graft selection but also for optimal deployment. One must consider the method of access, device delivery, management of large branches, graft orientation, and contralateral limb deployment. Once deployed, the graft must be assessed for endoleaks and limb compression before arteriotomy and wound closure. Failure to understand these EVAR techniques and inadequate planning for each step can result in endoleaks, visceral malperfusion, and extremity ischemia, precipitating the need for emergent complex open repair.

Keys to success include—appropriate patient selection, precise device placement with focus on good fixation and seal in proximal aortic neck and distal landing zone, appropriate and timely patient follow-up.

REFERENCES

1. Hirsch AT, Haskal ZJ, Hertzer NR, Bakal CW, Creager MA, Halperin JL, et al. ACC/AHA 2005 Practice Guidelines for the management of patients with peripheral arterial disease (lower extremity, renal, mesenteric, and abdominal aortic): A collaborative report from the American Association for Vascular Surgery/Society for Vascular Surgery, Society for Cardiovascular Angiography and Interventions, Society for Vascular Medicine and Biology, Society of Interventional Radiology, and the ACC/AHA Task Force on Practice Guidelines (Writing Committee to Develop Guidelines for the Management of Patients With Peripheral Arterial Disease): Endorsed by the American Association of Cardiovascular and Pulmonary Rehabilitation; National Heart, Lung, and Blood Institute; Society for Vascular Nursing; Trans-Atlantic Inter-Society Consensus; and Vascular Disease Foundation. Circulation. 2006;113:e463-e654.
2. Ouriel K, Green RM, Donayre C, Shortell CK, Elliott J, DeWeese JA. An evaluation of new methods of expressing aortic aneurysm size: Relationship to rupture. J Vasc Surg. 1992;15:12-8.
3. Greenhalgh RM, Powell JT. Endovascular repair of abdominal aortic aneurysm. N Engl J Med. 2008;358(5):494-501.
4. Naef AP. The mid-century revolution in thoracic and cardiovascular surgery: Part 5. Interact Cardiovasc Thorac Surg. 2004;3(3):415-22.
5. Volodos NL, Karpovich IP, Shekhanin VE, Troian VI, Iakovenko LF. A case of distant transfemoral endoprosthesis of the thoracic artery using a self-fixing synthetic prosthesis in traumatic aneurysm. Grudn Khir. 1988;(6):84-6.
6. Dake MD, Miller DC, Semba CP, Mitchell RS, Walker PJ, Liddell RP. Transluminal placement of endovascular stent-grafts for the treatment of descending thoracic aortic aneurysms. N Engl J Med. 1994;331(26):1729-34.
7. Jackson RS, Chang DC, Freischlag JA. Comparison of long-term survival after open vs endovascular repair of intact abdominal aortic aneurysm among Medicare beneficiaries. JAMA. 2012;307(15):1621-8.
8. Blum U, Voshage G, Lammer J, Beyersdorf F, Töllner D, Kretschmer G, et al. Endoluminal stent-grafts for infrarenal abdominal aortic aneurysms. N Engl J Med. 1997;336:13-20.
9. Criado FJ, Wilson EP, Fairman RM, Abul-Khoudoud O, Wellons E, et al. Update on the talent aortic stent-graft: A preliminary report from United States phase I and II trials. J Vasc Surg. 2001;33:S146-S9.
10. Elkouri S, Gloviczki P, McKusick MA, Panneton JM, Andrews JC, Bower TC, et al. Endovascular repair of abdominal aortic aneurysms: Initial experience with 100 consecutive patients. Mayo Clin Proc. 2003;78:1234-42.
11. Improve Trial, Powell JT, Thompson SG, Thompson MM, Grieve R, Nicholson AA, et al. The Immediate Management of the Patient with Rupture: Open Versus Endovascular repair (IMPROVE) aneurysm trial—ISRCTN 48334791 IMPROVE trialists. Acta Chir Belg. 2009;109(6):678-80.
12. Hoornweg LL, Wisselink W, Vahl A, Balm R. Amsterdam Acute Aneurysm Trial Collaborators. The Amsterdam Acute Aneurysm Trial: suitability and application rate for endovascular repair of ruptured abdominal aortic aneurysms. Eur J Vasc Endovasc Surg. 2007;33(6):679-83.
13. Greenhalgh RM, Brown LC, Kwong GP, Powell JT, Thompson SG; EVAR trial participants. Comparison of endovascular aneurysm repair with open repair

in patients with abdominal aortic aneurysm (EVAR trial 1), 30-day operative mortality results: Randomized controlled trial. Lancet. 2004;364:843-8.
14. Teufelsbauer H, Prusa AM, Wolff K, Polterauer P, Nanobashvili J, Prager M, et al. Endovascular stent grafting versus open surgical operation in patients with infrarenal aortic aneurysms: A propensity score-adjusted analysis. Circulation. 2002;106:782-7.
15. National Institute for Health and Clinical Excellence. Endovascular stent-grafts for the treatment of abdominal aortic aneurysms [TAG167]. London: National Institute for Health and Clinical Excellence; 2009.
16. Harris PL, Buth J. An update on the important findings from the EUROSTAR EVAR registry. Vascular. 2004;12:33-8.
17. United Kingdom EVAR Trial Investigators, Greenhalgh RM, Brown LC, Powell JT, Thompson SG, Epstein D, et al. Endovascular versus open repair of abdominal aortic aneurysm. N Engl J Med. 2010;362:1863-71.
18. De Bruin JL, Baas AF, Buth J, Prinssen M, Verhoeven EL, Cuypers PW, et al. Long-term outcome of open or endovascular repair of abdominal aortic aneurysm. N Engl J Med. 2010;362:1881-9.
19. Lederle FA, Freischlag JA, Kyriakides TC, Matsumura JS, Padberg FT Jr, Kohler TR, et al. Long-term comparison of endovascular and open repair of abdominal aortic aneurysm. N Engl J Med. 2012;367:1988-97.
20. Guo D, Hasham S, Kuang S-Q, Vaughan CJ, Boerwinkle E, Chen H, et al. Familial thoracic aortic aneurysms and dissections. Circulation. 2001;103:2461-8.
21. Milewicz DM, Chen H, Park E-S, Petty EM, Zaghi H, Shashidhar G, et al. Reduced penetrance and variable expressivity of familial thoracic aneurysms/dissections. Am J Cardiol. 1998;82:474-9.
22. Hasham SN, Willing MC, Guo DC, Muilenburg A, He R, Tran VT, et al. Mapping a locus for familial thoracic aortic aneurysms and dissections (TAAD2) to 3p24–25. Circulation. 2003;107:3184-90.
23. Ashton HA, Buxton MJ, Day NE, Kim LG, Marteau TM, Scott RA, et al. The Multicentre Aneurysm Screening Study (MASS) into the effect of abdominal aortic aneurysm screening on mortality in men: a randomised controlled trial. Lancet. 2002;360(9345):1531-9.
24. Brady AR, Thompson SG, Fowkes FG, Greenhalgh RM, Powell JT. Participants UK Small Aneurysm Trial Participants. Abdominal aortic aneurysm expansion: risk factors and time intervals for surveillance. Circulation. 2004;110(1):16-21.
25. Chaikof EL, Brewster DC, Dalman RL, Makaroun MS, Illig KA, Sicard GA, et al. The care of patients with an abdominal aortic aneurysm: The society for vascular surgery practice guidelines. J Vasc Surg. 2009;50:S2-49.
26. Gadowski GR, Pilcher DB, Ricci MA. Abdominal aortic aneurysm expansion rate: effect of size and beta-adrenergic blockade. J Vasc Surg. 1994;19:727-31.
27. Davies RR, Goldstein LJ, Coady MA, Tittle SL, Rizzo JA, Kopf GS, et al. Yearly rupture or dissection rates for thoracic aortic aneurysms: simple prediction based on size. Ann Thorac Surg. 2002;73:17-28.
28. LaRoy LL, Cormier PJ, Matalon TA, Patel SK, Turner DA, Silver B. Imaging of abdominal aortic aneurysms. AJR Am J Roentgenol. 1989;152:785-92.
29. US Preventive Services Task Force. Screening for abdominal aortic aneurysm: Recommendation statement. Ann Intern Med. 2005;142:198-202.

30. Schanzer A, Greenberg RK, Hevelone N, Robinson WP, Eslami MH, Goldberg RJ, et al. Predictors of abdominal aortic aneurysm sac enlargement after endovascular repair. Circulation. 2011;123(24):2848-55.
31. Vallabhaneni SR, Harris PL. Lessons learnt from the EUROSTAR registry on endovascular repair of abdominal aortic aneurysm repair. Eur J Radiol. 2001;39(1):34-41.
32. EVAR Trial Participants. Endovascular aneurysm repair versus open repair in patients with abdominal aortic aneurysm (EVAR trial 1): randomised controlled trial. Lancet. 2005;365(9478):2179-86.
33. Prinssen M, Verhoeven EL, Buth J, Cuypers PW, van Sambeek MR, Balm R, et al. A randomized trial comparing conventional and endovascular repair of abdominal aortic aneurysms. N Engl J Med. 2004;351(16):1607-18.
34. Pearce BJ, Jordan WD. Using IVUS during EVAR and TEVAR: improving patient outcomes. Semin Vasc Surg. 2009;22(3):172-80.
35. Brewster DC, Cronenwett JL, Hallett JW Jr, Johnston KW, Krupski WC, Matsumura JS. Joint Council of the American Association for Vascular Surgery and Society for Vascular Surgery. Guidelines for the treatment of abdominal aortic aneurysms: report of a subcommittee of the Joint Council of the American Association for Vascular Surgery and Society for Vascular Surgery. J Vasc Surg. 2003;37:1106-17.
36. Greenberg RK, Sternbergh WC, Makaroun M, Ohki T, Chuter T, Bharadwaj P, et al. Intermediate results of a United States multicenter trial of fenestrated endograft repair for juxtarenal abdominal aortic aneurysms. J Vasc Surg. 2009; 50:730-7.e1.
37. Mertens R, Bergoeing M, Mariné L, Valdés F, Krämer A, Vergara J. Ventana fenestrated stent-graft system for endovascular repair of juxtarenal aortic aneurysms. J Endovasc Ther. 2012;19:173-8.
38. Carpenter JP, Cuff R, Buckley C, Healey C, Hussain S, Reijnen MM, et al. Thirty-day results of the Nellix system investigational device exemption pivotal trial for endovascular aneurysm sealing. J Vasc Surg. 2016;63(1):23-31.e1.
39. Mangialardi N, Ronchey S, Malaj A, Fazzini S, Alberti V, Ardita V, et al. Value and limitations of chimney grafts to treat arch lesions. J Cardiovasc Surg (Torino). 2015;56:503-11.
40. Khanna NN, Henry M. Handbook of Interventions for Structural Heart and Peripheral Vascular Disease, 1st edition. New Delhi: Jaypee Brothers Medical Publisher; 2016.
41. Bown MJ, Jones GT, Harrison SC, Wright BJ, Bumpstead S, Baas AF, et al. Abdominal aortic aneurysm is associated with a variant in low-density lipoprotein receptor-related protein 1. Am J Hum Genet. 2011;89(5):619-27.

CHAPTER 48

Superficial Femoral Artery Interventions: Practical-based Approach

J Ezhilan

INTRODUCTION

Peripheral arterial disease (PAD) is defined as the deposition of atherosclerosis, causing blocks in any vessel in the body other than the coronaries and intracranial brain vessels. About 11.7% of people above 40 have PAD, and globally 113 million people have peripheral vascular disease (PVD). In PAD what we see clinically is only the tip of the iceberg.

Peripheral arterial disease (PAD) based on the body part and vascular territory can be classified as shown in **Box 1**.

Among various types of PAD, lower extremity artery disease is more common, and in LEAD, superficial femoral artery (SFA) disease is more common.

SUPERFICIAL FEMORAL ARTERY

The SFA is the most common site of PAD and also is the leading cause of claudication. The SFA artery extends from the groin to the knee and is 30 cm in length. The most common place of involvement in SFA is in the adductor canal. Occlusions are three times more common in SFA and often tend to be bilateral. Unlike any other artery, the body of the SFA is subjected to flexion, compression, torsion, extension, and contraction all of which make angioplasty of this vessel difficult **(Fig. 1)**. In SFA disease, the profunda femoris branch well collateralizes the SFA; hence, acute limb threat is very rare.

It is more than 55 years since the first SFA angioplasty was done by Charles Dotter. Initial results with plain balloon angioplasty were not good because of the inherent problems with SFA leading to high rates of restenosis, but now with advances in the technique of SFA angioplasty, the procedural success

BOX 1: Peripheral arterial disease based on the body part and vascular territory.

- *Neck:* Carotid and Vertebral artery disease (CVAD)
- *Upper limb:* Upper extremity artery disease (UEAD)
- *Abdomen:*
  - Mesenteric artery disease (MAD)
  - Renal artery disease (RAD)
- *Lower limb:* Lower extremity disease (LEAD)

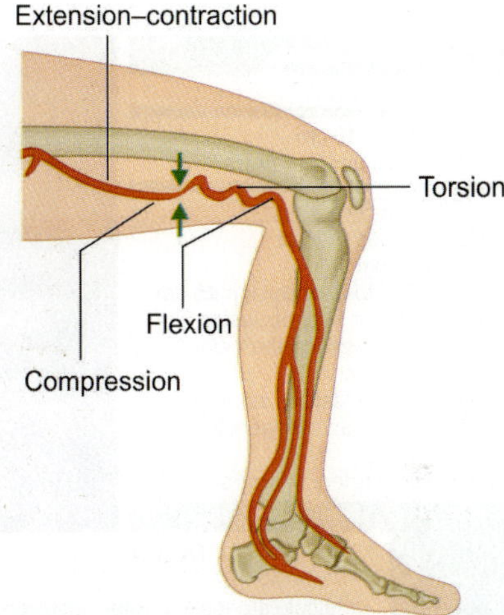

Fig. 1: Biomechanical forces acting on superficial femoral artery.

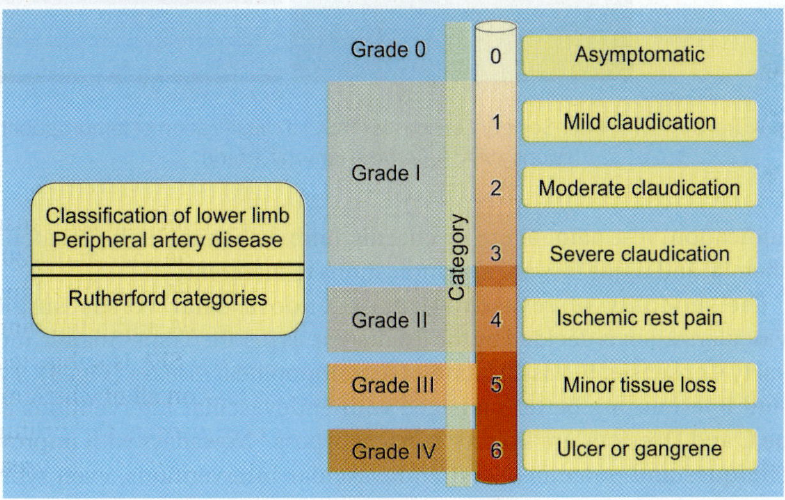

Fig. 2: Rutherford's classification of chronic limb ischemia.

has increased significantly, and the morbidity and mortality have also come down drastically. Nowadays more endovascular procedures are being done for SFA disease than open surgical procedures.

INDICATIONS FOR SUPERFICIAL FEMORAL ARTERY ANGIOPLASTY

The indication to intervene in a patient with SFA disease is based on the stage of the patient's presentation. If the patient is in Rutherford's class 4–6 **(Fig. 2)**, he can be taken up for revascularization.[1] The presence of severe

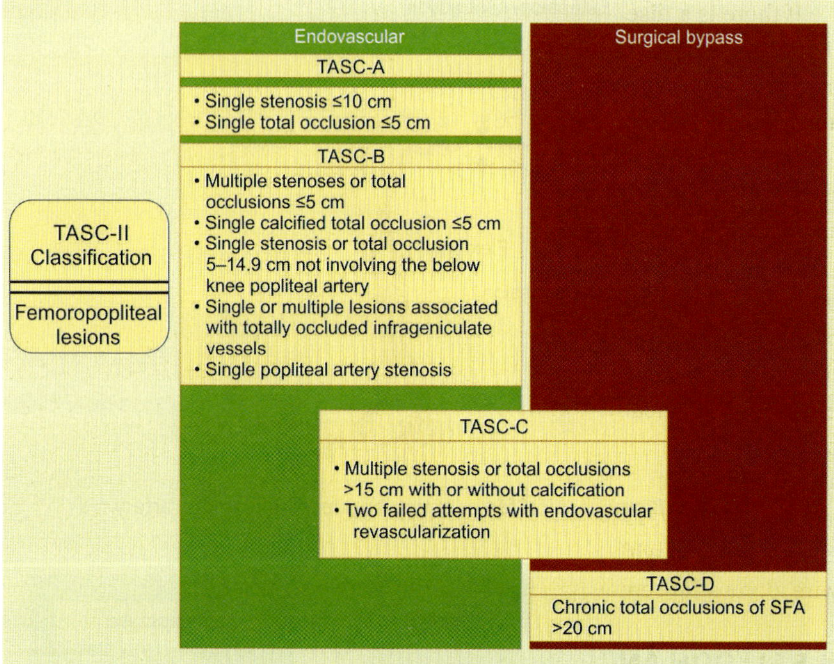

Fig. 3: Trans-Atlantic Inter-Society Consensus (TASC) II classification of femoropopliteal lesions. (SFA: superficial femoral artery)

claudication, rest pain, acute or chronic limb ischemia, limb-threatening ischemia, and tissue loss are also indications to intervene.

The modality of revascularization endovascular versus surgical revascularization is decided by the lesion type as per the Trans-Atlantic Inter-Society Consensus II classification of femoropopliteal disease **(Fig. 3)**. Type A and B lesions are better managed with endovascular interventions and type C and D lesions are sent for surgical bypass.[2] Nowadays with improved techniques and outcomes with endovascular interventions, even type C lesions can be dealt with endovascular interventions.

VASCULAR ACCESS TECHNIQUES

Vascular access for SFA interventions can be one of the following four routes:

1. Contralateral retrograde common femoral artery (CFA) access
2. Ipsilateral antegrade CFA access
3. Brachial/axillary approach
4. Retrograde popliteal/distal SFA/tibioperoneal/pedal arteries

An ultrasound-guided puncture is the best way to gain access and is very useful, especially if the artery is not palpable.[3] If ultrasound guidance is not available, fluoroscopic guidance can be utilized and a micropuncture needle is preferred for gaining access.

If there is a disease in proximal SFA, the antegrade puncture is avoided. If the aortic bifurcation angle is narrow (<80°), the antegrade approach is preferred as it will be difficult to cross over and work by the contralateral approach, or one can come down from the brachial or axillary approach.

In suprainguinal and SFA combined lesions where you need to work retrogradely for the iliacs and antegradely for the CFA, both can be done by a single puncture of the CFA.

In this technique, the CFA is accessed retrogradely first and a wire is placed in the aorta following which a sheath is inserted. After completion of the iliac angioplasty, 0.028″ guide wire is placed retrogradely from the puncture site into the aorta. One more 0.025″ or 0.028″ guide wire is inserted into the same sheath. The second wire was manually shaped with a U bend before insertion. Then gradually the CFA sheath is withdrawn till the puncture site. The wire with a U bend was gradually withdrawn till it engages the CFA in a antegrade way. This is called as reverse wiring technique. Then the sheath is removed and with a dilator the sheath is inserted only over the antegrade wire alone after removing the retrograde wire.

BALLOON ANGIOPLASTY

After gaining arterial access, a sheath is placed in the artery ranging from 4 to 7 French. The patient is then heparinized to achieve an activated clotting time (ACT) of 250 seconds or more. The lesion is then crossed with a 0.035″ or 0.018″ guide wire and the catheter is placed proximal to the lesion, providing support to track the balloon and stent.[4]

If the lesion is a chronic total occlusion, devices like FRONTRUNNER and QUICKCROSS are available which maintains the wire in the center and helps to cross the lesion. If the wire does not cross through true lumen, subintimal tracking of the wire can be done. After crossing the lesion reentry into the true lumen can be done with devices like OUTBACK or PIONEER.

Balloon angioplasty has been the most common technique used to open SFA for nearly five decades, but now plain balloon angioplasty is being slowly given up due to the availability of better options. However, it is still useful in discrete, less complex lesions, when used in complex lesions it might be complicated by dissection, residual stenosis, vessel recoil, or abrupt closure. The data from three randomized controlled trials showed in lesion length up to 8 cm, the 1-year patency rate for balloon angioplasty was 28%.

Techniques to achieve better results with balloon angioplasty are one should use noncompliant balloons for angioplasty, the diameter of the balloon should not increase the diameter of the vessel with a 1:1 ratio, one should not go above the rated burst pressure and the time of balloon inflation should be at least 2–3 minutes.

STENTING

In the early RCTs comparing balloon angioplasty to stenting did not show any benefit, but that was with the use of stainless-steel bare metal stents (BMSs). Now the following stents are available for SFA stenting:

- Stainless steel stents
- Nitinol stents
- Covered stents
- Drug-eluting stents
- Biodegradable stents

Nitinol Stents

The change in platform from stainless steel to nitinol showed better results with stenting compared to balloon angioplasty. The FAST trial showed that nitinol stents versus balloon angioplasty was comparable.[5] Later the VIENNA-ABSOLUTE study and the RESILIANT trial showed significant superiority of stenting versus balloon angioplasty, and the patency at 1 year was 75–80%.[6]

Covered Stents

Stent grafts were developed to overcome in-stent restenosis by creating a mechanical barrier to the ingress of the hyperplastic growth, and several studies were conducted however edge restenosis and stent graft thrombosis complications did not give better results with stent grafts. The Viabahn is one such covered self-expanding stent, which has a patency rate of 74% at 2 years.

Drug-eluting Stents

With the development of drug-eluting stents (DESs) for coronaries, the same was applied to peripheral arteries. Initial trials such as SIROCCO and STRIDES failed to show the advantage of DES over BMSs in SFA. Later the Zilver PTX study which randomized patients to Zilver PTX versus balloon angioplasty in one arm and Zilver PTX versus Zilver BMS in the other arm. Zilver PTX stent did better than balloon angioplasty or BMS.[7]

However, a recent trial of BMS versus paclitaxel-eluting stent in femoropopliteal lesions (BATTLE TRIAL) randomized to Zilver PTX DES versus Misago BMS found no difference in patency rates.[8]

The paclitaxel in Zilver PTX was released rapidly within 24 hours of implantation and probably because of early elution did not protect from late restenosis. With the intention of improving the drug delivery time ELUVIA stent was designed which involves a durable polymer and elutes the drug for months to years. In the IMPERIAL trial, the Eluvia stent was compared with Zilver PTX head to head and showed improved patency at 1 year. The subsequent CAPSICUM study which was IVUS-guided implantation of Eluvia stent in femoropopliteal lesions showed aneurysmal degeneration in 16.8% of patients.

DRUG-COATED BALLOONS

The drug-coated balloons (DCBs) are coated with antiproliferative drugs that inhibit neointimal hyperplasia and decrease in-stent restenosis. Meta-analysis of 13 randomized controlled trials and 9 global registries showed better outcomes for DCBs in terms of primary patency, target lesion revascularization, and late lumen loss.

All the initial trials comparing DCB with plain balloon angioplasty such as LEVANT-I, LEVANT-II, ILLUMINATE, and IN-PACT ADMIRAL™ used paclitaxel as the drug. A 2018 meta-analysis of these trials showed a link between paclitaxel-coated devices and increased late mortality.[9] The FDA had given a warning and advised judicious use of the device, which was still available in the market. Later on, meta-analysis, observational data, and interim studies of RCT data did not corroborate the link between paclitaxel devices and late mortality, which made FDA withdraw its warning.

Because of the above controversy, the industry started looking for alternative drugs such as sirolimus. Two sirolimus-coated DCBs available for SFA interventions are Magic Touch DCB and Selution DCB. All the DCB trials showed a primary patency rate of 88% much higher than plain balloon angioplasty or stents.

ATHERECTOMY

Balloon expansion in the diseased artery causes barotrauma, leading to increased restenosis.

Changing the arterial compliance by debulking has shown to increase the patency rate.

There are three atherectomy devices available for peripheral interventions: (1) Directional atherectomy, (2) rotational atherectomy, and (3) orbital atherectomy. These devices by debulking the plaque have shown to improve vessel compliance, improve vessel patency, and decrease complications. Silver Hawk directional atherectomy device was studied in the TALON registry which showed that in complex subset patients with SFA disease freedom from revascularization at one year was seen in 80%.

However, 25–50% of subjects who underwent atherectomy will also require adjunctive angioplasty or stenting. A potential complication seen with atherectomy was distal embolization; hence, distal embolic filter protection will be helpful to capture debris.

INTRAVASCULAR LITHOTRIPSY

Intravascular lithotripsy (IVL) is a novel balloon that uses acoustic waves to fracture calcium and improve compliance of the vessel to give better outcomes after stenting. This balloon was studied, both in the coronaries and peripheral vessels.

The DISRUPT PAD II STUDY enrolled 60 patients with severely calcified femoropopliteal lesions going for SFA angioplasty, and the study showed a 12-month primary patency of 54.5%, bail out stenting requirement was only 1.7%, and freedom from CD-TLR of 79.3%.

Subsequently, the DISRUPT PAD III STUDY randomized 306 patients to IVL + DCB versus DCB alone and found lower rates of residual stenosis and dissections in the IVL arm.[10] These short-term findings will translate into long-term benefits on follow-up.

COMPLICATIONS

The various complications that one can face while performing an SFA angioplasty are shown in **Table 1**, and one has to be vigilant to avoid each and every complication.

FUTURE DIRECTIONS

The future for endovascular interventions in SFA looks promising with many newer innovations around the corner.

- The Supera Stent (Abbott Vascular) has a novel woven design with improved radial strength, more flexibility, better radial strength, and resistance to fracture. This stent showed a primary patency rate of 86% in the SUPERB study.
- Abbott Vascular is studying the ESPRIT BVS biovascular scaffold for SFA and Iliac arteries in the ESPIRIT I TRIAL.
- Recently lipophilic nanocarriers and amphiphilic sirolimus-based formulations have been developed to overcome prior limitations.
- Adventitial delivery of dexamethasone is being tried to prevent vessel inflammation and intimal hyperplasia. DANCE TRIAL is a single-arm study of adventitial dexamethasone therapy after PTA of femoropopliteal

TABLE 1: Incidence of complications during superficial femoral artery angioplasty.

Contrast allergy	0.1%
Access site complications	2.3–33%
Pseudoaneurysm	0.2–2%
Distal thromboembolism	1.6–2.4%
Contrast nephropathy	2–20%
Arteriovenous fistula	0–0.7%
Acute thrombosis	<1%
Major amputation	0.6–2.2%
Death	0–1%

lesions. The trial saw high rates of primary patency of 75.5% and low rates of CD-TLR of 11%.

- Finally percutaneous femoropopliteal bypass may become a viable option for femoropopliteal disease bypassing the need for surgical revascularization. The DETOUR System utilizes the ipsilateral femoral vein to place covered stents as a conduit bypassing the SFA lesion. The DETOUR I trial showed the safety and efficacy of this device with a primary patency rate of 81%. The promising result is awaiting FDA approval for the device and the larger-scale DETOUR II study is now ongoing.[11]

CONCLUSION

Interventions for SFA did not have a good prognosis in the past because of the anatomical factors. Now with newer innovations like DCB, DES, imaging, and atherectomy devices, the outcomes for SFA angioplasty has improved remarkably.

REFERENCES

1. Rutherford RB, Baker JD, Johnston KW, Johnston KW, Porter JM, Ahn S, et al. Recommended standards for reports dealing with lower extremity ischemia: Revised version. J Vasc Surg. 1997;26:517-38.
2. Norgren L, Hiatt WR, Dormandy JA, Nehler MR, Harris KA, Fowkes FG, et al. Inter-Society Consensus for the Management of Peripheral Arterial Disease (TASC II). J Vasc Surg. 2007;45(Suppl S):S5-67.
3. Marcus AJ, Lotzof K, Howard A. Access to the superficial femoral artery in the presence of a "hostile groin": a prospective study. Cardiovasc Interv Radiol. 2007;30:351-4.
4. Tadros RO, Vouyouka AG, Ting W, Teodorescu V, Kim SY, Marin ML, et al. A review of superficial artery angioplasty and stenting. J Vasc Med Surg. 2015;3(1):1-5.
5. Krankenberg H, Schulter M, Steinkamp HJ, Burgelin K, Scheinert D, et al. Nitinol stent implantation versus percutaneous transluminal angioplasty in superficial femoral artery lesions up to 10 cm in length: The femoral artery stenting trial (FAST). Circulation. 2007;116:285-92.
6. Laird JR, Katzen BT, Scheinert D, Lammer J, Carpenter J, Buchbinder M, et al. Nitinol stent implantation versus balloon angioplasty for lesions in the superficial artery and proximal popliteal artery: twelve month results from the RESILENT randomized trial. Circ Cardiovasc Interv. 2010;3:267-76.
7. Dake MD, Ansell GM, Jaff MR, Ohki T, Saxon RR, Smouse HB, et al. Paclitaxel-eluting stents show superiority to balloon angioplasty and bare metal stents in femoropopliteal disease: twelve month Zilver PTX randomized study results. Circ Cardiovasc Interv. 2011;4:495-504.
8. Goueffic Y, Sauguet A, Desgranges P, Feugier P, Rosset E, Ducasse E, et al. A polymer-free paclitaxel-eluting stent versus a bare metal stent for de novo femoropopliteal lesions: the BATTLE trial. JACC Cardiovasc Interv. 2020;13(4):447-57.

9. Katsanos K, Spiliopoulous S, Kitrou P, Krokidis M, Karnabatidis D. Risk of death following application of paclitaxel coated balloons and stents in the femoropopliteal artery of the leg: a systematic review and meta-analysis of randomized controlled trials. J Am Heart Assoc. 2018;7(24):e011245.
10. Tepe G, Brodmann M, Werner M, Bachinsky W, Holden A, Zeller T, et al. Intravascular lithotripsy for peripheral artery calcification: 30 day outcomes from the randomized Disrupt PAD III trial. JACC Cardiovasc Interv. 2021;14(12):1352-61.
11. Mosarla RC, Armstrong E, Bitton-Faiwiszewski Y, Schneider PA, Secemsky EA. State-of-the-Art Endovascular Therapies for the Femoropopliteal Segment: Are We There Yet? J Soc Cardiovasc Angiogr Interv. 2022;1(5):100439.

CHAPTER 49

Management of Infrageniculate (Infrapopliteal) Peripheral Arterial Disease

Ashish Kumar Mandalay

INTRODUCTION

Peripheral arterial disease (PAD) is a clinical disorder associated with stenosis or occlusion in the aorta or the arteries of the limbs. It is one of the leading causes of limb loss and disability across the globe. It can either present as acute limb ischemia or chronic limb threatening ischemia (CTLI). The lack of adequate expertise and knowledge about the pathophysiology and natural history of peripheral arterial disease adds to the increase in the burden of the disease and its poor outcomes. Treatment of lower extremity arterial disease (LEAD) especially small arterial disease is always a challenge to the treating physician or surgeon especially when it is complicated by rest pain, nonhealing ulcers, and gangrene. Identification and addressing the problem early would lead to better patient outcomes and enhanced quality of life. Mortality and major amputations are common in patients who have untreated critical limb ischemia (CLI) during a median follow-up of 1 year, although these outcomes have improved in recent times after the advent of better endovascular techniques and expertise. In this chapter, we shall be mainly discussing CTLI and its management.

APPROACH TO INFRAGENICULATE DISEASE (INFRAPOPLITEAL VESSELS)

Etiology and the Real Problem of Peripheral Arterial Disease

Atherosclerosis is the leading cause of PAD after the 4th decade of life. The other important causes are thromboembolism, fibromuscular dysplasia, entrapment syndromes, vasculitis, trauma, and rarely cystic adventitial disease. Atherosclerotic PAD usually involves arterial branches which are associated with increased turbulence and altered shear stress resulting in intimal injury and disease.

Peripheral arterial disease is strongly associated with coronary artery disease (CAD) and cerebrovascular disease (CVD). Up to one half of patients with PAD have significant CAD on coronary angiograms. 5-year mortality rate of patients with PAD is 15–25%. The risk of death from CAD is twofold to sixfold.[1]

Major risk factors associated with atherosclerotic PAD are systemic hypertension, diabetes mellitus, dyslipidemia, atrial fibrillation, left ventricular dysfunction, chronic kidney disease (CKD), advanced age, sedentary life, male sex, smoking, and other hypercoagulable states and should be addressed effectively.

Clinical Presentation of Symptomatic Lower Extremity Arterial Disease

- Claudication
- CLI

In cases of symptomatic LEAD, aorta and iliac arteries are involved in one-third, femoropopliteal vessels in 80–90%, and infrapopliteal vessels in up to a half of cases.

Diagnosis

History and General Examination

A thorough historical review would help in identifying the risk factors for PAD and the stages of the disease-Fontaine and Rutherford classification **(Table 1)**.[2]

Meticulous examination would help in picking up loss of limb pulses in particularly asymptomatic patients. Presentations may be acute and abrupt in onset with pain, paralysis, paresthesias, pallor or blue-black

TABLE 1: Fontaine and Rutherford classification.

Fontaine classification			***Rutherford classification***			
Stage		***Symptoms***		***Grade***	***Category***	***Symptoms***
I		Asymptomatic	↔	0	0	Asymptomatic
II	IIa	Nondisabling intermittent claudication	↔	I	1	Mild claudication
				I	2	Moderate claudication
	IIb	Disabling intermittent claudication	↔	I	3	Severe claudication
III		Ischemic rest pain	↔	II	4	Ischemic rest pain
IV		Ulceration or gangrene	↔	III	5	Minor tissue loss
				III	6	Major tissue loss

Source: Aboyans V, Ricco JB, Bartelink MEL, Björck M, Brodmann M, Cohnert T, et al. 2017 ESC guidelines on the diagnosis and treatment of peripheral arterial diseases. Eur Heart J. 2018;39(9):763-816.

TABLE 2: ABI interpretation and initial treatment plan.

ABI value	*Interpretation*	*Recommendation*
>1.4	Calcification/vessel hardening	Refer to vascular specialist
1.0–1.4	Normal	None
0.9–1.0	Acceptable	
0.8–0.9	Some arterial disease	Treat risk factors
0.5–0.8	Moderate arterial disease	Refer to vascular specialist
<0.5	Severe arterial disease	Refer to vascular specialist

(ABI: ankle brachial index)
Source: https://stanfordmedicine25.stanford.edu/the25/ankle-brachial-index.html.

discoloration of limbs. These may be secondary to acute embolic occlusions or in situ thrombus formation inside a chronic lesion. Subacute or chronic presentations include nonhealing ulcers secondary to trauma. Nonhealing ulcers are primarily ischemic in origin in the vast majority of cases, other contributing causes being secondary to venous stasis, infection, and peripheral neuropathy.

Workup

Ankle brachial index (ABI): The ABI is the first investigation ordered in the evaluation of LEAD **(Table 2 and Fig. 1)**. High ABI values may be (>1.40) due to medial calcification and alternative tests such as Toe systolic BP, Toe Brachial Index (TBI), transcutaneous oxygen saturation ($TcPO_2$), or Doppler waveform analysis of ankle arteries may be useful during evaluation. ABI can also be used during patient follow-up and for cardiovascular risk stratification. Segmental pressure and pulse volume recordings can help in ascertaining the area of maximum stenosis by evaluating the pressure gradients.

Exercise test: Exercise test (Strandness protocol at a speed of 3 km/h and 10% slope[2]) is used for objective functional assessment, to ascertain whether the limb pain is secondary to vascular claudication and during exercise rehabilitation on follow-up.

The end point of exercise testing is limiting limb claudication which defines maximal walking distance (WD). A postexercise ankle systolic blood pressure decrease >30 mm Hg or a postexercise ABI decrease >20% confirms LEAD.[2]

Imaging tests: Duplex ultrasound (DUS) which is B mode ultrasound combined with Doppler velocity is the primary noninvasive imaging modality that is performed during evaluation. Full-leg DSA down to the plantar arches is mandatory to explore all revascularization options. Similarly computed

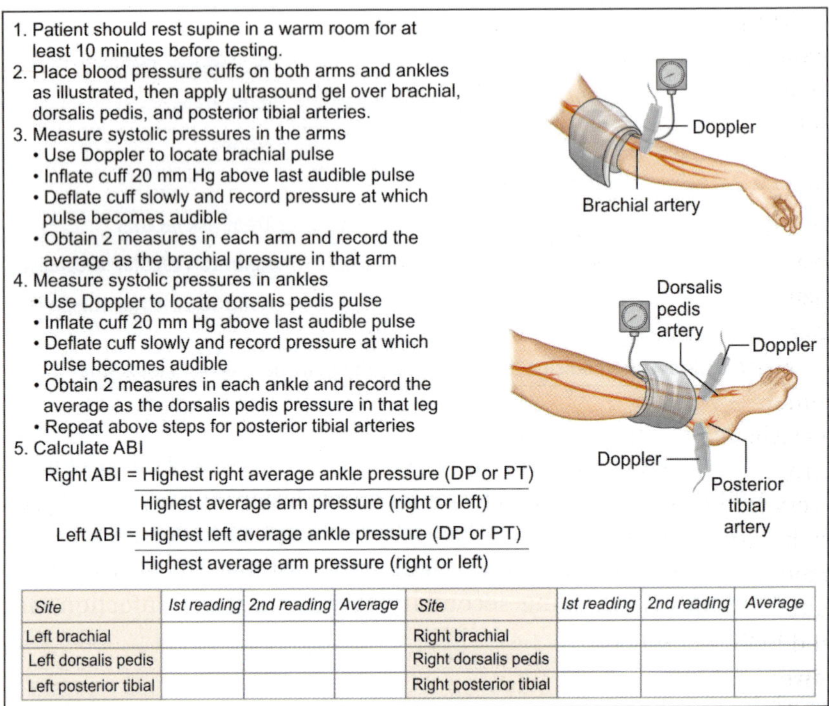

1. Patient should rest supine in a warm room for at least 10 minutes before testing.
2. Place blood pressure cuffs on both arms and ankles as illustrated, then apply ultrasound gel over brachial, dorsalis pedis, and posterior tibial arteries.
3. Measure systolic pressures in the arms
   - Use Doppler to locate brachial pulse
   - Inflate cuff 20 mm Hg above last audible pulse
   - Deflate cuff slowly and record pressure at which pulse becomes audible
   - Obtain 2 measures in each arm and record the average as the brachial pressure in that arm
4. Measure systolic pressures in ankles
   - Use Doppler to locate dorsalis pedis pulse
   - Inflate cuff 20 mm Hg above last audible pulse
   - Deflate cuff slowly and record pressure at which pulse becomes audible
   - Obtain 2 measures in each ankle and record the average as the dorsalis pedis pressure in that leg
   - Repeat above steps for posterior tibial arteries
5. Calculate ABI

$$\text{Right ABI} = \frac{\text{Highest right average ankle pressure (DP or PT)}}{\text{Highest average arm pressure (right or left)}}$$

$$\text{Left ABI} = \frac{\text{Highest left average ankle pressure (DP or PT)}}{\text{Highest average arm pressure (right or left)}}$$

Site	*Ist reading*	*2nd reading*	*Average*	*Site*	*Ist reading*	*2nd reading*	*Average*
Left brachial				Right brachial			
Left dorsalis pedis				Right dorsalis pedis			
Left posterior tibial				Right posterior tibial			

Fig. 1: Method of ABI measurement and reporting. (ABI: ankle brachial index)
Source: https://www.acpjournals.org/doi/10.7326/0003-4819-146-5-200703060-01003

tomography angiography (CTA) and magnetic resonance angiography (MRA) should only be used when considering revascularization options. Carbon dioxide angiography and intervention (zero-iodine) should be performed in selected subjects who are at high risk for renal insufficiency. Cardiovascular screening for other diseases like aortic aneurysms, coronary and cerebrovascular disease should also be performed to ascertain the extent of disease during the evaluation of PAD as these coexisting conditions may contribute to future outcomes.

Therapeutic Considerations: Holistic Approach to Treatment of CLTI

Lifestyle Modification and Pharmacological Therapy

The majority of treatment strategies during the initial stages of infrageniculate or below knee (BK) arterial disease are aimed at impeding disease progression and improving blood flow and should be based on the relief of clinical symptoms (claudication), improve quality of life, and short- and long-term prognosis.

The main focus should be on reducing risk factors by healthy diet, smoking cessation, improving exercise performance, and medications such as antiplatelets (clopidogrel and/or aspirin), lipid-lowering agents (statins), antihypertensive agents, and oral hypoglycemic drugs or insulin. Of late the importance of anticoagulation in lower extremity vascular disease is gaining importance.[3] Smoking cessation provides the most noticeable improvement in walking distance when combined with regular exercise, especially when lesions are located below the femoral arteries. In patients with intermittent claudication, the natural history is deteriorated by ongoing tobacco use, with increased risk of amputation.

More than two-thirds of patients with below knee arterial disease remain stable or improve with conservative management comprising lifestyle modifications and pharmacologic agents.[4] Disease progression and symptomatic worsening occur in the remainder with 1–2% developing CLI every year. One-third of patients with CLI undergo amputation within a year with worse prognosis in smokers and diabetics. Interventional strategies should be contemplated when features of critical limb ischemia set in and it is very crucial to pick up subtle findings in the early stages for optimal results and limb salvage **(Flowchart 1 shows the basic algorithm of approach to lower extremity arterial disease).**[4]

In the last decade, endovascular revascularization for patients with infrapopliteal/infrageniculate arterial disease has evolved rapidly. Currently, due to low morbidity and mortality as compared with vascular surgery, many clinical centers prefer endovascular approaches and the role of surgery is limited to debridement and limb salvage procedures.

Flowchart 1: Algorithm of lower extremity arterial disease management.

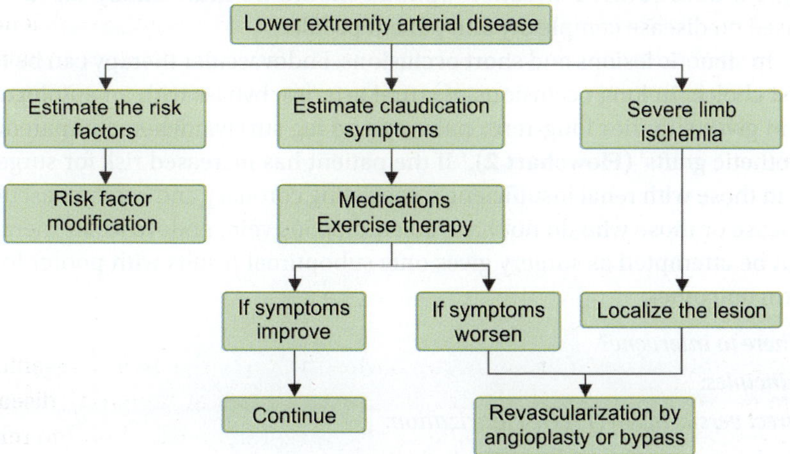

Source: Alyavi B, Uzokov J. Peripheral artery disease in the lower extremities. Eur Soc Cardiol. 2018;16(9):1-15.

Limb Revascularization in CLI: When, How, and Where?

When to intervene?

Patients with critical limb ischemia involving lower limbs frequently present with severe LEAD predominantly involving the infrapopliteal vessels. Diffuse, multilevel, and multivessel disease is very common and calcific involvement contributes to the burden of disease further. *Intervention is warranted as already discussed when the patients do not improve with exercise and pharmacological treatment and have intractable symptoms suggestive of critical limb ischemia (rest pain, nonhealing wound/ulcer, and gangrene) or in cases where a major amputation can be prevented by timely revascularization.*

How to intervene?

Endovascular versus surgical: Bypass versus Angioplasty in Severe Ischemia of the Leg (BASIL)[2] is a randomized control trial (RCT) that has directly compared endovascular therapy to open surgery in CLTI patients. At 2 years, there was no significant difference between endovascular therapy and surgery regarding amputation-free survival. In survivors after 2 years, bypass surgery was associated with improved survival. Best Endovascular versus Best Surgical Therapy in Patients with Critical Limb Ischemia[2] (BESTCLI) trial showed that among patients with CTLI who had a great saphenous vein adequate for surgical revascularization, clinical outcomes with an initial treatment of surgery were superior to those with endovascular therapy; however, in patients who required an alternative bypass conduit, outcomes were similar with the two procedures. However, these data are challenged by more recent endovascular therapy techniques. In BASIL-2[2] trial, a best endovascular treatment first revascularization strategy was associated with a better amputation-free survival, which was largely driven by fewer deaths in the best endovascular treatment group. Meanwhile, in each anatomical region, both revascularization options should be individually discussed based on disease complexity and patient profile.

In stenotic lesions and short occlusions, endovascular therapy can be the first choice. In long occlusions of crural arteries, bypass with an autologous vein gives superior long-term patency and leg survival when compared to synthetic grafts[1] **(Flowchart 2)**.[2] If the patient has increased risk for surgery as in those with renal insufficiency, coexisting coronary and cerebrovascular disease or those who do not have an autologous vein, endovascular therapy can be attempted as surgery gives only suboptimal results with poorer long term outcomes.

Where to intervene?

Principles:

Direct versus indirect revascularization:

Single versus multivessel revascularization:

There is still considerable debate regarding which vessel to revascularize in infrapopliteal disease of the lower extremity who present with nonhealing

Flowchart 2: Management of patients with chronic limb-threatening ischemia (CLTI).

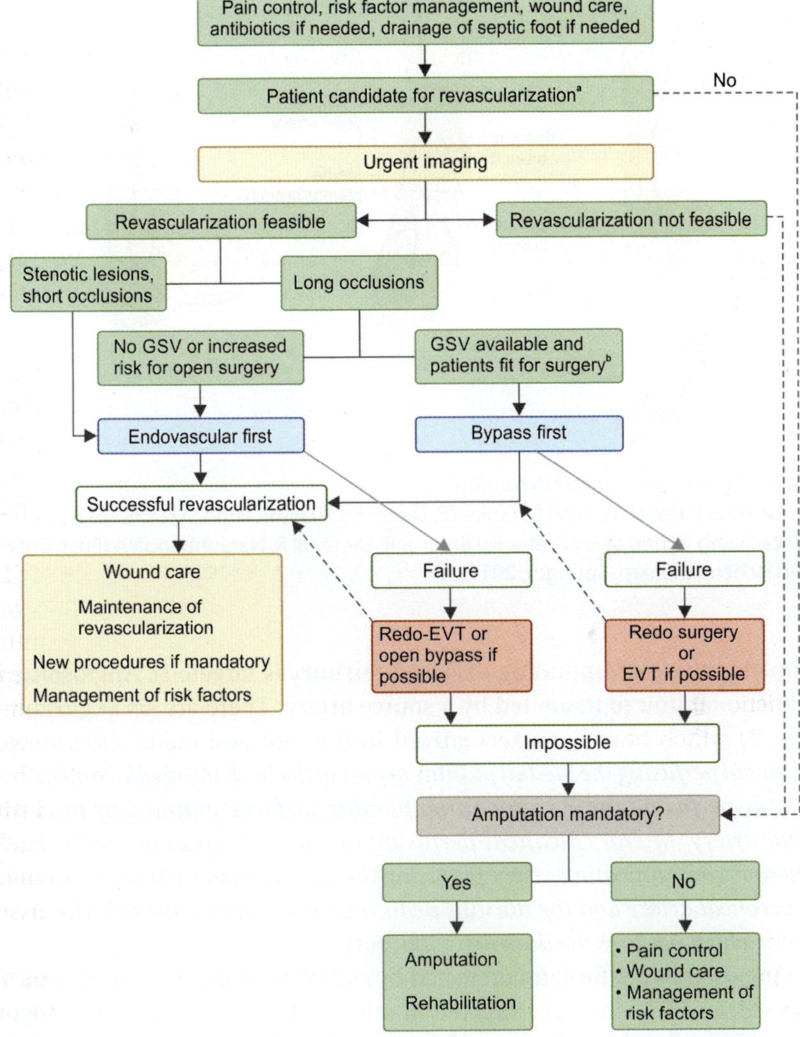

Note:

[a]In bedridden, demented and/or frail patients, primary amputation should be considered.

[b]In the absence of contraindication for surgery and in the presence of adequate target for anastomosis/runoff.

(EVT: endovascular therapy; GSV: great saphenous vein)

Source: Aboyans V, Ricco JB, Bartelink MEL, Björck M, Brodmann M, Cohnert T, et al. 2017 ESC guidelines on the diagnosis and treatment of peripheral arterial diseases. Eur Heart J. 2018;39(9):763-816.

wound. Despite aggressive revascularization, amputation still occurs in a fifth of patients with CLI and tissue loss. This has led to the suggestion of an *angiosome-based revascularization strategy*[5,6] (where the specific artery

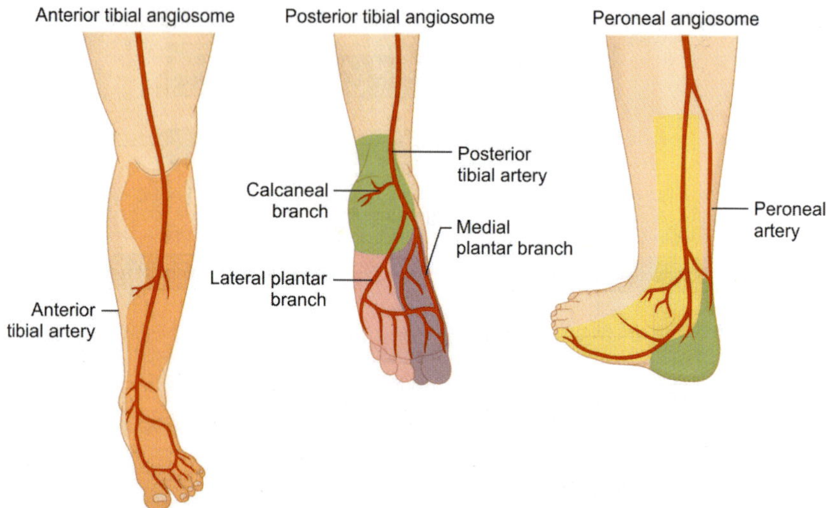

Fig. 2: Angiosomes of lower extremity.
Source: Hirai T, Dayal AS, Hirai R, Tanke TE, Dieter RS. Classification Systems for Acute and Chronic Limb Ischemia. In: Dieter R, Dieter Jr R, Dieter III R, Nanjundappa A (Eds). Critical Limb Ischemia. Cham: Springer; 2017.

supplying the corresponding diseased territory is targeted). Angiosome is a functional unit of tissue fed by a source artery. There are six angiosomes **(Fig. 2)** which have been recognized in the foot and ankle[6] (*the medial calcaneal perfusing the medial plantar aspect of the heel; the medial and lateral plantar perfusing the corresponding plantar surfaces supplied by posterior tibial artery; lateral calcaneal perfusing the lateral aspect of the heel and anterior communicating artery perfusing the anterior aspect of ankle supplied by peroneal artery and the dorsalis pedis angiosome fed by the anterior tibial artery which perfuses the dorsum of the foot*).

Angiosomes are further connected by collateral channels (PRIME zones:[6] **Figs. 3A and B**) which get affected in atherosclerosis and diabetes. Direct revascularization of angiosome of the wound in the limb provides pulsatile, inline flow which helps in better healing and limb salvage rates. In cases where there is severe disease of the angiosome perfusing the disease area (multilevel, multivessel, and calcific lesions) and direct revascularization may not be feasible or may not provide optimal results, indirect revascularization should be attempted which provides similar outcomes to direct revascularization[7] provided collateral flow to the angiosome is adequate. Multiple vessel approach[8] utilizing collateral and plantar arch vessels improves wound healing, clinical success and amputation-free survival by several mechanisms. It provides more inflow vessels and conduits to the foot and improves

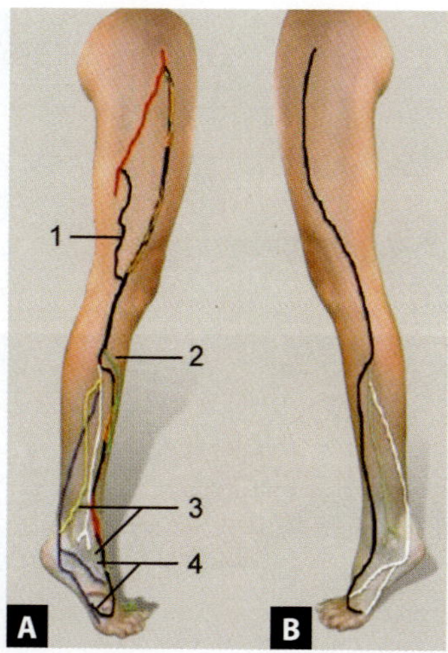

Figs. 3A and B: (A) PRIME collateral zones that keep the limbs intact while metabolic supply and demand are balanced (stable state): (1) the collateral path from the profunda to the popliteal and genicular branches; (2) the collateral path from the popliteal and genicular branches to the tibial arteries; (3) the collateral path from the proximal tibialis to the distal tibialis; (4) the pedal loop's collateral paths. (B) Normal, expected, infrainguinal runoff.
Source: Mustapha JA, Diaz-Sandoval LJ, Saab F. Angiosome Directed Therapy for the CLI Patient. Endovasc Today. 2014;13(5):65-70.

perfusion to an incomplete pedal arch making use of the principle of volume concept [The "volume concept"[6] states that increasing the volume of blood perfusing the affected limb helps in better wound healing **(Figs. 4A and B)** even if the affected angiosome is not directly addressed]. Restenosis is delayed and perfusion is maintained for a longer duration. Another important thing to consider is the need to address upstream stenosis in the iliac, femoral, and popliteal vessels as well if found during the evaluation process for optimal results.

The risks of multivessel and indirect revascularization include renal impairment due to increased contrast volume, increased radiation exposure resulting in operator fatigue and increased procedure time which may lead to patient instability and potential complications during revascularization.

However, in spite of all these measures, those undergoing indirect revascularization can still have poorer outcomes due to other comorbidities and adverse risk factors which can act as confounding factors. However, some studies have shown the theory of angiosome-based revascularization not holding true after surgical bypass in some subset of patients.[9]

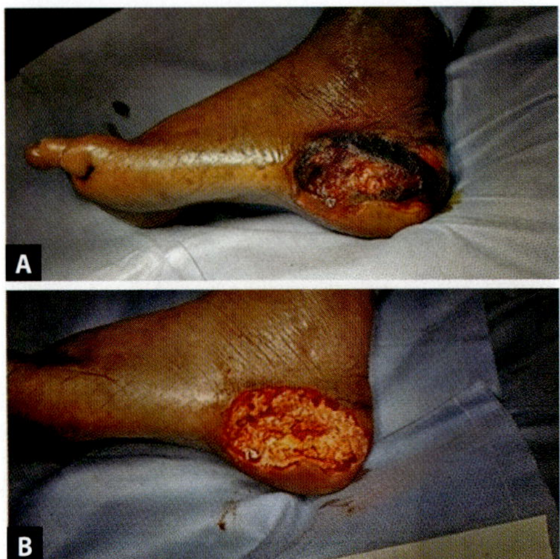

Figs. 4A and B: Pre- and postballoon angioplasty wound appearance: (A) Preballoon angioplasty impending gangrene; (B) Note the improved wound perfusion with good granulation necessary for wound healing.

Strategies of Endovascular Revascularization

Access

- *Retrograde femoral*
- *Antegrade femoral and superficial femoral*
- *Pedal*

Femoral artery is the most common access vessel employed for endovascular revascularization. Retrograde or contralateral femoral access needs the placement of crossover sheath across the aortoiliac bifurcation and other support hardware. The presence of coexisting significant iliac artery disease may act as a hindrance. Retrograde femoral approach also involves use of more contrast when compared with antegrade approach. **Figures 5A to D** shows antegrade superficial femoral artery and pedal puncture.

In our center, we prefer the antegrade femoral artery access to deal with infrapopliteal lesions. It helps in better maneuverability and support while performing procedures and decreases the procedure time, radiation exposure, and contrast volume when compared with retrograde femoral artery access. Ultrasound-guided micropuncture is the best method with less chance of major complications. Fluoroscopy-guided micropuncture may also be employed. Difficulty arises in high bifurcation of common femoral artery where tracking into the superficial femoral artery may be cumbersome. Long sheaths help to decrease contrast volume and gives better control during hardware exchanges.

Pedal artery puncture with retrograde crossing **(Figs. 6A to F)** may be tried in cases involving femoropopliteal disease where upstream access is

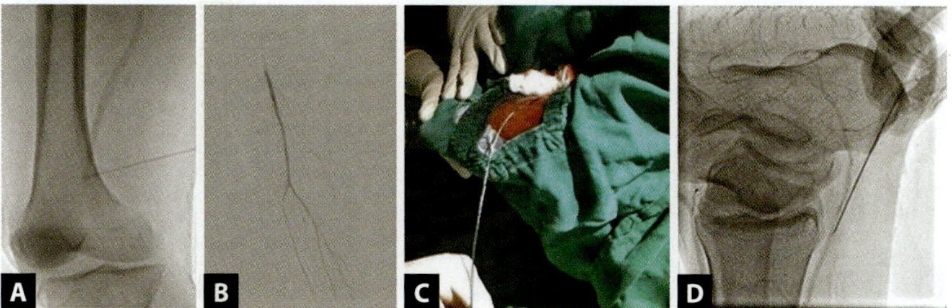

Figs. 5A to D: (A and B) Lower superficial femoral artery puncture and angiogram; (C and D) Pedal artery puncture and angiogram.

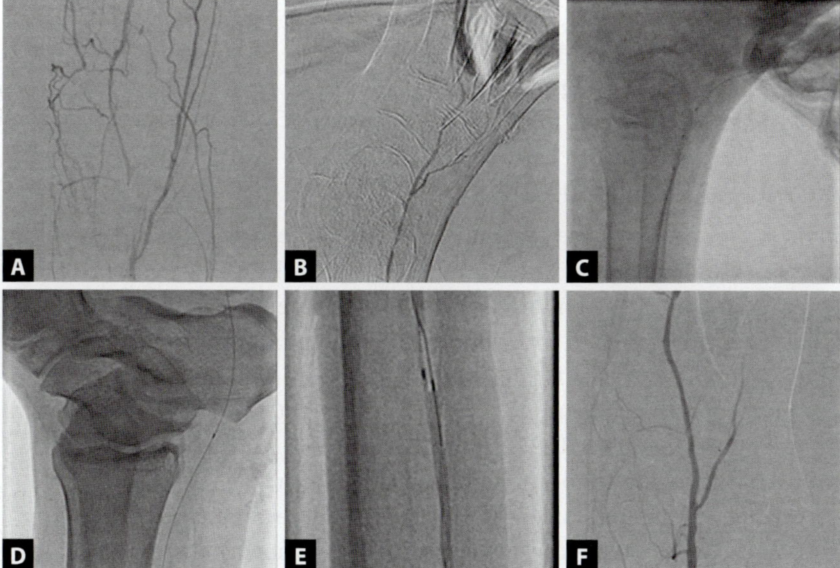

Figs. 6A to F: Pedal artery intervention: (A) Preintervention angiogram; (B) Pedal artery puncture; (C) Tracking microcatheter (Rubicon); (D) Balloon tracking; (E) Crossing from below and above; (F) Postintervention angiogram.

not feasible. Sheathless technique is employed. The disadvantage with pedal artery puncture is the possibility of the access vessel going into spasm which may result in procedural failure. Pedal punctures can rarely cause access site nonhealing. The presence of pre-existing foot ulcers may sometimes complicate things further.

Lesion Crossing Techniques

Target vessels can be approached directly or indirectly depending on the lesion characteristics and feasibility.

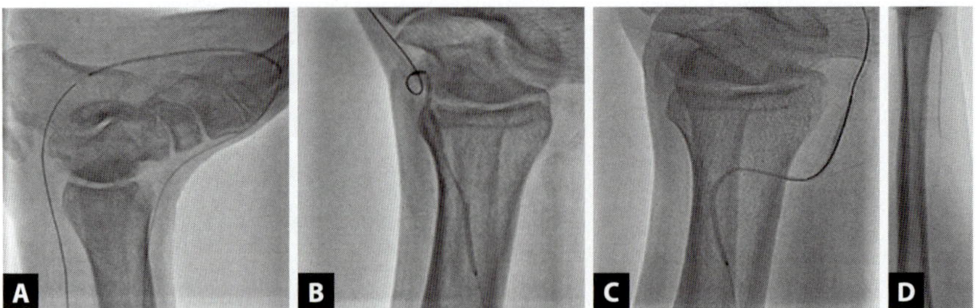

Figs. 7A to D: Pedoplantar and collateral angioplasty: (A) Pedo-plantar loop angioplasty; (B and C) Transcollateral angioplasty into plantar arch vessels; (D) Intertibial collateral angioplasty.

- *Direct antegrade*
- *Transcollateral* ***(Figs. 7A to D)***
- *Pedoplantar arch* ***(Figs. 7A to D)***
- *Pedal artery puncture and retrograde crossing*

Methods of Tackling the Lesion

Plain balloon angioplasty is the standard and most preferred modality for treatment of below knee interventions and gives excellent results **(Figs. 8 and 9)**. The Achilles' heel of below knee interventions, however, is the need for repeated procedures till healing of an ulcer is completed. Long segment and calcific disease are more prone for recoil and abrupt vessel closure. Hence to improve vessel patency rates and outcomes, several other options like BMS, DES and DEB have been studied comparing head to head with plain balloon angioplasty.[10,11] Severe below knee disease is associated with poorer outcomes whatever be the revascularization strategy.[12] DEB and DES in below-the-knee disease have shown no superiority over plain balloon angioplasty in multiple trials in diabetic and nondiabetic subgroups.[13-16] In our center, we use only balloon angioplasty for infrapopliteal disease with good results.

ACHILLES, YUKON, and DESTINY trials which randomized patients to treatment with a sirolimus/everolimus-eluting stent or percutaneous transluminal angioplasty (PTA) or BMS showed improved primary patency rates at the end of 12 months. Meta-analyses have showed that treatment with DES in focal disease of the infrapopliteal arteries results in improved angiographic outcomes compared to PTA or BMS.[17] The use of paclitaxel-eluting balloons and stents has been paused of late due to adverse data.

Hardware Selection

Appropriate use of the right hardware **(Fig. 10)** is key to successful outcomes and prevention of complications. The right combination of access sheaths,

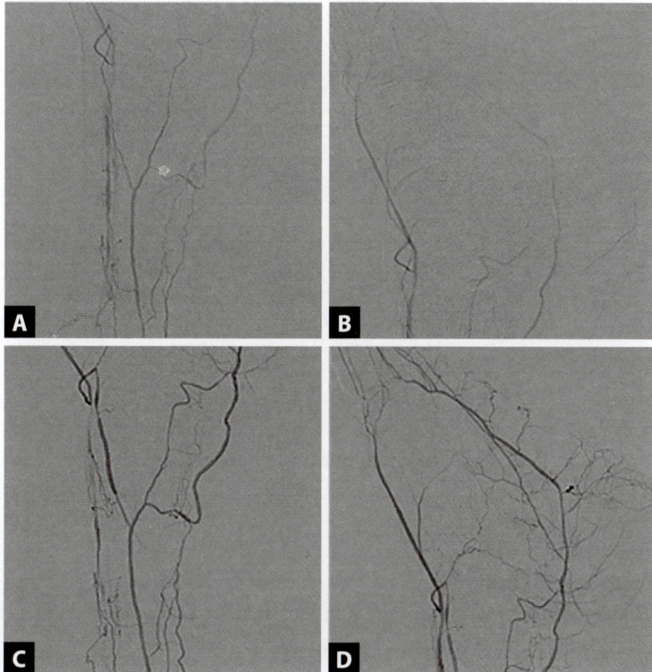

Figs. 8A to D: Pre- and postballoon angioplasty: (A and B) Pre infrapopliteal balloon angioplasty; (C and D) Post infrapopliteal balloon angioplasty: Note the blush in the foot vessels which would promote wound healing. Multiple, prolonged (>3 minutes up to 5 minutes) low pressure inflations are performed. Inflation end point is uniform balloon dilatation till lesion yields completely or limiting pain reported by the patient.

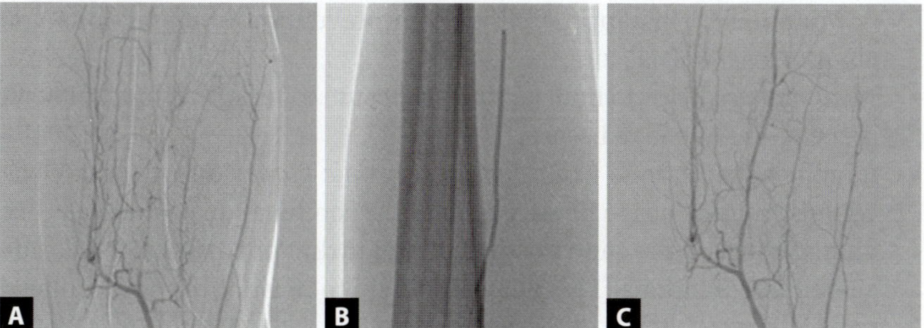

Figs. 9A to C: Drug-eluting balloon (DEB) intervention in infrapopliteal disease: (A) Pre-DEB angiogram; (B) DEB inflation. Note the uniform dilatation; (C) Post-DEB angiogram.

glide catheters, wires, microcatheters, and peripheral balloons gives the best results.

- Micropuncture (Cook)
- Long sheaths
- *Basic platform:* 0.014″

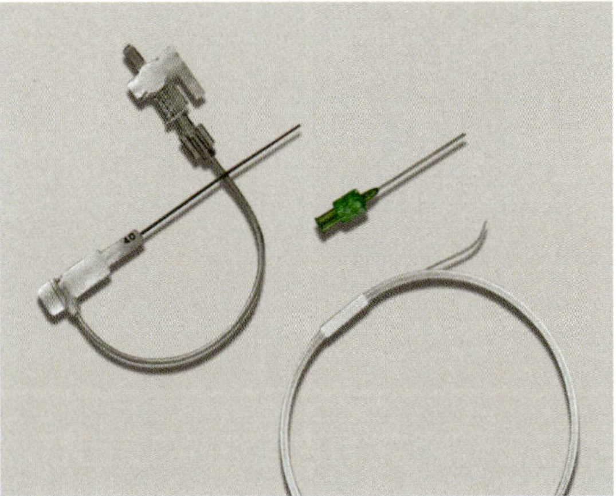

Fig. 10: Pedal puncture hardware.

- Workhorse guidewire
- Guidewire escalation
- *Support catheters:* Rubicon series
- *Peripheral balloons:* Mustang series

Adjuvant Strategies and Role of Technology and Research

- *Low pressure dilatation with prolonged inflation time:* Long-term outcomes and vessel patency rates are found to be better when low pressure dilatations with longer balloon inflation time (>3 minutes) are used rather than high pressure dilatations and lower inflation time (<3 minutes). This approach helps in prevention of dissections and abrupt vessel wall closure.[18]
- *Roadmap* use helps to limit contrast exposure especially in long, difficult procedures and renal disease.
- In clinical conditions like *advanced chronic kidney disease* where the contrast volume has to be very minimal, a combination of strategies like diluted contrast, pre- and postprocedural hydration and carbon-dioxide guided interventions **(Fig. 11)** would help to prevent contrast-induced renal injury.
- *Robotic cardiac catheterization lab (Zeego)* in peripheral interventions has come a long way in limiting radiation and contrast exposure in view of its superior specifications.
- *Newer technologies like shockwave lithoplasty and pantheris lumivascular atherectomy system* are now being used increasingly in difficult to treat cases associated with calcium.
- *Upcoming options for CLI patients unsuitable for revascularization:* Multiple regenerative and adjunctive therapies like angiogenic gene

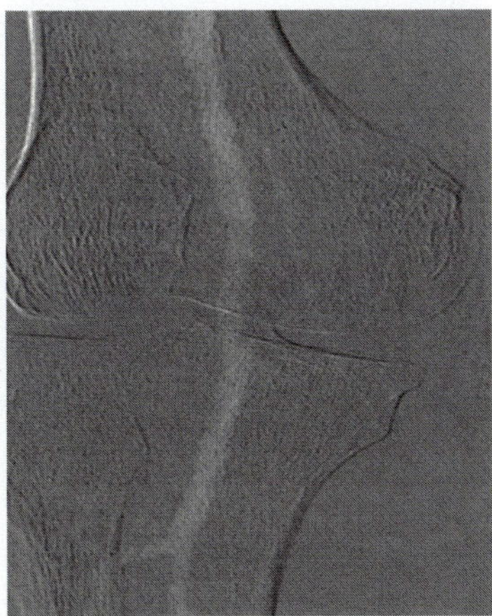

Fig. 11: Carbon dioxide (zero iodine contrast) angiogram.

TABLE 3: Clinical categories of acute limb ischemia (Rutherford grades).

Grade	*Category*	*Sensory loss*	*Motor deficit*	*Prognosis*
I	Viable	None	None	No immediate threat
IIA	Marginally threatened	None or minimal (toes)	None	Salvageable if promptly treated
IIB	Immediately threatened	More than toes	Mild/moderate	Salvageable if promptly revascularized
III	Irreversible	Profound, anesthetic	Profound, paralysis (rigor)	Major tissue loss, permanent nerve damage inevitable

Source: Aboyans V, Ricco JB, Bartelink MEL, Björck M, Brodmann M, Cohnert T, et al. 2017 ESC guidelines on the diagnosis and treatment of peripheral arterial diseases. Eur Heart J. 2018;39(9):763-816.

therapy and autologous cell-based therapies are being evaluated in CLI patients.

Other Clinical Scenarios Encountered in the Setting of Lower Limb Ischemia

- *Acute limb ischemia:*[2] Basic approach to management is detailed in **Table 3** and **Flowchart 3**.
- *Blue toe syndrome:* Another particular clinical presentation is blue toe syndrome. This is characterized by a sudden cyanotic discoloration of one or more toes. It is usually due to embolic atherosclerotic debris from the proximal arteries.
- *Thromboangiitis obliterans **(Fig. 12)**:* Characterized by cork screw type of vessels

Flowchart 3: Management of acute limb ischemia.

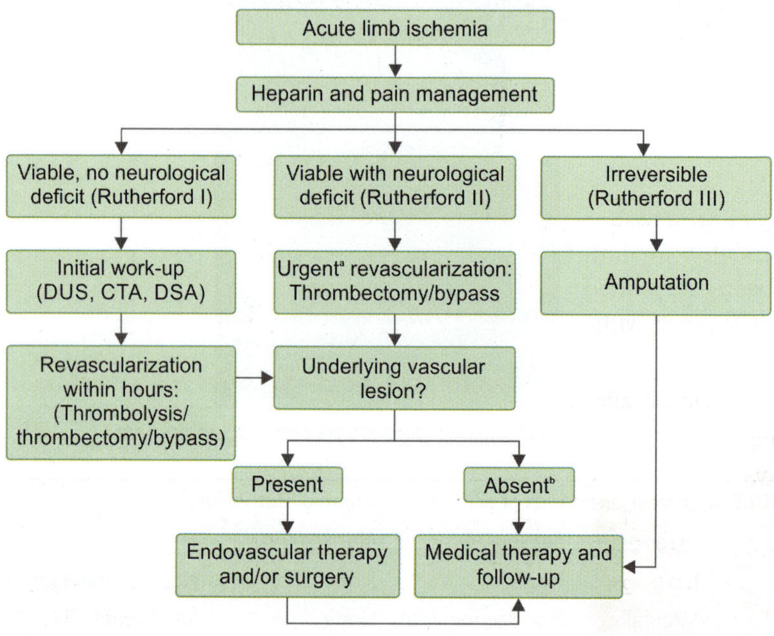

Note:

[a]Imaging should not delay revascularization.

[b]Specific etiological work-up is necessary (cardiac, aorta).

(CTA: computed tomography angiography; DSA: digital subtraction angiography; DUS: duplex ultrasound)

Source: Aboyans V, Ricco JB, Bartelink MEL, Björck M, Brodmann M, Cohnert T, et al. 2017 ESC guidelines on the diagnosis and treatment of peripheral arterial diseases. Eur Heart J. 2018;39(9):763-816.

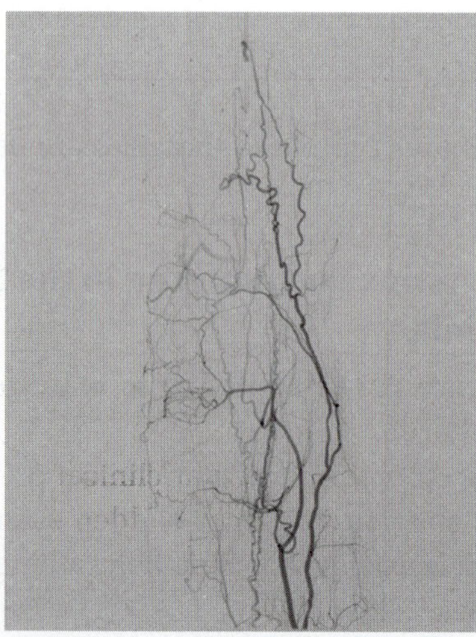

Fig. 12: Thromboangiitis obliterans. Angiogram in a case of probable thromboangiitis obliterans—note the corkscrew nature of vessels.

Limb Salvage and Role of Multidisciplinary Team: The Idea of Advanced Foot Care Center

Management of infrageniculate disease (infrapopliteal) needs a dedicated and multidisciplinary team effort (physicians, diabetologists, peripheral interventional specialists, vascular surgeons, podiatrists, nutritionists, and dedicated nurses) where each person has their own role to play. Early recognition of tissue loss and/or infection and referral to a vascular specialist is mandatory for limb salvage. The Advanced Foot Care Centre at our Institute has been established with the vision of providing comprehensive high end care to subjects with PAD and limb threatening ischemia.

TABLE 4: WIfI classification.

Component	*Score*	*Description*		
W (Wound)	0	No ulcer (ischemic rest pain)		
	1	Small, shallow ulcer on distal leg or foot without gangrene		
	2	Deeper ulcer with exposed bone, joint or tendon ± gangrenous changes limited to toes		
	3	Extensive deep ulcer, full thickness heel ulcer ± calcaneal involvement ± extensive gangrene		
I (Ischemia)		ABI	Ankle pressure (mm Hg)	Toe pressure or $TcPO_2$:
	0	≥0.80	>100	≥60
	1	0.60–0.79	70–100	40–59
	2	0.40–0.59	50–70	30–39
	3	<0.40	<50	<30
fI (foot Infection)	0	No symptoms/signs of infection		
	1	Local infection involving only skin and subcutaneous tissue		
	2	Local infection involving deeper than skin/subcutaneous tissue		
	3	Systemic inflammatory response syndrome		

Example: A 65-year-old male diabetic patient with gangrene of the big toe and a <2 cm rim of cellulitis at the base of the toe, without any clinical/biological sign of general infection/inflammation, whose toe pressure is at 30 mm Hg would be classified as Wound 2, Ischemia 2, foot Infection (WIfI 2-2-1). The clinical stage would be 4 (high risk of amputation). The benefit of revascularization (if feasible) is high, also depending on infection control.

(ABI: ankle brachial index)

Source: Aboyans V, Ricco JB, Bartelink MEL, Björck M, Brodmann M, Cohnert T, et al. 2017 ESC guidelines on the diagnosis and treatment of peripheral arterial diseases. Eur Heart J. 2018;39(9):763-816.

Chronic limb-threatening ischemia specifies clinical patterns with a vulnerable limb viability related to several factors. Without successful revascularization, those with critical ischemia have a limb loss (amputation) rate of 80–90% in 1 year. The WIfI system[19] **(Table 4)**[2] is followed for chronic limb-threatening ischemia while planning treatment strategies.

Amputation up to forefoot level may be needed to remove necrotic tissues in CLTI. Below knee angioplasty especially before amputation improves wound healing—higher rate of wound healing and shorter time to wound healing.[20] Patients who are nonambulatory with extensive necrosis or infectious gangrene may need primary major amputation. Secondary amputation should be performed when revascularization has failed and the limb continues to deteriorate because of infection or necrosis. Below knee amputation should be preferred, because it promotes ambulation and quality of life. However, above knee amputation may be the best option for bed ridden patients.

CONCLUSION

Most patients with infrapopliteal disease are asymptomatic and exercise testing must be performed to detect clinically silent disease. Even asymptomatic patients are at high risk of cardiovascular events and will benefit from lifestyle modification. Ankle-brachial index is the initial screening test for the diagnosis of infrapopliteal disease. Duplex ultrasound is the first imaging modality. Behavioral changes, pharmacological therapy, and exercise training help to limit intermittent claudication. Revascularization along with exercise therapy is the treatment strategy in severe limiting disease. Chronic limb-threatening ischemia has to be recognized early and referred to a vascular specialist. Revascularization is indicated to improve limb perfusion. Endovascular treatment scores over surgical options in infrapopliteal disease and angiosome-directed revascularization should be aimed at as far as possible. Limb preservation should be attempted as far as possible and managed by a multidisciplinary team. Acute limb ischemia is an emergency. Continuing medical education and translational research are the need of the hour and more evidence in this area would help to improve limb salvage rates and quality of life in the long run.

REFERENCES

1. Creagar MA, Loscalzo J. Arterial disease of the Extremities—Peripheral arterial disease. Loscalzo J (Ed). Harrison's™ Principles of Internal Medicine, 20th edition. New Delhi: McGraw-Hill Education. 2018. pp. 1923-30.
2. Aboyans V, Ricco JB, Bartelink MEL, Björck M, Brodmann M, Cohnert T, et al. 2017 ESC guidelines on the diagnosis and treatment of peripheral arterial diseases, in collaboration with the European Society for Vascular Surgery (ESVS): document covering atherosclerotic disease of extracranial carotid and

vertebral, mesenteric, renal, upper and lower extremity arteries. Eur Heart J. 2018;39:763-816.

3. Bonaca MP, Bauersachs RM, Anand SS, Debus ES, Nehler MR, Patel MR, et al. Rivaroxaban in Peripheral Artery Disease after Revascularization. N Engl J Med. 2020;382:1994-2004.
4. Alyavi B, Uzokov J. (2018). Peripheral artery disease in the lower extremities: indications for treatment. [online] Available from https://www.escardio.org/Journals/E-Journal-of-Cardiology-Practice/Volume-16/Peripheral-artery-disease-in-the-lower-extremities-indications-for-treatment. [Last accessed October 2024].
5. Kinlay S, Bhat DL. Treatment of Noncoronary Obstructive Vascular Disease. In: Braunwald E (Ed). Braunwald's Heart Disease, 11th edition. Philadelphia, PA: Elsevier; 2018. pp. 1365-82.
6. Mustapha JA, Diaz-Sandoval LJ, Saab F. Angiosome-directed therapy for the CLI patient. Endovasc Today. 2014;13(5):65-70.
7. Fioole B, Bekken JA, Verhagen H. Where Do We Stand on Data Collection? An overview of the current evidence and perspectives on what data are still needed. CLI Trial Update. Endovasc Today. 2019;18(5):41-9.
8. Biagioni RB, Biagioni LC, Nasser F, Burihan MC, Ingrund JC, Neser A, et al. Infrapopliteal angioplasty of one or more than one artery for critical limb ischaemia: a randomised clinical trial. Eur J Vasc Endovasc Surg. 2018; 55:518-27.
9. Azuma N, Uchida H, Kokubo T, Koya A, Akasaka N, Sasajima T. Factors Influencing Wound Healing of Critical Ischaemic Foot after Bypass Surgery: Is the Angiosome Important in Selecting Bypass Target Artery? Eur J Vasc Endovasc Surg. 2012;43:322-8.
10. Siablis D, Kitrou PM, Spiliopoulos S, Katsanos K, Karnabatidis D. Paclitaxel-coated balloon angioplasty versus drug-eluting stenting for the treatment of infrapopliteal long-segment arterial occlusive disease the IDEAS randomized controlled trial. JACC Cardiovasc Interv. 2014;7(9):1048-56.
11. Bosiers M, Scheinert D, Peeters P, Torsello G, Zeller T, Deloose K, et al. Randomized comparison of everolimus-eluting versus bare-metal stents in patients with critical limb ischemia and infrapopliteal arterial occlusive disease. J Vasc Surg. 2012;55(2):390-8.
12. Singh GD, Brinza EK, Hildebrand J, Waldo SW, Foley TR, Laird JR, et al. Midterm outcomes after infrapopliteal interventions in patients with critical limb ischemia based on the TASC II classification of below-the-knee arteries. J Endovasc Ther. 2017;24(3):321-30.
13. Zeller T, Baumgartner I, Scheinert D, Brodmann M, Bosiers M, Micari A, et al. Drug-eluting balloon versus standard balloon angioplasty for infrapopliteal arterial revascularization in critical limb ischemia: 12-month results from the IN.PACT DEEP randomized trial. J Am Coll Cardiol. 2014;64:1568-76.
14. Cassese S, Ndrepepa G, Liistro F, Fanelli F, Kufner S, Ott I, et al. Drug-coated balloons for revascularization of infrapopliteal arteries: a meta-analysis of randomized trials. JACC Cardiovasc Interv. 2016;9:1072-80.
15. Ipema J, Huizing E, Schreve MA, de Vries JPM, Ünlü Ç. Drug coated balloon angioplasty vs. standard percutaneous transluminal angioplasty in below the knee peripheral arterial disease: a systematic review and meta-analysis. Eur J Vasc Endovasc Surg. 2020;59:265-75.

16. Liu X, Zheng G, Wen S. Drug-eluting stents versus control therapy in the infrapopliteal disease: a meta-analysis of eight randomized controlled trials and two cohort studies. Int J Surg. 2017;44:166-75.
17. Fusaro M, Cassese S, Ndrepepa G, Tepe G, King L, Ott I, et al. Drug-eluting stents for revascularization of infrapopliteal arteries: updated meta-analysis of randomized trials. JACC Cardiovasc Interv. 2013;6:1284-93.
18. Rockley M, Jetty P, Radonjic A, Rockley K, Wells G, Fergusson D. Prolonged versus brief balloon inflation during arterial angioplasty for de novo atherosclerotic disease: a systematic review and meta-analysis. CVIR Endovasc. 2019;2:29.
19. Mills JL Sr, Conte MS, Armstrong DG, Pomposelli FB, Schanzer A, Sidawy AN, et al. The Society for Vascular Surgery Lower Extremity Threatened Limb Classification System: risk stratification based on wound, ischemia, and foot infection (WIfI). J Vasc Surg. 2014;59:220-34.
20. Nakama T, Watanabe N, Haraguchi T, Sakamoto H, Kamoi D, Tsubakimoto Y, et al. Clinical Outcomes of Pedal Artery Angioplasty for Patients With Ischemic Wounds Results From the Multicenter RENDEZVOUS Registry. JACC Cardiovasc Interv. 2017;10(1):79-90.

CHAPTER 50

Carotid Stenting: Step-by-Step Approach

Atul Mathur

INTRODUCTION

About 20–25% of ischemic stroke is accounted for by carotid stenosis (CS).[1] Various studies in the past have established the benefits of carotid endarterectomy (CEA) over the best medical therapy (BMT).[2-6] With significant technical advances made, carotid artery stenting (CAS) is now emerged as an alternative to CEA. Carotid artery angioplasty and its stenting require careful selection of patient, counseling, and procedural planning.

PATIENT SELECTION

Success entirely depends on the appropriate selection of the patient. Prior to the planned procedure, stroke risk stratification should be performed. Candidates for carotid revascularization would be symptomatic patients (neurological event that has occurred in preceding 6 months) and asymptomatic patients with >50% stenosis and >70% stenosis, respectively. The choice between CAS and CEA would depend on patient factors as well as operator's preference. High-risk candidates would be the ones having unstable angina, left ventricular ejection fraction <30%, congestive cardiac failure in NYHA III/IV, recent myocardial infarction, previous CEA with restenosis, and history of radiation therapy to the neck. Regardless of the intent for revascularization, risk factor modifications include control of hypertension, diabetes, dyslipidemia, and cessation of smoking **(Table 1)**.[7]

TABLE 1: Indications and contraindications for CAS.

Indication for CAS	*Contraindication for CAS*
Inability to tolerate general anesthesia	History of allergic reaction to IV contrast
History of contralateral vocal cord damage (prior neck surgery/CEA)	Unfavorable anatomy
Previous neck surgery on the ipsilateral side	Unstable carotid artery plaque
Neck irradiation	Unstable aortic arch plaque
Restenosis after CEA	

(IV: intravenous; CAS: carotid artery stenting; CEA: carotid endarterectomy)

PATIENT PREPARATION

Once a detailed informed consent has been taken, the patient should be started on oral clopidogrel antiplatelet therapy 5 days prior to the planned procedure. If not feasible, then the patient can be loaded with 300 mg of loading clopidogrel dose to 4–5 hours prior to the procedure. Baseline neurological evaluation should be performed and documented. Bilateral inguinal area should be prepared for access.

ARCH ANATOMICAL CONSIDERATION

In reference to the origin of the great vessels from the convexity of arch of aorta, the aortic arch has been classified into three types. Type I is defined as the arch where the great vessels arise at the level of the upper convexity; Type II is when these great vessels arise between the upper and lower convexity; and it is Type III when great vessels originate caudally to the lower convexity **(Figs. 1A to C)**. The catheter selection for common carotid artery (CCA) catheterization depends on the type of aortic arch that is met with.

DIAGNOSTIC ANGIOGRAM

The preferred artery access for CAS is right common femoral artery; if suboptimal, then left common femoral artery and brachial access can be considered. The transfemoral approach is done under local anesthesia, helps in monitoring the neurological status during and as well as postprocedure period. If general anesthesia is needed, then use of intraoperative electroencephalogram (EEG)/brain mapping should be considered. Once the access is taken, a 5F vascular sheath is placed and subsequently heparinized to maintain activated clotting time (ACT) of 250–350 seconds.

Cervical arch aortogram is obtained at an approximate 35° left anterior oblique projection; this would help in profiling the ostia of great vessels.

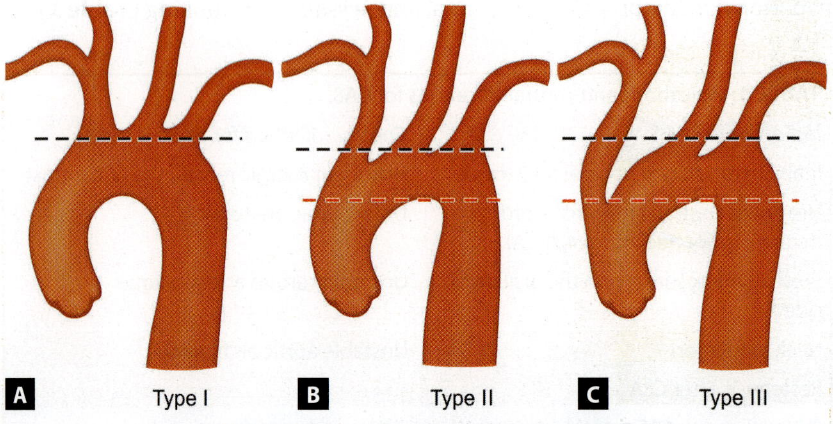

Figs. 1A to C: Arch of aorta classification.

An angled 5F glide diagnostic catheter, (usually Judkins right), is used with a 0.035" Glidewire (Terumo Medical Corporation, Somerset, NJ) to cannulate the carotid vessels **(Fig. 2)**. If faced with difficult anatomies, a reverse curve catheter can be used, including Vitek, Simmons-1, Berenstein, or Amplatz **(Fig. 3)**. Road mapping the angiogram helps during the guide catheter cannulation. A close watch must be kept on Glidewire as it could inadvertently cross the lesion.

After a suitable catheter position is achieved, the lesion visualization is done in multiple views; the best exposure being wherein the origins of internal carotid artery (ICA) and external carotid artery (ECA) are seen.

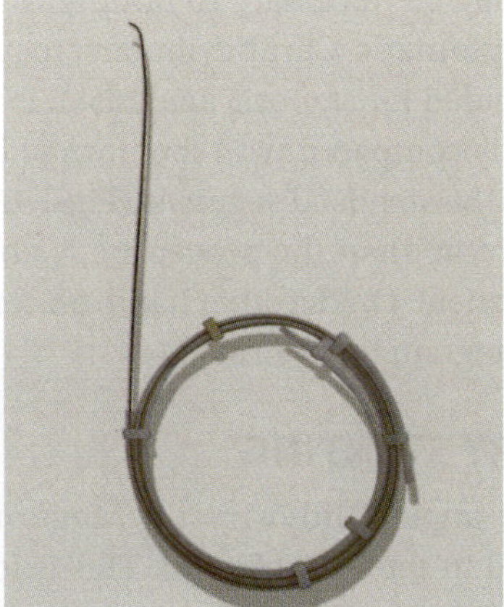

Fig. 2: 0.035"Terumo Glidewire.

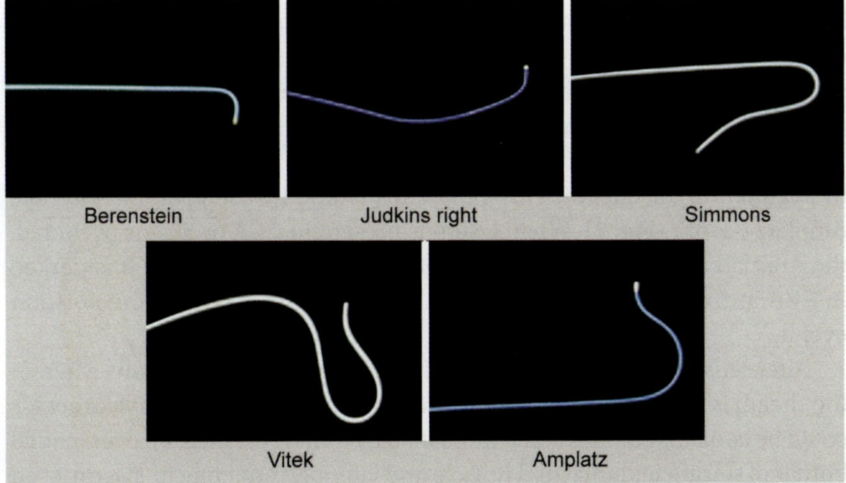

Fig. 3: Various catheters used for carotid angiograms.

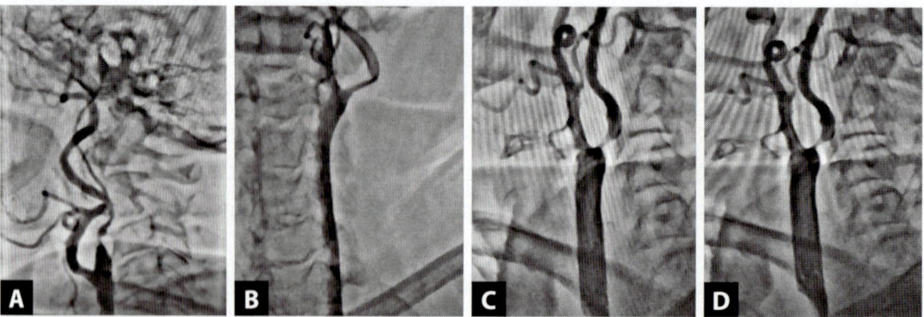

Figs. 4A to D: Picture showing critical stenosis of internal carotid artery (ICA). Percentage of stenosis is calculated using the diameter of the normal distal cervical ICA.

Oblique projections may be necessary to optimally visualize the stenosis. North American Symptomatic Carotid Endarterectomy Trial (NASCET) technique is recommended for stenosis analysis; it is the narrowest portion of the stenosis, which is compared with the normal diameter of the vessel immediate cephalic to the stenosed segment **(Figs. 4A to D)**. If the stenosis does not meet the criteria, then the procedure is abandoned and BMT is recommended to the patient. On the other hand, on confirmation of stenosis, ipsilateral cerebral angiogram is performed.

CAROTID ARTERY STENTING

The exchange length angle Glidewire tip/Magic torque wire (Boston Scientific) is positioned in the ECA **(Fig. 5)**. This is followed by placement of the sheath, commonly 90 cm 6 F sheath, in the CCA. This sheath could be Judkin's Right or Shuttle (Cool Medical Inc.) **(Fig. 6)**.

With the shuttle sheath advancement into CCA, precaution should be taken with its dilator as it is lengthy and nonradio opaque. Hence, care should be taken not to inadvertently advance the dilator into the stenosis. Care should also be taken with the Tuohy-Borst sidearm system provided with the shuttle sheath, as it can lead to significant back-bleed during the exchanges as well as stent deployment.

In situations when there is tortuosity met at CCA, there could be hindrance in negotiating the sheath. This can be overcome by use of stiffer wire like Amplatz (Cook) **(Fig. 7)**. When lesion is present in CCA or ECA is occluded, the Amplatz wire with J tip and a shot floppy segment is used. It is parked in CCA, proximal to stenosis and the sheath is advanced into the position over it.

Alternatively, in situations with difficulty anatomy or conditions wherein the sheath is not able to traverse the arch (or occluded aorta), cervical access could be considered. This is accomplished by transverse incision over medial border of sternocleidomastoid muscle and laterally retracting it. The exposed CCA is then accessed with 6 F introducer sheath.

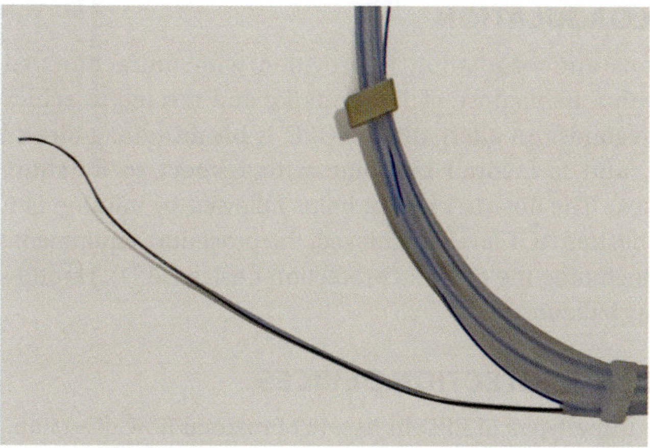

Fig. 5: Magic torque wire (Boston Scientific).

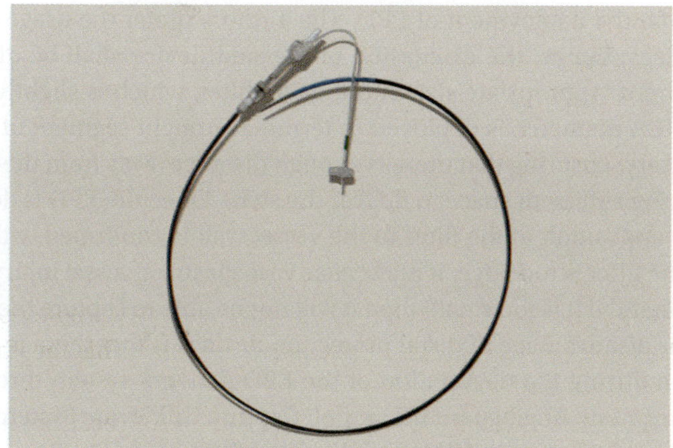

Fig. 6: Shuttle sheath with dilator in situ.

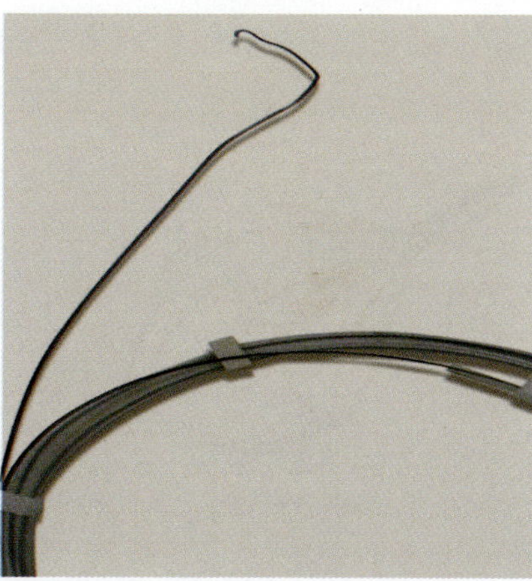

Fig. 7: Amplatz wire with J tip and a shot floppy segment.

ANTICOAGULATION

Intravenous anticoagulation is provided with unfractionated heparin (UFH), with a bolus dose of 100 units/kg and titrated to achieve ACT of 250–300 seconds. An alternative to UFH is bivalirudin, a direct thrombin inhibitor, and is favored by some with respect to its short half-life (25 minutes). The dose is 1 mg/kg bolus followed by infusion of 0.2 mg/kg. Once the desired ACT level is achieved, the procedure equipment should be prepped including the embolic protection device (EPD), carotid stent, and angioplasty balloon.

EMBOLIC PROTECTION DEVICES

There are three types of EPD in use: (1) Proximal flow diversion, (2) distal occlusion balloon, and (3) distal filter device. All three EPDs have their own advantages and disadvantages. Careful assessment of the ICA needs to be done before the deployment of EPD. The authors prefer the usage of distal filter devices; hence, the discussion of the said device shall be discussed in detail here. Appropriate size of the distal filter, which is slightly greater than the ICA diameter, is deployed in terminal straight segment of cervical carotid artery; ensuring that there is enough distance away from the stenosis and allowing sufficient space to deliver the stent. Once the EPD is deployed, adequate apposition of the filter to the vessel wall is confirmed with angiogram. If the filter is too large, it may cause vasospasm or vessel injury and on the other hand if it is too small, then it will not be able to capture the emboli. The major disadvantage of distal protection devices is that there is a lack of protection during the negotiation of the EPD delivery system through the stenosis segment. Angioguard RX Emboli Capture Guidewire System (Cordis Corporation, Bridgewater, NJ) is one the distal filter used **(Fig. 8)**.

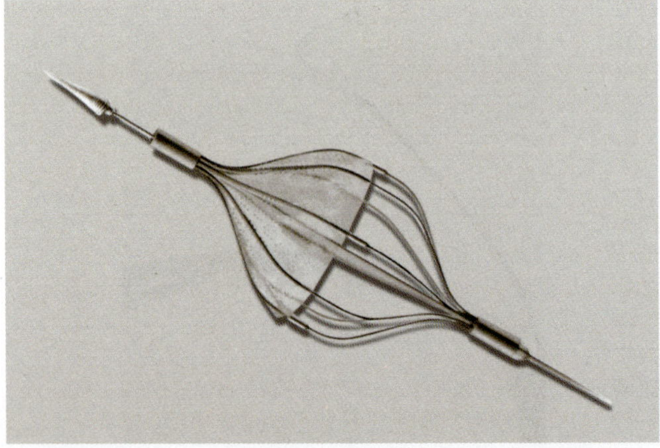

Fig. 8: Angioguard RX Emboli Capture Guidewire System.

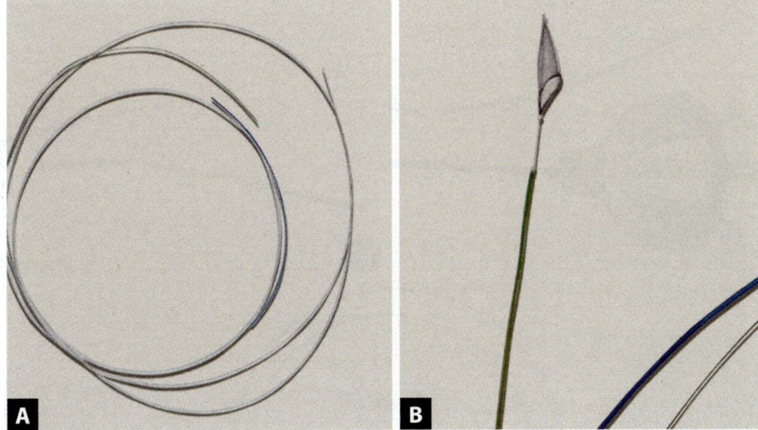

Figs. 9A and B: (A) Spider FX Embolic protection device. Green colored port houses the filter in it, the blue port helps in retrieving the filter at the end of procedure; (B) Spider FX Filter exposed outside the green port of the device.

In situation where the stenosis is complex or too severe, such that the leading wire of the EPD may not be able to sufficiently traverse the stenotic segment safely, in that case a 0.014" coronary guidewire can be used to cross the stenosis. In these circumstances, SpiderFx Embolic Protection Device (Covidien, Mansfield, MA) can be used **(Figs. 9A and B)**. The filter is housed inside the "garage", and it is distal to the monorail exit port. Once the 0.014" guidewire has crossed the stenosis, the delivery system is advanced beyond the stenosis over this wire, and thereafter the wire is removed via the monorail exit port. Now the filter is advanced from the garage over the delivery system and uncovered and deployed.

In comparison to the distal filter devices, the proximal protection devices provide an additional advantage in which the stenotic lesion is not crossed with any device until the protection is engaged, thereby making the entire procedure safe. The proximal devices include Mo.Ma Ultra proximal cerebral protection device (Medtronic, Inc., Minneapolis, MN) and Gore Flow Reversal (Gore & Associates, Flagstaff, AZ) **(Figs. 10A to C)**.

Nonetheless, these proximal devices require the use of 9F sheath, and few numbers of patients may not tolerate the occlusion due to insufficient collateral circulation. Like the proximal devices, the disadvantage of using the distal occlusion type of devices is that minority of patients may develop neurological symptoms during the distal balloon occlusion, thereby precluding its usage.

PREDILATATION

Once the deployment of the EDP takes place, predilatation of the stenotic segment is considered controversial. The advantage includes less traumatic

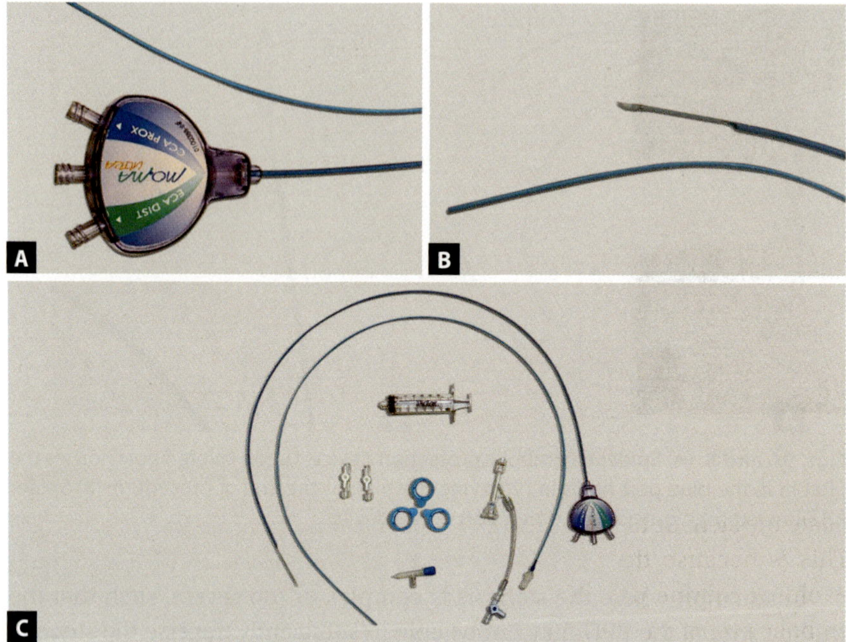

Figs. 10A to C: Mo.Ma Ultra proximal cerebral protection device.

stent delivery system as well as it reduces the requirement of poststent dilatation. On the other hand, the disadvantage includes the risk of plaque rupture and distal embolization. If predilatation is performed, then use of noncompliant balloon of 3.5–4 mm is used for the same. One must be ready with 0.6 mg atropine, should there be ensuing bradycardia postpredilatation.

CAROTID ARTERY STENT PLACEMENT

For CAS, nitinol or elgiloy based self-expanding stents are used. The length of the stent is sufficient that it extends from distal CCA to ICA. For the optimal wall apposition, the stent diameter needs to match that of distal CCA. The stent should be advanced slightly beyond the stenotic segment and prior to its deployment, it is retracted **(Figs. 11A to C)**. This helps in reducing the redundancy or slack that might have caused the stent to migrate forward. If there is incomplete coverage of the stenotic area, a second stent may be required to cover it. One should be ready to give atropine, should there be a bradycardia event poststent deployment.

POSTDILATATION

Once the stent is deployed, there may be a requirement of postdilatation, if the stent is not adequately expanded. However, the temptation to over

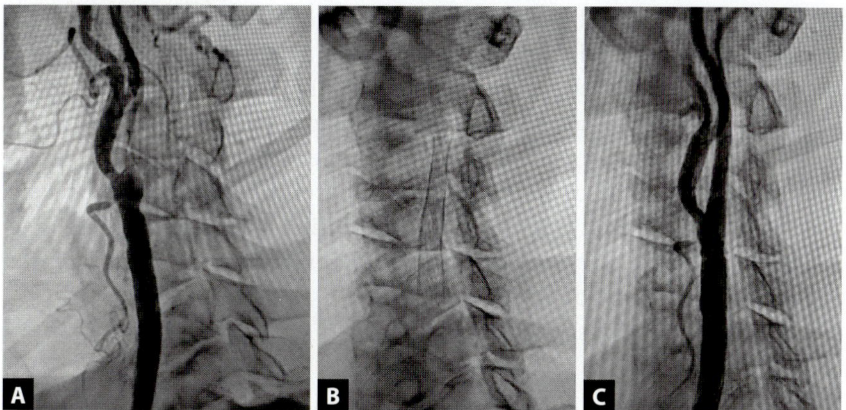

Figs. 11A to C: (A) Stenotic ICA; (B) Post-CAS; (C) Post-CAS.

dilate the stent or to make it look "cosmetically perfect" needs to be curbed. This is because the carotid stents have shown to expand overtime.[8,9] Avoiding routine postdilatation also ensures that there is less chance of embolic events. In conditions where heavy calcific CS is met with, judicious balloon postdilatation is preferred when the luminal diameter of the stent is inadequate. The usual postdilatation balloon diameter used is 5 mm, and gentle dilatation is recommended. Here too atropine may be required if there is significant bradycardia.

REMOVAL OF EMBOLIC PROTECTION DEVICE

After the stent deployment as well as postdilatation (if required) is completed, the EPD is evaluated for the embolic load. If the embolic burden is high, then aspiration catheter is used to aspirate the trapped debris. In most cases, there is minimal embolic load, and the EPD is safely recaptured and removed under fluoroscopic guidance. Care must be taken during its removal, as EPD may get engaged with margin of the stent while withdrawing through it. After the EPD is removed successfully, a complete angiogram is performed which includes the visualization of the cervical ICA as well as intracranial circulation. This helps to evaluate the residual stenosis, look for vasospasm or dissections, and assess the intracranial blood flow. After final angiogram, basic neurological evaluation is done, by asking the patient simple questions and performing basic maneuvers. Finally, hemostasis is achieved by manual compression or using a closure device.

POSTPROCEDURAL CARE

After the procedure, the patient's serial neurological assessment is performed and documented. Access site evaluation is a must. Serial hemodynamic monitoring is essential, postprocedural hypotension is common. Volume resuscitation is typically adequate in such a situation; if still persistent, then pharmacological support is initiated. On the other hand, in the setting of hypertension, it is essential to keep the systolic pressure below 150 mm Hg.

Most of the patients are discharged the next day on dual antiplatelet therapy (aspirin and clopidogrel). Clopidogrel is continued for at least 45 days, and after that, it is stopped and aspirin is continued for life long. Follow-up is recommended at 3 months, then 6 months, and thereafter yearly with ultrasound of the carotids.

CONCLUSION

Traditionally, the primary method to treat high-grade symptomatic as well as asymptomatic carotid artery stenosis has been CEA. However, with continuous evolution in endovascular technology and with growing experience with CAS, this minimally invasive procedure has become an alternative to endarterectomy for treating carotid artery disease patients. In the last two decades, CAS has undergone a significant evolutionary leap; despite that, it continues to be under much scrutiny and debate. Large studies till date have shown that CAS, when performed by skilled operators, is a safe and durable revascularization option in CS patients. CAS especially has already proven its mettle in high-risk patients as a standard of care. In comparison to CEA, with further improvements in the procedure as well as advancement in operator's skill, CAS is likely to become equivalent or standard of care for all patients.

REFERENCES

1. Miniño AM, Murphy SL, Xu J, Kochanek KD. Deaths: final data for 2008. Natl Vital Stat Rep. 2011;59(10):1-126.
2. Barnett HJM, Taylor DW, Haynes RB, Sackett DL, Peerless SJ, Ferguson GG, et al.; North American Symptomatic Carotid Endarterectomy Trial Collaborators. Beneficial effect of carotid endarterectomy in symptomatic patients with high-grade carotid stenosis. N Engl J Med. 1991;325(7):445-53.
3. National Institute of Neurological Disorders and Stroke. Carotid endarterectomy for patients with asymptomatic internal carotid artery stenosis. J Neurol Sci. 1995;129(1):76-77.
4. Randomised trial of endarterectomy for recently symptomatic carotid stenosis: final results of the MRC European Carotid Surgery Trial (ECST). Lancet. 1998;351(9113):1379-87.
5. Hobson RW II, Weiss DG, Fields WS, Goldstone J, Moore WS, Towne JB, et al. Efficacy of carotid endarterectomy for asymptomatic carotid stenosis. N Engl J Med. 1993;328(4):221-7.
6. Endarterectomy for asymptomatic carotid artery stenosis. Executive Committee for the Asymptomatic Carotid Atherosclerosis Study. JAMA. 1995;273(18):1421-8.
7. Furie KL, Kasner SE, Adams RJ, Albers GW, Bush RL, Fagan SC, et al. Guidelines for the prevention of stroke in patients with stroke or transient ischemic attack:

a guideline for healthcare professionals from the American Heart Association/American Stroke Association. Stroke. 2011;42(1):227-76.

8. Lownie SP, Pelz DM, Lee DH, Men S, Gulka I, Kalapos P. Efficacy of treatment of severe carotid bifurcation stenosis by using self-expanding stents without deliberate use of angioplasty balloons. AJNR Am J Neuroradiol. 2005;26(5):1241-8.
9. Maynar M, Baldi S, Rostagno R, Zander T, Rabellino M, Llorens R, et al. Carotid stenting without use of balloon angioplasty and distal protection devices: preliminary experience in 100 cases. AJNR Am J Neuroradiol. 2007;28(7):1378-83.

CHAPTER 51

Techniques of Pericardiocentesis

Ramesh Natarajan

INTRODUCTION

Cardiac tamponade can be a life-threatening condition that requires urgent pericardiocentesis. On the other hand, the pericardiocentesis procedure, although life-saving, may be associated with serious complications. With the introduction of image-guided procedures, safety and feasibility of pericardiocentesis have improved significantly allowing the possibility of choosing the best anatomical approach among apical, subcostal, and parasternal approaches.

Pericardiocentesis is the most useful therapeutic procedure for the early management of large, symptomatic pericardial effusion and cardiac tamponade.[1] The first description of cardiac decompression was in 1653, when Riolanus suggested sternal trephination to relieve pericardial pressure. In 1911, Marfan first described the subxiphoid approach, which had been used for the blind pericardiocentesis procedure for decades, despite the significant morbidity and mortality rates (50% and 6%, respectively).[2] In subsequent years, with the introduction of fluoroscopic, electrocardiographic, and echocardiographic guidance[3] and with the description of approaches other than the substernal one like the apical and parasternal, the safety of the procedure has improved dramatically.

PATHOPHYSIOLOGY OF CARDIAC TAMPONADE

Cardiac tamponade involves a slow or rapid compression of the heart due to increasing pericardial fluid. The pericardium can stretch to accommodate fluid accumulation, but when the pericardial compliance cannot increase any further, an equalization of intrapericardial pressures (central venous, right and left cardiac chambers) occurs, typically around 15–20 mm Hg. At this point, the right ventricle collapses and hypotension becomes severe. The hemodynamic effect of significant pericardial effusion is a continuum because a small increase in pericardial content couples the pericardium to the heart, significantly increasing atrial and especially ventricular interaction. Such phenomena exaggerate the normal reciprocal respiratory effects on the right and left sides of the heart. In the first steps of the hemodynamic impairment of pericardial effusion, patients may show only echocardiographic findings of heart chamber compression (right and left atrial collapse, right ventricle collapse, swinging heart, leftward of interventricular septum motion, inferior vena cava congestion) without clinical signs and symptoms (subclinical tamponade). In these cases, echocardiographic findings are very sensitive and raise suspicion of cardiac tamponade in patients with only subtle evidence of hemodynamic compromise.[4,5]

TECHNIQUES OF PERICARDIAL ASPIRATION

Fluoroscopy-guided Technique

The fluoroscopic approach was the first imaging system used for percutaneous pericardiocentesis. It is performed through the subxiphoid approach with a needle containing a contrast medium, directed toward the left shoulder at an angle of 30° to the skin. Needle position in the pericardial space is confirmed by the contrast agent medium injection: the inferior position appearance of a sluggish layering of the contrast medium indicates the correct position and that a soft J-tip guidewire can be introduced. It is essential to check the guidewire position in at least two angiographic projections (lateral view and anterior–posterior view).[6]

This procedure is standardized and effective, but it can only be performed in cardiac catheterization laboratories and it implies an exposure to radiation for both the patient and the physician. However, this procedure could be very useful to treat iatrogenic tamponade during percutaneous procedures. An echocardiographic examination to assess the distribution and amount of pericardial effusion should always precede the fluoroscopy-guided procedure, whenever possible.

Computed Tomography-guided Technique

In recent years, evidence of the feasibility of pericardiocentesis under computed tomography (CT) guidance has been reported. Through the planning CT scan, the full extension of the pericardial effusion is evaluated and the optimal entrance point is defined and marked on the skin. Next, the needle is advanced into the pericardial effusion and a single CT scan is used for verification of the needle position. This technique does not allow a continuous visualization of the needle and it implies a significant exposure to radiation for the patient. In addition, it is not widely available and logistically feasible, and is time-consuming (median duration of 65 minutes).[7] However, it can be successfully used in patients with a poor ultrasound window and can show loculated effusion very effectively, allowing identification of the best entry site. Moreover, a CT scan can measure the density of the pericardial effusion, thus avoiding a procedure failing in case of highly viscous effusions, such as purulent ones and intrapericardial hematoma.[6] Finally, a CT scan allows assessment of the entire chest and detection of associated abnormalities, which is useful in identifying the underlying disease.[8]

Echo-guided Technique

Echocardiography-guided pericardiocentesis is a safe and simple technique, introduced at the Mayo Clinic in 1979 and widely used nowadays.[3] The echocardiography-guided approach allows defining the position of the effusion, the ideal entry site and needle trajectory for pericardiocentesis. There are two different approaches to echo guidance: the first (described by the Mayo Clinic) is the echo-assisted method, in which the operator memorizes the optimal needle trajectory and advances the needle toward the pericardial space without a continuous ultrasound visualization.[3] The second approach is the echo-guided method with a continuous echocardiographic monitoring. It has also been proposed to use a needle carrier mounted on the ultrasound transducer to advance the needle to the pericardial space.[9]

PUNCTURE SITE

Three main approaches can be used for pericardiocentesis: the apical, the subcostal, or the parasternal approach.

Traditionally, a subcostal approach has been preferred, largely because it was considered the safest route without image guidance. However, pericardial effusion is not always circumferential and equally distributed; consequently, an ultrasound evaluation of the ideal entry site for drainage is fundamental for procedural success. The Mayo Clinic advocates selecting the approach based purely on echocardiographic findings and defines the optimal entry site as the point where the pericardial space is closest to the probe and the fluid accumulation is maximal, with no intervening vital organs. This site is more often para-apical than subcostal.[3] Furthermore, an observational series on echo-guided pericardiocentesis demonstrated a greater success rate and a minor complication rate when the entry site was echocardiographically selected rather than when the subxiphoid approach was routinely used **(Table 1 and Fig. 1)**.[3,9,10]

TECHNICAL ASPECTS OF ECHO-GUIDED PROCEDURE

Prior preparation is essential for the safe performance of pericardiocentesis. The platelet count and coagulation profile should be checked. Electrocardiographic monitoring is required in an appropriate environment with resuscitation equipment. A central venous catheter is essential for rapid infusion of fluids and drugs if indicated. Continuous arterial pressure monitoring if available can detect the presence of pulsus paradoxus and to detect and rapidly correct sudden hemodynamic instability.

A preliminary echocardiographic evaluation is recommended to assess the size and distribution of the effusion, to select the proper entry site and also to monitor the procedure. The patient should be placed in a semireclining position at an angle of about 30° and slightly rotated leftwards to enhance

TABLE 1: Characteristics of the different pericardiocentesis approaches.

Place of puncture	*Description*	*Disadvantages*	*Advantages*
Apical	The needle insertion site is 1–2 cm lateral to the apex beat within the fifth, sixth, or seventh intercostal space. Advance the needle over the superior border of the rib to avoid intercostal nerves and vessels	• Risk of ventricular puncture due to the proximity to the left ventricle • Increased risk for pneumothorax for the proximity to the left pleural space	• The thicker left ventricle wall is more likely to self-seal after puncture • Due to ultrasound not penetrating air, using echocardio-graphic guidance ensures avoidance of the lung • The path to reach the pericardium is shorter
Parasternal	The needle insertion site is in the fifth left intercostal space close to the sternal margin. Advance the needle perpendicular to the skin (at the level of the cardiac notch of the left lung)	Risk of pneumothorax and puncture of the internal thoracic vessels (if the needle is inserted >1 cm laterally)	Echocardiographic guidance, also with phase array probe, provides a good visualization of pericardial structures
Subxiphoid	The needle insertion site is between the xiphisternum and left costal margin. Once beneath the cartilage cage, lower the needle to a 15–30° angle, with the abdominal wall directed toward the left shoulder	• A steeper angle may enter the peritoneal cavity, and a medial direction increases the risk of right atrial puncture. In some cases, the left liver lobe may be transversed intentionally if an alternative site is not available • The path to reach the fluid is longer	Lower risk of pneumothorax

fluid collection in the inferior–anterior part of the chest. After appropriate disinfection of the operative field, a local anesthetic is administered at the puncture site. The trajectory of the needle is defined by the angle between

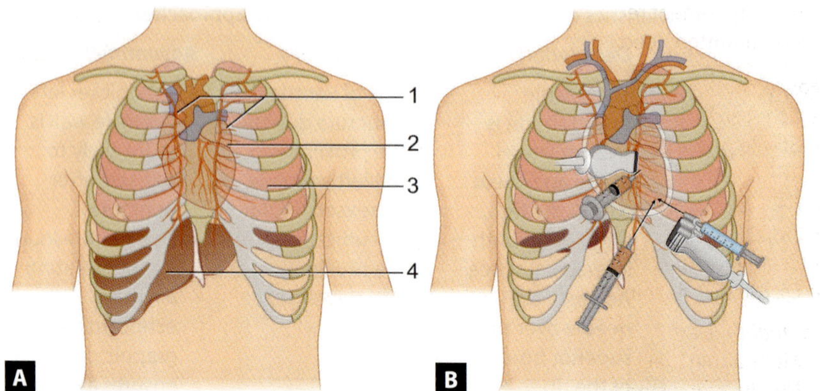

Figs. 1A and B: Pericardiocentesis: Anatomical structures and approaches. (A) Anatomical structures to bear in mind during pericardiocentesis: 1. Internal mammary artery, 2. Heart, 3. Lung, 4. Liver; (B) Three main approaches to pericardiocentesis: 1. Parasternal, 2. Substernal, 3. Apical.

the probe and the chest wall. The optimal needle trajectory should be visualized in the operator's mind, and then a 16–18 gauge, Teflon-sheathed needle with an attached saline-filled syringe advanced in the direction of the fluid-filled space. When fluid is aspirated, the needle should be advanced approximately 2 mm further. The sheath should be advanced over the needle and the steel core withdrawn, maintaining only the sheath in the pericardial space. A guidewire should be advanced through the sheath, which can then be removed. A bloody aspirate may indicate myocardial puncture or hemorrhagic pericardial effusion. The extracardiac position of the tip can be confirmed by injecting 5 mL of agitated saline infusion: the bubbles can be visualized through echocardiography in the pericardial space. A small incision should be made at the entry site followed by the introduction of a sheathed dilator (6–8 Fr) over the guide. The dilator should be removed and a pigtail catheter inserted directly into the sheath. The pericardial effusion is aspirated by syringe suction and the catheter is closed after flushing with 5 mL of heparinized saline **(Box 1)**.

A different approach utilizes a needle carrier mounted on the transducer to advance the needle under continuous visualization (real-time, echo-monitored procedure). In most cases, the procedure is carried out by two physicians—one who performs the echocardiogram and another who performs the puncture and drainage.

COMPLICATIONS

The rate of major complications reported in large observational studies for echo-guided or fluoroscopic pericardiocentesis is 0.3–3.9%, and the rate of minor complications is 0.4–20%.[9,11,12]

BOX 1: Equipment required to perform echo-guided pericardiocentesis with or without probe-mounted needle system.

For echo-guided pericardiocentesis:
- Echocardiography with a cardiac probe
- Sterile probe cover and sterile echo gel
- 16–18 gauge, Teflon-sheathed needle
- 6–8 Fr dilator and introducer sheath
- J-tipped guidewire
- *Drainage catheter:* Pigtail angio catheter 6–8 Fr or specific pericardial drainage set
- Disposable flushing system to maintain patency of the catheter

For real-time echo-monitored procedure:
- Multi-angle bracket to be mounted on the echo probe
- Needle guide sterile kit
- 18-gauge, 9 cm needle (or 15 cm for subxiphoid approach)
- 6–8 Fr dilator

The most serious complications include injury of the cardiac chambers, laceration of the coronary arteries or intercostal vessels, puncture of the abdominal viscera or peritoneal cavity, pneumothorax requiring chest tube placement, pneumopericardium, ventricular arrhythmias and pericardial decompression syndrome. Myocardial and coronary puncture may initially be silent and present with delayed hemopericardium or intrapericardial thrombus.

Pericardial decompression is a rare, potentially life-threatening syndrome characterized by wide clinical scenarios (from pulmonary edema to cardiogenic shock). It generally develops after a successful pericardial drainage, from a few hours to days later. The mechanism of this situation is not yet well understood. However, the simplest explanation is an acute left ventricular overload due to an increased right-sided preload associated with a persistent catecholaminergic peripheral vasoconstriction. To date, there are no effective recommendations to prevent this syndrome except to remove enough fluid to normalize the central venous and systemic blood pressure (not >1 L) and to complete the removal in the subsequent few hours.[13]

Minor complications include transient vasovagal hypotension and bradycardia, supraventricular arrhythmias, pneumothorax without hemodynamic instability, and pleuropericardial fistulas.

Several authors have suggested that particular attention must be paid to periprocedural management of anticoagulant treatment and propose that in the presence of severe coagulation disorders, pericardiocentesis should be postponed until sufficient blood transfusion or other appropriate hematologic treatment is provided if overt tamponade is not present.[13] In the setting of iatrogenic pericardial effusion, full anticoagulation is considered as a major risk factor for both tamponade and its sequelae.

CONCLUSION

Pericardiocentesis is a lifesaving procedure for cardiac tamponade, and it has a high risk of complications. Proper puncturing techniques and imaging support help to perform the procedure with fewer complications.

REFERENCES

1. Adler Y, Charron P, Imazio M, Badano L, Barón-Esquivias G, Bogaert J, et al.; European Society of Cardiology (ESC). 2015 ESC guidelines for the diagnosis and management of pericardial diseases: The Task Force for the Diagnosis and Management of Pericardial Diseases of the European Society of Cardiology (ESC). Endorsed by the European Association for Cardio-Thoracic Surgery (EACTS). Eur Heart J. 2015;36(42):2921-64.
2. Krikorian JG, Mancock EW. Pericardiocentesis. Am J Med. 1978;65(5):808-14.
3. Tsang TS, Freeman WK, Sinak LJ, Seward JB. Echocardiographically-guided pericardiocentesis: evolution and state-of-the-art technique. Mayo Clin Proc. 1998;73(7):647-52.
4. Roy CL, Minor MA, Brookhart MA, Choudhry NK. Does this patient with a pericardial effusion have cardiac tamponade? JAMA. 2007;297(16):1810-8.
5. Singh V, Dwivedi SK, Chandra S, Sanguri R, Sethi R, Puri A, et al. Optimal fluid amount for haemodynamic benefit in cardiac tamponade. Acute Cardiovasc Care. 2014;3(2):158-64.
6. Maisch B, Ristić AD, Seferović PM, Tsang TSM. Interventional Pericardiology: Pericardiocentesis, Pericardioscopy, Pericardial Biopsy, Balloon Pericardiotomy and Intrapericardial Therapy. Heidelberg: Springer Medizin Verlag; 2011.
7. Neves D, Silva M, Morais G, Ferreira N, Carvalho M, Gama Ribeiro V, et al. Computed tomography-guided pericardiocentesis—A single center experience. Rev Port Cardiol. 2016;35(5):285-90.
8. Maggiolini S, De Carlini C, Ferri L, Colombo GI, Gentile G, Meles E, et al. The role of early contrast-enhanced chest computed tomography in the aetiological diagnosis of patients presenting with cardiac tamponade or large pericardial effusion. Eur Heart J Cardiovasc Imaging. 2016;17(4):421-8.
9. Maggiolini S, Gentile G, Farina A, De Carlini CC, Lenatti L, Meles E, et al. Safety, Efficacy and Complications of Pericardiocentesis by Real-Time Echo-Monitored Procedure. Am J Cardiol. 2016;117(8):1369-74.
10. Tsang TS, Seward JB. Pericardiocentesis under echocardiographic guidance. Eur J Echocardiogr. 2001;2(1):68-9.
11. Tsang TS, Enriquez-Sarano M, Freeman WK, Barnes ME, Sinak LJ, Gersh BJ, et al. Consecutive 1127 therapeutic echocardiographically guided pericardiocentesis: clinical profile, practice patterns, and outcomes spanning 21 years. Mayo Clin Proc. 2002;77:429-36.
12. Akyuz S, Zengin A, Arugaslan E, Yazici S, Onuk T, Ceylan US, et al. Echo-guided pericardiocentesis in patients with clinically significant pericardial effusion. Outcomes over a 10-year period. Herz. 2015;40 Suppl 2:153-9.
13. Ristić AD, Imazio M, Adler Y, Anastasakis A, Badano LP, Brucato A, et al. Triage strategy for urgent management of cardiac tamponade: a position statement of the European Society of Cardiology Working Group on Myocardial and Pericardial Diseases. Eur Heart J. 2014;35(34):2279-84.

Index

Page numbers followed by *b* refer to box, *f* refer to figure, *fc* refer to flowchart, and *t* refer to table.

A

B

C

D

E

G

H

I

M

N

O

P

Q

R

S

T

U

V

W

X

Z